CT of the Heart

CONTEMPORARY CARDIOLOGY

CHRISTOPHER P. CANNON, MD
SERIES EDITOR

CT of the Heart: Principles and Applications, edited by *U. Joseph Schoepf, MD, 2005*

Principles of Molecular Cardiology, edited by *Marschall S. Runge, MD and Cam Patterson, MD, 2005*

Heart Disease Diagnosis and Therapy: *A Practical Approach, Second Edition,* edited by *Gabriel M. Khan, MD, FRCP, FRCP (C), FACC, 2005*

Cardiovascular Genomics: *Gene Mining for Pharmacogenomics and Gene Therapy,* edited by *Mohan K. Raizada, PhD, Julian F. R. Paton, PhD, Michael J. Katovich, PhD, and Sergey Kasparov, MD, PhD, 2005*

Surgical Management of Congestive Heart Failure, edited by *James C. Fang, MD and Gregory S. Couper, MD, 2005*

Cardiopulmonary Resuscitation, edited by *Joseph P. Ornato, MD, FACP, FACC, FACEP and Mary Ann Peberdy, MD, FACC, 2005*

Cardiac Transplantation: The Columbia University Medical Center/New York-Presbyterian Hospital Manual, edited by *Niloo M. Edwards, MD, Jonathan M. Chen, MD, and Pamela A. Mazzeo, 2004*

Heart Disease and Erectile Dysfunction, edited by *Robert A. Kloner, MD, PhD, 2004*

Coronary Disease in Women: *Evidence-Based Diagnosis and Treatment,* edited by *Leslee J. Shaw, PhD and Rita F. Redberg, MD, FACC, 2004*

Complementary and Alternative Cardiovascular Medicine, edited by *Richard A. Stein, MD and Mehmet C. Oz, MD, 2004*

Nuclear Cardiology, The Basics: *How to Set Up and Maintain a Laboratory,* by *Frans J. Th. Wackers, MD, PhD, Wendy Bruni, BS, CNMT, and Barry L. Zaret, MD, 2004*

Minimally Invasive Cardiac Surgery, Second Edition, edited by *Daniel J. Goldstein, md, and Mehmet C. Oz, MD 2004*

Cardiovascular Health Care Economics, edited by *William S. Weintraub, MD, 2003*

Platelet Glycoprotein IIb/IIIa Inhibitors in Cardiovascular Disease, Second Edition, edited by *A. Michael Lincoff, MD, 2003*

Heart Failure: *A Clinician's Guide to Ambulatory Diagnosis and Treatment,* edited by *Mariell L. Jessup, MD and Evan Loh, MD, 2003*

Management of Acute Coronary Syndromes, Second Edition, edited by *Christopher P. Cannon, MD 2003*

Aging, Heart Disease, and Its Management: *Facts and Controversies,* edited by *Niloo M. Edwards, MD, Mathew S. Maurer, MD, and Rachel B. Wellner, MPH, 2003*

Peripheral Arterial Disease: *Diagnosis and Treatment,* edited by *Jay D. Coffman, MD and Robert T. Eberhardt, MD, 2003*

Cardiac Repolarization: *Bridging Basic and Clinical Science,* edited by *Ihor Gussak, MD, phd, Charles Antzelevitch, phd, Stephen C. Hammill, MD, Win K. Shen, MD, and Preben Bjerregaard, MD, DMSC, 2003*

Essentials of Bedside Cardiology: *With a Complete Course in Heart Sounds and Murmurs on CD, Second Edition,* by *Jules Constant, MD, 2003*

Primary Angioplasty in Acute Myocardial Infarction, edited by *James E. Tcheng, MD, 2002*

Cardiogenic Shock: *Diagnosis and Treatment,* edited by *David Hasdai, MD, Peter B. Berger, MD, Alexander Battler, MD, and David R. Holmes, Jr., MD, 2002*

Management of Cardiac Arrhythmias, edited by *Leonard I. Ganz, MD, 2002*

Diabetes and Cardiovascular Disease, edited by *Michael T. Johnstone, md and Aristidis Veves, MD, DSc, 2001*

Blood Pressure Monitoring in Cardiovascular Medicine and Therapeutics, edited by *William B. White, MD, 2001*

Vascular Disease and Injury: *Preclinical Research,* edited by *Daniel I. Simon, MD, and Campbell Rogers, MD, 2001*

Preventive Cardiology: *Strategies for the Prevention and Treatment of Coronary Artery Disease,* edited by *JoAnne Micale Foody, MD, 2001*

CT of the Heart

Principles and Applications

Edited by

U. Joseph Schoepf, MD

Department of Radiology,
Medical University of South Carolina,
Charleston, SC

Foreword by

Alexander R. Margulis, MD, DSc (hon)

Clinical Professor of Radiology,
Weill Medical College of Cornell University,
New York, NY

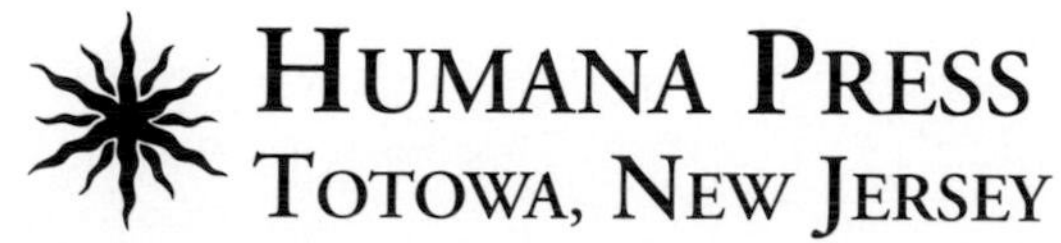

999 Riverview Drive, Suite 208
Totowa, New Jersey 07512
www.humanapress.com

For additional copies, pricing for bulk purchases, and/or information about other Humana titles, contact Humana at the above address or at any of the following numbers: Tel.: 973-256-1699; Fax: 973-256-8341; E-mail:humana@humanapr.com; Website: humanapress.com

Cover illustration: figure 6D from chapter 25, "CT Angiography for Assessment of Coronary Artery Anomalies," by Steffen C. Froehner, Matthias Wagner, Juergen Brunn, and Rainer R. Schmitt; figures 13 and 14 from chapter 3, "Scan Techniques for Cardiac and Coronary Artery Imaging With Multislice CT," by Bernd M. Ohnesorge, Brian R. Westerman, and U. Joseph Schoepf; figure 13 from chapter 4, "Image Reconstruction for ECG-Triggered and ECG-Gated Multislice CT," by Thomas Flohr and Tinsu Pan; figure 13 from chapter 24, "Visualization Techniques for Contrast-Enhanced CT Angiography of Coronary Arteries," by Jean-Louis Sablayrolles and Pascal Giat; and figure 9 from chapter 18, "Multidetector-Row CT Assessment of Left-Ventricular Function," by Kai Uwe Juergens and Roman Fischbach.

Production Editor: Tracy Catanese
Cover design by Patricia F. Cleary

This publication is printed on acid-free paper. ∞
ANSI Z39.48-1984 (American National Standards Institute) Permanence of Paper for Printed Library Materials.

e-ISBN: 1-59259-818-8

Printed in China 10 9 8 7 6 5 4 3 2 1

Library of Congress Cataloging-in-Publication Data

CT of the heart : principles and applications / edited by U. Joseph Schoepf.
p. ; cm. -- (Contemporary cardiology)
Includes bibliographical references and index.
ISBN 1-58829-303-3 (alk. paper)
1. Heart--Tomography.
[DNLM: 1. Heart--radiography. 2. Tomography, X-Ray Computed. WG 141.5.T6 C959 2004] I. Schoepf, U. J. (U. Joseph), 1969- II. Series: Contemporary cardiology (Totowa, N.J. : Unnumbered)
RC683.5.T66C785 2004
616.1'20757--dc22

2004003443

Foreword

Radiologic technology has made dramatic advances in the last 25 years, and none have been more impressive than those in computed tomography (CT). The progress in the speed of obtaining images, computing, postprocessing, and spatial resolution has been incredible. The result is that CT has moved from displaying purely morphologic information to providing valuable physiologic data as well. Whether with electron beam or multidetector-row CT, advances are impressive and nowhere have the applications been more useful and dramatic than in the heart.

This multiauthored book, *CT of the Heart*, edited by U. Joseph Schoepf, MD, is a splendid rendition of the state-of-the-art in CT imaging of the heart; however, where appropriate, it also features comparisons with other technical approaches, such as magnetic resonance and ultrasound. The contributors are leading radiologists, cardiologists, physicists, engineers, and basic and clinical scientists from Europe, the United States, Israel, and Japan.

The entire contents are meticulous and comprehensive, from the introduction about the past, present, and future of CT of the heart, through the technical underpinning of the method and the various clinical, physiologic, and pathologic applications of CT in studying the heart.

This book fills an immense need, particularly at a time when cardiac screening with CT, whether one agrees with this practice or not, is a reality. Furthermore, with the rapid increase of aging populations in the industrialized world, noninvasive diagnostic approaches are increasingly needed. As technology continues to advance and applications of CT to heart studies expand, it is my hope that the editor will bring this book up to date with a new edition.

Alexander R. Margulis, *MD, DSc (HON)*
Clinical Professor of Radiology
Weill Medical College of Cornell University

Preface

Through the ages of exploration and enlightenment the heart has kept its fascination as the metaphor of life. Its firm entrenchment in human emotion and consciousness and the overwhelming socioeconomic importance of its diseases make noninvasive visualization and diagnosis of the heart and its diseases the coveted "holy grail" of medical imaging.

Imaging of the heart has always been technically challenging, because of the heart's continuous motion. The introduction and ongoing technical improvement of fast ECG-synchronized computed tomography (CT) scanning of the heart has enabled imaging of the elusive but cardinal cardiac anatomy and pathology with a combination of speed and spatial resolution that is hitherto unparalleled by other noninvasive imaging modalities. Accordingly, considerable interest has been directed in recent years at the beneficial utilization of CT for noninvasive interrogation of the coronary arteries and for imaging studies of anatomic and functional sequelae of ischemic heart disease, such as cardiac perfusion, motion, and viability. The current and potential future roles of CT for these and other applications are the subject matter of this book.

CT of the Heart, however, does not claim to have all of the answers. CT of the heart is a nascent but rapidly evolving field, and the act of condensing expert knowledge and experience in the format of a book can only result in a snapshot of the status quo at a certain point in time. Novel iterations of existing technology and profoundly new concepts of medical imaging are already on the horizon. The benefits and indications of integrating CT into the diagnostic algorithm of heart disease is intensely researched and discussed: to date, the diagnostic value of CT coronary calcium measurements and the exact role of this marker for cardiac risk stratification remain unclear and controversial. We are only beginning to understand the usefulness and potential clinical application of CT angiography for noninvasive detection of coronary artery stenosis. Cross-sectional assessment of the coronary artery wall for noninvasive identification, characterization, and quantification of atherosclerotic lesions and disease burden is a promising and exciting but yet untested concept.

Within *CT of the Heart*, the reader will be exposed to a variety of expert opinions on the respective topics. Some authors will assume a more optimistic or a more conservative perspective on cardiac CT applications. Because of the lack of large-scale clinical studies, only future experience will show who may be right. It is a declared goal of this book to showcase the full scope of current developments, research, and scientific controversy regarding the principles and applications of CT of the heart. Truth is most likely to be found in the equilibrium of opinions. The publisher and I have striven to maintain this equilibrium by providing a platform for differing opinions and for different technical approaches to CT of the heart. To mitigate commercial overtones and bias, which so often accompany the first steps of a potentially important new technology, contributions of users and/or developers of all cardiac CT manufacturers were included. Scientists representing different companies graciously disregarded commercial divisions and agreed to co-author chapters in order to provide the reader with a truly balanced view on cardiac CT technology.

Accordingly, *CT of the Heart* is the work of many. I am indebted to Dr. Christopher Cannon, the series editor, and to Paul Dolgert of Humana Press for entrusting me with the role of editor. I am grateful to my chairman, Dr. Philip Costello, for his unfailing guidance, support, and friendship. I feel very, very honored by all the kindness that my many friends in the cardiac imaging community have shown me by volunteering their time, their knowledge, their experience, and the vision that went into their respective contributions. All authors are highly respected experts in their fields and this book would never have come to pass without their incredible support, for which I am so grateful. Finally I would like to thank Tracy Catanese and Craig Adams of Humana Press for so efficiently and expertly steering the production of *CT of the Heart*.

U. Joseph Schoepf, MD
Charleston, South Carolina

Contents

Contributors

Masanori Aikawa, MD, PhD, *Cardiovascular Division, Department of Medicine, Brigham and Women's Hospital and Harvard Medical School, Boston, MA*

Christoph R. Becker, MD, *Department of Clinical Radiology, University of Munich, Munich, Germany*

Juergen Brunn, MD, *Department of Diagnostic and Interventional Radiology, Herz- und Gefaess-Klinik GmbH, Bad Neustadt an der Saale, Germany*

Allen P. Burke, MD, *Department of Cardiovascular Pathology, Armed Forces Institute of Pathology, Washington, DC*

Filippo Cademartiri, MD, *Department of Radiology, Erasmus Medical Center, Rotterdam, The Netherlands*

J. Jeffrey Carr, MD, MSCE, *Division of Radiological Sciences and Public Health Sciences, Wake Forest University School of Medicine, Winston-Salem, NC*

Marcello De Santis, MD, *Department of Radiology, S. Andrea Hospital, Rome, Italy*

Selami Dogan, MD, *Department of Thoracic and Cardiovascular Surgery, J. W. Goethe University, Frankfurt, Germany*

Raimund Erbel, MD, *Department of Cardiology, University Clinic Essen, Essen, Germany*

Andrew Farb, MD, *Department of Cardiovascular Pathology, Armed Forces Institute of Pathology, Washington, DC*

Zahi Fayad, MD, *Zena and Michael A. Wiener Cardiovascular Institute, Mount Sinai School of Medicine, New York, NY*

Roman Fischbach, MD, *Department of Clinical Radiology, University of Muenster, Muenster, Germany*

Aloke V. Finn, MD, *Cardiac Unit, Department of Internal Medicine, Massachusetts General Hospital, Boston, MA*

Thomas Flohr, *Division of Computed Tomography, Siemens Medical Solutions, Forchheim, Germany*

Steffen C. Froehner, MD, *Department of Diagnostic and Interventional Radiology, Herz- und Gefaess-Klinik GmbH, Bad Neustadt an der Saale, Germany*

Kunihiko Fukuda, MD, *Department of Radiology, The Jikei University School of Medicine, Tokyo, Japan*

Pascal Giat, PhD, *Division of Computed Tomography, General Electric Medical Systems, Buc, France*

Herman Gold, MD, *Cardiac Unit, Department of Internal Medicine, Massachusetts General Hospital, Boston, MA*

Reinhard Groell, MD, *Department of Radiology, Medical University Graz, Graz, Austria*

Christopher Herzog, MD, *Institute for Diagnostic and Interventional Radiology, J. W. Goethe University, Frankfurt, Germany*

David G. Hill, PhD, *General Electric Medical Systems, South San Francisco, CA*

Udo Hoffmann, MD, *Department of Radiology, Massachusetts General Hospital and Harvard Medical School, Boston, MA*

Armin Huber, MD, *Department of Clinical Radiology, University of Munich, Munich, Germany*

Kai Uwe Juergens, MD, *Department of Clinical Radiology, University of Muenster, Muenster, Germany*

Marc Kachelriess, PhD, *Institute of Medical Physics, University of Erlangen-Nürnberg, Nürnberg, Germany*

Willi A. Kalender, PhD, *Institute of Medical Physics, University of Erlangen-Nürnberg, Nürnberg, Germany*

Birgit Kantor, MD, *Division of Cardiovascular Diseases and Internal Medicine, Mayo Clinic College of Medicine, Rochester, MN*

Frank D. Kolodgie, PhD, *Department of Cardiovascular Pathology, Armed Forces Institute of Pathology, Washington, DC*

Yasushi Koyama, MD, *Department of Cardiology, Ehime Prefectural Imabari Hospital, Ehime, Japan*

Axel Kuettner, MD, *Department of Radiology, University of Tübingen, Tübingen, Germany*

Alexander W. Leber, MD, *Medizinische Klinik I, University Hospital Clinic Munich-Grosshadern, Ludwig Maximilians University, Munich, Germany*

Cynthia H. McCollough, PhD, *Department of Radiology, Mayo Clinic College of Medicine, Rochester, MN*

David Maintz, MD, *Department of Clinical Radiology, University of Muenster, Muenster, Germany*

Alexander R. Margulis, MD, DSc (HON), *Department of Radiology, Weill Medical College of Cornell University, New York, NY*

Teruhito Mochizuki, MD, *Department of Radiology, Ehime University School of Medicine, Ehime, Japan*

Stefan Möhlenkamp, MD, *Department of Cardiology, University Clinic Essen, Essen, Germany*

Koen Nieman, MD, *Department of Cardiology (Thoraxcenter) and Department of Radiology, Erasmus Medical Center, Rotterdam, The Netherlands*

Konstantin Nikolaou, MD, *Department of Clinical Radiology, University of Munich, Munich, Germany, and Zena and Michael A. Wiener Cardiovascular Institute, Mount Sinai School of Medicine, New York, NY*

Christopher J. O'Donnell, MD, MPH, *National Heart, Lung, and Blood Institute's Framingham Heart Study, Framingham, MA, and Cardiology Division, Department of Medicine, Massachusetts General Hospital and Harvard Medical School, Boston, MA*

Bernd M. Ohnesorge, PhD, *Division of Computed Tomography, Siemens Medical Solutions, Forchheim, Germany*

Tinsu Pan, *General Electric Medical Systems, Waukesha, WI*

Jean-François Paul, MD, *Radiology Unit, Marie Lannelongue Hospital, Plessis Robinson, France*

Heiko Pump, MD, *Institute of Diagnostic and Interventional Radiology, University of Witten-Herdecke, Witten-Herdecke, Germany*

Erik L. Ritman, MD, PhD *Physiological Imaging Research Laboratory, Department of Physiology and Biomedical Engineering, Mayo Clinic College of Medicine, Rochester, MN*

Jean-Louis Sablayrolles, MD, *Centre Cardiologique du Nord, Saint Denis, France*

Toru Sakuma, MD, *Department of Radiology, The Jikei University School of Medicine, Tokyo, Japan*

Axel Schmermund, MD, *Department of Cardiology, University Clinic Essen, Essen, Germany*

Rainer R. Schmitt, MD, *Department of Diagnostic and Interventional Radiology, Herz- und Gefaess-Klinik GmbH, Bad Neustadt an der Saale, Germany*

U. Joseph Schoepf, MD, *Department of Radiology, Medical University of South Carolina, Charleston, SC*

Stephen Schroeder, MD, PhD • Division of Cardiology, Eberhard-Karls-Universität, Tübingen, Germany

Rainer Seibel, MD, *Institute of Diagnostic and Interventional Radiology, University of Witten-Herdecke, Witten-Herdecke, Germany*

Kaiss Shanneik, MSc, *Institute of Medical Physics, University of Erlangen-Nürnberg, Nürnberg, Germany*

Joseph Shemesh, MD, *Department of Cardiology, The Grace Ballas Cardiac Research Unit, Sheba Medical Center, Sackler School of Medicine, Tel Aviv, Israel*

William Stanford, MD, *Division of Chest and Cardiovascular Radiology, Department of Radiology, Ray J. and Lucille A. Carver University of Iowa College of Medicine, Iowa City, IA*

Stefan Ulzheimer, PhD, *Division of Computed Tomography, Siemens Medical Solutions, Forchheim, Germany*

Robert J. M. van Geuns, MD, *Department of Radiology, Erasmus Medical Center, Rotterdam, The Netherlands*

Renu Virmani, MD, *Department of Cardiovascular Pathology, Armed Forces Institute of Pathology, Washington, DC*

Thomas J. Vogl, MD, *Institute for Diagnostic and Interventional Radiology, J. W. Goethe University, Frankfurt, Germany*

Matthias Wagner, MD, *Department of Diagnostic and Interventional Radiology, Herz- und Gefaess-Klinik GmbH, Bad Neustadt an der Saale, Germany*

Dominik Weishaupt, MD, *Institute of Diagnostic Radiology, University Hospital Zurich, Zurich, Switzerland*

Brian R. Westerman, PhD, *Division of Computed Tomography, Toshiba Medical Solutions, Los Angeles, CA*

Jürgen K. Willmann, MD, *Institute of Diagnostic Radiology, University Hospital Zurich, Zurich, Switzerland*

Bernd J. Wintersperger, MD, *Department of Clinical Radiology, University of Munich, Munich, Germany*

INTRODUCTION AND HISTORICAL BACKGROUND

I

1 CT of the Heart

Past, Present, and Future

William Stanford, MD

INTRODUCTION

Imaging of the heart and great vessels has previously been done with plain film, cardiac catheterization, nuclear medicine, and echocardiography as the primary imaging modalities. The recent newer advances in the computed tomography (CT) and magnetic resonance imaging (MRI) technologies, however, have dramatically changed our approach to imaging cardiac disease. CT and MRI, supplemented by CT angiography and MRI angiography, are increasingly replacing the chest film, as well as nuclear and—to some extent—echo imaging as the primary modalities in evaluating heart disease.

CT images, which initially took over 4 min to generate, can now be obtained in 50–100 ms with electron beam imaging and in 125–500 ms with helical imaging. Importantly, these advances in temporal resolution are rapid enough to essentially stop cardiac motion, and thus visualization of extremely small structures such as calcium deposits within the walls of the coronary arteries is now possible. Along with this increased temporal resolution has come a concomitant increase in spatial resolution, and isotropic voxels as small as 0.5 mm^3 are now identifiable. These advances, along with the increasing use of 3D reconstruction techniques, have revolutionized cardiac imaging and have moved CT from only anatomic visualization into the arena of functional and perfusion imaging.

HISTORICAL

CT was first introduced by Sir Godfrey Hounsfield in the 1970s—a short 30 yr ago *(1,2)* (Fig. 1). Hounsfield was an electrical engineer working for EMI, an electronics firm in England. While there, he conceived the idea of taking cross-sectional X-ray data and reformatting these data into images. For this, he and Alan M. Cormack, a Tufts professor of mathematics working independently, received the Nobel Prize in medicine in 1979.

Hounsfield's first-generation scanner used a translate/rotate technology. In this methodology, an X-ray source moving laterally activated a series of single detectors before moving to another position and repeating the process. This translate/rotate process was repeated until the entire circumference of the patient was scanned (Fig. 2A). Scan times of 4.5 min per image were required.

The technology was then advanced with the addition of fan beam architecture to the translate/rotate process. With this refinement, each radiation beam activated multiple detectors rather than a single detector. Thus increased numbers of images were possible from each tube activation. With this upgrade, imaging times were reduced to approx 2.5 min per image (Fig. 2B).

The next advance was the introduction of a continuously rotating X-ray tube coupled with a continuously rotating detector array. This further decreased scan times to approx 18 s (Fig. 2C).

Around 1978, the rotating detector array concept was changed to that of a fixed detector array, and this further decreased scan times to approx 2 s per image, and this is the configuration present in many of our conventional CT scanners in operation today (Fig. 2D). As a consequence of these advances, CT was able to become a major workhorse for whole-body imaging, which included many cardiac applications. However, although the excellent resolution and absence of overlying structures allowed visualization of the pericardium and many of the relatively static abnormalities such as intracardiac filling defects from thrombi and tumors, the contracting heart was not well visualized.

An additional problem with this conventional technology was that the scanner cabling restricted tube movement and allowed for only a single tube rotation to a fixed point before the tube had to be returned to its original position. Thus a continuous tube movement was not possible and scan times were relatively fixed. Because of this, cardiac applications were restricted to a 2-s-per-image acquisition time. Yet, the ability to visualize not only the vessel lumina and cardiac chamber endocardium but also the vessel wall and the surrounding myocardium were important applications not heretofore possible. Thus CT provided a more comprehensive view of cardiovascular pathology.

In the early 1980s, an important advance moved CT into the realm of cardiac imaging. This was the introduction of the electron beam technology concept by Dr. Douglas Boyd of the University of California, San Francisco *(3)*. The electron beam scanner, while having an appearance similar to a conventional CT scanner, did not have an X-ray tube rotating around the patient. Instead, electrons were generated by a source and then

From: *Contemporary Cardiology: CT of the Heart: Principles and Applications*
Edited by: U. Joseph Schoepf © Humana Press, Inc., Totowa, NJ

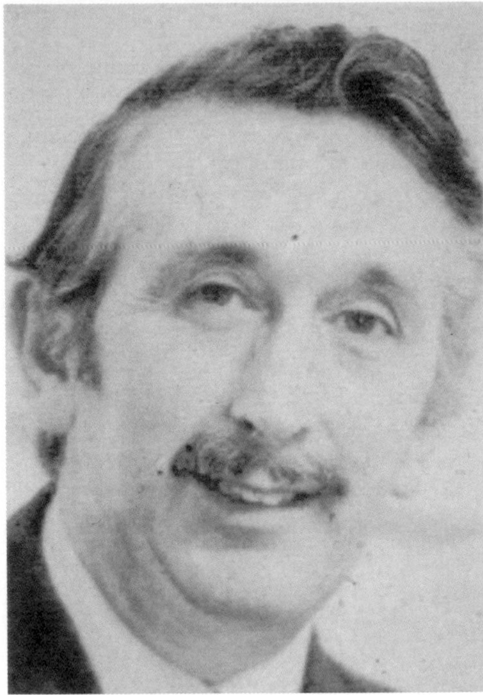

Fig. 1. Godfrey N. Hounsfield, the father of computed tomography. For their achievements, Hounsfield and Alan M. Cormack were awarded the Nobel Prize in medicine in 1979.

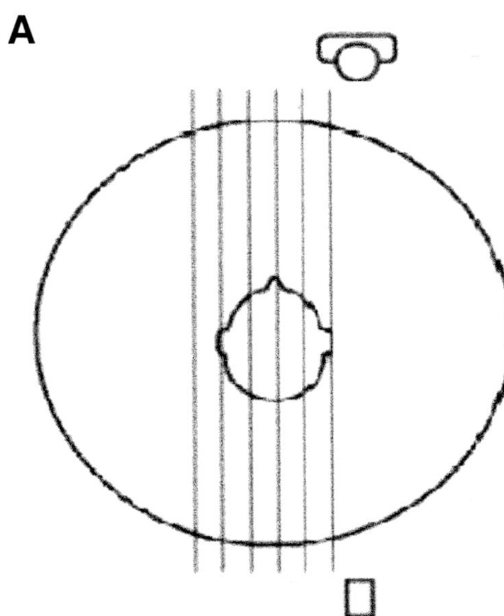

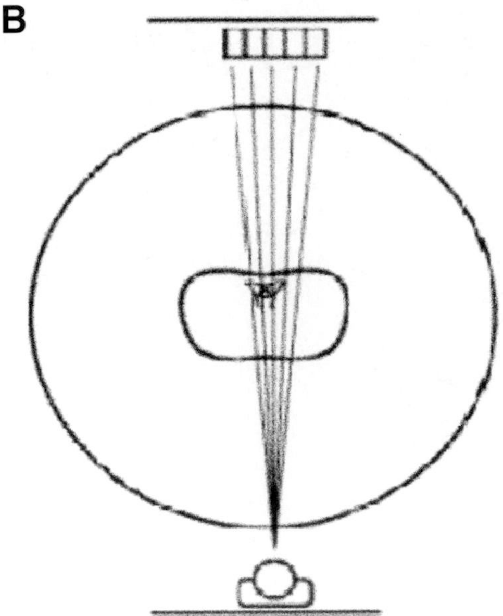

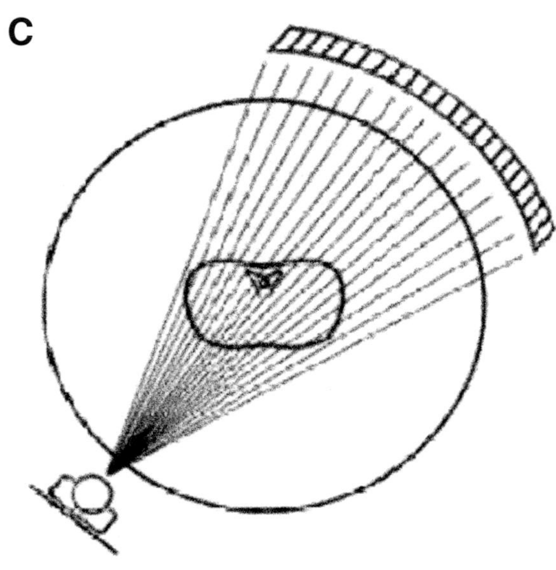

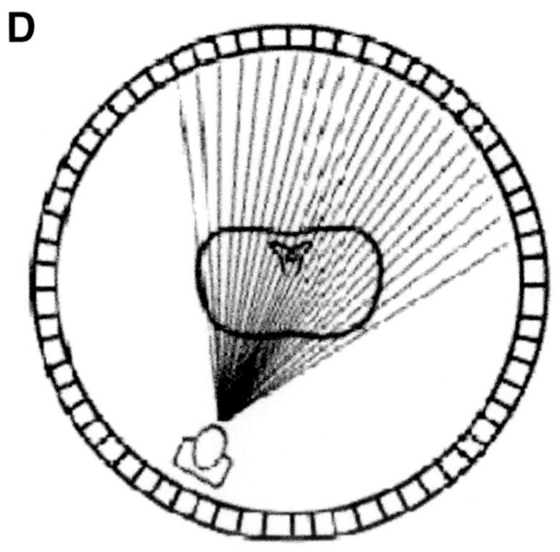

Fig. 2. **(A)** Diagram of the first-generation translate/rotate CT scanner. To create the image, a series of exposures were taken as the X-ray source moved a short distance laterally. The tube then rotated to a different position and the sequence was repeated. A single image required 4.5 min exposure time. **(B)** A later modification of the translate/rotate sequence introduced fan beam architecture to activate multiple detectors before moving to a new position. With this modification, scan times were reduced to 2.5 min/image. **(C)** The next generation of scanners used a rotating X-ray source coupled to rotating detectors. Scan times were reduced to 18 s/image. **(D)** Subsequent modifications used a rotating X-ray source with a fixed detector sarray. Scan times were 2 s/image.

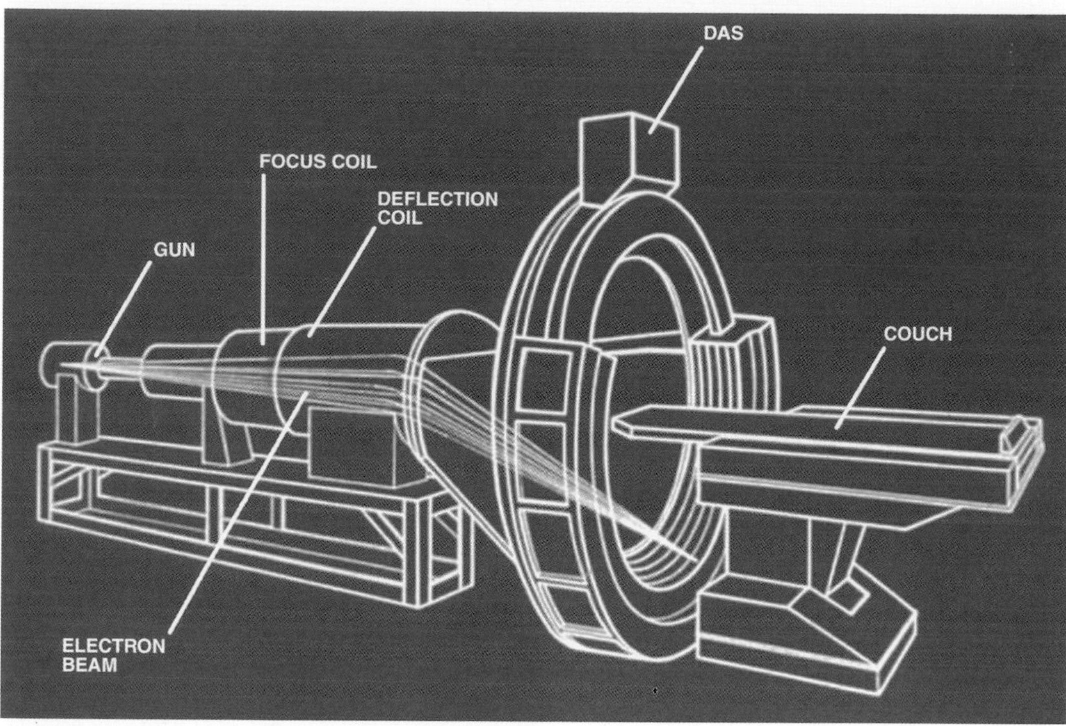

Fig. 3. Cross-sectional diagram of the GE-Imatron C150 XP electron beam scanner. Electron sweeps of tungsten target rings generate X-rays that traverse the patient to activate detectors in the gantry over the patient. With this development, imaging times were reduced to 50–100 ms. (Courtesy GE-Imatron Inc.)

bent electromagnetically to sweep tungsten target rings located in the gantry beneath the patient. The X-rays produced by the electron sweep traversed the patient and were collected by fixed solid-state detectors located in the gantry above the patient (Fig. 3). This technology decreased scan times to 50–100 ms, which essentially froze cardiac motion and thus dramatically changed our ability to image the beating heart. For the first time it was possible to view cardiac contractions and to visualize small structures such as calcium deposits within the walls of the coronary artery.

An additional major advance in CT imaging came in the early 1990s with the introduction of helical/spiral CT imaging and its slip-ring technology *(4)* (Fig. 4). With these advances, the X-ray beam was able to continuously rotate around the patient as the patient moved through the scanner gantry. These innovations decreased scan times to approx 500–1000 ms and ultimately produced data sets with spatial resolutions as small as 0.5 mm^3. The initial platform for helical CT scanners consisted of a single X-ray source and a single detector ring; however, subsequent developments in helical CT technology have enlarged imaging platforms from a single detector to 4 rows and now 16 rows, and in the future 32-, 64-, and 256-row detectors are expected. Along with the increase in numbers of detector rows were advances in the temporal resolution, and now imaging times now as fast as 420 ms are possible. These and other innovations in multislice helical CT have allowed the entire heart to be scanned within a 20–30 s breath-hold, and do so with excellent spatial resolution *(5)*.

THE PRESENT

CONVENTIONAL CT

The design of our current conventional CT scanners is that of a rotating X-ray source activating fixed detectors in the gantry surrounding the patient. The tube movement is limited by cables so that once the tube rotates around the patient, it has to stop and rewind. This constrained tube travel is a major limitation of conventional CT; however, the cross-sectional image detail is excellent and spatial resolutions of 9–12 line pairs (lp)/cm are possible.

ELECTRON BEAM CT

The electron beam CT (EBCT) scanner (GE-Imatron) works on a different principle than does conventional CT. With EBCT, electrons sweep tungsten target rings to produce X-rays that enter from beneath the patient, and are attenuated and collected by solid-state detectors in the gantry above the patient. The technology, because of the absence of moving parts, dramatically decreases scan times to 50–100 ms, which is rapid enough to essentially freeze cardiac motion.

There are several different EBCT scanner models in operation. The older C150 and C300 scanners operate at 130 kV, 625 mA, 83 kW to produce 100-ms, 1.5-, 3-, and 6-mm slice thickness images at resolutions of 9.5 lp/cm. The technology also makes it possible to generate flow and movie mode 50-ms, 8-mm dual slice thickness images from four target rings. The latter ability is important in functional imaging; its spatial resolution is limited at 4.5 lp/cm.

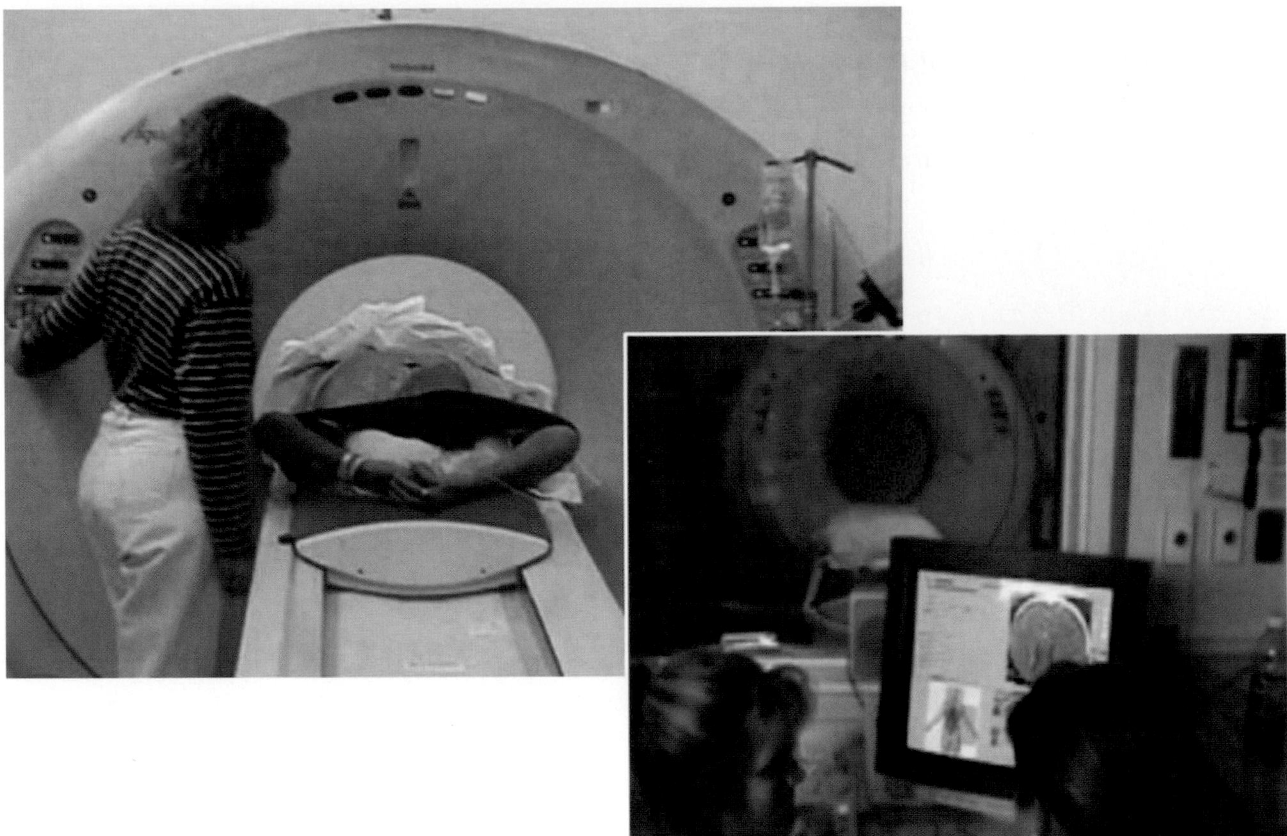

Fig. 4. A modern helical CT imaging suite.

The newer EBCT e-Speed™ version operates at 140 kV, 1000 mA, 140 kW. It can generate dual 1.5-, 3-, and 8-mm slices, at 50 ms temporal resolution. The spatial resolution is 10 lp/cm. This version also has a 100-ms mode for higher spatial resolution and a 33-ms mode for higher temporal resolution. Both are significant advances in EBCT technology.

Flow Mode

EBCT uses several sequences to image the heart. In the flow mode sequence, the C150 and C300 scanners generate eight 8-mm images in 224 ms. Then, following an 8-ms delay to reset the beam, an additional eight 8-mm slices can be generated in another 224 ms. The advantage of this configuration is that a stack of multilevel images can be obtained almost simultaneously, thus allowing visualization of a contrast bolus as it enters, peaks, and washes out of a region of interest (Fig. 5). This sequence is similar to the first-pass studies used in nuclear medicine. Flow mode sequences are useful in evaluating coronary artery bypass graft patency, intracardiac shunts, and arteriovenous malformations, as well as identifying bolus arrival times in aberrant vessels.

Movie Mode

A more commonly used EBCT sequence is the movie (cine) sequence. In this configuration, the C150 and C300 scanners can generate images of the contracting heart every 58 ms (17 images per second). These images can be acquired during systole and diastole, which allows visualization during a cardiac contraction (Fig. 6). This sequence, usually consisting of 10–12 same-level images, is triggered off the R wave of the ECG. Once completed, it then takes 8 ms for the scanner to reset, and another 10–12 image data set at the same or usually a different level can be obtained. The spatial resolution in the flow and movie modes is moderate at 4.5 lp/cm; however, with the new e-Speed model, resolutions of 10 lp/cm are possible. Movie sequences are important in quantifying cardiac function and in evaluating abnormal contraction patterns, such as those seen post myocardial infarction. Also, by completely opacifying the cardiac chambers, filling defects such as thrombi or tumors are readily identified.

Step Volume and Continuous Volume Scans

Lastly, in the step volume scan (SVS) and continuous volume scan (CVS) modes, 1.5-, 3-, or 6-mm single-slice thicknesses are obtainable. In the SVS sequence, the temporal resolution of the C150 and C300 platforms is 100 ms, which is 9 images per second, with the pixel sizes varying from 0.06 to 1 mm^2. With the e-Speed, 50-ms volume scan sequences at 17 or 34 images per second are possible, depending upon whether one or two detectors are used. The SVS images can be triggered at preset intervals from the ECG signal. The maximal resolution is 10 lp/cm, depending upon the field of view and the reconstructive algorithm selected. In the SVS mode, images are acquired in a manner similar to that of conventional CT scanners—i.e., a single target ring is swept to produce an image and then the table moves and a second image is generated. Multiple sweeps of the same target can be taken and volume averaged if

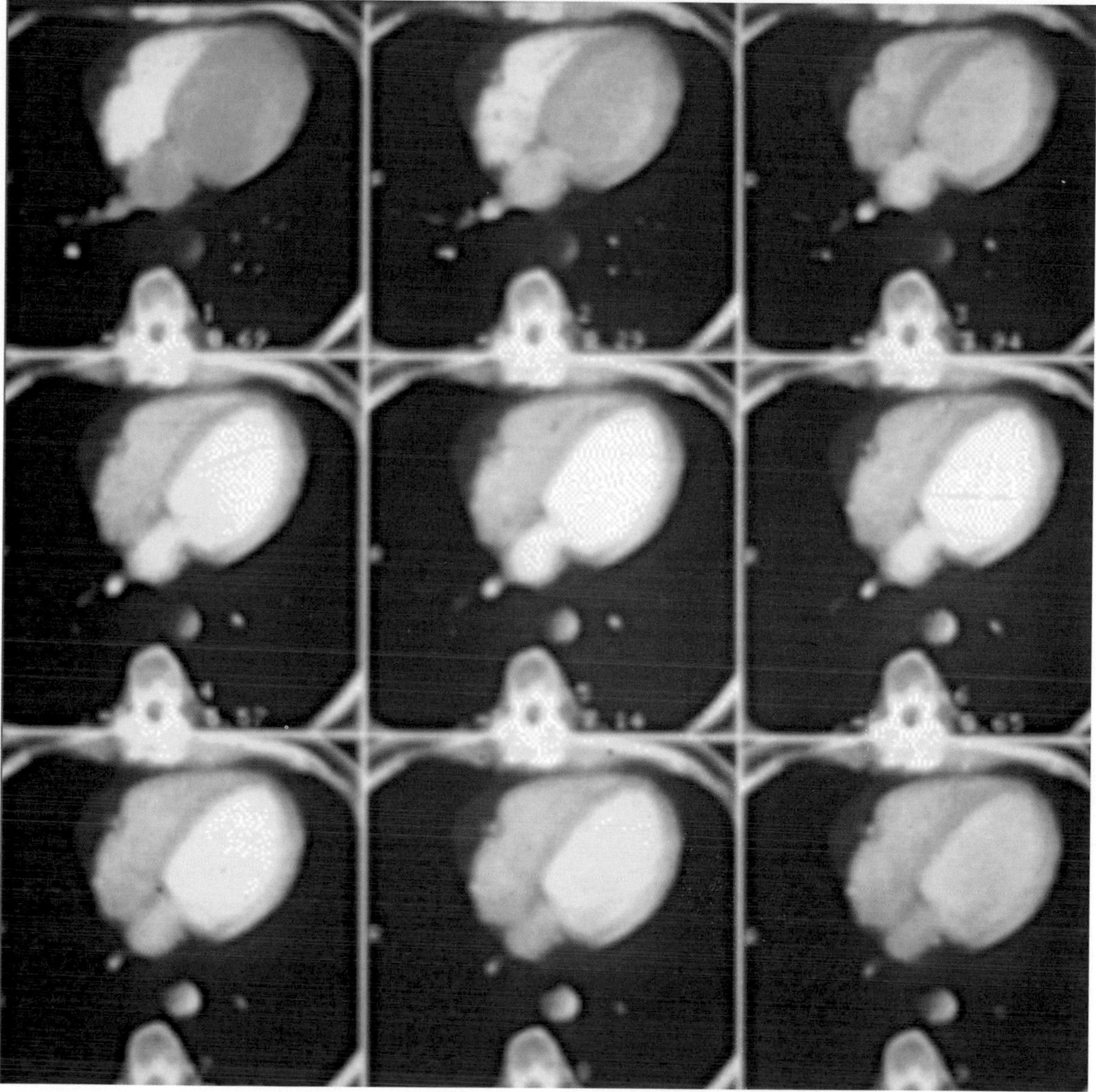

Fig. 5. An electron beam CT flow mode sequence showing a contrast bolus opacifying the right atrium and ventricle, and then washing out and later appearing in the left ventricle. This sequence is useful in evaluating bypass graft patency, intracardiac shunts, and arteriovenous malformations, as well as identifying contrast arrival in aberrant vessels.

additional resolution is required; however, this comes at the price of increased radiation exposure.

The continuous volume mode (CVS) is similar to that of spiral or helical CT methodologies, with up to 140 images on the C150, up to 280 images on the C300, and 400 images on the e-Speed scanners possible during an acquisition period of about 33 s. The minimum exposure time is 100 ms (33 ms on e-Speed) and the images can be contiguous or overlapped. On the C150 or C300 scanners, this mode allows a complete 140-slice, 3-mm thick data set to be acquired during a 17-second breath-hold. Scan widths of 1.5–10 mm are possible.

HELICAL CT

Current-generation helical/spiral CT scanners have multirow detectors capable of generating 1 to 16 slices of varying thickness with each gantry rotation. Technological advances have reduced gantry rotation times from 1 s to 420 ms, and with segmented reconstruction, image times approximating 100 ms are possible. An additional advantage of the helical technology is that the detector information is generated as a volumetric data set, and this permits later reformations of different slice thickness that allows 3D reconstructions. Helical CT images are commonly ECG gated, and this further decreases motion artifacts by being able to restrict image acquisition to the quiet phase of the cardiac cycle. The latter is particularly important in coronary calcification screening.

Helical/Spiral CT Sequence

In cardiac imaging, helical CT scanners are operated in two basic modes, both gated from the patient's ECG. The first mode, designated *prospective gated scanning*, activates the X-ray tube for only the time needed to acquire a partial image. This is

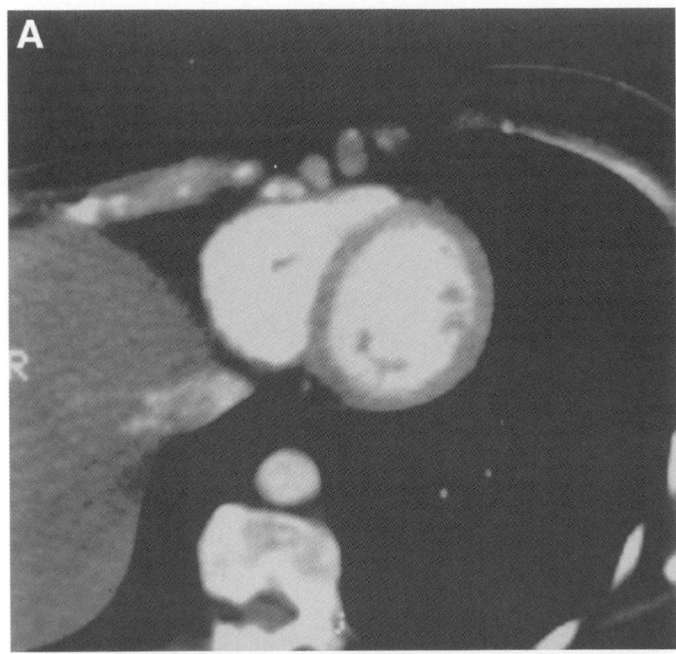

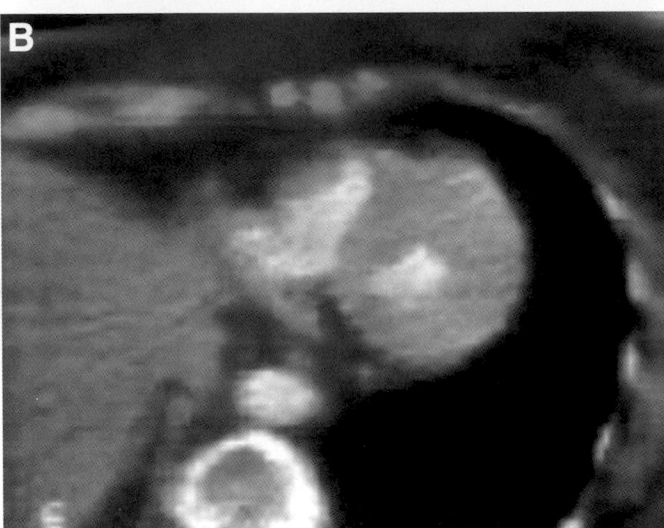

Fig. 6. Electron-beam short axis movie mode images at the mid-left-ventricular level in diastole (**A**) and systole (**B**). This sequence is useful in quantifying cardiac function and evaluating abnormalities of wall motion.

roughly half the gantry rotation time, or as short as 200–250 ms. The time of data collection is measured from the R wave, and the operator selects this delay. This mode is frequently used for coronary artery calcium imaging, because the radiation dose to the patient is kept to a minimum. However, rapid or irregular patient heart rates can affect image quality and the reproducibility of the study. Data collection periods that extend beyond diastole may exhibit motion artifacts that can reduce accuracy. A 4-detector ring scanner rotating at 0.5 s and programmed to provide 3-mm slices can acquire a data set in about 20 s, a reasonable breath-hold for most patients. Sixteen-row detector scanners in the same study reduced scanning times to roughly 8–12 s.

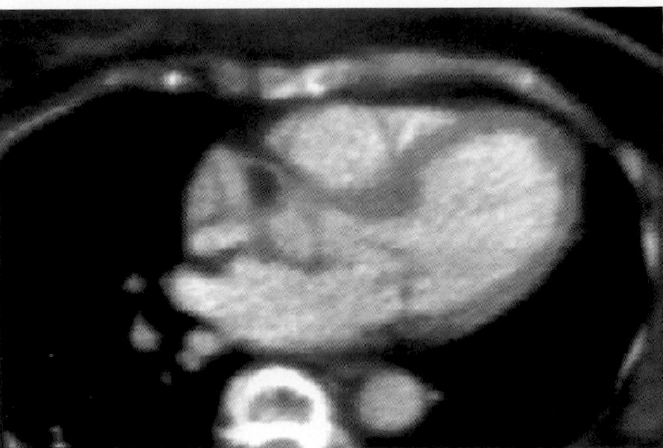

Fig. 7. Electron beam CT long axis (four-chamber) view image showing the left and right atria, left and right ventricles, and left-ventricular outflow tract.

Retrospective gated scanning is the other operating mode of helical scanners. This sequence involves the helical scanning of the entire heart while at the same time recording the patient's ECG. After the scan, images are reconstructed at a preselected phase of the cardiac cycle. This mode is commonly used for coronary artery angiography and for cardiac functional analysis. In order to avoid anatomical gaps in the data set, the helical pitch is set lower than that used for general body imaging. Thus the dose to the patient is higher. Nevertheless, the ability to reconstruct images in multiple phases from the same high-resolution data set can provide important information. Submillimeter slices, as small as 0.5 mm, can be used to achieve a high spatial resolution, and cardiac data collection can be accomplished in about 30 s. However, the patient's heart rate is again a major factor in maintaining high image quality. If the heart rate exceeds 70 beats per minute (bpm), segmented image reconstruction can be used. This algorithm uses data from two, three, or four consecutive cardiac cycles to reconstruct a single image, thus improving the temporal resolution significantly and extending the range of heart rates that can be scanned with high-quality images.

ADDITIONAL CONSIDERATIONS

IMPORTANCE OF TEMPORAL RESOLUTION

Although conventional, helical, and EBCT are able to identify cardiac anatomy, motion artifacts can still remain a problem. With contrast enhancement, conventional CT can image cardiac chambers and great vessel anatomy extremely well. However, helical/spiral CT and EBCT, because of their faster scan times, are suited better for imaging moving structures. In a typical cardiac sequence, the superior and inferior vena cavae, pulmonary arteries, and aorta are routinely visualized, as are the right and left atria and ventricles, and their outflow tracts (Fig. 7). With CT, the interfaces between the contrast-enhanced cardiac chambers and myocardium are usually well defined, especially if the image is acquired during diastole; in systole this interface may be partially degraded by motion. Overall, both helical/spiral CT and EBCT, because of their faster scan times, generally better define struc-

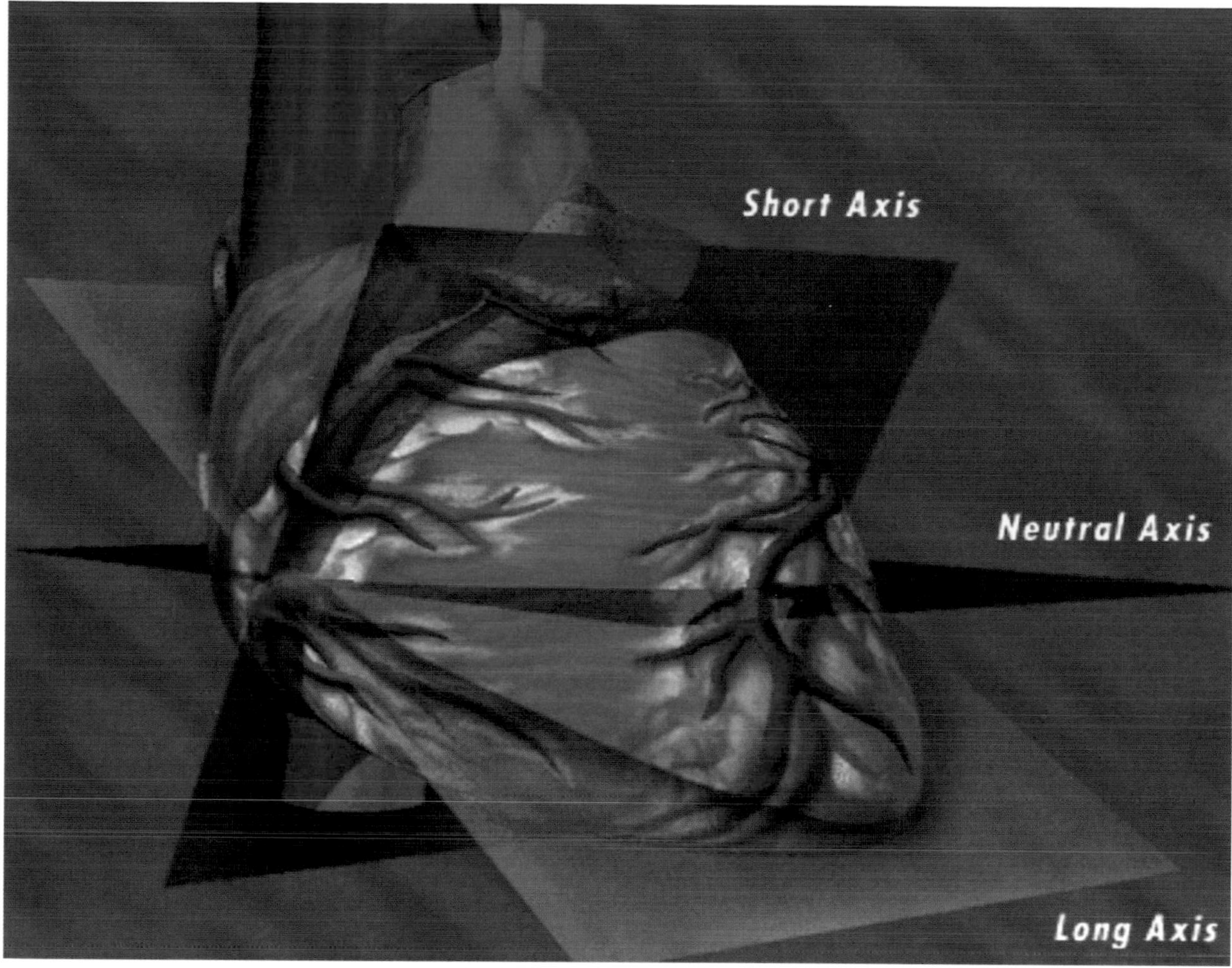

Fig. 8. Heart model showing the cross-sectional planes used in cardiac imaging.

tural detail *(5)*. Although it is important that the patient remain quiet and suspend respiration, often it is still possible with the EBCT and helical/spiral CT scanners to obtain satisfactory images, even if the individual is unable to hold his or her breath.

CONTRAST CONSIDERATIONS

In cardiac imaging, contrast administration is often necessary. The contrast material is usually administered as a bolus or as a continuous infusion, but because of the speed of the scanners, contrast arrival times become critical. Commonly, volumes of 80–150 mL of contrast material, varying from 240 to 370 mg of iodine per mL, are administered. Generally, the contrast material is infused at a rate of 1–4 mL/s using a power injector.

For contrast administration, timing methodologies become important to ensure contrast optimization. One method is to administer a test bolus of 10 mL of contrast material and perform repeated imaging over the area of interest to determine contrast bolus arrival time. Another is to perform a circulation time using either cardiogreen dye or a solution of 0.5% magnesium sulfate. Both are injected at approx 4 mL/s. With magnesium sulfate, approx 10 mL of 0.5% solution is commonly administered, with bolus arrival being manifested by a warm sensation in the back of the tongue or throat. With cardiogreen dye, an earlobe densitometer records the arrival of the bolus. Other techniques are the "sure start" technologies, where the scanner monitors the rise in contrast attenuation over the area of interest. When the attenuation approaches the preselected threshold, the scanner is triggered automatically. Alternatively, a fixed delay of 15–30 s may be used.

POSITIONAL CONSIDERATIONS

Cardiac CT scanning, especially in evaluating cardiac function, requires imaging in planes less familiar to radiologists. The oblique position of the heart requires modifications to our traditional scanning planes. The two configurations commonly used in cardiac imaging are the short axis view, wherein the ventricle is "bread-loafed" (Fig. 8), and the "four-chamber view," which slices the heart longitudinally from top to bottom and produces images that are similar to those familiar to our echocardiology colleagues (Fig. 7).

RADIATION DOSAGE

The effective dose is the overall radiation exposure to the patient. This is designated in mSv, and is frequently equated to months of background exposure. For an EBCT calcium study, the effective dose would be 1.0 mSv in males and 1.3 mSv in women (4.0 and 5.2 mo of background radiation, respectively) *(6)*.

3 Scan Techniques for Cardiac and Coronary Artery Imaging With Multislice CT

Bernd M. Ohnesorge, PhD, Brian R. Westerman, PhD,
and U. Joseph Schoepf, MD

INTRODUCTION

Cardiac imaging is a demanding application for any noninvasive imaging modality. On the one hand, high temporal resolution is needed to virtually freeze cardiac motion and thus avoid motion artifacts in the images. On the other hand, sufficient spatial resolution—at best submillimeter—is required to adequately visualize small and complex anatomical structures like the coronary arteries. The complete heart volume has to be examined within a single short breath-hold time to avoid breathing artifacts and to limit the amount of contrast agent, if necessary. The motion of the heart is both complex and very fast. Some estimates of the temporal resolution needed to freeze cardiac motion in any phase of the cardiac cycle are as low as 10 ms. In 1984, electron beam computed tomography (EBCT) was introduced as a noninvasive imaging modality for the diagnosis of coronary artery disease *(1–4)*. Its temporal resolution of 100 ms allows for relatively motion-free imaging of the cardiac anatomy in the diastolic phase, even at higher heart rates. Because the EBCT at that time was limited to axial scanning for electrocardiogram (ECG)-synchronized cardiac investigations, a single breath-hold scan of the heart required slice widths of at least 3 mm. The resulting axial resolution was therefore limited and not adequate for 3D visualization of the coronary arteries. With the advent of subsecond rotation, combined with prospective and retrospective ECG-gating, mechanical single-slice helical or spiral CT systems with superior general image quality entered the realm of cardiac imaging *(4,5)*. Since 1999, 4-slice CT systems, which have the potential to overcome some of the limitations of single-slice cardiac CT scanning, have been used to establish ECG-triggered or ECG-gated multislice CT (MSCT) examinations of the heart and the coronary arteries in clinical use *(6–10)*. As a result of the increased scan speed with four simultaneously acquired slices, coverage of the entire heart volume with thin slices within one breath-hold became feasible. The improved axial resolution provided much more accurate CT imaging of the heart and the coronary arteries *(11–14)*. Recent clinical studies have demonstrated the potential of MSCT to differentiate and classify lipid, fibrous, and calcified coronary plaques *(15)*. Despite these promising advances, the 4-slice CT scanner technology still faces some challenges and limitations with respect to motion artifacts in patients with higher heart rates, limited spatial resolution, and long breath-hold times *(12)*. In 2001, a new generation of MSCT systems with simultaneous acquisition of up to 16 slices was introduced *(16,17)*. With submillimeter slice acquisition and gantry rotation times shorter than 0.5 s, both spatial and temporal resolution are improved, while examination times are considerably reduced.

In this chapter, we present the basic technology of MSCT cardiac scanning with a special focus on recommended scan techniques for different clinical applications. We will also discuss the technology advances and improved clinical performance of state-of-the-art 16-slice CT equipment compared with 4-slice CT scanners.

TECHNOLOGY PRINCIPLES

TECHNOLOGY OVERVIEW

CT examinations of the heart should be performed in a single, short breath-hold scan with high temporal resolution to eliminate cardiac motion and high, preferably isotropic, spatial resolution. It has become increasingly apparent that submillimeter slices are necessary to adequately visualize small and complex cardio-thoracic anatomy and the coronary arteries.

In 1984, EBCT was introduced as the first cross-sectional noninvasive imaging modality that could visualize the cardiac anatomy and the coronary arteries *(1)*. During this period, mechanical scanners typically had single-slice detectors and a minimum gantry rotation time of 0.75–1.0 s, and were not considered of value for strictly cardiac imaging. With presently available EBCT scanners, temporal resolution of 100 ms provides motion-free images of the cardiac anatomy in the diastolic phase of the cardiac cycle even at higher heart rates *(2)*. Cardiac anatomy can be covered in a single breath-hold of 30–40 s with slice widths of 3 mm, but this limits the diagnostic

From: *Contemporary Cardiology: CT of the Heart: Principles and Applications*
Edited by: U. Joseph Schoepf © Humana Press, Inc., Totowa, NJ

accuracy of coronary artery visualization *(3)*. In 1998, spiral/helical CT systems with simultaneous acquisition of four detector slices and rotation time of 500 ms were introduced *(6,7,10)*, which provided a substantial performance increase over the single- and dual-slice spiral CT systems that had been available until then. These MSCT scanners can cover larger scan volumes with slice collimation down to 0.5 mm and thus provide higher spatial resolution for improved visualization of small and complex anatomy.

Detector configurations in use today enable simultaneous collimation of four slices with different slice widths. In the "fixed array" design, detector rows with equal spacing are used, while the "adaptive array" and "hybrid" detector designs consist of fewer detector rows, containing elements that become wider away from the center of the detector (Fig. 1A,B). In all designs the thinnest slices result from collimation of the inner four detector rows, and thicker slices are generated by electronic combination of adjacent detector rows.

Regardless of detector design, it was apparent from the operation of the 4-slice scanners that no fundamental barrier prevented the construction of CT scanners that could acquire more slices simultaneously, and indeed this quickly came to pass. Systems capable of eight slices became available in 2000, with commensurate increases in exam speed. Meanwhile, 8- and 10-slice CT scanners are being used that provide further improved volume coverage with about 1-mm slice width and 500 ms rotation time *(18)*. The first 16-slice CT scanners, introduced in early 2002, provide faster rotation time (down to 400 ms) and submillimeter detector collimation for routine volume imaging *(16,17)*. The 16-slice systems are sufficiently fast to cover the entire heart, scanning with submillimeter slices, in a reasonable breath-hold. All of the 16-slice scanners have adopted a detector design with elements of two sizes. In the examples given (SOMATOM Sensation 16, Siemens, and Aquillion 16, Toshiba Medical) (Fig. 1C,D) the 16 central rows define submillimeter detector acquisition. By adding outer detector rows on both sides, wider slices of 1 mm and above can be achieved.

Higher temporal resolution than the older mechanical CT scanners is provided by a combination of faster gantry rotation speed, with rotation times down to 500 ms, and specialized reconstruction algorithms *(10)*. As of 2002, the shortest gantry rotation time was reduced to 400 ms, and more recently even to 370 ms, thus further improving temporal resolution *(16,17)*. The combination of fast rotation time and multislice acquisition with submillimeter spatial resolution has proved to be of particular importance for improved cardiac image quality *(17,19–21)*.

Motion artifacts caused by cardiac pulsation can be minimized in high-resolution CT studies by limiting image reconstruction to those parts of the cardiac cycle associated with the least motion, typically during diastole. The heart phases can be determined from a simultaneously recorded ECG signal. Two different ECG synchronization techniques are most commonly employed for cardiac CT scanning—prospective ECG triggering and retrospective ECG gating.

ECG-TRIGGERED MSCT IMAGING

Prospective ECG triggering has long been used in conjunction with EBCT and single-slice spiral CT *(1–4)*. A trigger signal is derived from the patient's ECG based on a prospective estimation of the present RR interval, and the scan is started at a user-defined time after a detected R wave, usually during diastole. MSCT allows simultaneous acquisition of several slices in one heartbeat with a cycle time that usually allows scanning in every other heartbeat (Fig. 2A). Thus shorter breath-hold times are required compared to single-slice scanners, and respiratory artifacts can be virtually eliminated. To achieve the best possible temporal resolution, scan data are acquired only during a partial gantry rotation (approximately two thirds of a rotation with 240–260° projection data) that covers the minimum amount of data required for image reconstruction. Conventional partial image reconstruction based on fan beam projection data results in a temporal resolution equal to the acquisition time of the partial scan. Optimized temporal resolution can be achieved with parallel-beam-based "half-scan" reconstruction algorithms that provide a temporal resolution of half the rotation time in a central area of the scan field of view *(6,7,10,16)*. Thus, prospective ECG triggering is also the most dose-efficient method of ECG-synchronized scanning, as only the very minimum of scan data needed for image reconstruction are acquired. However, usually only relatively thick slices (3 mm with EBCT, 2.5–3 mm with 4-, 8-, and 16-slice CT) are used for prospectively triggered acquisition, to maintain a reasonably short single breath-hold. Thus, resulting data sets are often not suitable for 3D or multiplanar reformation (MPR) reconstruction of small cardiac anatomy. In addition, prospective ECG-triggered scans are sensitive to changes in heart rate during acquisition, so significant fluctuation or arrhythmia can have a severe effect on image quality.

ECG-GATED MSCT SCANNING AND IMAGE RECONSTRUCTION

Retrospective ECG gating overcomes the limitations of prospective ECG triggering with regard to scan time and spatial resolution, and can provide more consistent image quality for examination of patients with changing heart rate during the scan. This technique requires multislice spiral scanning with slow table speed and simultaneous recording of the ECG trace that is used for retrospective assignment of image reconstruction *(8–10)*. Phase-consistent coverage of the heart requires a highly overlapping spiral/helical scan with a table feed adapted to the heart rate in order to avoid gaps between image stacks that are reconstructed in consecutive heart cycles. The image stacks are reconstructed at exactly the same phase of the heart cycle and cover the entire heart and adjacent anatomy (Fig. 2B). To achieve gapless coverage of the entire heart over a wide range of heart rates, pitch values between 0.2 and 0.4 are employed (pitch equals table feed per rotation, divided by the nominal width of the X-ray beam—equal to all slices combined). Images are reconstructed during every heart beat, and somewhat faster scan coverage is possible as compared to prospective ECG triggering. Moreover, the continuous spiral acquisition enables reconstruction of overlapping image slices,

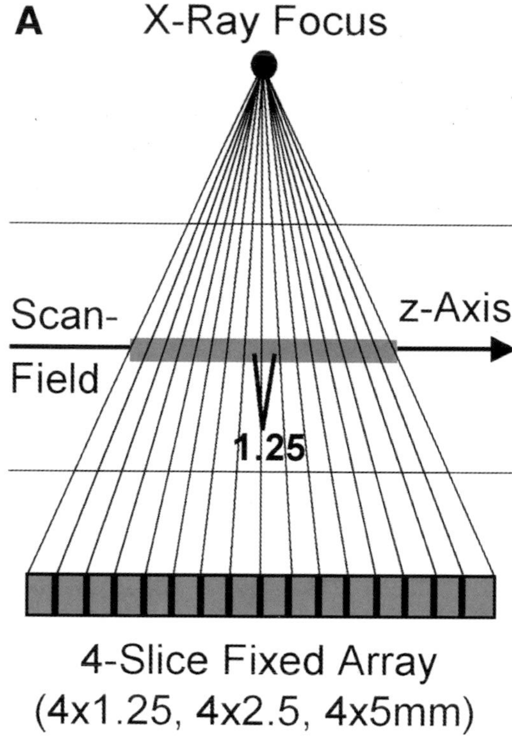

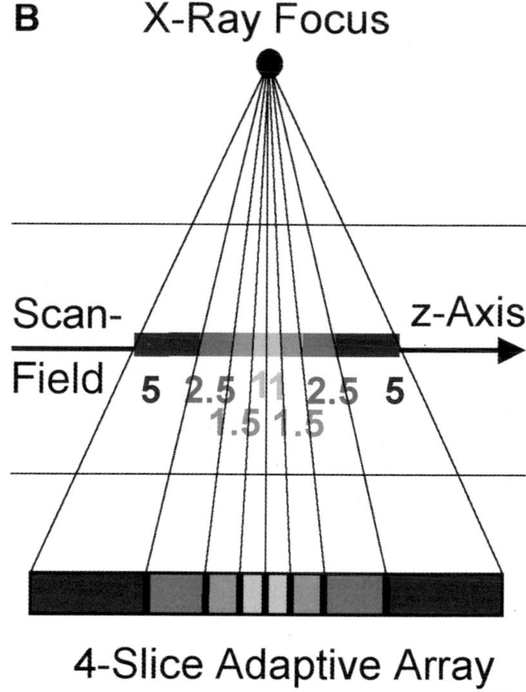

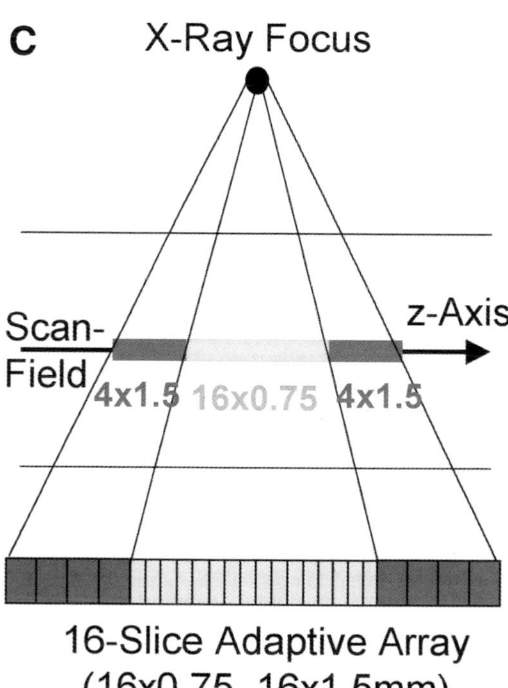

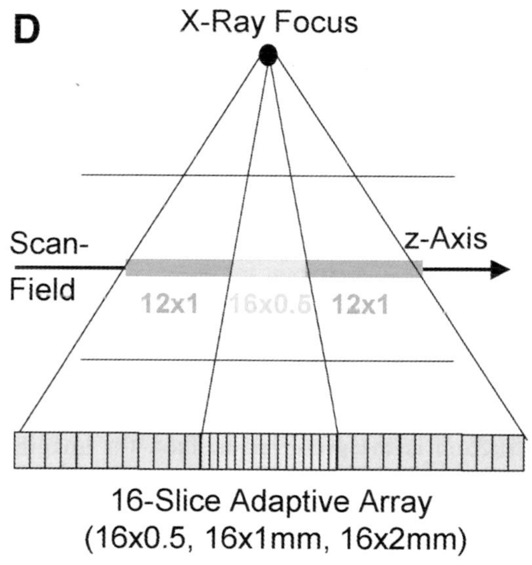

Fig. 1. (**A**) Equally spaced detector elements build the fixed array detector (FAD) for a 4-slice system. Different 4-slice collimation settings (4 × 1.25, 4 × 2.5, 4 × 3.75, 4 × 5 mm) are produced by electronic combination of adjacent elements. (**B**) Differently sized detector elements build the adaptive array detector (AAD) for a 4-slice system. Different 4-slice collimation settings (4 × 2.5, 4 × 5 mm) are produced by electronic combination of adjacent elements. For 4 × 1 mm collimation, partial shielding of the elements with 1.5-mm width is required. Partial illumination of the inner two detector elements allows for 2 × 0.5-mm collimation for high-resolution scanning. (**C**) The latest 16-slice CT scanners are also based on the AAD design with differently sized detector elements. 16-slice collimation settings 16 × 0.75 mm and 16 × 1.5 mm are produced by equally spaced 16 × 0.75-mm detector elements in the center, eight additional 1.5-mm detector elements (four on each side), and electronic combination of adjacent elements. (**D**) Other 16-slice CT designs allow for illumination of 16 × 0.5-mm slices in the detector center and up to 16 × 2.0-mm slices via adding detector elements with 1.0-mm detector spacing on each side that are also electronically combined.

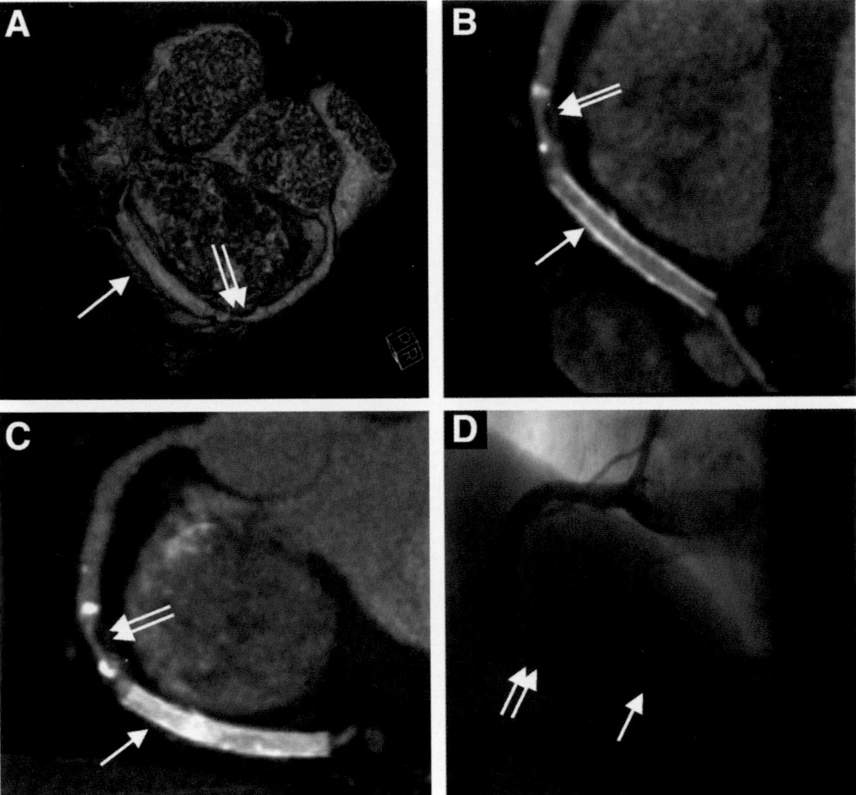

Fig. 11. Coronary CT angiography examination of a patient after percutaneous transluminal coronary angioplasty with stent in the distal right coronary artery, using a 16-slice CT scanner. Scan protocol: 16 × 0.75-mm detector collimation, 0.75-mm reconstructed slice width, 420-ms rotation speed, 12-cm scan range covered in 16 s (SOMATOM Sensation 16, Siemens). The patient presented for follow-up examination after the intervention and was examined to rule out re-stenosis. Coronary CT angiography reveals a patent stent lumen (arrow) but calcified and noncalcified atherosclerotic lesions and high-grade lumenal narrowing of about 70% proximal to the stent (double arrow). **(A)** The lumenal narrowing can be readily displayed with 3D volume-rendering technique in combination with cut planes that remove overlying anatomy. **(B)** Multiplanar reformation allows for visualization of the open in-stent lumen and of the narrowed lumen proximal to the stent. **(C)** Additional display of the same anatomy with maximum intensity projection provides clear assessment of the calcified and noncalcified atherosclerotic lesions related to the stenotic lesion. **(D)** Conventional angiography confirms the patent stent and the 70% stenosis, which was successfully dilated in the same session (case courtesy of Dr. C. S. Soo, HSC Medical Center, Kuala Lumpur, Malaysia).

applied for high-resolution reconstruction of small high-contrast structures (e.g., coronary stents and calcified coronary segments) in a limited range (Figs. 11 and 12).

Rotation times down to 370 ms and the extended number of slices, up to 16, result in a reduced scan time of 15–20 s (*see also* Table 1). Thus, 16-slice CT can also cover larger scan ranges of 18–20 cm with ECG-gated thin-slice spiral scan protocols in a reasonably short breath-hold of 25–30 s that enables high-resolution imaging of most parts of the great thoracic vasculature and coronary bypass grafts over their entire course (Fig. 13).

Optimization of scan protocols in terms of radiation exposure is particularly important for contrast-enhanced CT imaging of the coronary arteries. Sufficiently high spatial resolution and low-contrast resolution has to be achieved in patients of all sizes at the lowest possible radiation exposure. For tube voltage of 120 kV and 500 ms rotation time, tube current of approx 300 mA should be used for imaging 4- and 8-slice CT with slice width of 1 to 1.25 mm. The tube current may need to be increased to approx 350–400 mA for 16-slice CT using submillimeter slices and faster rotation time. ECG-gated scan acquisition with highly overlapping helical/spiral pitch (i.e., pitch much less than 1) in a 10-cm scan range results in an effective dose of approx 7–8 mSv for males and approx 9–11 mSv for female patients (based on protocol examples in Table 1). Despite increased tube current and spatial resolution with 16-slice CT scanners, radiation exposure does not considerably increase, due to better dose utilization of 16-slice detector geometry *(16,17)*. However, radiation exposure increases with reduced spiral pitch and with extension of the scan range. Using ECG-gated dose modulation, radiation exposure can be reduced by 30–50% depending on heart rate, provided that images do not need to be reconstructed over a wide range of the RR interval. ECG-gated dose modulation can reduce radiation exposure to approx 3.5–6.0 mSv for male and to approx 4.5–8.0 mSv for female patients, and works best in patients with a reasonably stable heart rate during the scan.

The overall diagnostic quality of coronary CT angiography largely depends on choice of the appropriate reconstruction time point within the cardiac cycle, the rate and stability of the patient's heart rate during the examination, and the effectiveness of contrast enhancement. The motion pattern of the left

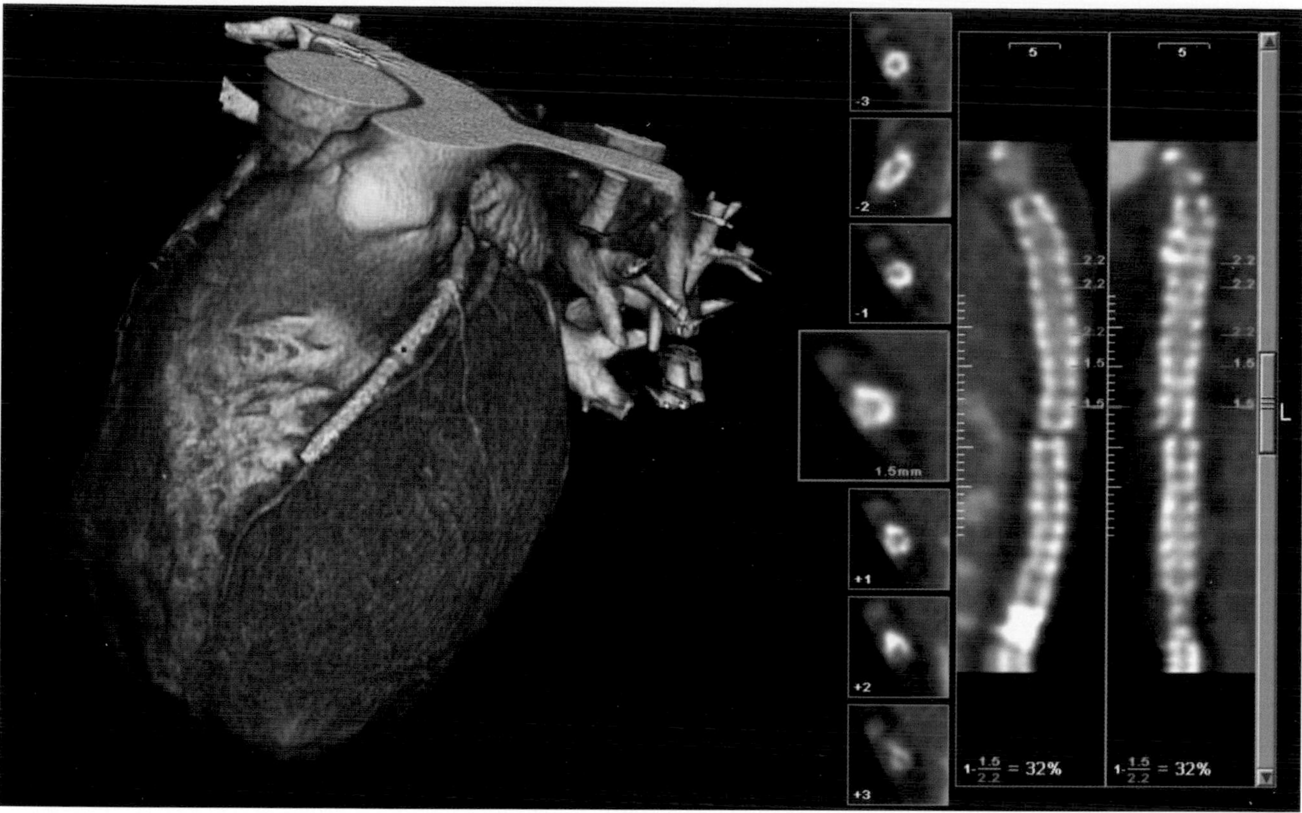

Fig. 12. Coronary CT angiography examination of a patient after percutaneous transluminal coronary angioplasty with two stents in the left descending coronary artery using a 16-slice CT scanner. Scan protocol: 16 × 0.5-mm detector collimation, 0.6-mm reconstructed slice width, 400-ms rotation speed, 12-cm scan range covered in 32 s (Aquillion 16, Toshiba Medical). Cross-sectional reconstruction of orthogonal multiplanar reformations and longitudinal visualization of the vessel based on automatic center-line detection and data segmentation shows both stents open (Vessel Probe, Vital Images) (case courtesy of Dr. Strobie, Florida Institute for Advanced Diagnostic Imaging).

heart and the left anterior descending and circumflex coronary arteries follows the left-ventricular contraction, whereas the right coronary artery moves synchronously with the right heart, i.e., the right atrium. Because of these different motion patterns, different reconstruction time points over the cardiac cycle are frequently necessary in order to display the different coronary vessels with a minimum of motion artifact *(26,27)*. Most studies agree that patient heart rate is inversely related to image quality of cardiac and coronary CT angiography *(12–14,26,27)* because of motion artifacts. It has been shown that MSCT provides better diagnostic accuracy and reliability of results in patients with slow heart rates. Study data based on 4-slice CT with 500-ms rotation time indicates that an upper limit to achieve consistently appropriate image quality lies between 65 and 75 beats per minute (bpm) *(26,27)*. At higher heart rates, adequate image quality can be achieved by using segmented image reconstruction, but overall results may be less consistent and reproducible. Even with the recent reduction of gantry rotation times to as little as 370 ms (Fig. 14), heart rate still remains the crucial factor in determining motion artifact and thus image quality. In those patients with heart rates above the 75–80 bpm threshold, the practical options are use of segmented reconstruction to improve temporal resolution where possible, or reduction of the heart rate pharmacologically by administering beta-blockers. Reliable evaluation of larger cardiac morphology, such as the cardiac chambers and the great vessels, is possible in patients who present with higher heart rates without resorting to drugs, although some image artifacts may be present.

The reliability of multislice cardiac and coronary CT angiography in patients with arrhythmias is limited. However, misinterpretations of the ECG signal can be partially compensated by retrospective editing of the ECG trace. Persistent irregular heart rates, such as in patients with atrial fibrillation, are contraindications for coronary CTA, but the assessment of the greater cardiac morphology such as the ventricles and atria usually remains possible.

The presence of heavy coronary calcification may limit the value of CT coronary imaging, because beam hardening and partial volume effects, and an inability to distinguish between calcium and contrast, can completely obscure the coronary lumen. Metal objects such as stents, surgical clips, and sternal wires can also obscure the evaluation of underlying structures. Use of the thinnest possible slice width reduces partial-volume artifacts and improves visualization of calcified coronary segments. Additionally, dedicated filtering could be beneficial to the imaging of calcified vessels.

Optimization of contrast media injection protocols for cardiac and coronary CT angiography is aimed at providing homogenous enhancement within the entire course of the coro-

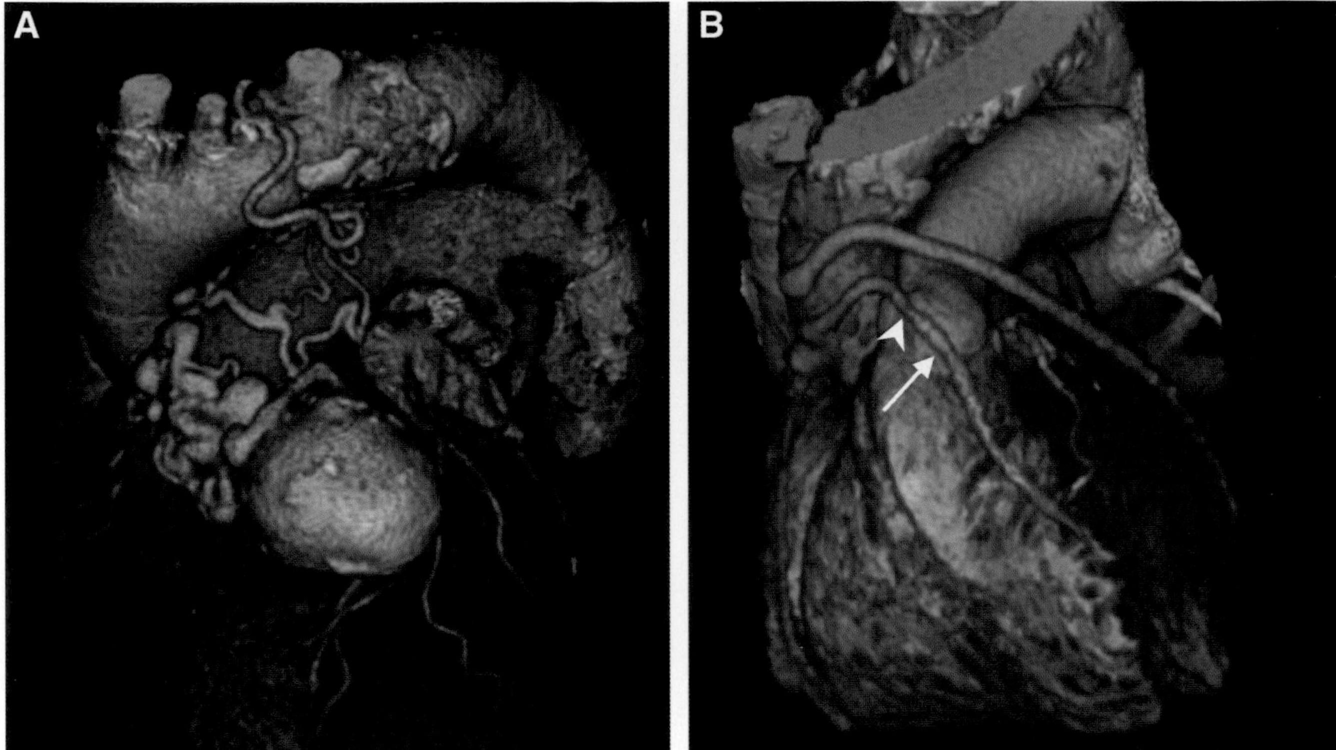

Fig. 13. Coronary CT angiography examination of two patients using a 16-slice CT scanner. with 16 × 0.75-mm detector collimation, 420-ms rotation speed, and extended volume coverage of 15 cm in order to visualize the heart, the ascending aorta, and the pulmonary vessels (SOMATOM Sensation 16, Siemens). **(A)** The first case demonstrates abnormal anatomy of the left descending coronary artery, including multiple fistula. Real-time 3D rendering is of advantage for assessment of the complex anatomy conditions. **(B)** In the second case, three bypasses to right coronary artery, left anterior descending coronary artery, and marginal branch are visualized with 3D volume-rendering technique. The bypass to the left anterior descending coronary artery (arrow) shows a patent proximal and distal anastomosis. However, a 50% stenosis (arrow head) is present in the proximal part of the bypass. The other two bypasses reveal open lumen over the entire course (cases courtesy of Dr. G. Lo, Department of Radiology, Hongkong Sanatorium Hospital [A] and the departments of Radiology and Cardiology, Rhön-Klinikum Bad Neustadt, Germany [B]).

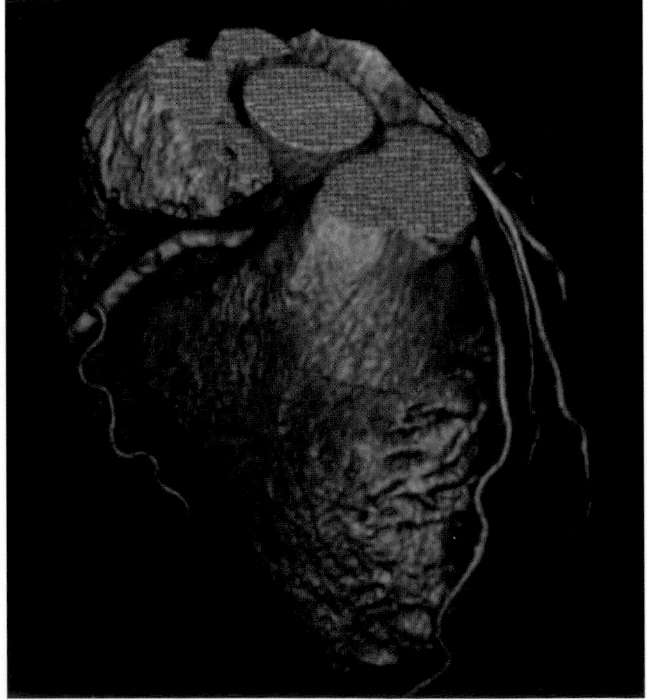

nary arteries in order to facilitate density-threshold-dependent 2 and 3D visualization. Contrast attenuation within the vessel should be high enough to allow for lesion detection, but not high enough to obscure calcified coronary artery wall lesions. Adequate opacification can be achieved in the majority of patients over the course of a 40-s scan with 140 mL of 300 mg/mL iodinated contrast material injected at a flow rate of 3.5 mL/s. Owing to increased acquisition speed with 16-slice CT (approx 20 s scan time) the amount of contrast media can be reduced to 80–100 mL, but the injection rate will need to be increased to 4 to 5 mL/s. The use of reliable contrast-tracking software remains the best option for achieving the desired opacification

Fig. 14. (*left*) Coronary CT angiography examination to rule out coronary artery disease using a 16-slice CT scanner. Scan protocol: 16 × 0.75-mm detector collimation, 1.0-mm reconstructed slice width, 370-ms rotation speed, 12-cm scan range covered in 16 s (SOMATOM Sensation 16 Cardiac, Siemens, Germany). Display of the coronary tree with 3D volume-rendering technique in combination reveals all main coronary segments normal. Also the rapidly moving right coronary artery can be displayed free of motion owing to the fast rotation speed (case courtesy of Department of Cardiology, University of Erlangen, Germany).

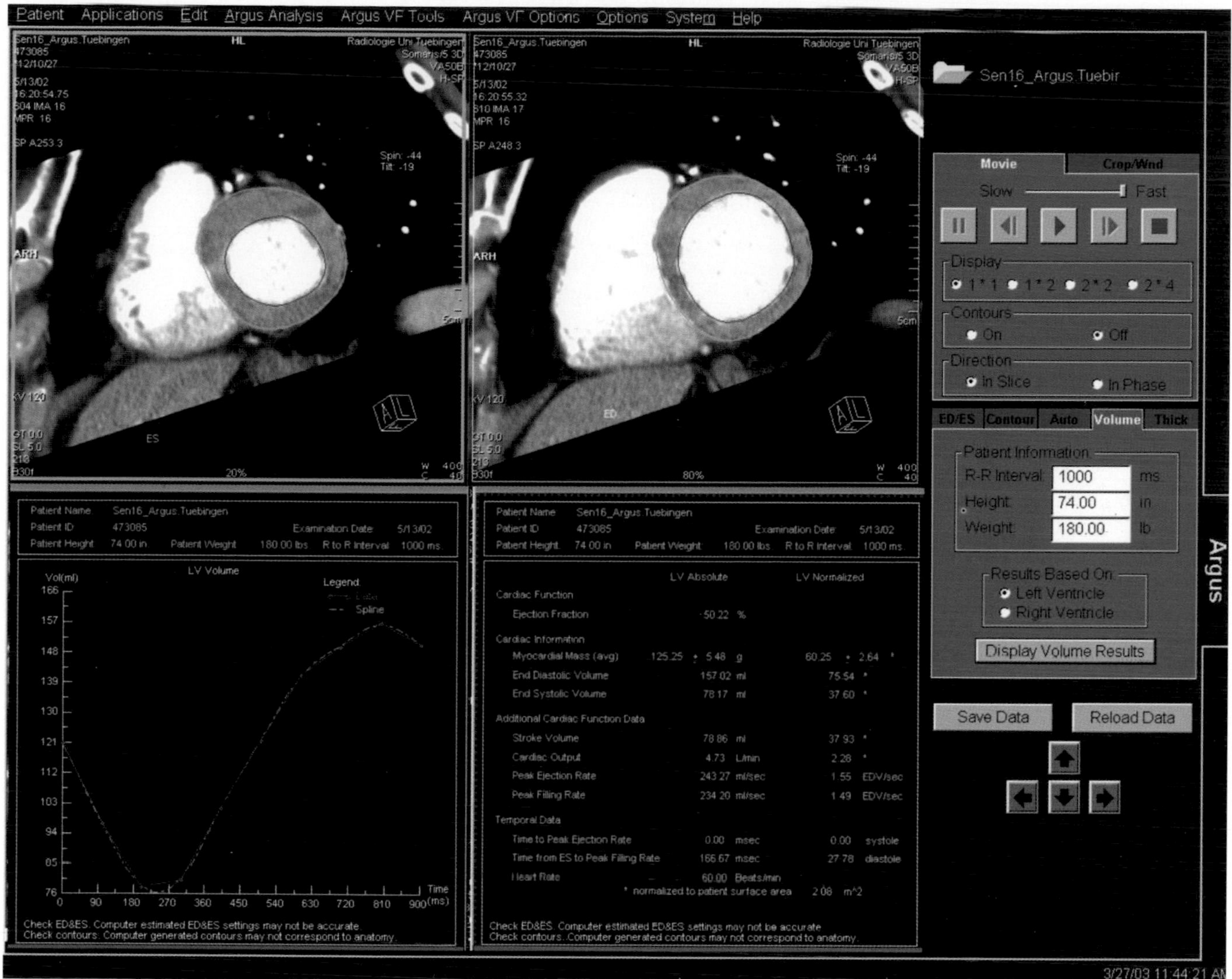

Fig. 15. CT angiographic examination of a patient with an occlusion of the left anterior descending coronary artery using a 16-slice CT scanner. Scan protocol: 16 × 0.75-mm detector collimation, 1.0-mm reconstructed slice width, 420-ms rotation speed, 12-cm scan range covered in 16 s (SOMATOM Sensation 16, Siemens). In addition to reconstruction of the coronary artery tree, ECG-gated spiral image reconstruction was performed in 10 different time points during the cardiac cycle with a distance of 10% of the RR interval to provide input data for cardiac function evaluation. End-diastolic volume and end-systolic volume of the left ventricle as well as ejection fraction can be readily assessed based on short axis and long axis multiplanar reformations with 5-mm thickness that are loaded into a dedicated functional evaluation software (syngo Argus, Siemens) (case courtesy of the Department of Radiology, Tübingen University, Germany).

in patients with a wide range of cardiac output. Use of saline chasing technique (e.g., with a bolus of 50 mL of saline injected immediately after the iodine bolus) may be helpful for better contrast bolus utilization and for reducing streak artifacts arising from dense contrast material in the superior vena cava and the right heart. In order to minimize the likelihood of the latter effect, the injection site should be considered carefully. Thorough patient preparation remains an integral part of achieving consistent results.

EVALUATION OF CARDIAC FUNCTION

In addition to the diagnosis of cardiac and coronary morphology, evaluation and quantification of cardiac function provides important information for the assessment of cardiac and coronary diseases. Because ECG-gated helical/spiral scanning permits retrospective reconstruction of images at all phases of the cardiac cycle, it is a relatively simple matter to automatically segment the chamber and generate left-ventricular ejection fractions and wall motion using the same data set collected for coronary CTA. Thus, the diagnosis of cardiac and coronary morphology and also of basic cardiac function parameters can be derived from a single contrast-enhanced ECG-gated spiral examination with thin-section acquisition. Standard analysis techniques yield most of the metrics associated with cardiac function, including ejection fraction, end-diastolic and end-systolic volumes, stroke volume, and cardiac output. Left-ventricular regional function can also be quickly displayed on polar maps of percent wall thickness, wall motion, and ejection fraction (Figs. 15 and 16).

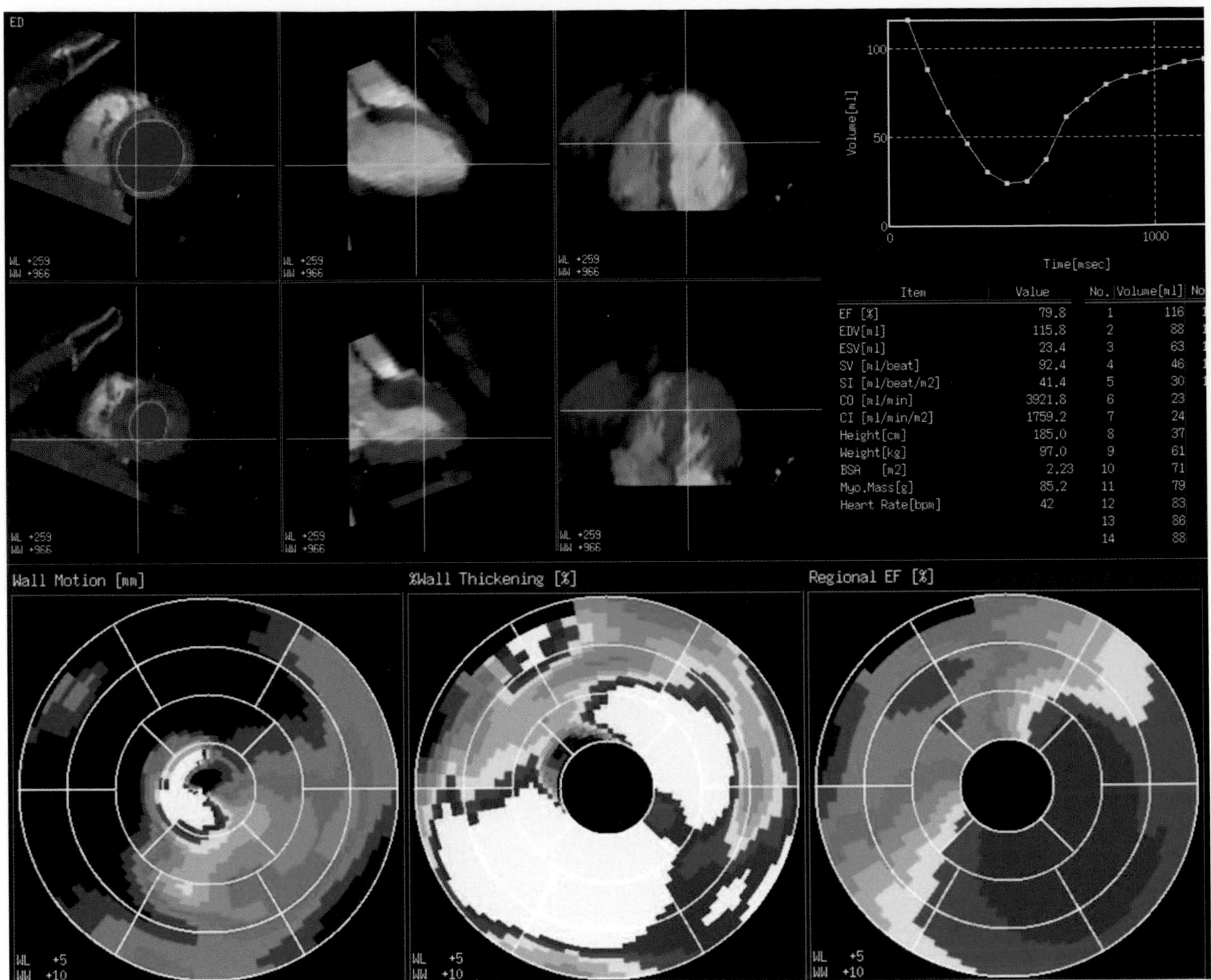

Fig. 16. Cardiac Function Analysis software (Toshiba Medical Systems) reconstructs short- and long-axis images of the heart at multiple phases of the cardiac cycle. From this data set, ejection fraction, cardiac output, wall motion, and other parameters are calculated and displayed. This provides additional diagnostic information without any additional radiation to the patient (case courtesy of Dr. Shapiro, Johns Hopkins University, Baltimore).

First study results *(54)* show that basic cardiac function parameters derived with 4-slice CT correlate well with the gold-standard techniques MRI and coronary angiography, based on a standardized heart phase selection for end-diastolic and end-systolic CT reconstruction and semi-automated evaluation tools (Figs. 15 and 16).

Although dose is significantly reduced during end diastole and systole with ECG-controlled tube current modulation, sufficient contrast resolution can still be obtained for functional evaluation. Use of MPRs in short and long heart axis with thickness of 5–8 mm enables appropriate delineation of the ventricle wall in both end-diastolic and end-systolic reconstruction. Automated direct 3D reconstruction of oblique planes in predefined views such as short and long heart axis and in multiple phases of the cardiac cycle will enable a more efficient workflow for cardiac function analysis in the future.

Rapid cardiac motion during the systolic phase of the cardiac cycle can cause motion artifacts in the end-systolic reconstructions. However, correct delineation of the ventricle walls is usually still possible with sufficient accuracy. The latest 16-slice CT scanners have the potential to further improve the accuracy of cardiac function measurement as compared to 4- and 8-slice CT scanners, based on increased gantry rotation speed.

CARDIO-THORACIC IMAGING

Thoracic CT studies are frequently degraded by motion artifacts caused by transmitted cardiac pulsation. Typical diagnostic pitfalls related to this effect are false-positive findings of aortic dissection and distortion of paracardiac lung segments. Suppression of cardiac pulsation artifacts improves image quality in CT studies of the thorax, including the heart. Important indications are the planning and follow-up of surgical proce-

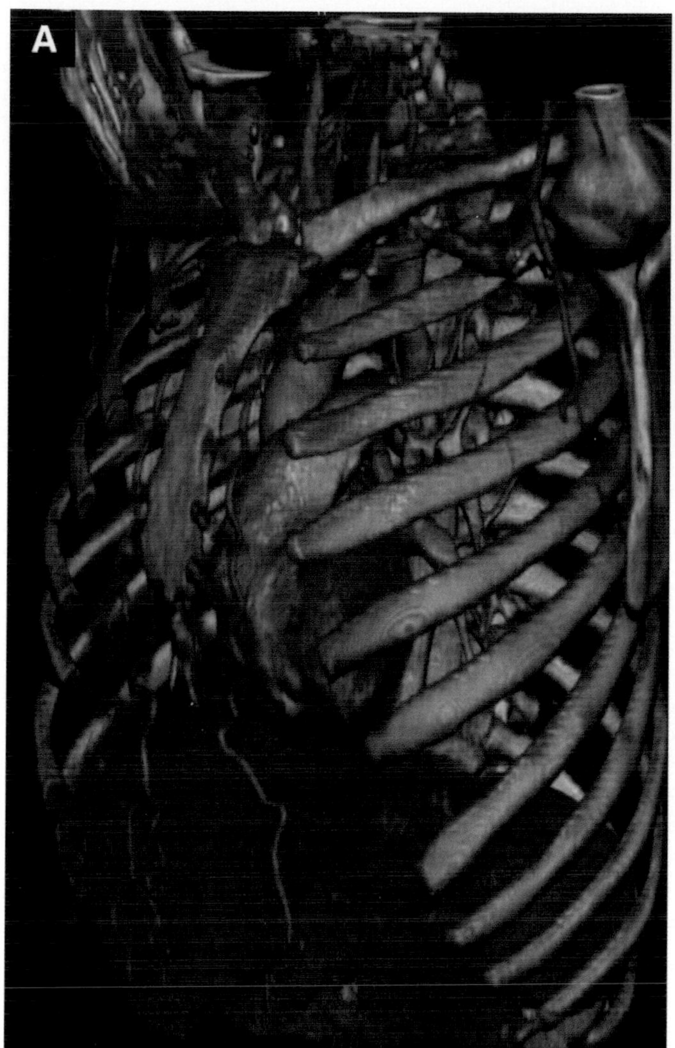

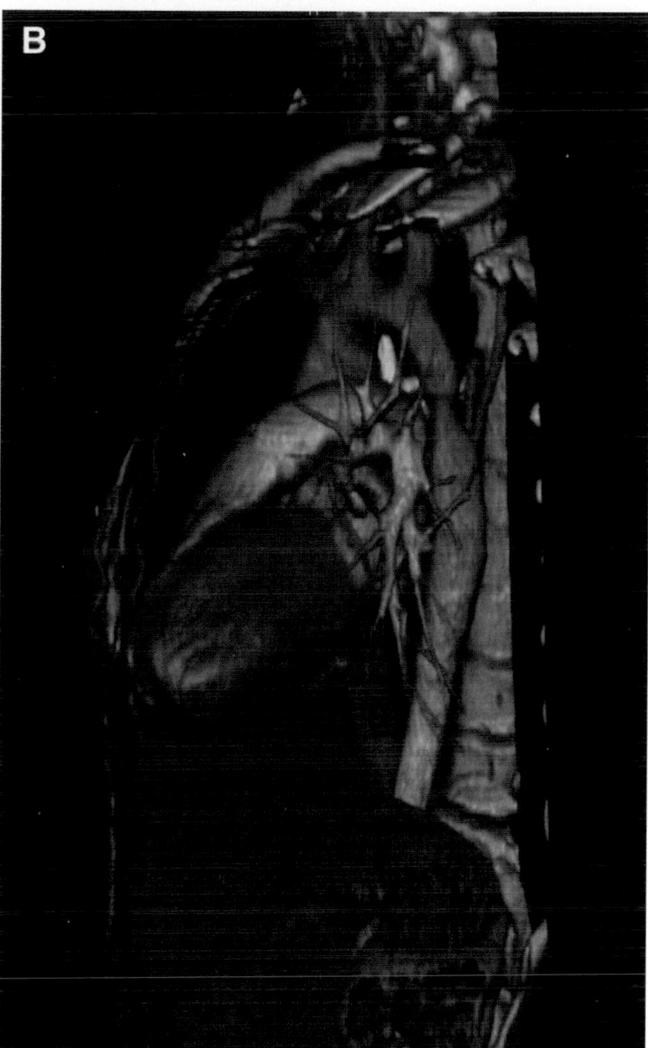

Fig. 17. Electrocardiogram (ECG)-gated examination of the thoracic aorta in a 30-s breath-hold using a 16-slice CT scanner with 16 × 0.75-mm detector collimation and 420-ms rotation speed. The thoracic vasculature is displayed with 3D volume-rendering technique. Based on ECG-gated reconstruction that suppresses cardiac pulsation, the entire thoracic aorta can be evaluated free of pulsation artifacts (case courtesy of the Department of Radiology, Cleveland Clinic Foundation, USA).

dures, diagnosis or exclusion of aortic dissection and aortic aneurisms, detection of pulmonary embolism, assessment of congenital heart and vessel disease, and early detection and reliable diagnosis of paracardiac lung nodules.

Prospectively ECG-triggered and retrospectively ECG-gated protocols have been successfully applied to suppress cardiac-related motion artifacts in thoracic studies. With 4-slice CT, ECG-triggered or ECG-gated thin-slice scanning of the thorax is usually not possible within a single breath-hold, but can be used for re-scanning that part of the thorax where most pulsation is present. With the substantial performance increase of 16-slice CT, retrospectively ECG-gated coverage of the thorax is feasible in a single breath-hold and with a single contrast injection (Fig. 17). Thus, this technique now has the potential to be used as a standard examination for multislice spiral examination of the lung and thoracic vasculature. As a future step, ECG-gated thoracic imaging may become possible even with submillimeter resolution owing to 16-slice CT in combination with specialized ECG-gated cone-beam reconstruction techniques that enable faster volume coverage *(30)*.

FUTURE PERSPECTIVE

Further CT technology enhancements are required for accurate and consistent diagnosis of cardiac and coronary diseases, including the detection and quantification of coronary artery stenosis and coronary atherosclerotic lesions. Detection and quantification of the degree of lumen narrowing with the ability to differentiate a 10–20% change in vessel cross-sectional area represents a future goal for cardiac CT imaging. To meet this goal, future CT systems need to achieve a spatial resolution in all three dimensions (isotropic voxels) of 0.4–0.5 mm for visualization of the main coronary vessels and 0.3 mm or better for smaller branches. A recent study indicates that a heart-rate-independent temporal resolution of 100 ms or less allows for virtual elimination of motion artifacts in phases of the cardiac cycle with limited motion, with heart rates up to approx 100

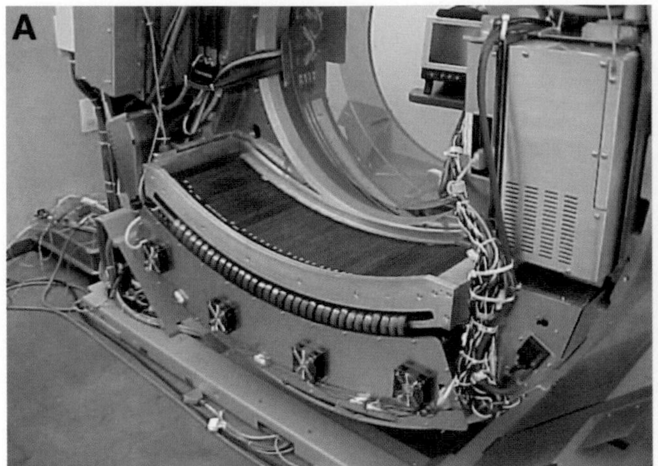

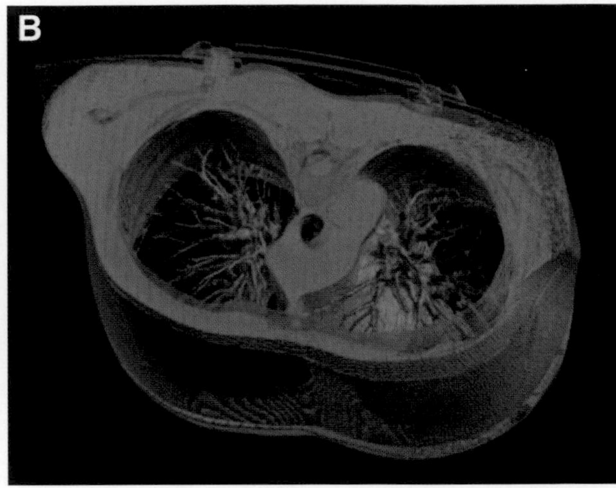

Fig. 18. **(A)** Illustration of a prototype system with large-area detector technology, capable of acquiring 256 0.5-mm slices simultaneously (Toshiba Medical Systems). Experimental ex vivo and human studies demonstrate the potential of such future CT scanners to cover large patient volumes with a single gantry rotation. **(B)** The 3D scan of the chest demonstrates the potential for capturing the heart in one rotation (images courtesy of Y. Saito, Toshiba Medical Systems).

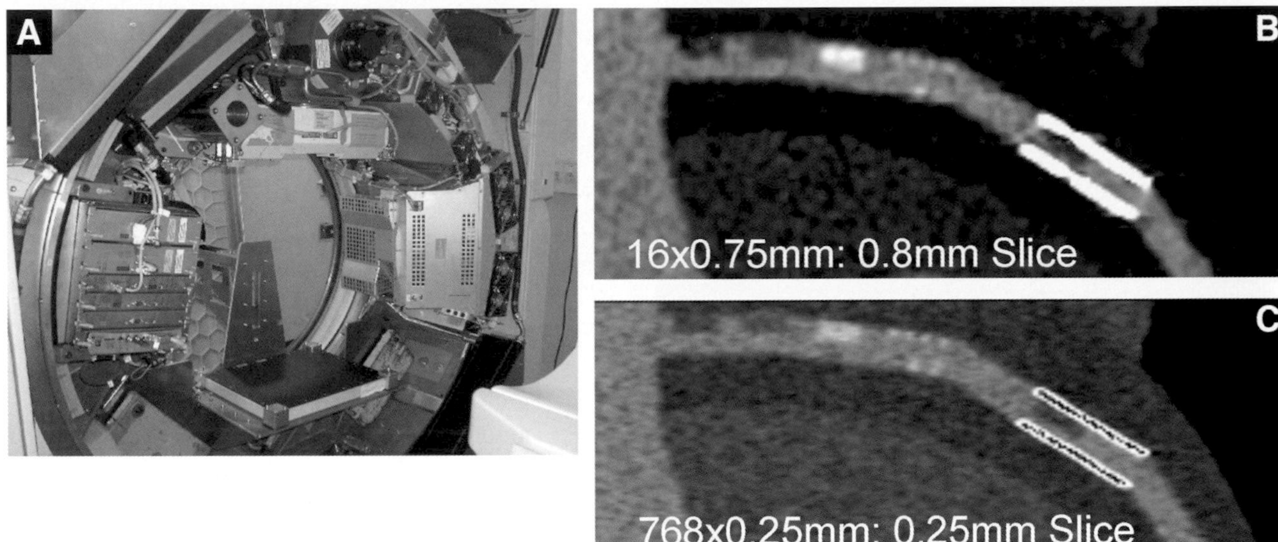

Fig. 19. The anthropomorphic heart and coronary artery phantom displayed in Fig. 6 was used to compare the maximum possible spatial resolution of 16-slice CT with future area detector CT systems **(A)** that may provide detector pixel sizes below 0.5 mm (CT prototype with flat-panel detector system, Siemens). Such systems may be able to cover the heart in a single scanner rotation with isotropic resolution of 0.25 mm. Extremely high spatial resolution can improve visualization of in-stent lumen and small coronary segments compared to 16-slice CT **(B)**, but do not necessarily provide improved delineation of noncalcified coronary lesions because of compromised signal-to-noise ratio **(C)**.

bpm *(55)*. For motion-free imaging at very high heart rates and in phases with rapid cardiac motion for analysis of cardiac function, a temporal resolution of 50 ms or less might be required *(56)*. Scan acquisition within a single, short breath-hold is mandatory for minimized contrast-medium injection and to avoid respiratory artifacts. Breath-hold times of 15 s or less are appropriate for stable patients, but breath-hold times of 10 s or less are advisable for patients who are ill or uncooperative. Ideally, all data of the complete heart anatomy would be acquired within a single heart cycle or less without patient movement. All these requirements related to spatial resolution, temporal resolution, and scan time have to be achieved without substantial increase of radiation exposure, which should not exceed the amount of invasive diagnostic coronary angiography.

The very short acquisition times of EBCT, down to 50 ms, combined with prospectively ECG-triggered scanning, enable motion-free imaging of the coronary arteries for patients with moderate and higher heart rates and stable sinus rhythm. However, the restrictions in spatial resolution and contrast-to-noise ratio as well as rather long breath-hold times limit the ability of EBCT today to reliably visualize all main coronary artery segments and noncalcified atherosclerotic plaques. New EBCT detectors are under evaluation that allow for simultaneous acquisition of two 1.5-mm slices and increased in-plane spatial

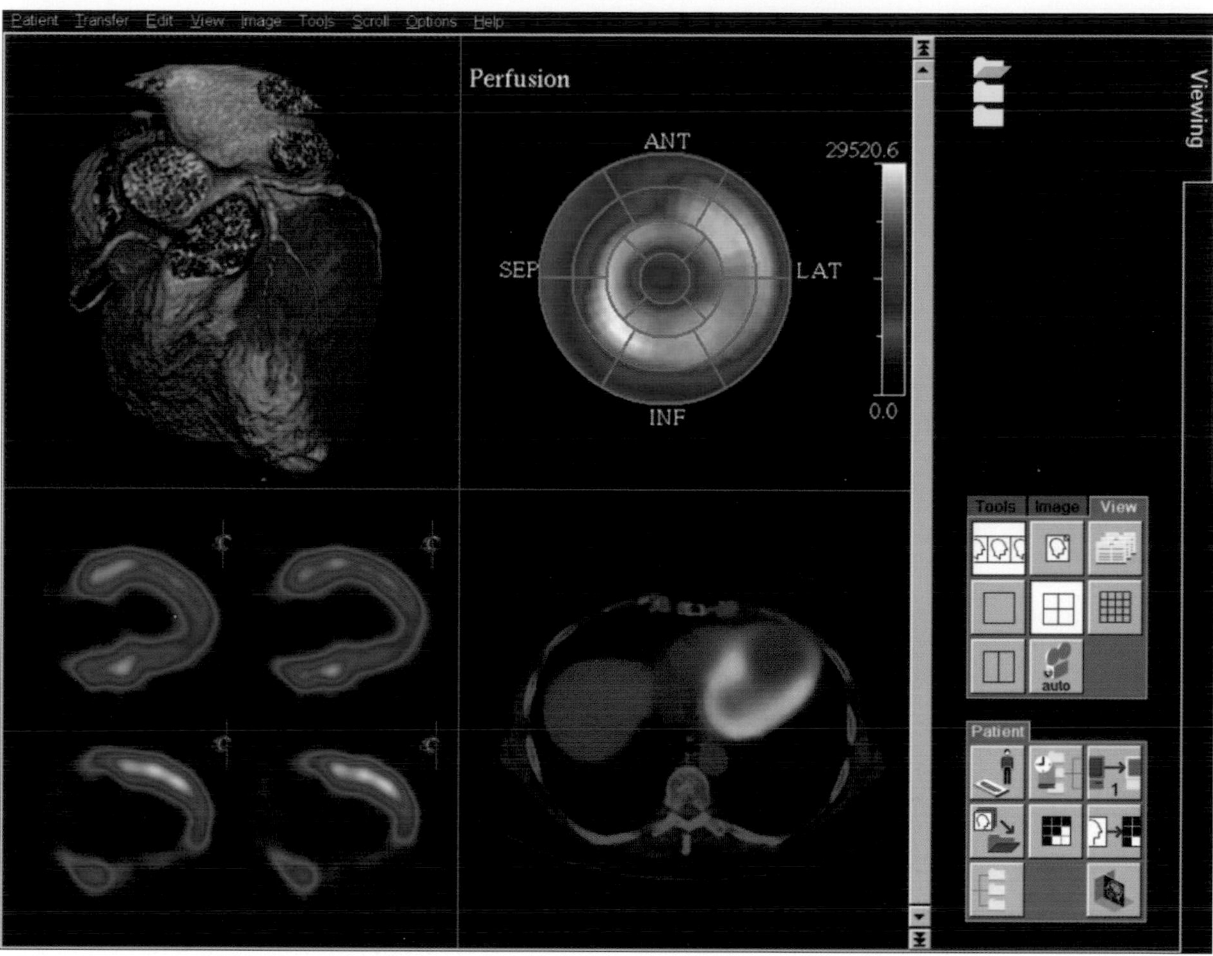

Fig. 20. CT/positron emission tomography (PET) examination of a patient with a known occlusion of the left anterior descending coronary artery and history of myocardial infarction (biograph Sensation 16, Siemens). The 3D volume-rendering reconstruction of the ECG-gated 16-slice CT scan reveals the occluded coronary vessel and a related infarct scar. The PET scan demonstrates a perfusion defect and necrotic myocardium at the anterior wall (case courtesy of the Department of Radiology of Tübingen University, Germany, and the Department of Nuclear Medicine of the Technical University of Munich, Germany).

resolution via finer structuring of the elements of the fixed detector ring. With these detectors, the heart can be scanned with 1.5-mm slices in a 30–40-s breath-hold. However, limited signal-to-noise ratio will remain a major challenge for EBCT technology for high-resolution cardiac and coronary artery imaging.

The temporal resolution of current multislice mechanical CT scanners needs to be improved to provide motion-free and robust coronary imaging also for moderate and high heart rates. Since the introduction of CT in 1972, there has been a persistent and successful effort to reduce gantry rotation times, reaching a remarkable 0.4 . Further increased rotation speed is still a very real goal; however, the rotational forces on the gantry components (tube, generator, and detector) increase as the square of the rotation speed.

Thinner slices, leading to improved z-axis resolution, are technically feasible, but require a higher radiation dose to maintain a high contrast-to-noise ratio, and more detector-slices to maintain a short scan time (<20s). As a complement to further increased spatial resolution, advanced beam-hardening and metal artifact reduction algorithms can be developed that improve imaging of calcified and stented coronary vessels; use of these algorithms to date is restricted to cerebral and bone imaging. Practical cardiac imaging has also benefited tremendously from the development of advanced software, particularly with regard to image reconstruction. Another approach to improved temporal resolution may lie with advances in segmented image reconstruction. While current algorithms are robust, using as many as four cardiac cycles, these and related techniques may develop to further extend the range of patient heart rates that can reliably be imaged.

Area detector technology and related new cone beam reconstruction techniques are being researched that may allow the entire coronary anatomy to be covered in a single heartbeat without movement of the table. Prototype systems with large area detectors exist, capable of acquiring as many as 256 slices of 0.5 mm simultaneously. Alternative designs can provide in-plane and through-plane spatial resolution even up to 0.2 mm using flat-panel detector technology (Figs. 18 and 19). With these CT scanners, imaging of high-resolution morphology as well as dynamic and functional information via repeated scanning of the same scan range may become possible. The application potential of such technology is being evaluated with experimental systems using phantom models and post mortem hearts. Initial experience shows that today's area detector technology is still too limited in contrast resolution, and the high radiation dose that is needed to provide adequate signal-to-noise ratio even for high-contrast studies is unacceptable for use in human subjects.

The latest MSCT scanners also allow combining 16-slice CT with PET cameras. These systems may allow for a clinical combination of cardiac CT imaging and cardiac PET scans in a single examination and subsequent fusion of the information on cardiac morphology and myocardial function and metabolism (Fig. 20). The clinical potential of these scanners is currently under evaluation, and initial study data can be expected in the near future.

REFERENCES

1. Boyd DP, Lipton MJ. Cardiac computed tomography. Proc IEEE 1982;71:298–307
2. Agatston AS, Janowitz WR, Hildner FJ, Zusmer NR, Viamonte M, Detrano R. Quantification of coronary artery calcium using ultrafast computed tomography. JACC 1990;15:827–832.
3. Achenbach S, Moshage W, Ropers D, Nössen J, Daniel WG. Value of electron-beam computed tomography for the non-invasive detection of high-grade coronary artery stenoses and occlusions. N Engl J Med 1998;339:1964–1971.
4. Becker CR, Jakobs TF, Aydemir S, et al. Helical and single-slice conventional CT versus electron beam CT for the quantification of coronary artery calcification. AJR 2000;174:543–547.
5. Bahner ML, Böse J, Lutz A, Wallschläger H, Regn J, van Kaick G. Retrospectively ECG-gated spiral CT of the heart and lung. Eur Radiol 1999;9:106–109.
6. Ohnesorge B, Flohr T, Schaller S, et al. Technische Grundlagen und Anwendungen der Mehrschicht CT. Radiologe 1999;39:923–931.
7. Taguchi K, Aradate H. Algorithm for image reconstruction in multi-slice helical CT. Med Phys 1998;25(4):550–561.
8. Ohnesorge B, Flohr T, Becker CR, et al. Cardiac imaging by means of electrocardiographically gated multisection spiral CT: initial experience. Radiology 2000;217:564–571.
9. Kachelriess M, Ulzheimer S, Kalender WA. ECG-correlated image reconstruction from subsecond multi-row spiral CT scans of the heart. Med Phys 2000;27:1881–1902.
10. Ohnesorge B, Becker CR, Flohr T, Reiser MF. Multi-Slice CT in Cardiac Imaging—Technical Principles, Clinical Application and Future Developments. Springer, New York: 2002.
11. Knez A, Becker CR, Leber A, Ohnesorge B, Reiser MF, Haberl R. Non-invasive assessment of coronary artery stenoses with multidetector helical computed tomography. Circulation 2000;101: e221–e222.
12. Niemann K, Oudkerk M, Rensing BJ, et al. Coronary angiography with multi-slice computed tomography. Lancet 2001;357:599–603.
13. Knez A, Becker CR, Leber A, et al. Usefulness of multislice spiral computed tomography angiography for determination of coronary artery stenoses. Am J Cardiol 2002;88:1191–1194.
14. Kopp AF, Schröder S, Küttner A, et al. High resolution multi-slice computed tomography with retrospective gating for angiography in coronary arteries: results in 102 patients. Eur Heart J 2002;23: 1714–1725.
15. Schröder S, Kopp AF, Baumbach A, et al. Non-invasive detection and evaluation of atherosclerotic plaque with multi-slice computed tomography. JACC 2001;37:1430–1435.
16. Flohr T, Stierstorfer K, Bruder H, Simon J, Schaller S. New technical developments in multislice CT, part 1: approaching isotropic resolution with sub-mm 16-slice scanning. Fortschr Röntgenstr 2002;174:839–845.
17. Flohr T, Stierstorfer K, Bruder H, Simon J, Schaller S, Ohnesorge B. New technical developments in multislice CT, part 2: sub-millimeter 16-slice scanning and increased gantry rotation speed for cardiac imaging. RöFo, Fortschr Röntgenstr 2002;174:1022–1027.
18. Funabashi N, Komiyama N, Yanagawa N, et al. Coronary artery patency after metallic stent implantation evaluated by multislice computed tomography. Circulation 2003;107:147–148.
19. Kopp AF, Küttner A, Heuschmid M, Schröder S, Ohnesorge B, Claussen CD. Multidetector-row CT cardiac imaging with 4 and 16 slices for coronary CTA and imaging of atherosclerotic plaques. Eu Radiol 2002;12(Suppl 2): S17–S24.
20. Flohr TG, Küttner A, Bruder H, et al. Performance evaluation of a multi-slice CT system with 16-slice detector and increased gantry rotation speed for isotropic submillimeter imaging of the heart. Herz 2003;28:7–19.
21. Flohr TG, Schoepf UJ, Küttner A, et al. Advances in cardiac imaging with 16-slice CT-systems. Acad Radiol 2003;10:386–401.
22. Flohr T, Ohnesorge B. Heart-rate adaptive optimization of spatial and temporal resolution for ECG-gated multi-slice spiral CT of the heart. J Comp Assist T 2001;25:907–923.
23. Flohr T, Stierstorfer K, Bruder H, et al. New technical developments in multislice CT—part 1: approaching isotropic resolution with sub-millimeter 16-slice scanning. Fortschr Röntgenstr (RöFo) 2002; 174:1022–1027.
24. Flohr T, Ohnesorge B, Bruder H, et al. Image reconstruction and performance evaluation for ECG-gated spiral scanning with a 16-slice system. Med Phys 2003;30(10):2650–2662.
25. Bruder H, Flohr TG, Stierstorfer K, Rauscher A, Hölzel A, Schaller S. ECG-gated dynamic cardiac volume imaging with CT area detectors (abstract). Radiology 2002;225(P):310.
26. Hong C, Becker CR, Huber A, et al. ECG-gated reconstructed multi-detector row CT coronary angiography: effect of varying trigger delay on image quality. Radiology 2001;220:712–717.
27. Kopp AF, Schröder S, Küttner A, et al. Coronary arteries: retrospectively ECG-gated multi-detector row CT angiography with selective optimization of the reconstruction window. Radiology 2001;221: 683–688.
28. Jakobs T, Becker CR, Ohnesorge B, Flohr T, Schoepf UJ, Reiser MF. Reduction of radiation exposure with ECG-controlled tube current modulation for retrospectively ECG-gated helical scans of the heart. Eur Radiol 2002;12:1081–1086.
29. Flohr T, Prokop M, Schöpf, et al. A new ECG-gated multislice spiral CT scan and reconstruction technique with extended volume coverage for cardio-thoracic applications. Eur Radiol 2002;12: 1527–1532.
30. Flohr T, Bruder H, Küttner A, Heuschmid M, Schaller S, Ohnesorge BM. ECG-gated spiral scanning of the lung and mediastinal vessels with optimized temporal resolution and cone-correction on a 16-slice CT system: performance evaluation and initial clinical results (abstract). Radiology 2002;225(P):449.
31. Kopp AF, Ohnesorge B, Becker C, et al. Reproducibility and accuracy of coronary calcium measurement with multidetector-row versus electron beam CT. Radiology 2002;225:113–119.
32. Ulzheimer S, Halliburton SS, McCollough CH, Becker CR, White RD, Kalender WA. Evaluation of image quality and calcium scoring performance in multislice cardiac computed tomography (abstract). Radiology 2002;221(P):458.
33. Hunold P, Vogt FM, Schmermund A, Kerkhoff G, Debatin JF, Barkhausen J. Radiation exposure during noninvasive coronary artery imaging: comparison of multislice CT and electron beam CT. Radiology 2002;221(P):503–504.
34. Schoepf UJ, Becker CR, Ohnesorge BM, Yucel EK (2003). CT of coronary artery disease. Radiology, in press.
35. Kalender WA, Schmidt B, Zankl M, Schmidt M. A PC program for estimating organ dose and effective dose values in computed tomography. Eur Radiol 1999;9:555–562.
36. Schmidt B, Ulzheimer S, Kalender WA. Dose in multi-slice cardiac CT: assessment of organ effective dose values with Monte Carlo methods (abstract). Radiology 2001;221(P):414.
37. Hong C, Becker CR, Schoepf UJ, Ohnesorge B, Brüning R, Reiser MF. Absolute quantification of coronary calcification in non-con-

trast and contrast-enhanced multislice CT studies. Radiology 2002;223:474–480.

38. Fleischmann D, Rubin GD, Bankier AA, Hittmair K. Improved uniformity of aortic enhancement with customized contrast medium injection protocols at CT angiography. Radiology 2000;214:363–371.
39. Schweiger GD, Chang PJ, Brown BP. Optimizing contrast enhancement during helical CT of the liver: a comparison of two bolus tracking techniques. Am J Roentgenol 1998;171:1551–1558.
40. Becker CR, Kleffel T, Crispin A, et al. Coronary artery calcium measurement: agreement of multirow detector and electron beam CT. Am J Roentgenol 2001;176:1295–1298.
41. Achenbach S, Ropers D, Mohlenkamp S, et al. Variability of repeated coronary artery calcium measurements by electron beam tomography. Am J Cardiol 2001;87:210–213.
42. Achenbach S, Ropers D, Pohle K, et al. Influence of lipid-lowering therapy on the progression of coronary artery calcification—a prospective study. Circulation 2002;106:1077–1082.
43. Shemesh J, Apter S, Stroh CI, et al. Tracking coronary calcification by using dual-section spiral CT: a 3-year follow-up. Radiology 2000;217:461–465.
44. Daniell A, Friedman J, Berman D, et al. Concordance of coronary calcium estimation between multi-detector and electron beam CT (abstract). Circulation 2002(Suppl. II);106(19):II–479.
45. Stanford W, Thompson B, Burns TL, Heery S, Burr M. Multi-detector helical CT versus electron beam CT in the quantification of coronary artery calcification: emphasis on lower calcium scores. Radiology 2004;230:397–402.
46. Ohnesorge B, Flohr T, Heuschmid M, Becker C. Evaluation of different examination protocols for coronary artery calcium quantification with ECG-gated 16-slice spiral CT (abstract). Radiology 2002;225(P):239.
47. Ohnesorge B, Kopp AF, Fischbach R, et al. Reproducibility of coronary calcium quantification in repeat examinations with retrospectively ECG-gated multislice spiral CT. Eur Radiol 2002;12:1532–1540.
48. Moser K, Bateman T, Case J, et al. The influence of acquisition mode on the reproducibility of coronary artery calcium scores using multi-detector computed tomography (abstract). Circulation 2002(Suppl. II);106(19):II–479.
49. Hong C, Bae KT, Pilgram TK, et al. Coronary artery calcium measurement with multi-detector row CT: in vitro assessment of effect of radiation dose. Radiology 2002;225:901–906.
50. Ulzheimer S, Kalender WA. Assessment of calcium scoring performance in cardiac computed tomography. Eur Radiol 2003;13:484–497.
51. Becker CR, Schöpf UJ, Reiser MF. Coronary calcium scoring: medicine and politics. Eur Radiol 2003;13:445–447.
52. Nieman K, Cademartiri F, Lemos PA, et al. Reliable noninvasive coronary angiography with fast submillimeter multislice spiral computed tomography. Circulation 2002;106:2051–2054.
53. Ropers D, Baum U, Pohle K, et al. Detection of coronary artery stenoses with thin-slice multi-detector row spiral computed tomography and multiplanar reconstruction. Circulation 2003;107:664–666.
54. Juergens KU, Grude M, Fallenberg EM, Heindel W, Fischbach R. Using ECG-gated multidetector CT to evaluate global left ventricular myocardial function in patients with coronary artery disease. AJR Am J Roentgenol 2002;179:1545–1550.
55. Achenbach S, Ropers D, Holle J, et al. In-plane coronary arterial motion velocity: measurement with electron beam CT. Radiology 2000;216:457–463.
56. Wang Y, Watts R, Mitchell I, et al. Coronary MR angiography: selection of acquisition window of minimal cardiac motion with electrocardiography-triggered navigator cardiac motion prescanning—initial results. Radiology 2001;218:580–585.

4 Image Reconstruction for ECG-Triggered and ECG-Gated Multislice CT

THOMAS FLOHR AND TINSU PAN

INTRODUCTION

Computed tomography (CT) imaging of the heart and the coronary anatomy requires high temporal resolution to avoid motion artifacts and to achieve sufficient spatial resolution—at best submillimeter—to adequately visualize small anatomical structures such as the coronary arteries. Furthermore, the complete heart volume has to be examined within the time of one breath-hold. First attempts to use single-slice spiral CT systems for cardiac scanning were not convincing because of poor temporal resolution and insufficient volume coverage with thin slices *(1,2)*. Since 1999, 4-slice CT systems with higher volume coverage speed and improved temporal resolution thanks to faster gantry rotation (rotation time down to 0.5 s) have been clinically used for electrocardiogram (ECG)-triggered or ECG-gated multislice CT (MSCT) examinations of the cardiac anatomy *(3–9)*. Coverage of the entire heart volume with thin slices (4 × 1-mm/4 × 1.25-mm collimation) within one breath-hold period became feasible, allowing for new applications such as high-resolution CT angiographies of the coronary arteries *(6–9)*. First clinical studies have demonstrated the ability of MSCT to characterize lipid, fibrous, and calcified coronary plaques *(10)*. Despite all promising advances, challenges and limitations remain for cardiac MSCT with 4-slice detectors. Spatial resolution is still not sufficient to clearly depict stents or severely calcified coronary arteries *(6,7)*. Temporal resolution is not yet adequate for patients with higher heart rates, and a diagnostic outcome cannot be guaranteed in these cases despite careful selection of the reconstruction interval *(11,12)*. The scan time of about 40 s required to cover the entire heart volume (approx 12 cm) with 4 × 1-mm, 4 × 1.25-mm collimation is at the limit for a single breath-hold scan. In 2000, a shorter scan time was realized with 8 × 1.25-mm collimation, cardiac MSCT, which enables scan times of about 20 s. In 2001, a new generation of MSCT systems was introduced. With simultaneous acquisition of up to 16 submillimeter slices and gantry rotation times down to 0.4 s, spatial resolution in the transverse direction and temporal resolution are further improved, while examination times are considerably reduced *(13,14)*. Sixteen-slice systems have the potential to overcome the limitations of established 4-slice/8-slice CT scanners, and first clinical studies have already demonstrated enhanced clinical performance *(15,16)*. While system properties such as gantry rotation time and detector slice width determine the intrinsic temporal and spatial resolution of the data, dedicated scan and image reconstruction techniques are needed to optimize the outcome of cardiac CT examinations. In this chapter, we present the basics of ECG-triggered and ECG-gated MSCT scanning. We give an overview on image reconstruction techniques, starting with single-segment partial scan reconstruction and ending with multisegment approaches. We discuss the pros and cons of single- and multisegment reconstruction. We demonstrate the properties of reconstruction algorithms with patient scans, and end with a short summary and discussion.

From: *Contemporary Cardiology: CT of the Heart: Principles and Applications*
Edited by: U. Joseph Schoepf © Humana Press, Inc., Totowa, NJ

SCAN TECHNIQUES FOR ECG-CONTROLLED MULTISLICE CT: ECG-TRIGGERED AXIAL AND ECG-GATED SPIRAL SCANNING

For ECG-synchronized examinations of the cardio-thoracic anatomy, either ECG-triggered axial scanning or ECG-gated spiral scanning can be used. The most basic approach is prospectively ECG-triggered axial scanning, which was previously introduced with electron beam CT. The patient's ECG signal is monitored during examination, and axial scans are started with a predefined temporal offset relative to the R waves, which can be either relative (given as a certain percentage of the RR interval time) or absolute (given in ms), and either forward or reverse *(5)*. Data acquisition is therefore "triggered" by the R waves of the patient's ECG signal. A schematic illustration of absolute and relative phase setting is given in Fig. 1. The principle of ECG-triggered multislice axial scanning is illustrated in Fig. 2. The coordinate system in Fig. 2 shows the patient's ECG-signal as a function of time on the horizontal axis and the position of the detector slices relative to the patient on the vertical axis (in this example, four detector slices are indicated). Usually, partial scan data intervals (180° + detector fan angle) are acquired. Thanks to optimized half-scan reconstruction algorithms with adequate data weighting, a temporal resolution up to half the gantry rotation time per image (250 ms for 0.5 s gantry rotation) can be achieved in a sufficiently centered region of interest. The number of images acquired with every scan corresponds to the number of active detector slices. In between the individual axial scans, the table moves to the next z position; the heart

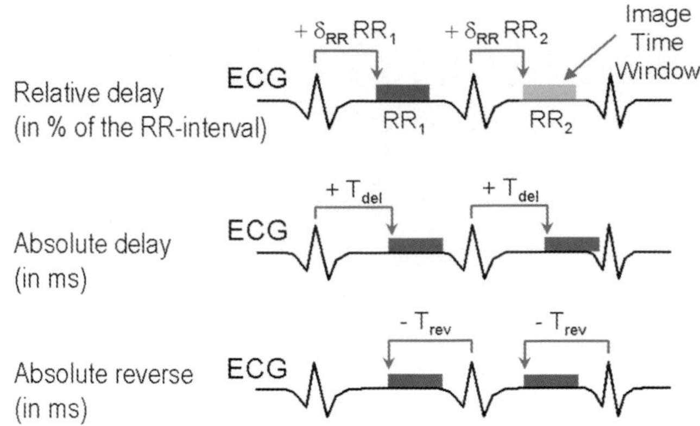

Fig. 1. Schematic illustration of absolute and relative phase setting for electrocardiogram (ECG)-controlled CT examinations of the cardiothoracic anatomy.

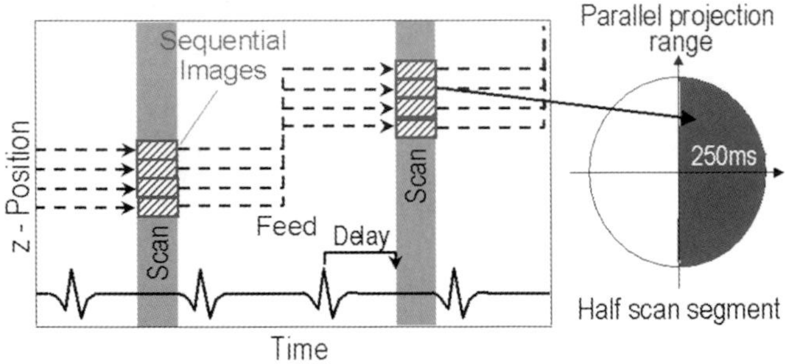

Fig. 2. Principle of electrocardiogram (ECG)-triggered multislice axial scanning. The patient's ECG signal is indicated as a function of time on the horizontal axis. The position of the detector slices relative to the patient (four slices in this example) is shown on the vertical axis. Usually, partial scan data intervals (180° + detector fan angle) are acquired, which are marked as boxes.

volume is therefore covered in a "step and shoot" technique. As a result of the time necessary for table motion, only every second heart beat can be used for data acquisition, which limits the minimum slice width to 2.5 mm with 4-slice or 1.25 mm with 8-slice CT systems if the whole heart volume has to be covered within one breath-hold period.

With retrospective ECG gating, the heart volume is covered continuously by a spiral scan. The patient's ECG signal is recorded simultaneously to allow for a retrospective selection of the data segments used for image reconstruction. The principle of retrospectively ECG-gated spiral scanning is illustrated in Fig. 3. Similar to Fig. 2, the patient's ECG signal is indicated as a function of time on the horizontal axis, and the position of the detector slices relative to the patient is shown on the vertical axis. The table moves continuously, and continuous spiral scan data of the heart volume are acquired. Only scan data acquired in a predefined cardiac phase, usually the diastolic phase, are used for image reconstruction *(5,17)*. These scan data segments are indicated as boxes in Fig. 3. A variety of dedicated reconstruction approaches for ECG-gated spiral MSCT have been introduced with 4-slice CT scanners *(3–5,17)*, resulting in a temporal resolution of half the gantry rotation time (250 ms for 0.5 s gantry rotation time) or better, thanks to multisegment

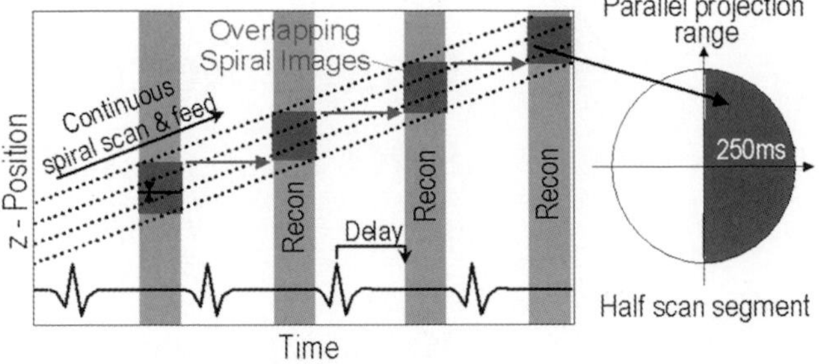

Fig. 3. Principle of retrospectively electrocardiogram (ECG)-gated spiral scanning. The patient's ECG signal is indicated as a function of time on the horizontal axis, and the position of the detector slices relative to the patient is shown on the vertical axis. The table moves continuously, and continuous spiral scan data of the heart volume are acquired. Only scan data acquired in a pre-defined cardiac phase, usually the diastolic phase, are used for image reconstruction, which are marked as boxes.

reconstruction. Different from ECG-triggered axial scanning, scan data from every heart cycle can be used for image reconstruction; therefore, the entire heart volume can be covered with a 4-slice system within one breath-hold period using 1-mm or 1.25-mm slices. Image reconstruction during different heart phases is feasible by shifting the start points of the data segments used for image reconstruction relative to the R waves. For a given start position, a stack of images at different z positions covering a small subvolume of the heart can be reconstructed thanks to the multislice data acquisition *(4,5,17)*.

Prospective ECG triggering combined with "step and shoot" acquisition of axial slices has the benefit of smaller patient dose than ECG-gated spiral scanning, since scan data are acquired in the previously selected heart phases only. It does not, however, provide continuous volume coverage with overlapping slices, and misregistration of anatomical details cannot be avoided. Furthermore, reconstruction of images in different phases of the cardiac cycle for functional evaluation is not possible. Because ECG-triggered axial scanning depends on a reliable prediction of the patient's next RR interval by using the mean of the preceding RR intervals, the method encounters its limitations for patients with severe arrhythmia. To maintain the benefits of ECG-gated spiral CT but reduce patient dose, ECG-controlled dose-modulation has been developed *(18)*. During the spiral scan, the output of the X-ray tube is modulated according to the patient's ECG. It is kept at its nominal value during a user-defined phase of the cardiac cycle—in general, the mid- to end-diastolic phase. During the rest of the cardiac cycle, the tube output is reduced. Clinical studies with 4-slice CT systems have demonstrated dose reduction by 30–50%, depending on the patient's heart rate, using ECG-controlled dose modulation *(18)*.

IMAGE RECONSTRUCTION FOR ECG-TRIGGERED MULTISLICE AXIAL SCANNING

Using prospective ECG-triggering, axial scan data are acquired. Since the table is stationary for each individual scan and moves only between scans, no multislice spiral interpolation is necessary. In general, partial scans are performed, with

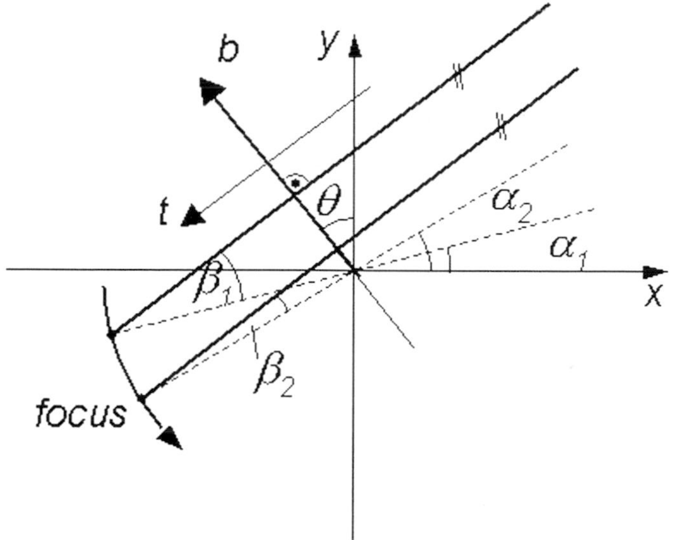

Fig. 4. Geometry of CT data acquisition. A modern CT scanner acquires data in "fan beam geometry," characterized by the projection angle α and by the fan angle β within a projection. Another set of variables serving the same purpose is θ and *b*. *b* denotes the distance of a ray from the iso-center. θ and *b* are the coordinates of a ray in "parallel geometry."

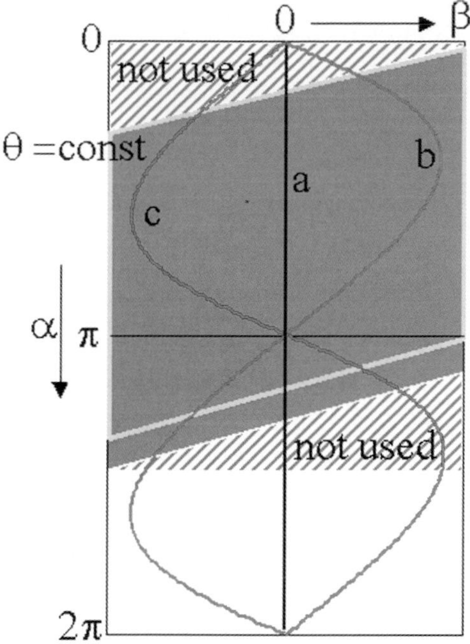

Fig. 5. Sinogram illustrating parallel rebinning according to Eq. 1 for the partial scan data segment. The sinogram curves for three image points *a*, *b*, and *c* at different positions within the scan field of view are indicated.

a scan data segment covering 180° plus the detector fan angle (about 50–60°, depending on system geometry). Including some additional data for smooth transition weighting of complementary rays to avoid streaking artifacts resulting from data inconsistencies at the beginning and at the end of the scan interval, the total scan interval of a partial scan is $\Delta\alpha_p$ = 240–260°. This is the minimum necessary for image reconstruction throughout the entire scan field of view (SFOV) of usually 50-cm diameter. The temporal resolution at a certain point in the SFOV is determined by the acquisition time window of the data contributing to the reconstruction of that particular image point. Similar to slice sensitivity profiles (SSP), temporal resolution may be characterized by time sensitivity profiles (TSP). The temporal resolution ΔT_{ima} assigned to an image is the full width at half maximum (FWHM) of the TSP. In a conventional approach, the entire partial scan data segment is used for image reconstruction in any point of the SFOV. Redundant data are weighted using algorithms such as the one described by Parker *(19)*. The temporal resolution ΔT_{ima} in this case is $\Delta\alpha_p/360°$ times the rotation time of the scanner; for 0.5 s rotation, ΔT_{ima} = 0.33–0.36 s. To improve temporal resolution, modified reconstruction approaches for partial scan data have been proposed *(5,17)*, which are best explained in parallel geometry. A modern CT scanner acquires data in fan beam geometry, characterized by the projection angle α and by the fan angle β within a projection. Another set of variables serving the same purpose is θ and *b*. θ is the azimuthal angle and *b* denotes the distance of a ray from the iso-center (*see* Fig. 4). θ and *b* are used to label rays when projection data are in the form of parallel projections. A simple coordinate transformation relates the two sets of variables:

$$\theta = \alpha + \beta,\ b = R_F \sin\beta. \quad (1)$$

Using this equation, the measured fan beam data can be transformed to parallel data, a procedure called "rebinning." In parallel geometry, 180° of scan data are necessary for image reconstruction. For data acquisition in fan beam geometry, a partial scan interval larger than 180°, namely 180° plus the detector fan angle, is necessary to provide 180° of parallel data for any image point within the SFOV. In the center of rotation, for β = 0, 180° of the acquired fan beam data are sufficient to provide 180° of parallel data; *see* Eq. (1). If all redundant data are neglected, temporal resolution in the center of rotation can be as good as 180°/360° times the rotation time of the scanner; for 0.5 s rotation, ΔT_{ima} = 0.25 s. As a consequence of the rebinning Eq. (1), data with different fan beam projection angles α and hence different acquisition times contribute to a parallel projection at projection angle θ. Fig. 5 is a sinogram and illustrates the rebinning procedure. Obviously, the temporal resolution is not constant, but depends on the position of the image point in the SFOV. This is illustrated in Fig. 5 for the example of three different image points *a*, *b*, and *c*. Measurement values contributing to point *a* in the iso-center are located on a straight vertical line in the sinogram (β = 0). Hence, the temporal resolution for this particular point is half the rotation time of the scanner. Data contributing to points *b* and *c* are located on sinosoidal curves in the sinogram. A measure for temporal resolution is given by the path lengths of the sinosoidal curves within the gray shaded parallel sinogram. Obviously, the total acquisition time of the data for point *b* is longer than for the central point *a*, whereas it is even shorter for point *c*. For clinical applications, the heart should be sufficiently centered within the SFOV to maintain a stable temporal resolution of half the gantry rotation time. It is not possible to make use of the areas

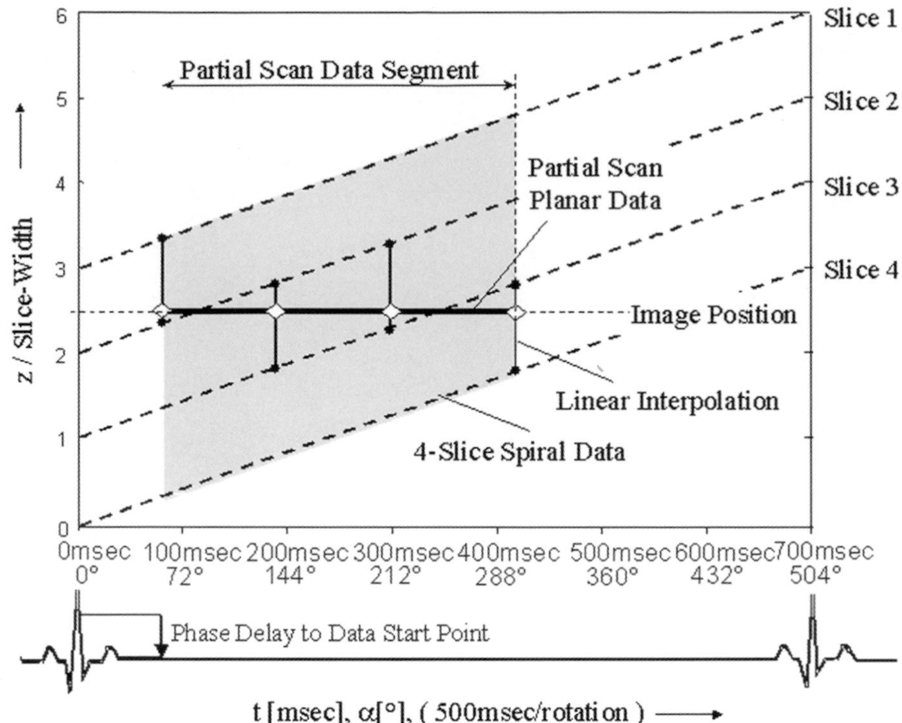

Fig. 6. Spiral interpolation scheme for a four-slice scanner using one segment of multislice data for image reconstruction. The z position of the four detector slices changes linearly relative to the patient due to the constant spiral feed. The spiral interpolation is indicated for some representative projection angles α. Please note that in general no interpolation between projections measured at different projection angles, i.e., different acquisition times, is performed, even in cases where this would be possible (180°-type interpolation). On the bottom, the electrocardiogram signal is shown schematically.

with better temporal resolution, as start and end position of the X-ray source during ECG-triggered acquisition depend on the patient's heart rate and cannot be fixed.

IMAGE RECONSTRUCTION FOR ECG-GATED MULTISLICE SPIRAL SCANNING

Using ECG-gated multislice spiral scanning, the heart volume is covered continuously by a spiral scan. Image reconstruction for ECG-gated multislice spiral scanning therefore consists of two parts: multislice spiral interpolation to compensate for the continuous table movement and to obtain scan data at the desired image z position, followed by a partial scan reconstruction of the axial data segments as described above. A "single-slice" partial scan data segment is generated for each image using a partial rotation of the multislice spiral scan that covers the given z position. For each projection angle within the multislice data segment, a linear interpolation is performed between the data of those two detector slices that are in closest proximity to the desired image plane z_{ima}. The temporal resolution, which is limited to half the gantry rotation time for prospective ECG triggering, can be improved up to $1/(2N)$ times the rotation time by using scan data of N subsequent heart cycles for image reconstruction *(17)*. With increased N, better temporal resolution is achieved, but at the expense of reduced volume coverage within one breath-hold time or loss of transverse resolution. To maintain good transverse resolution and thin-slice images, every z position of the heart has to be seen by a detector slice at every time during the N heart cycles. As a consequence, the larger the N and the lower the patient's heart rate, the more the spiral pitch has to be reduced. If the pitch is too high, there will be z positions which are not covered by a detector slice in the desired phase of the cardiac cycle. To obtain images at these z positions, far-reaching spiral interpolations have to be performed, which degrade SSPs and reduce transverse resolution.

SINGLE-SEGMENT RECONSTRUCTION

At low heart rates, a single-segment reconstruction ($N = 1$) yields the best compromise between sufficient temporal resolution on the one hand and adequate volume coverage with thin slices on the other. For $N = 1$, consecutive multislice spiral data from the same heart period are used to generate the single-slice partial scan data segment for an image. The spiral interpolation scheme for a 4-slice scanner using one segment of multislice data is illustrated in Fig. 6, together with the calculation of the spiral interpolation weights for some representative projection angles. In general, no interpolation between projections measured at different projection angles, i.e., different acquisition times, is performed, even in cases where this would be possible (180°-type interpolation). The temporal resolution is constant and equals half the gantry rotation time of the scanner using optimized partial scan reconstruction techniques as described above. For 0.5-s gantry rotation time, temporal resolution is

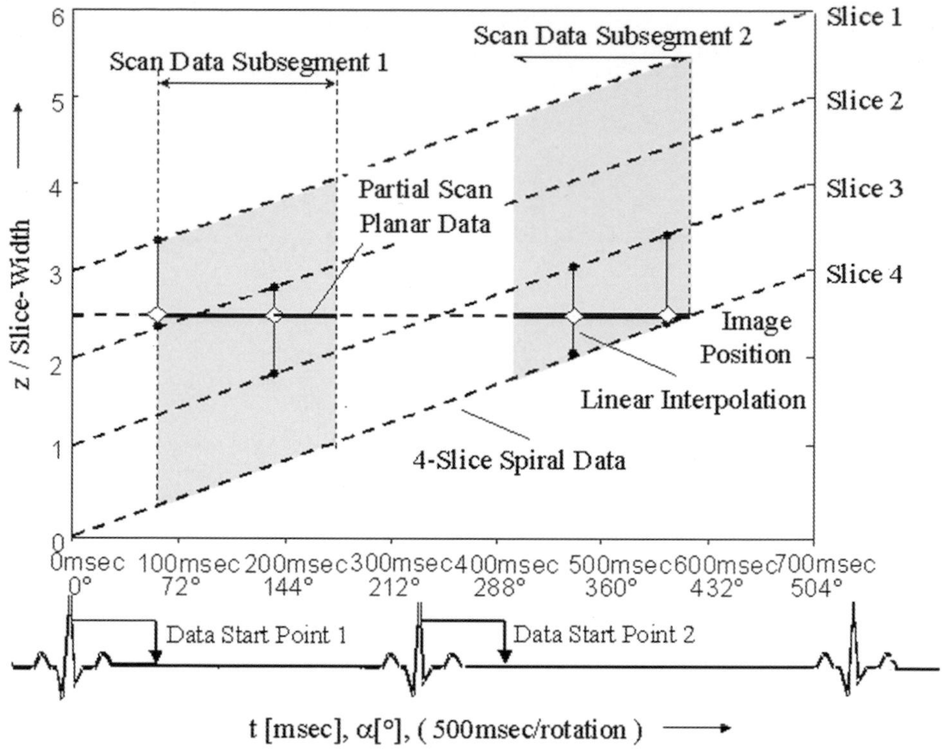

Fig. 7. Spiral interpolation scheme for a four-slice scanner using $N = 2$ subsegments of multislice data from consecutive heart periods for image reconstruction. Both subsegments have to fit together to build up a partial scan data interval. The spiral interpolation is indicated for some representative projection angles α.

$\Delta T_{ima} = 0.25$ s. Some of the recently introduced 16-slice CT systems offer gantry rotation times even shorter than 0.5 s, such as 0.42 s or 0.4 s. In this case, temporal resolution can be as good as $\Delta T_{ima} = 0.21$ s or 0.2 s.

MULTISEGMENT RECONSTRUCTION

At higher heart rates, temporal resolution can be improved by dividing the partial scan data segment used for image reconstruction into $N = 2–4$ subsegments acquired in subsequent heart cycles. Each subsegment is generated by using data from one heart period only, and there are temporal gaps between the multislice data segments used for image reconstruction. Similar to the case $N = 1$, for each projection angle α within subsegment *j*, a linear interpolation is performed between the data of those two detector slices that are in closest proximity to the desired image plane. The result are *N* single-slice partial scan subsegments located at the given image z position z_{ima} (*see* Fig. 7 for the example $N = 2$).

With this technique, the patient's heart rate and the gantry rotation time of the scanner have to be properly desynchronized to allow for an improved temporal resolution. Two requirements have to be met: firstly, start- and end-projection angles of the subsegments have to fit together to build up a full partial scan interval (*see* Fig. 8). As a consequence, the start projections of subsequent subsegments have to be shifted relative to each other. Secondly, all subsegments have to be acquired in the same relative phase of the patient's heart cycle to reduce the total time interval contributing to an image. If the patient's heart cycle and the rotation of the scanner are completely synchronous, the two requirements are contradictory. For instance, for a heart rate of 60 beats per minute (bpm) and a 360° rotation time of 0.5 s, the same heart phase always corresponds to the same projection angle segment, and a partial scan interval cannot be divided into smaller subsegments acquired in successive heart periods. Then no better temporal resolution than half the gantry rotation time is achieved. In the best case, when the patient's heart cycle and the rotation of the scanner are optimally desynchronized, the entire partial scan interval may be divided into *N* subsegments of equal length, and each subsegment is restricted to a data time interval of $1/(2N)$ times the rotation time within the same relative heart phase. Generally, depending on the relation of rotation time and patient heart rate, temporal resolution is not constant but varies between one half and $1/(2N)$ times the gantry rotation time. There are "sweet spots," heart rates with optimum temporal resolution, and heart rates where temporal resolution cannot be improved beyond half the gantry rotation time. Multisegment approaches rely on a complete periodicity of the heart motion, and they encounter their limitations for patients with arrhythmia or patients with changing heart rates during examination. In general, clinical practice suggests the use of $N = 1$ segment at lower heart rates and $N \geq 2$ segments at higher heart rates. In some CT scanners,

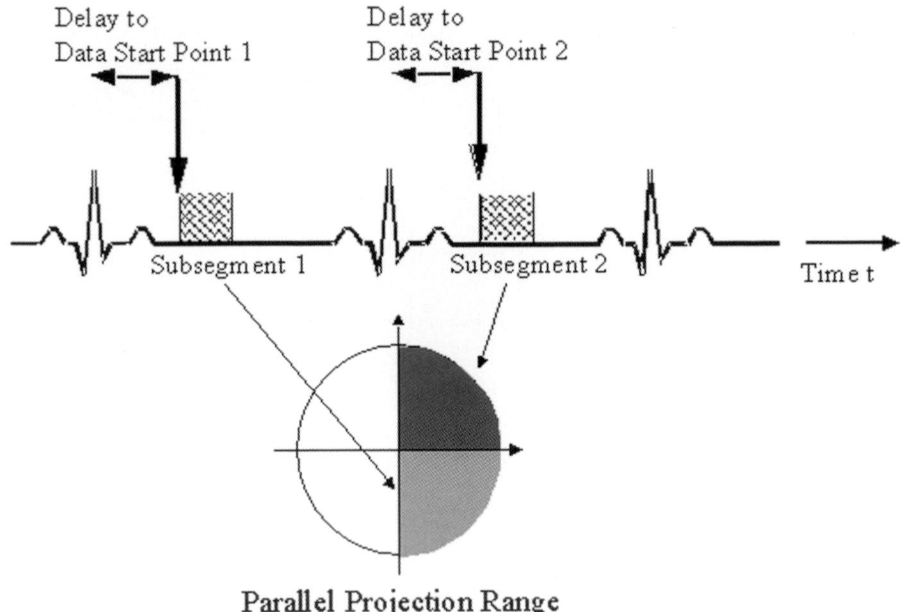

Fig. 8. Schematic illustration of the two-segment cardio reconstruction approach. The circular graph represents the full partial scan interval in parallel geometry (180° of parallel data), which is composed of two subsegments acquired in subsequent heart cycles. These two subsegments have to be measured in the same phase of the cardiac cycle, and start- and end-projections have to fit together. To fulfill both requirements, the patient's heart cycle and the rotation of the scanner have to be asynchronous.

the partial scan data segment is automatically divided into one or two subsegments depending on the patient's heart rate during examination (Adaptive Cardio Volume ACV algorithm *[17]*). At heart rates below a certain threshold, one subsegment of consecutive multislice spiral data from the same heart period is used. At higher heart rates, two subsegments from adjacent heart cycles contribute to the partial scan data segment. In some other CT scanners, the single-segment partial scan images are reconstructed prospectively as baseline images, followed by a two-segment reconstruction retrospectively for a potential gain of temporal resolution for higher heart rates. Alternatively, a two-segment prospective reconstruction can be prescribed with a slower table feed for scanning the same cardiac anatomy in two heart cycles, followed by a retrospective single-segment reconstruction for comparison with the two-segment reconstruction. A single-segment reconstruction is usually preferred for its reliability, even though a two-segment reconstruction may yield a better image quality.

Another approach is to prospectively adjust the rotation time of the scanner to the heart rate of the patient to obtain best possible temporal resolution for a multisegment reconstruction. The range of heart rates is preferred to cover 15 bpm for each selected gantry cycle, to account for the patient's heart rate variation during a scan. Figure 9 shows an example of using 0.5-s and 0.6-s gantry rotation time for this implementation. The 0.5-s two-segment reconstruction covers low 60s to 75 bpm, followed by 0.6-s three- to four-segment reconstruction for 75–90 bpm, and 0.5-s three- to four-segment reconstruction for the heart rates of over 90 bpm. Figure 10 shows another example of using 0.42-s and 0.5-s gantry rotation time in combination with an automatic selection of one- and two-segment reconstruction (ACV algorithm). The 0.5-s two-segment reconstruction covers 64–73 bpm, whereas the 0.42-s two-segment reconstruction is preferable for 73–90 bpm. Figures 11 and 12 show examples of patient scans at higher heart rates, to illustrate the potential of multisegment reconstruction to improve image quality in selected cases. Again, prospectively adapting the rotation time of the scanner and exploiting multisegment reconstruction requires a stable and predictable heart rate during examination and complete periodicity of the heart motion.

DISCUSSION AND SUMMARY

We have reviewed the scanning and reconstruction techniques for ECG-controlled MSCT. Two basic scanning techniques are discussed: ECG-triggered axial scanning and ECG-gated spiral scanning. For ECG-triggered axial scanning, the X-ray will be turned on only for the duration of the data for image reconstruction; therefore, the dose to the patient can be kept to a minimum. For ECG-gated spiral scanning, the dose is higher, since the X-ray is turned on for the whole duration of the scanning. Ways of reducing the X-ray dose have been proposed, such as ECG-controlled dose modulation *(18)*. There are two major reconstruction techniques associated with spiral scanning: one is single-segment reconstruction, where each image is reconstructed with the data from a single cardiac cycle; the other is *N*-segment reconstruction, where each image is reconstructed with the data from *N* contiguous cardiac cycles. The two-segment reconstruction has the advantage of extending from single-segment reconstruction without changing the gantry rotation cycle. The three- and four-segment reconstructions can be used when the heart rate is becoming too high (>75

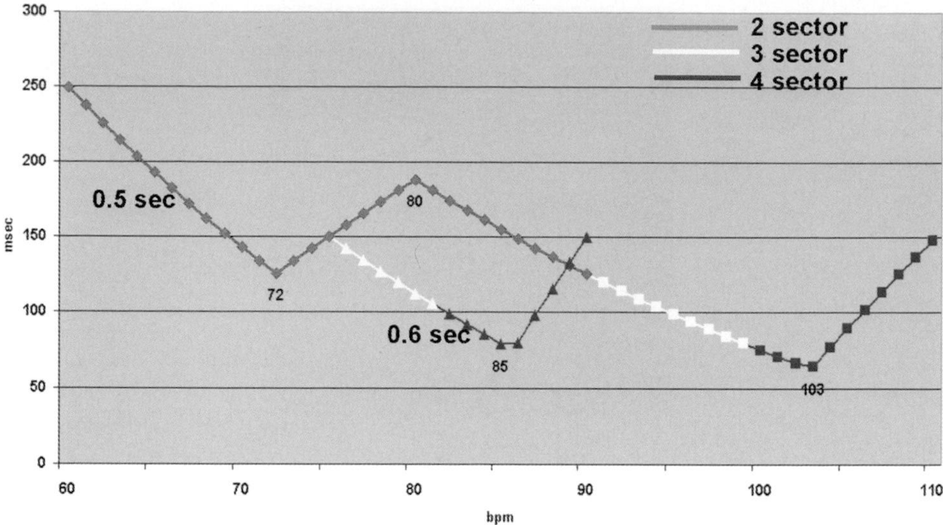

Fig. 9. A design of *N*-segment reconstruction with gantry cycles of 0.5 and 0.6 s to improve temporal resolution for higher heart rates. The 0.5-s two-segment reconstruction covers from the low 60s to 75 bpm, followed by 0.6-s three- to four-segment reconstruction for 75–90 bpm, and 0.5-s three- to four-segment reconstruction for heart rates of over 90 bpm.

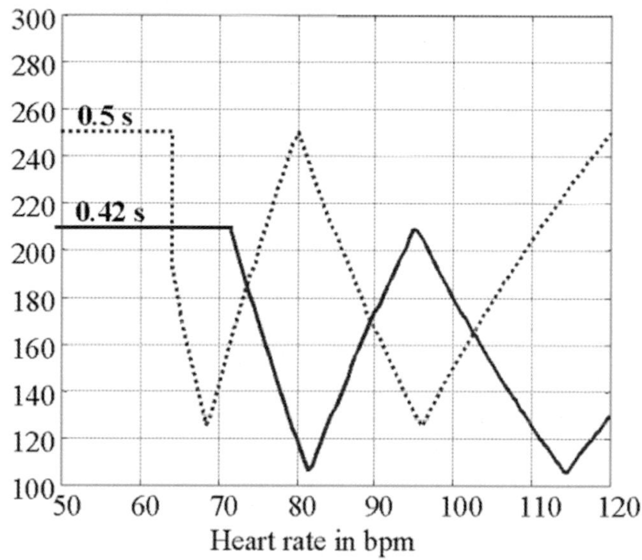

Fig. 10. A design of automatic selection of single- and two-segment reconstruction (ACV algorithm) with gantry cycles of 0.42 and 0.5 s. 0.42-s gantry rotation is preferable for low heart rates (single-segment reconstruction) and for 73–90 bpm (two-segment reconstruction). The 0.5-s two-segment reconstruction yields better temporal resolution for 64–73 bpm.

bpm), and a slower gantry cycle of 0.6 s can be used to optimize the temporal resolution. Single-segment reconstruction is the clinically most robust reconstruction technique. The reliability of obtaining good quality images with *N*-segment reconstruction generally goes down when *N* becomes larger from 2, to 3, to 4. Multisegment reconstruction requires a stable heart rate during examination and complete periodicity of the heart motion. The cardiac MSCT has also benefited significantly from the advancements of 4 × 1-mm/4 × 1.25-mm to 16 × 0.75-mm/16 × 0.625-mm collimation and faster gantry speeds of 0.5 s to 0.42 s or 0.4 s. The wider coverage with thinner slices (16 × 0.75 mm/16 × 0.625 mm) has improved the spatial resolution in the cranio-caudal direction (or Z coordinate) to submillimeter, with already submillimeter resolution in the in-plane direction (or X and Y coordinates); this is critical for coronary artery imaging, and has shortened the scan time of 40 s (4-slice) to 20 s (8- or 16-slice) or even 10 s (16-slice), which is well under a single breath-hold. The gantry rotation cycle of 0.5 s to 0.42 or 0.4 s has improved the temporal resolution of 0.25 s to 0.21 and 0.2 s, which will help the MSCT become a scanner for most patients. The image quality that can be obtained in clinical routine is demonstrated in Fig. 13. Meanwhile, first clinical experience has demonstrated the potential of 16-slice technology for cardiac imaging *(15,16,20)*.

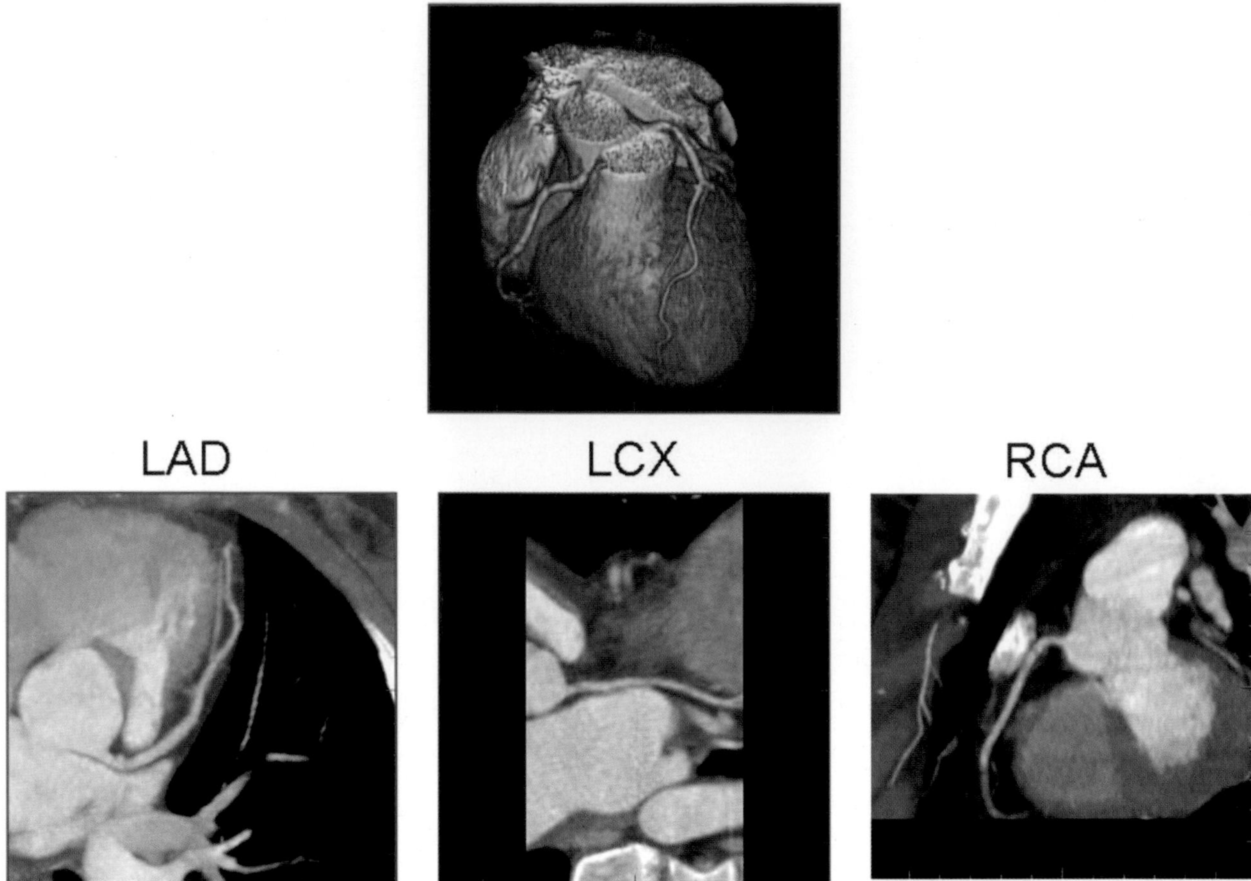

Fig. 11. A patient study with heart rates of 97–101 bpm with three- to four-segment reconstruction. Shown here are the volume-rendered image, and the curved reformatted images of the left anterior descending (LAD), left circumflex (LCX), and right coronary artery (RCA). It demonstrates the potential for three- to four-segment reconstruction to improve the temporal resolution for higher heart rates.

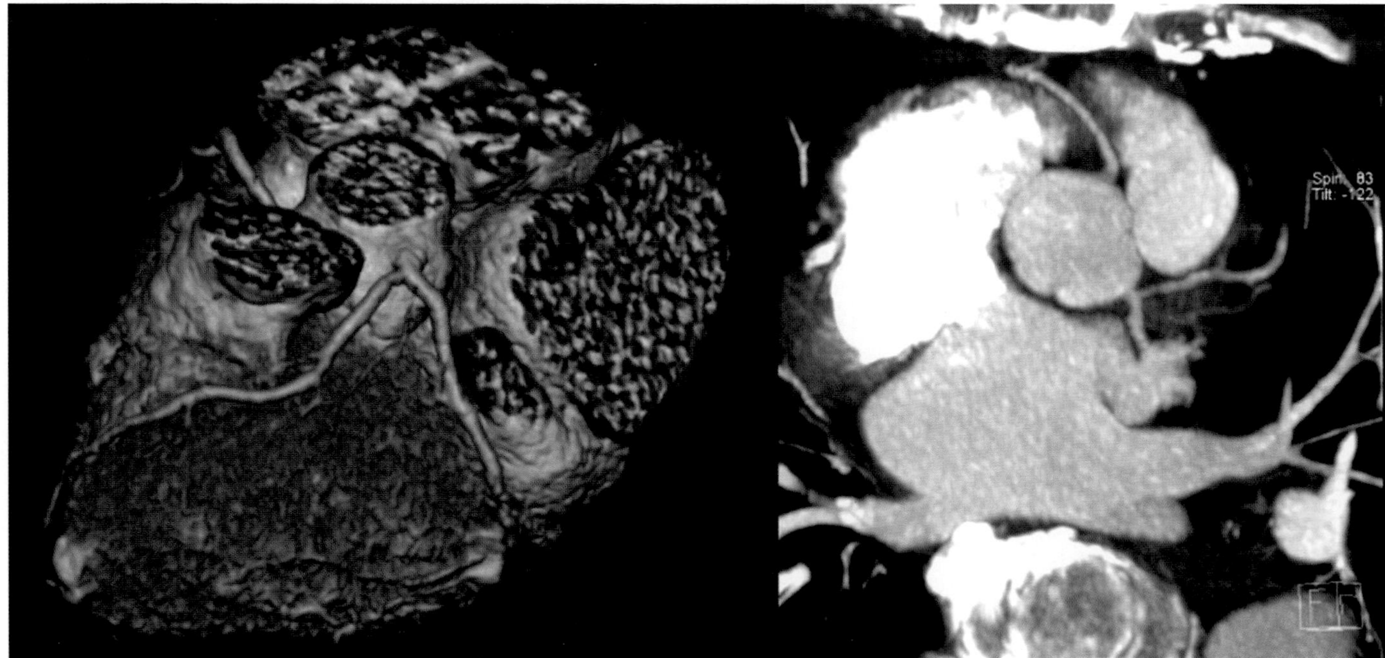

Fig. 12. A patient study of heart rates of around 92 bpm with two-segment reconstruction. Shown here are the volume-rendered image, and a "spider view" maximum intensity projection showing the origins of left anterior descending, left circumflex, and right coronary artery (courtesy of Dr. Ropers, Erlangen University, Germany).

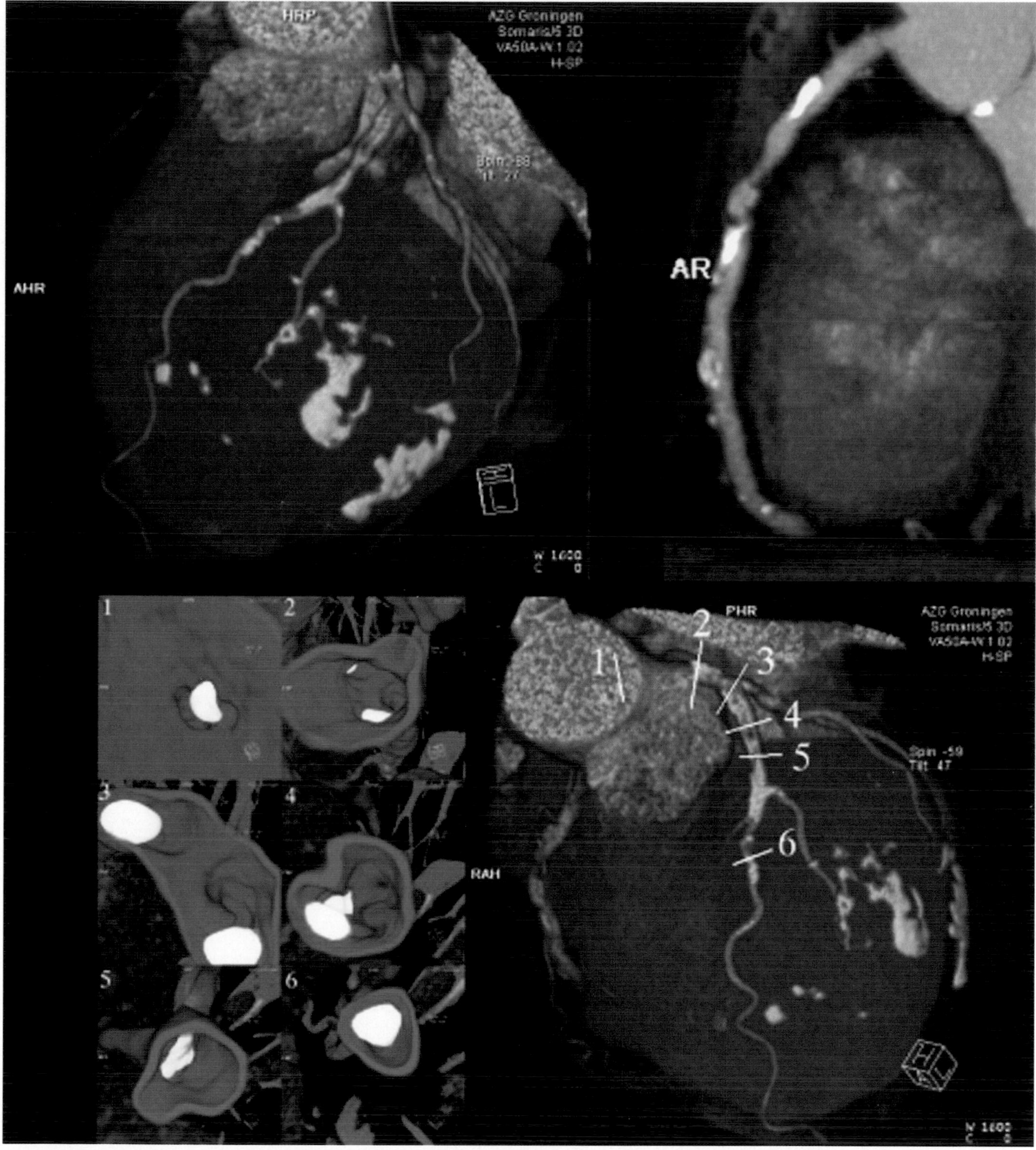

Fig. 13. Case of a 68-yr-old male patient with a history of stroke secondary to a bilateral carotid obstruction. The CT scan was obtained on a 16-slice CT system. The images show severe calcification in the left anterior descending (LAD) and right coronary artery (RCA), as well as large pericardial calcifications. The calcifications are displayed in endoscopic and maximum intensity projection viewing techniques. Corresponding to the coronary angiogram, a 40% stenosis of the left main (LM) and 80% stenosis of the LAD and RCA were found (courtesy of Prof. Oudkerk, Groningen University, Groningen, the Netherlands).

REFERENCES

1. Bahner M, Boese J, Lutz A, et al. Retrospectively ECG-gated spiral CT of the heart and lung. Eur Radiol 1999;9:106–109.
2. Kachelriess M, Kalender W. Electrocardiogram-correlated image reconstruction from subsecond spiral computed tomography scans of the heart. Med Phys 1998;25:2417–2431.
3. Kachelriess M, Ulzheimer S, Kalender W. ECG-correlated image reconstruction from subsecond multi-slice spiral CT scans of the heart. Med Phys 2000;27:1881–1902.
4. Taguchi K, Anno H. High temporal resolution for multi-slice helical computed tomography. Med Phys 2000,27(5):861–872.
5. Ohnesorge B, Flohr T, Becker C, et al. Cardiac imaging by means of electro-cardiographically gated multisection spiral CT—initial experience. Radiology 2000;217:564–571.
6. Achenbach S, Ulzheimer S, Baum U, et al. Noninvasive coronary angiography by retrospectively ECG-gated multi-slice spiral CT. Circulation 2000;102:2823–2828.
7. Becker C, Knez A, Ohnesorge B, Schöpf U, Reiser M. Imaging of non calcified coronary plaques using helical CT with retrospective EKG gating. AJR 2000;175:423–424.
8. Knez A, Becker C, Leber A, Ohnesorge B, Reiser M, Haberl R. Noninvasive assessment of coronary artery stenoses with multidetector helical computed tomography. Circulation 2000;101:e221–e222.
9. Nieman K, Oudkerk M, Rensing B, et al. Coronary angiography with multi-slice computed tomography. Lancet 2001;357:599–603
10. Schroeder S, Kopp A, Baumbach A, et al. Noninvasive detection and evaluation of atherosclerotic coronary plaques with multi-slice computed tomography. JACC 2001;37(5):1430–1435.
11. Hong C, Becker C, Huber A, et al. ECG-gated reconstructed multidetector row CT coronary angiography: effect of varying trigger delay on image quality. Radiology 2001;220:712–717.
12. Kopp A, Schröder S, Küttner A, et al. Coronary arteries: retrospectively ECG-gated multi-detector row CT angiography with selective optimization of the image reconstruction window. Radiology 2001;221:683–688.
13. Flohr T, Stierstorfer K, Bruder H, Simon J, Schaller S. New technical developments in multislice CT, part 1: approaching isotropic resolution with sub-mm 16-slice scanning. Fortschr Röntgenstr 2002;174:839–845.
14. Flohr T, Bruder H, Stierstorfer K, Simon J, Schaller S, Ohnesorge B. New technical developments in multislice CT, part 2: sub-millimeter 16-slice scanning and increased gantry rotation speed for cardiac imaging. Fortschr Röntgenstr 2002;174:1022–1027.
15. Kopp AF, Küttner A, Heuschmid M, Schröder S, Ohnesorge B, Claussen CD. Multidetector-row CT cardiac imaging with 4 and 16 slices for coronary CTA and imaging of atherosclerotic plaques. Eu Radiol 2002;12(Suppl 2):S17–S24.
16. Nieman K, Cademartiri F, Lemos PA, Raaijmakers R, Pattynama PMT, de Feyter PJ. Reliable noninvasive coronary angiography with fast submillimeter multislice spiral computed tomography. Circulation 2002;106:2051–2054.
17. Flohr T, Ohnesorge B. Heart rate adaptive optimization of spatial and temporal resolution for ECG-gated multi-slice spiral CT of the heart. JCAT 2001;25(6):907–923.
18. Jakobs TF, Becker CR, Ohnesorge B, et al. Multislice helical CT of the heart with retrospective ECG gating: reduction of radiation exposure by ECG-controlled tube current modulation. Eur Radiol 2002;12:1081–1086.
19. Parker D. Optimal short scan convolution reconstruction for fanbeam CT. Med Phys 1982;9(2):254–257.
20. Ropers D, Baum U, Pohle K, et al. Detection of coronary artery stenosis with thin-slice multi-detector row spiral computed tomography and multiplanar reconstruction. Circulation 2003;107:664–666.

5 Phase-Correlated Image Reconstruction Without ECG

MARC KACHELRIESS, PhD AND WILLI A. KALENDER, PhD

INTRODUCTION

Improvements in computed tomography (CT) technology such as the introduction of spiral CT, subsecond rotation times, and multislice data acquisition have stimulated cardiac CT imaging within the last decade (Fig. 1). Cardiac spiral CT started with the introduction of dedicated phase-correlated reconstruction algorithms for single-slice spiral CT in 1997 *(1–3)*. These approaches have been generalized to the case of multislice spiral CT (MSCT) acquisition *(2,4–6)* to process data of 4-slice scanners. Since then, the algorithms have been extended to the case of cone-beam scanning with 16 slices *(7–10)* and to scanners with far more than 16 slices *(11)*. Vendor-specific implementations that take into account the cone angle have not been announced yet.

What all cardiac reconstruction algorithms have in common is the need to synchronize the reconstruction with heart motion. With this synchronization, the algorithms seek to use projection data from a temporal window (allowed data ranges) aligned to the synchronization points. The size of these allowed data ranges determines the temporal resolution of the reconstruction and thus the level of motion-artifact reduction. The position of the windows determines the motion phase that is visible in the reconstruction. The most elaborate phase-weighting strategy currently available is the cardio-interpolation (CI) method, which is an adaptive multiphase weighting: minimal-width allowed data ranges of all heart cycles contributing to a given z position are determined to form a 180° complete high temporal resolution data set ready for reconstruction. Inter-segment combination artifacts are eliminated by applying a multi-triangular weighting function to each data segment followed by proper normalization. Other known methods such as single- and bi-phase weighting restrict the image contributions to one or two heart cycles, respectively, depending on the local heart rate, and are a subset of CI.

The synchronization signal traditionally stems from the patient's electrocardiogram (ECG), which is simultaneously recorded during the scan. In those cases, the reconstruction procedure is termed *ECG-correlated reconstruction*. Note that the origin of the sync signal is not a property of the phase-correlated reconstruction algorithm itself; it can be easily substituted by any other appropriate synchronization measure.

There are several reasons to look into alternative synchronization approaches. Recording the ECG requires additional hardware and additional patient-handling effort. Further, extra systoles that do not necessarily correspond to cardiac motion are interpreted as valid signals and may therefore impair image quality in the reconstructions. Sometimes the ECG signal is corrupted due to hardware failure, is unavailable, or totally useless. A fallback solution is desired in such cases. Additionally, for some applications that may profit from cardiac motion reduction, such as thoracic imaging, applying the ECG leads is inconvenient or not desired.

KYMOGRAM DETECTION

Recently, a hardware-independent synchronization method, the *kymogram*, has become available *(12–14)*. The method in its present implementation consists of a raw data-based center of mass (COM) detection of the patient cross-section currently scanned. Since the heart is in permanent motion, the detected COM will vary with the tube position, and the synchronization information can be derived from these variations.

The COM detection is illustrated in Fig. 2. The mathematical relations between object data and projection data state that the COM of the projection (at angle ϑ) of an object is equal to the projection (at angle ϑ) of the COM of the object. In our case this is illustrated with two small disks (Fig. 2A). The disk in the center of the heart is the patient's COM. The second disk is the COM of the projection data. The positions of the disks are related by projecting along the ray direction. The kymogram algorithm uses the acquired raw data and computes the projection COM for each view angle ϑ. Then, adjacent projections are used to compute the intersection of the corresponding lines of COM projection and the current patient COM results (Fig. 2B).

So far, the algorithm results in a COM curve similar to the plots on the right in Fig. 3. The curves are obscured by a dominant slowly varying bias; heart motion is not visible yet. The multiplanar reformations (MPRs) attached to the COM plots clarify the origin of the bias: the patient COM is dominated by large structures such as the overall thorax shape or the liver.

As soon as the bias is removed (e.g., by subtracting a running mean of appropriate length), the cardiac motion is restored and

From: *Contemporary Cardiology: CT of the Heart: Principles and Applications*
Edited by: U. Joseph Schoepf © Humana Press, Inc., Totowa, NJ

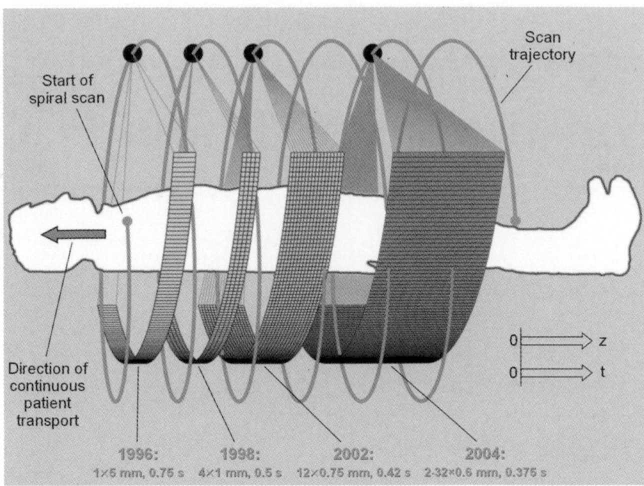

Fig. 1. Four generations of spiral CT scanners. Collimation and rotation times (bottom) are given for typical CT coronary angiography protocols.

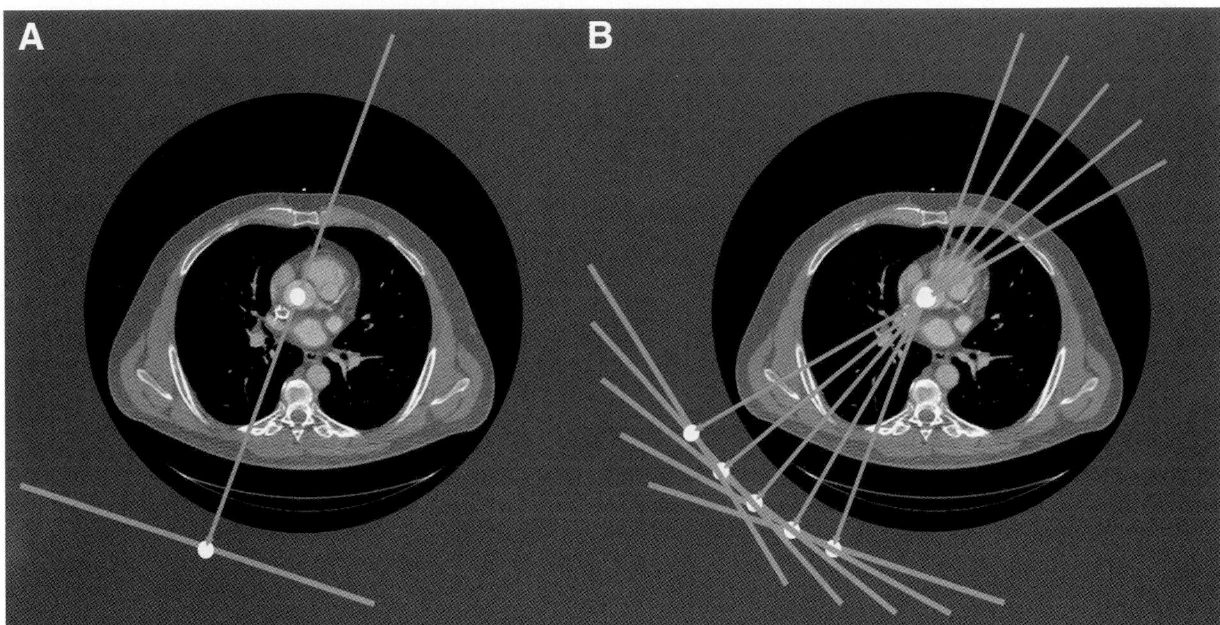

Fig. 2. (A) The center of mass (COM) of the current cross-section is projected onto the COM of the projection data. **(B)** Adjacent projection COMs can be used to find the object COM by simple intersection.

becomes visible. Figure 4 shows a plot of the unbiased heart COM motion. The dots' hue values are chosen as the cardiac ECG phase (relative to RR). The fact that dots of similar color are located close together indicates a correlation of the heart's COM and the ECG phase. For example, the upper right area corresponds to systolic, the lower left area to diastolic motion.

The two-dimensional signal can now be reduced to a one-dimensional function by projecting it onto the principal axis of cardiac in-plane motion (diagonal line in Fig. 4). An example of such a resulting kymogram function is given in Fig. 5. Visual inspection indicates a good correlation to the patient's ECG except for regions at scan start and end that correspond to anatomical levels above and below the heart. In analogy to the ECG's R peaks, the kymogram's maxima are called K peaks, and synchronization is performed with respect to the K peaks, just as it is done with the ECG's R peaks.

HEART IMAGING

Examples of kymogram-based reconstructions are given in Figs. 6, 7, and 8. The images clearly indicate the high quality of kymogram-based reconstruction. The patient shown in Fig. 8 is an example for an ECG-based reconstruction that failed. In this case, the ECG monitor reported twice as many R peaks as a result of a misinterpretation of the T waves. The kymogram-correlated reconstructions of this patient are therefore of higher quality than the ECG-correlated images.

It must be pointed out that the kymogram phase and the ECG phase are correlated up to an unknown scan- and patient-spe-

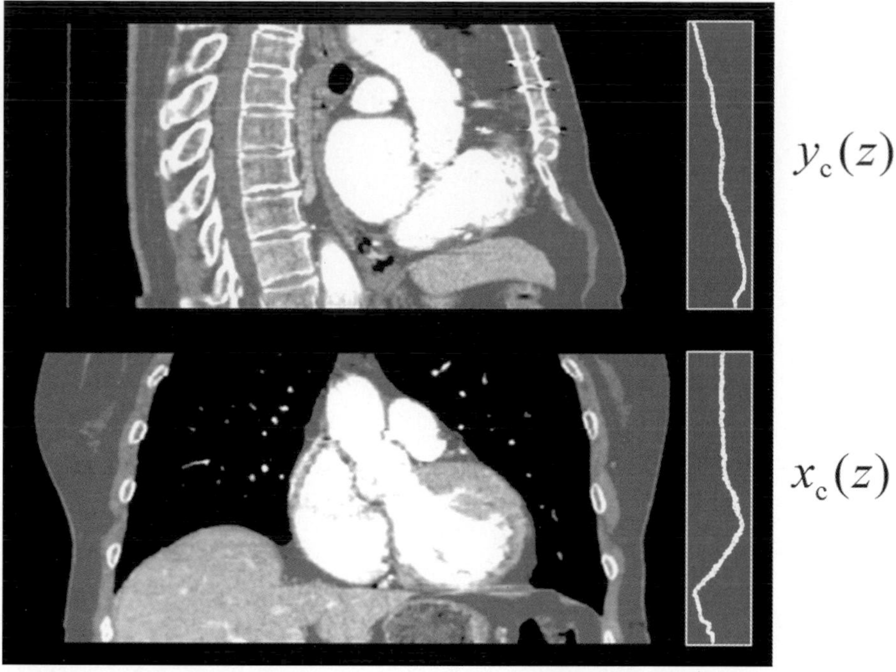

Fig. 3. The detected center of mass (COM) is a function of the z position (and thus of time). The plots show that the COM is dominated by global patient structures, and the heart motion cannot be readily deduced therefrom.

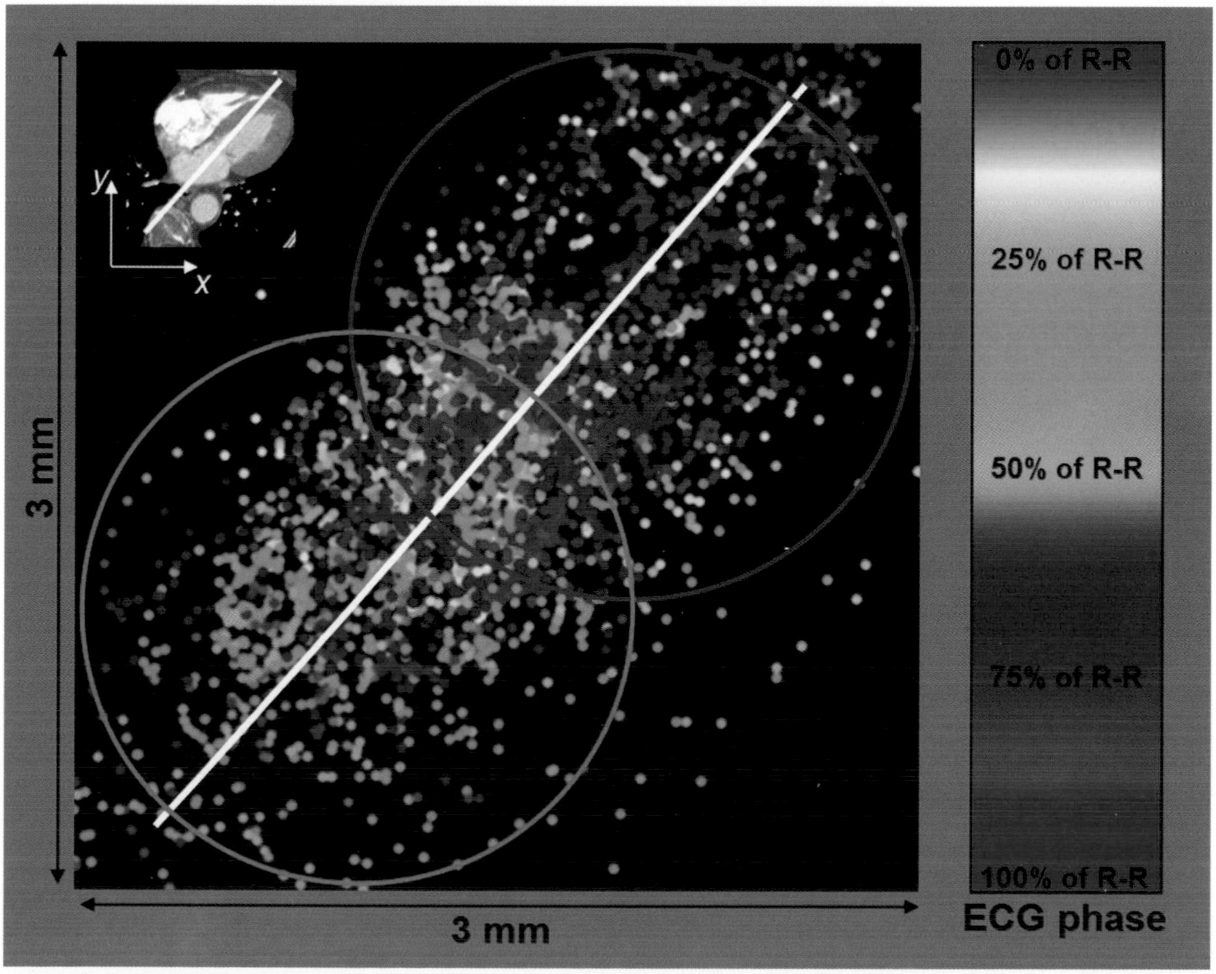

Fig. 4. Scatter plot showing the unbiased cardiac motion for a complete scan (about 30 s of cardiac motion). The dots are colored according to a simultaneously acquired electrocardiogram signal. Dots of similar hue are located close together.

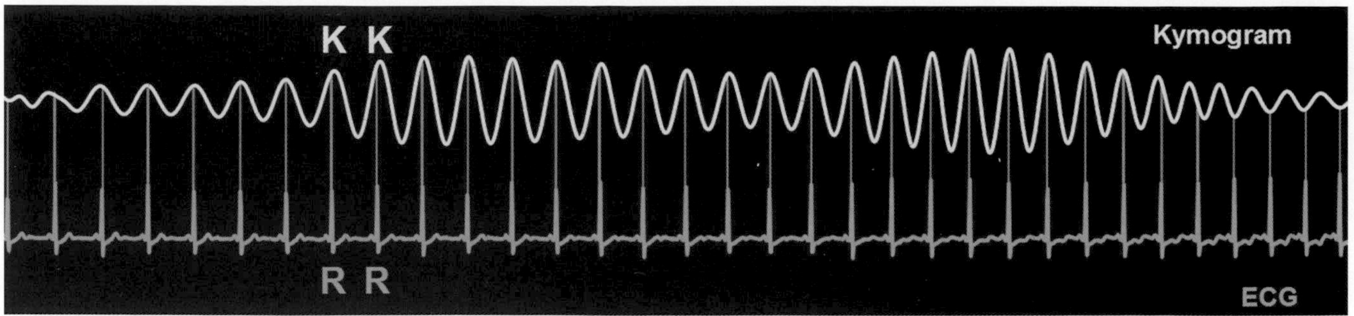

Fig. 5. The kymogram's K peaks are highly correlated to the electrocardiogram's R peaks. Correlation is less optimal at the start and end of the scan, i.e., above and below the heart, where hardly any cardiac motion can be detected.

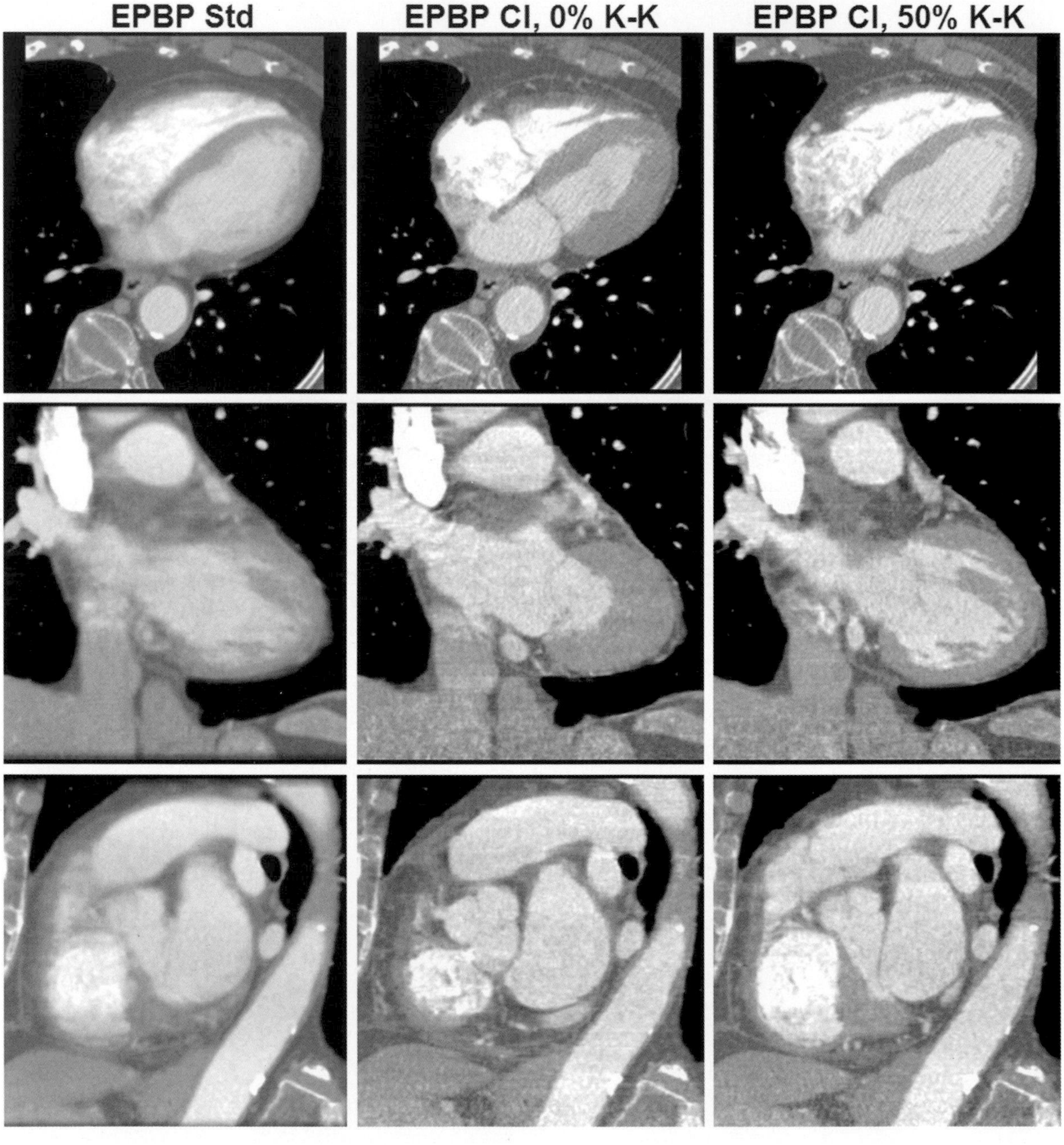

EPBP Std | EPBP CI, 0% K-K | EPBP CI, 50% K-K

Fig. 6. Patient example reconstructed with the standard reconstruction algorithm extended parallel backprojection (EPBP) Std and with the phase-correlated reconstruction algorithm EPBP cardio-interpolation (CI) at 0% and 50% of KK, respectively. Parameters: 12 × 0.75-mm collimation, 0.42 s per rotation, 3-mm table increment.

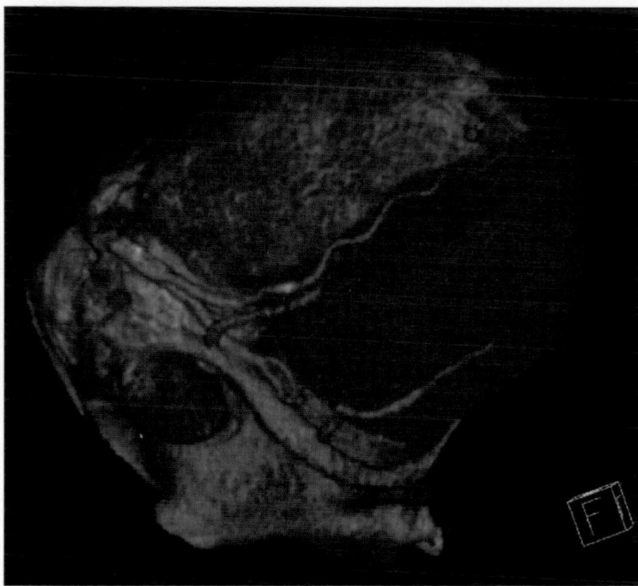

Fig. 7. Volume rendering of a kymogram-based volume reconstruction. The coronary arteries are depicted at great length.

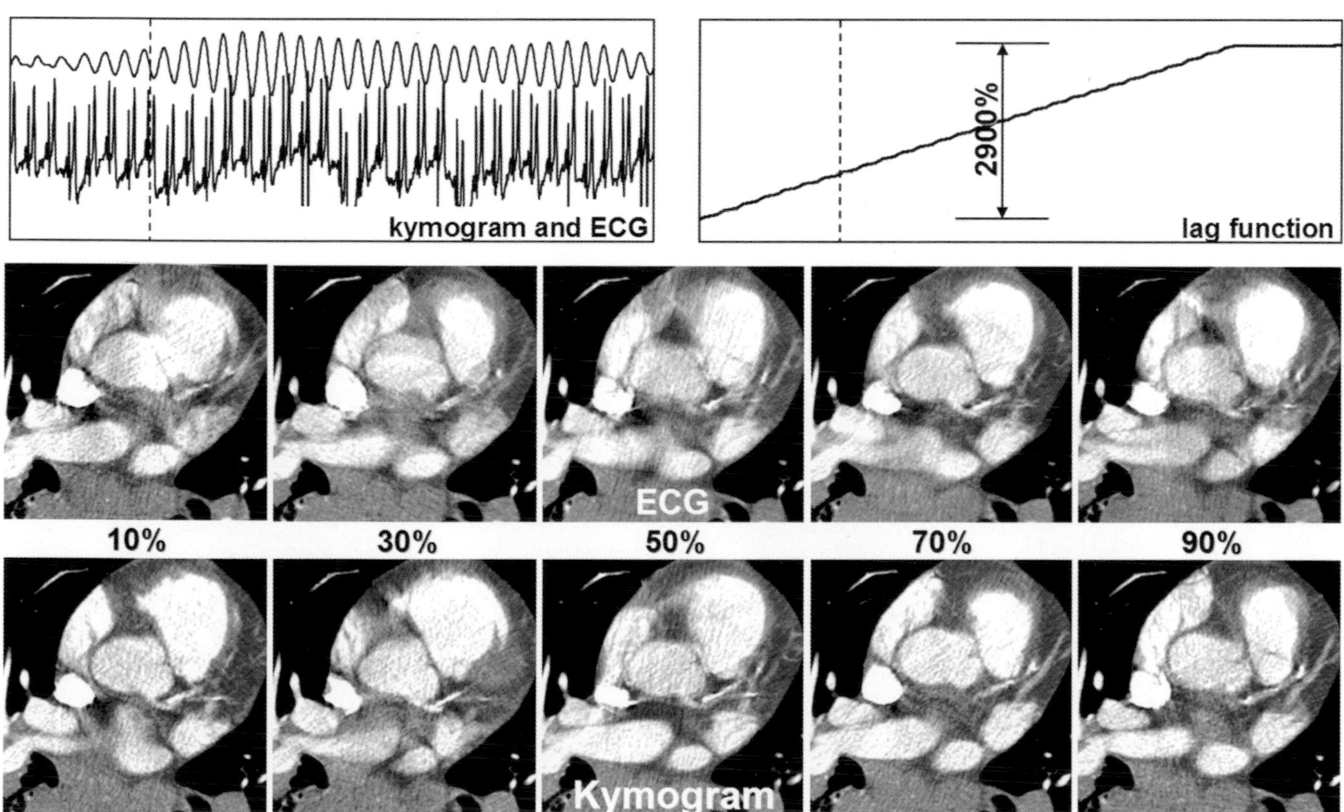

Fig. 8. Case where two R peaks per heart cycle were assumed by the electrocardiogram (ECG)-based reconstruction as a result of a misinterpretation of the ECG's T waves. The heart rate reported by the ECG monitor was 130 bpm, but the true heart rate was 65 bpm, and was detected by the kymogram algorithm. The images are reconstructed at a fixed z position (dashed lines in the plots above) at increments of 20% of RR and KK, respectively. Only the kymogram-based reconstructions show temporal contiguity.

cific constant, the so-called phase lag: Reconstructions at 0% of KK therefore do not necessarily correspond to reconstructions at 0% of RR. In cases with defect ECG signals, the phase lag is no longer constant (*see* Fig. 8).

THORACIC IMAGING

Imaging of pericardial lung areas usually suffers from motion artifacts and blurring as a result of cardiac motion. The use of phase-correlated reconstruction algorithms promises to

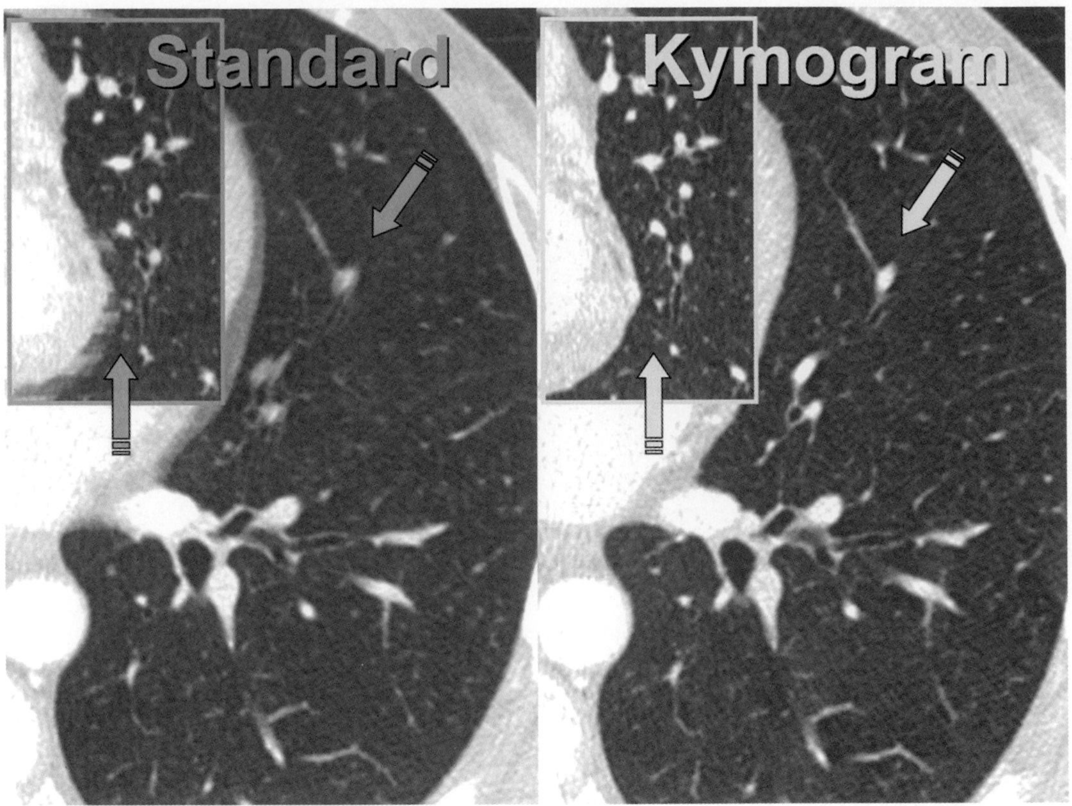

Fig. 9. Improved lung imaging using kymogram-correlated reconstruction for scans of the thorax. The motion artifacts at the borders of the heart and the double contours in the lung vanish using the kymogram.

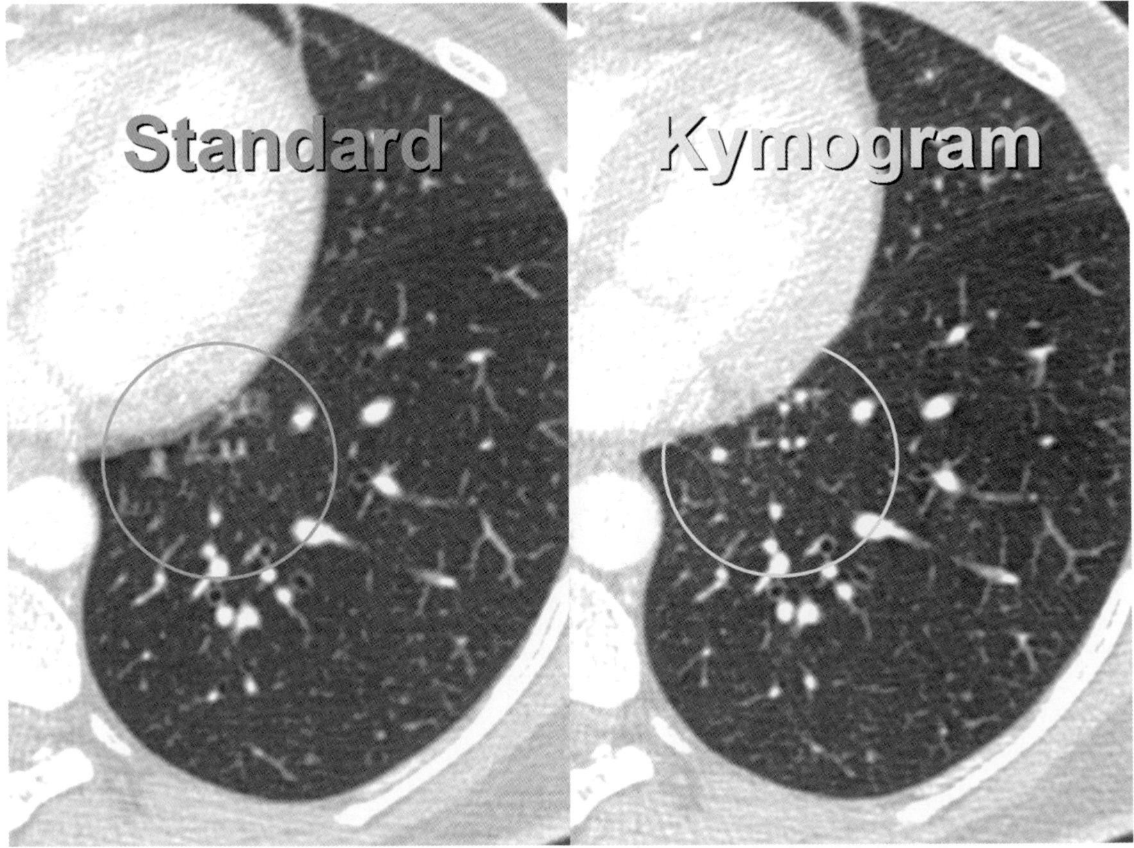

Fig. 10. Pericardial motion can be greatly reduced using kymogram-correlated reconstruction.

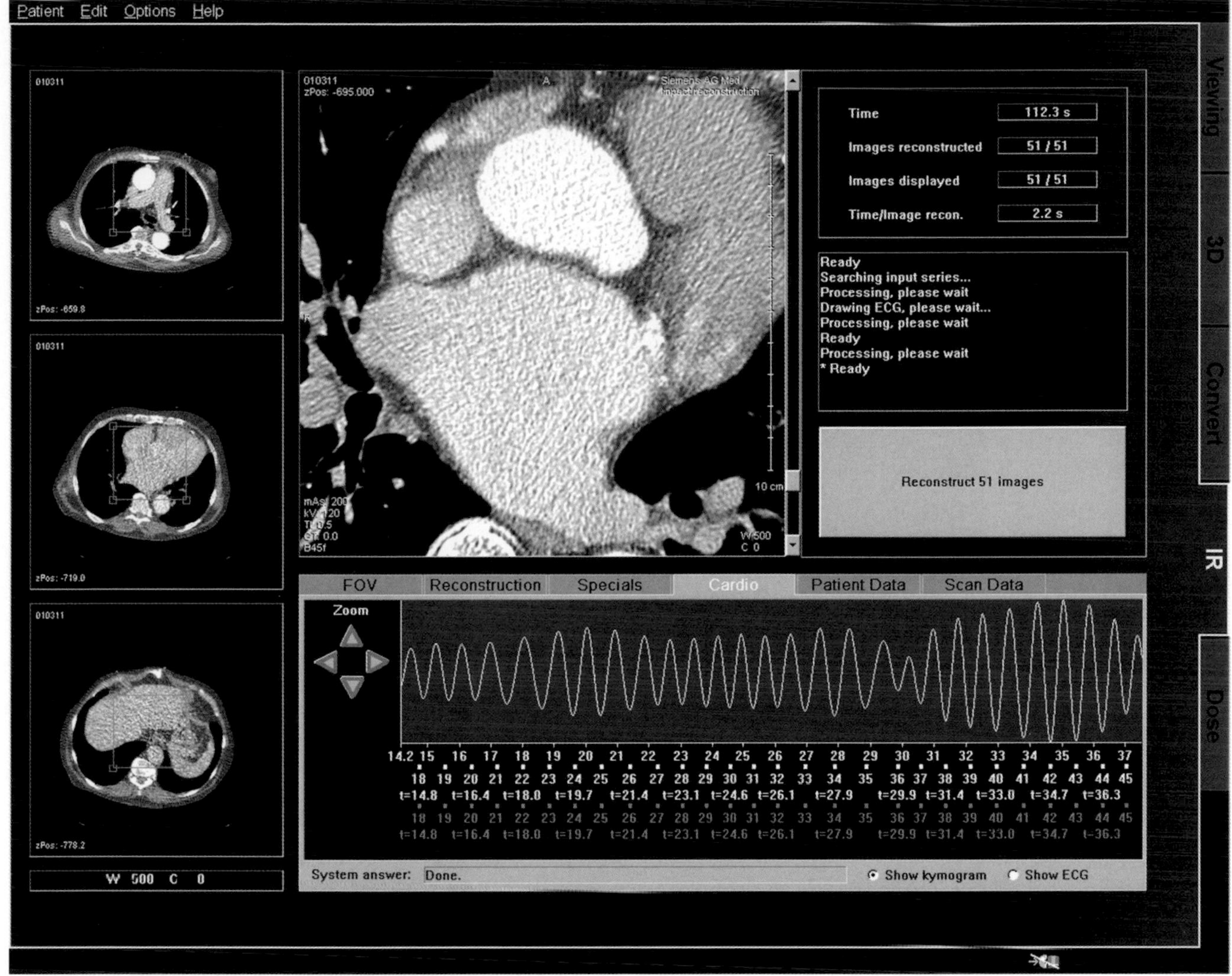

Fig. 11. The kymogram detection algorithm and complete reconstruction pipelines are available for clinical use, e.g., on the PC-based VAMP syngo Explorer workstation *(17)*.

improve the image quality in lung imaging. In general, no ECG is acquired for standard thorax scans, and the use of kymogram-based reconstruction approaches applied to lung images is the method of choice *(15,16)*. Figures 9 and 10 demonstrate results obtained from two patients scanned with a 16 × 0.75-mm collimation, a rotation time of 0.5 s, and a table increment of 6 mm per rotation (pitch 0.5). The scan mode allows us to cover a scan range of 40 cm during a single breath- hold. The potential for motion artifact reduction in the lung region can be seen in the axial displays and in the multiplanar reformations (inserts in Fig. 9). Blurring and double contours are greatly reduced by the kymogram-based approach.

CONCLUSIONS

Synchronization alternatives can be used for those imaging cases where applying the ECG leads is inconvenient, and they may further serve as a fallback solution in cases of corrupted ECG signals.

One particular alternative to ECG correlation is the kymogram algorithm (Fig. 11). It is based on a COM tracking of the cardiac motion. Kymogram-gated reconstruction has proven to be adequate to image the heart and adjacent lung areas with high quality. The results are comparable to those of ECG-based synchronization. Kymogram correlation also seems to be especially useful to improve thoracic imaging in general. Potentially, it may replace ECG-based approaches in general and thereby eliminate the need for ECG hardware and efforts by personnel to record high-quality ECG signals.

REFERENCES

1. Kachelriess M, Kalender WA. ECG-based phase-oriented reconstruction from subsecond spiral CT scans of the heart. Radiology 1997;205(P):215.
2. Kachelriess M, Kalender WA, Karakaya S, et al. Imaging of the heart by ECG-oriented reconstruction from subsecond spiral CT scans. In: Glazer G, Krestin G (eds), Advances in CT IV. Springer Verlag, New York: 1998;137–143.

3. Kachelriess M, Kalender WA. Electrocardiogram-correlated image reconstruction from subsecond spiral CT scans of the heart. Med Phys 1998;25(12):2417–2431.
4. Kachelriess M, Ulzheimer S, Kalender WA. ECG-correlated imaging of the heart with subsecond multi-slice spiral CT. IEEE Transactions on Medical Imaging 2000;19(9):888–901.
5. Taguchi K, Anno H. High temporal resolution for multislice helical computed tomography. Med Phys 2000;27(5):861–872.
6. Flohr T, Ohnesorge B, Kopp AF, Becker C, Halliburton SS, Knez A. A reconstruction concept for ECG-gated multi-slice spiral CT of the heart with pulse-rate adaptive optimization of spatial and temporal resolution. Radiology 2000;217(P):438.
7. Kachelriess M, Fuchs T, Lapp R, Sennst D-A, Schaller S, Kalender WA. Image to volume weighting generalized ASSR for arbitrary pitch 3D and phase-correlated 4D spiral cone-beam CT reconstruction. Proceedings of the 2001 Int. Meeting on Fully 3D Image Reconstruction 2001;179–182.
8. Kachelriess M, Sennst D-A, Kalender WA. 4D phase-correlated spiral cardiac reconstruction using image to volume weighting generalized ASSR for a 16-slice cone-beam CT. Radiology 2001; 221(P):457.
9. Kachelriess M, Kalender WA. Extended parallel backprojection for cardiac cone-beam CT for up to 128 slices. Radiology 2002;225(P):310.
10. Sourbelle K, Kachelriess M, Kalender WA. Feldkamp-type reconstruction algorithm for spiral cone-beam (CB) computed tomography (CT). Radiology 2002;225(P):451.
11. Kachelriess M, Knaup M, Kalender WA. Extended parallel backprojection for standard 3D and phase-correlated 4D axial and spiral cone-beam CT with arbitrary pitch and 100% dose usage. Med Phys 2004;31(6), in press .
12. Kalender WA, Kachelriess M. Computertomograph mit objektbezogener Bewegungsartefaktreduktion und Extraktion der Objektbewegungsinformation (Kymogramm). European Patent Office (Patent pending). 1999.
13. Kachelriess M, Kalender WA. Kymogram-correlated image reconstruction from subsecond multi-slice spiral CT scans of the heart. Radiology 2000;217(P):439.
14. Kachelriess M, Sennst D-A, Maxlmoser W, Kalender WA. Kymogram detection and kymogram-correlated image reconstruction from sub-second spiral computed tomography scans of the heart. Med Phys 2002;29(7):1489–1503.
15. Kachelriess M, Sennst D-A, Kalender WA. Reconstruction of motion-free pericardial lung images from standard spiral CT scans using kymogram correlation. Radiology 2002;225(P):403.
16. Lell M, Dassel M, Kalender WA, Bautz WA, Kachelriess M. Improvement of image quality in thoracic CT comparing standard reconstruction with kymogram-based reconstruction. Radiology 2002;225(P):567.
17. Sennst D-A, Kachelriess M, Leidecker C, Schmidt B, Watzke O, Kalender WA. Syngo explorer: an extensible software-based platform for reconstruction and evaluation fo CT images. RadioGraphics 2004;24:601–612.

6 Radiation Dose From CT of the Heart

CYNTHIA H. MCCOLLOUGH, PhD

INTRODUCTION

The issue of radiation dose from X-ray computed tomography (CT) has received much attention recently in both the popular media and scientific literature *(1–5)*. This is in part due to the fact that the dose levels from CT typically exceed those from conventional radiography and fluoroscopy, and that the use of CT continues to grow. Thus, CT contributes a significant portion of the total collective dose from ionizing radiation delivered to the public from medical procedures. It is important, therefore, that physicians ordering or performing these examinations have an understanding of the dose delivered from a cardiac CT, as well as how that amount of radiation compares to those from other imaging procedures that use ionizing radiation.

HOW TO DESCRIBE THE DOSE FROM A CT EXAMINATION: CTDI AND DLP

CT dose descriptors, the basic tools required for understanding radiation dose in CT, have been in existence for many years, yet continue to be refined as multidetector-row CT (MDCT) evolves. The primary measured value is known as the CT Dose Index (CTDI) and represents the integrated dose, along the z axis, from one *axial* CT scan (one rotation of the X-ray tube) *(6–8)* (Fig. 1). Typically, a 100-mm long ionization chamber is used for routine measurements. Thus, the subscript 100 is used to denote the measurement length. All other CT dose descriptors are derived from this primary measured value. It is important to note that the CTDI is always measured in the axial scan mode, and that doses for helical scan modes are calculated from the axial information. The equipment used to measure CTDI is shown in Fig. 2.

The CTDI varies across the field of view. For example, for body CT imaging, the CTDI is typically a factor or two higher at the surface than at the center of the field of view. The average CTDI across the field of view is given by the weighted CTDI (CTDIw), where CTDIw = 2/3 CTDI(edge) + 1/3 CTDI(center) *(9–10)*. Figure 3 gives the typical relative distribution of dose in the head and body phantoms. CTDIw is a useful indicator of scanner radiation output for a specific kVp and mAs. CTDIw is reported in terms of absorbed dose to air *(9–10)*.

To represent dose for a specific scan protocol, which almost always involves a series of scans, it is essential to take into account any gaps or overlaps between the radiation dose profiles from consecutive rotations of the X-ray source. This is accomplished with use of a dose descriptor know as the Volume CTDIw ($CTDI_{vol}$), where

$$CTDI_{vol} = [(N \times T)/\,I\,] \times CTDIw$$

and

N = the number of simultaneous axial scans per X-ray source rotation
T = the thickness of one axial scan (mm)
I = the table increment per axial scan (mm) *(10)*.

In helical CT, the ratio of the table travel per rotation (I) to the total nominal beam width ($N \times T$) is referred to as pitch *(10–11)*. Hence

$$CTDI_{vol} = (1/\text{pitch}) \times CTDIw.$$

So, whereas $CTDI_w$ represents the average radiation dose over the x and y directions, $CTDI_{vol}$ represents the average radiation dose over the x, y, and z directions. This provides a single CT dose parameter, based on a directly and easily measured quantity, which represents the average dose within the scan volume for a standardized (CTDI) phantom *(10)*. $CTDI_{vol}$ is a useful indicator of the dose for a specific exam protocol, because it takes into account protocol-specific information such as pitch. Its value may be displayed prospectively on the console of newer CT scanners, although it may be mislabeled on some systems as CTDIw. Recent consensus agreement on these definitions is reflected in newer scanner software releases *(10)*.

Thus, $CTDI_{vol}$ *estimates* the average radiation dose within the irradiated volume of a CT acquisition. The SI units are milliGray (mGy). It does not indicate, however, the total energy deposited into the scan volume. Its value remains unchanged whether there are 20 or 40 scans acquired.

To better represent the overall energy (or dose) delivered by a given scan protocol, the dose can be integrated along the scan length to compute the dose-length product (DLP), where

$$\text{DLP (mGy-cm)} = CTDI_{vol}\text{ (mGy)} \times \text{scan length (cm)}\ (9).$$

The DLP reflects the total energy absorbed (and thus the potential biological effect) attributable to the complete scan acquisition. Thus, a limited abdomen CT might have the same

From: *Contemporary Cardiology: CT of the Heart: Principles and Applications*
Edited by: U. Joseph Schoepf © Humana Press, Inc., Totowa, NJ

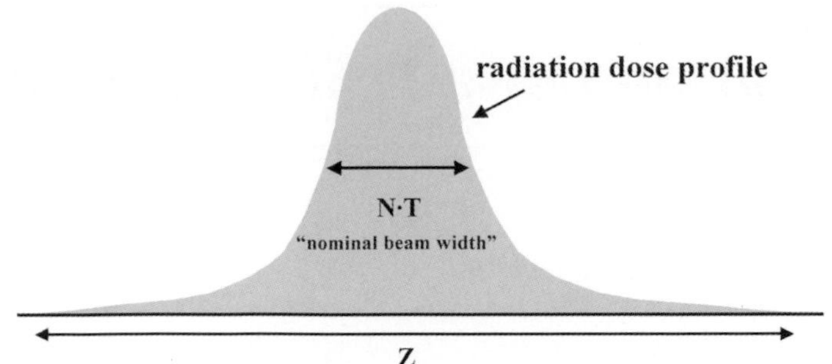

Fig. 1. Computed Tomography Dose Index (CTDI) is the integral under the radiation dose profile from a single axial scan.

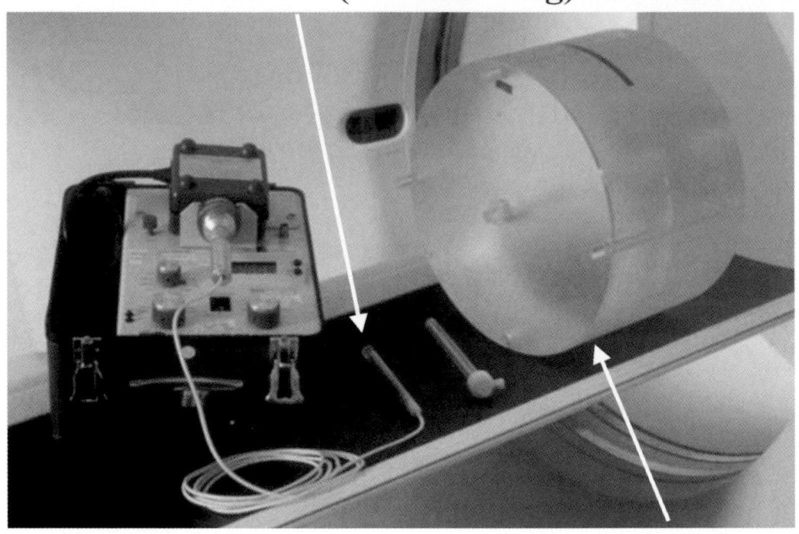

Fig. 2. Typical equipment used for measuring CT dose index.

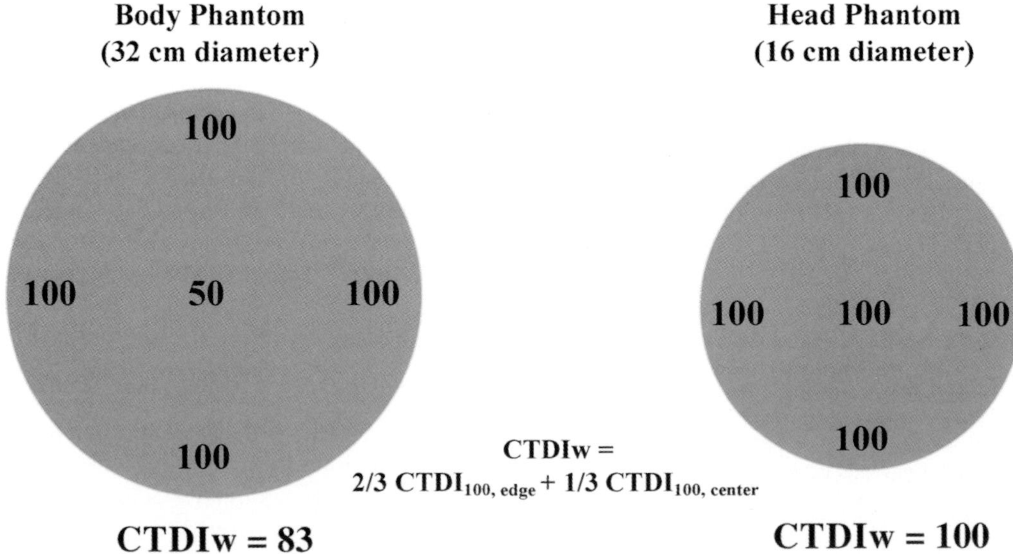

Fig. 3. Typical dose distributions (%) across the image field-of-view.

Table 1
Sample Volume CT Dose Index ($CTDI_{vol}$) and Dose Length Product (DLP) Values for Common CT Exams

	Chest	*Abdomen*	*Abdomen and pelvis*
Peak kilovotage (kVp)	120	120	120
Tube current (mA)	200	300	300
Exposure time (s)	0.5	0.5	0.5
Detector configuration ($N \times T$)	4 × 5 mm	4 × 5 mm	4 × 5 mm
Table index per rotation (I)	15 mm	15 mm	15 mm
Pitch ($I/N \times$ T)	0.75	0.75	0.75
Reconstructed scan width (mm)	5	5	5
Scan length (cm)	40	20	40
CTDIvol (mGy)	12.0	19.1	19.1
DLP (mGy × cm)	480	382	764

Table 2
Scan Acquisition Parameters, Volume CT Dose Index ($CTDI_{vol}$), and Dose Length Product (DLP) for Coronary Calcification Imaging (12-cm scan length)

	EBCT	*MDCT1*	*MDCT1*	*MDCT2*	*MDCT2*
Data acquisition method	Prospective triggering	Prospective triggering	Retrospective gating	Prospective triggering	Retrospective gating
Peak kilovotage (kVp)	130	120	120	120	120
Tube current (mA)[a]	630	140	100	150	150
Exposure time (s)	0.1	0.36	0.5	0.33	0.5
Detector configuration ($N \times T$)	1 × 3 mm	4 × 2.5 mm	4 × 2.5 mm	4 × 2.5 mm	4 × 2.5 mm
Table index per rotation (I)	3 mm	10 mm	3.75 mm	10 mm	3.75 mm
Pitch ($I/N \times$ T)	1	1	0.375	1	0.375
Reconstructed scan width (mm)	3	2.5	3	2.5	2.5
CTDIvol (mGy)	3.5	4.6	12.5	4.7	20.3
DLP (mGy × cm)	42	55	150	56	243
Effective dose[b] (mSv)	0.7	0.9	2.6	1.0	4.1

[a] mA can be increased in multidetector-row CT (MDCT) scanners for larger patients to avoid an increase in image noise. The mA values for MDCT 1 and MDCT 2 were provided by the respective manufacturers, and do not necessarily produce an identical level of image noise.

[b] Effective Dose estimate, with $k = 0.017$ mSv × (mGy × cm)$^{-1}$. This value is averaged between male and female models (*see* text and ref. 5).

EBCT, electron beam CT.

$CTDI_{vol}$ as an abdomen and pelvis CT, but the latter exam would have a greater DLP, proportional to the greater z extent of the scan volume.

Table 1 demonstrates the differences in $CTDI_{vol}$ and DLP for typical body CT exams. The values are for demonstration only; they can vary by scanner model, vendor, and image quality requirements. Note that a change in technique (mAs/rotation) affects the $CTDI_{vol}$, while a change in acquisition length (at the same technique) is reflected by the DLP.

In cardiac CT, the anatomic scan length is relatively constant (typically 12 cm); thus, the variability in $CTDI_{vol}$ and DLP is primarily a result of differences in scanner output and scan acquisition parameters. Tables 2 and 3 provide the scan acquisition parameters, $CTDI_{vol}$, and DLP for coronary calcification imaging and coronary angiography. Data are provided for an electron beam CT (EBCT) system as well as for MDCT systems from two different manufacturers.

AUTOMATIC EXPOSURE CONTROL

It is technologically feasible for CT systems to adjust the X-ray tube current (mA) in response to variations in X-ray intensity at the detector *(12–13)*, much as fluoroscopic X-ray systems adjust exposure automatically. This capability, in various implementations, is now available commercially on MDCT systems in response to wide interest from the radiology community. Some systems adapt the tube current based on changes in attenuation along the z axis, others adapt to changes in attenuation as the X-ray tube travels around the patient. The ideal is to combine both approaches with an algorithm that "chooses" the correct tube current to achieve a predetermined level of image noise.

With regard to cardiac CT, the radiation dose for a retrospectively gated exam, where the X-ray tube is kept continuously on throughout the acquisition, can be dramatically reduced if the tube current is reduced during portions of the cardiac cycle

Table 3
Scan Acquisition Parameters, Volume CT Dose Index ($CTDI_{vol}$) and Dose Length Product (DLP) for Coronary Angiography (12-cm Scan Length)

	EBCT	*MDCT1*	*MDCT2*
Data acquisition method	Prospective triggering	Retrospective gating	Retrospective gating
Peak kilovotage (kVp)	130	120	120
Tube current (mA)[a]	630	300	300
Exposure time (s)	0.1	0.5	0.5
Detector configuration ($N \times T$)	1 × 3 mm	4 × 1 mm	4 × 1.25 mm
Table index per rotation (I)	2 mm	1.5 mm	1.9 mm
Pitch ($I/N \times T$)	0.66	0.375	0.375
Reconstructed scan width (mm)	3	1.25	1.25
CTDIvol (mGy)	5.3	46	55
DLP (mGy × cm)	64	547	662
Effective dose[b] (mSv)	1.1	9.3	11.3

[a] mA can be increased in multidetector-row CT (MDCT) scanners for larger patients to avoid an increase in image noise. The mA values for MDCT 1 and MDCT 2 were provided by the respective manufacturers, and do not necessarily produce an identical level of image noise.

[b] Effective Dose estimate, with $k = 0.017$ mSv × (mGy × cm)$^{-1}$. This value is averaged between male and female models (*see* text and ref. *5*).

EBCT, electron beam CT.

that are not likely to be of interest for the reconstructed data. Thus, in addition to modulation of the tube current based on patient attenuation, the tube current can be modulated by the ECG signal. Since cardiac motion is least during diastole and greatest during systole, the projection data are least likely to be corrupted by motion artifact for diastolic-phase reconstructions. Accordingly, the tube current is reduced during systole. Dose reductions of approx 50% have been reported using such a strategy *(14)*. The implementation of these and other dose-reduction strategies is expected industry-wide over the next several years, in response to the strong concern about the radiation dose from CT.

EFFECTIVE DOSE

It is important to recognize that the potential biological effects from ionizing radiation depend not only on the radiation dose, but also on the biological sensitivity of the tissue or organ system irradiated. A 100-mGy dose to an extremity would not have the same potential biological effect (detriment) as a 100-mGy dose to the pelvis *(15)*. Effective dose (E) is a dose descriptor that reflects this difference in biologic sensitivity *(16–17)*. It is a single dose parameter that reflects the risk of a nonuniform exposure in terms of an equivalent whole-body exposure. The units of E are milliSieverts (mSv).

Although the concept of effective dose has some limitations when applied to medical populations, it does facilitate the comparison of biological effect between diagnostic exams of different types *(16,17)*. Published values of E per DLP *(9)* allow convenient *estimates* of E based on the DLP value provided at the CT scanner console. The use of E facilitates communication with patients regarding the potential harm of a medical exam that uses ionizing radiation. For example, when a patient inquires, "What dose will I receive from this exam," an answer in the units of mGy or mGy × cm will not likely answer the more fundamental, but perhaps unspoken, question, "What is the likelihood that I will be harmed from this exam." Characterizing the radiation dose in terms of E and comparing that value to some meaningful level—for instance, one year's E from naturally occurring background radiation—better conveys to the patient the relative potential for harm from the medical exam. Table 4 provides typical values of E for several common imaging exams, as well as the annual level of background radiation in the US (approx 3.6 mSv).

It is important to remember, however, that E describes the relative whole-body dose for a particular exam and scanner, but is *not* the dose for any one individual, as E calculations use many assumptions including a mathematical model of a "standard" human body that does not accurately reflect any one individual. Effective dose is best used to optimize exams and compare risks between proposed exams. It is a broad measure of risk, and as such should not be quoted with more than one or two significant digits.

Specific values of E can be calculated using several different software packages *(17)*, which are based on the use of data from one of two sources: the National Radiological Protection Board (NRPB) in the UK *(18)* or the Institute of Radiation Protection (GSF) in Germany *(19)*. To minimize controversy over differences in E values that are purely the result of calculation methodology and data sources, a generic estimation method was proposed by the European Working Group for Guidelines on Quality Criteria in CT *(9)*, where E is estimated from the non-controversial value of DLP: E = k × DLP, where the values of k are dependent only on the region of the body being scanned (head, neck, thorax, abdomen, or pelvis) (Table 5). The values of E predicted by DLP and the values of E estimated using more rigorous calculation methods are remarkably consistent, with a maximum deviation from the mean of approx 10–15%. Hence, the use of DLP to estimate E appears to be a reasonably robust

Table 4
Effective Dose Values for Common Imaging Examinations

Examination	*Effective dose (mSv)*
Head CT	1–2
Chest CT	5–7
Abdomen and pelvis CT	8–11
Selective coronary angiogram	3–5
Posterior-anterior and lateral chest X-ray	0.04–0.06
Average annual background radiation in the US	3.6

Table 5
Values of the Conversion Coefficient k for Use in Estimating Effective Dose (E) (mSv) From Dose Length Product (DLP) (in mGy × cm) According to the Formula E = k × DLP *(9)*

Anatomic region	*k* ($mSv \times mGy^{-1} \times cm^{-1}$)
Head	0.0023
Neck	0.0054
Chest	0.017
Abdomen	0.015
Pelvis	0.019

method for estimating E. The effective doses for several cardiac CT examinations, based upon values of DLP, are given in Tables 2 and 3.

SUMMARY

The fundamental dose parameter in CT, the CTDI, is measured at edge and center locations in an acrylic phantom for a given kVp, mAs, and scan width, and reported for a given exam protocol as the volume CTDI ($CTDI_{vol}$) in units of mGy. This value represents the average dose *in a standard acrylic phantom* for a given exam protocol. Another relevant dose parameter is that of effective dose, which is given in units of mSv. The effective dose is a single dose parameter that best represents the radiation detriment corresponding to a given exam protocol. Neither of these parameters is an estimate of radiation dose to any one individual, but rather should be used to optimize and compare exam protocols. E can be estimated with good accuracy from the DLP, which is equal to the $CTDI_{vol}$ multiplied by the total scan length (in cm).

Techniques to modulate the tube current as a function of patient attenuation or the time within the cardiac cycle are important innovations that will reduce the dose from cardiac CT by at about a factor of two. Hence, coronary artery calcium examinations, which currently have E values between 1 and 4 mSv, may be able to be conducted using retrospective gating techniques and an E of less than 2 mSv. CT coronary angiography, which currently requires an E of approx 10 mSv with retrospectively gated MDCT may be performed with approx 5 mSv if ECG tube current modulation is applied. These effective dose values are of similar magnitude to those from a chest CT examination (5–7 mSv) or a conventional (diagnostic) coronary angiogram (3–5 mSv).

Finally, as cardiac CT image quality, diagnostic accuracy, and availability all continue to improve, there will be more and more publications regarding the clinical efficacy of cardiac CT as compared to alternate imaging modalities. Discussions of patient safety and societal cost will include discussions of the radiation dose from the various procedures. To ensure that these discussions are accurate, it is essential that the dose information associated with specific techniques be reported in an accurate and complete fashion using standardized terminology.

REFERENCES

1. Brenner DJ, Elliston CD, Hall EJ, Berdon WE. Estimated risks of radiation-induced fatal cancer from pediatric CT. AJR 2001;176: 289–296.
2. Donnelly LF, Emery KH, Brody AS, et al. Minimizing radiation dose for pediatric body applications of single-detector helical CT: strategies at a large children's hospital. AJR 2001;176:303–306.
3. Haaga JR. Radiation dose management. AJR 2001;177:289–291.
4. Nickoloff EL, Alderson PO. Radiation exposure to patients from CT: reality, public perception, and policy. AJR 2001;177:285–287.
5. Pierce DA, Preston DL. Radiation-related cancer risks at low dose among atomic bomb survivors. Radiation Research 2000;154:178–186.
6. Shope TB, Gagne RM, Johnson GC. A method for describing the doses delivered by transmission x-ray computed tomography. Med Phys 1981;8:488–495.
7. American Association of Physicists in Medicine. Standardized methods for measuring diagnostic x-ray exposures. Report no. 31. AAPM, New York, 1990.
8. Nagel HD. Radiation exposure in computed tomography. Frankfurt: COCIR, 2000.
9. European guidelines for quality criteria for computed tomography. Luxembourg: European Commission, 2000.
10. International Electrotechnical Commission. Medical Electrical Equipment. Part 2–44: Particular Requirements for the Safety of X-ray Equipment for Computed Tomography. IEC publication No. 60601-2-44 Amendment 1.
11. McCollough CH, Zink FE. Performance evaluation of a multi-slice CT system. Medical Physics 1999;26:2223–2230.
12. Gies M, Kalender WA, Wolf H, Suess C, Madsen M. Dose reduction in CT by anatomically adapted tube current modulation I: simulation studies. Medical Physics 1999;26:2235–2247.
13. Kalender WA, Wolf H, Suess C. Dose reduction in CT by anatomically adapted tube current modulation II: phantom measurements. Medical Physics 1999;26:2248–2253.
14. Jakobs TF, Becker CR, Ohnesorge B, et al. Eur Rad 2002;12: 1081–1086.
15. Committee on the Biological Effects of Ionizing Radiation. Health effects of exposure to low levels of ionizing radiation, BEIR V. Washington, DC: National Academy, 1990.
16. International Commission on Radiological Protection (ICRP). 1990 Recommendations of the ICRP. Publication 60. ICRP, New York, NY, 1991.

17. McCollough CH, Schueler BA. Calculation of effective dose. Medical Physics 2000;27:828–837.
18. Jones DG, Shrimpton PC. Survey of CT practice in the UK. Part 3: Normalised organ doses calculated using Monte Carlo techniques, NRPB-250. Oxon, United Kingdom: National Radiological Protection Board, 1991.
19. Zankl M, Panzer W, Drexler G. The calculation of dose from external photon exposures using reference human phantoms and Monte Carlo methods. Part IV: Organ dose from computed tomographic examinations, GSF-Bericht 30/91. Neuherberg, Germany: GSF – Forschungszentrum fur Umwelt und Gesundtheit, Institut fur Strahlenschutz, 1991.

DETECTION AND QUANTIFICATION OF CORONARY CALCIUM

III

7 Coronary Calcium Screening

An Epidemiologic Perspective

Christopher J. O'Donnell, MD, MPH and Udo Hoffmann, MD

INTRODUCTION

Because coronary artery disease (CAD) is the most frequent cause of death in industrialized nations *(1)* and the available tools for prediction of CAD onset are imperfect, there is a need for new methods to screen apparently healthy individuals to identify those at increased risk. Current risk prediction of CAD is based on the patient's age and sex as well as on the presence and extent of established, modifiable coronary risk factors such as hypertension, hyperlipidemia, diabetes mellitus, and cigarette smoking. Risk prediction algorithms such as the Framingham Heart Study coronary risk score have been shown feasible and valid for CAD risk prediction in the United States population *(2)*. As a consequence, those traditional risk factors and/or risk-factor algorithms have been incorporated into treatment guidelines for hyperlipidemia *(3)* and hypertension.*(4)*. However, coronary risk scores can explain only 70% of the overall risk for CAD and are more sensitive than specific. Consequently, there is need to develop new strategies to identify patients at high risk, specifically among patients who appear to be at intermediate (i.e., 6–20% 10-yr risk) or low risk according to traditional risk factors *(5,6)*.

Recently developed fast computed tomography (CT) techniques such as multidetector-row CT (MDCT) and electron beam CT (EBCT) now offer the opportunity to noninvasively detect and quantify coronary artery plaque burden (Figs. 1–4). The conduct of both techniques and their similarities and differences are described in detail elsewhere in this book. These CT scanners are capable of nearly freezing the motion of the heart as a result of very fast image acquisition and synchronization to ECG signals. Both have been shown to be highly sensitive for the detection of calcified coronary atherosclerotic plaques. A typical report from either MDCT or EBCT contains the Agatston score, a semiquantitative measure that is based on the area and a weighted density factor for coronary calcium.

In the past decade, a large number of studies have been conducted to examine the predictive value of CT coronary artery calcium (CAC) as a predictor for coronary risk. In addition, this technique has been shown to be capable of following the natural history of coronary atherosclerosis and tracking the dynamics of coronary calcification under drug treatment. In this chapter, we review the strengths and limitations of available original research and discuss consensus statements of the American College of Cardiology/American Heart Association (ACC/AHA) regarding the use of CAC as an adjunct to established risk factors. We also provide insight into ongoing research and propose studies that could help to facilitate evidence-based practice guidelines.

CORONARY CALCIFICATION AND CORONARY ARTERY DISEASE

Experts agree that CT testing can determine whether calcifications are present in the walls of the coronary arteries. If calcification of any amount is present, it follows that atherosclerosis is present in the coronary artery. Hence, patients with no symptoms but with detectable calcification can be said to have coronary artery disease not detectable by the usual clinical tests ("subclinical atherosclerosis"). However, there is controversy regarding the relation of the calcification score to the prevalence of CAD and the incidence of cardiac events such as unstable angina, myocardial infarction, and sudden cardiac death.

Early studies by Rumberger *(6a)* showed that there is a linear relationship between the amount of calcium and the overall amount of atherosclerotic plaque. Logically, a number of studies have shown that high Agatston scores are associated with the presence and number of obstructive coronary artery lesions. While the technique appears to be quite sensitive, there is no one-to-one correlation, and the location of calcification and stenosis may be different. Two meta-analyses evaluated the diagnostic accuracy of CAC (EBCT) for the detection of significant coronary artery stenosis as compared to coronary angiography. In both studies, the overall sensitivity and specificity of CAC were 80–90% and 40–50%, with a maximum joint value of 75%, respectively *(7,8)*. Moreover, the summary odds ratios were increased 20-fold (95% confidence interval [CI], 5 to 88) indicating that the odds of having a significant coronary artery stenosis are 20 times higher if calcium was detected. However, the generalizability of these studies is limited—most of the patients were middle-aged men. Apart from a small number of studies where most patients were referred to angiography as a result of chest pain, the indication for coronary angiography was not specified. However, most likely almost all patients were symptomatic for CAD or had known

From: *Contemporary Cardiology: CT of the Heart: Principles and Applications*
Edited by: U. Joseph Schoepf © Humana Press, Inc., Totowa, NJ

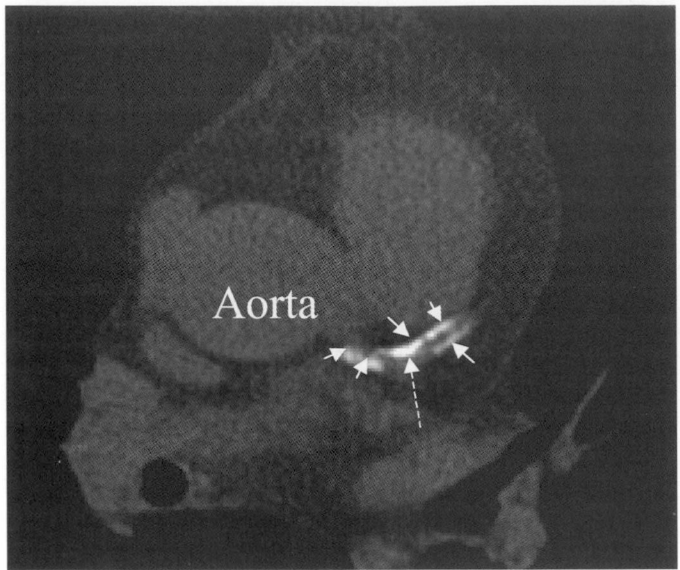

Fig. 1. A cross-sectional image through the aorta and the origin of the left coronary artery (dashed arrow). A moderate amount of calcification can be easily identified as bright signals (solid arrows).

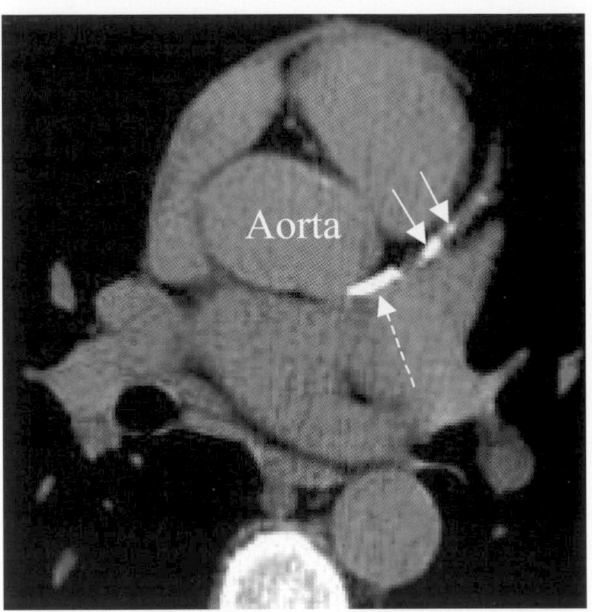

Fig. 2. A cross-sectional image through the aorta; a moderate amount of calcification can be easily identified as bright signals (arrows).

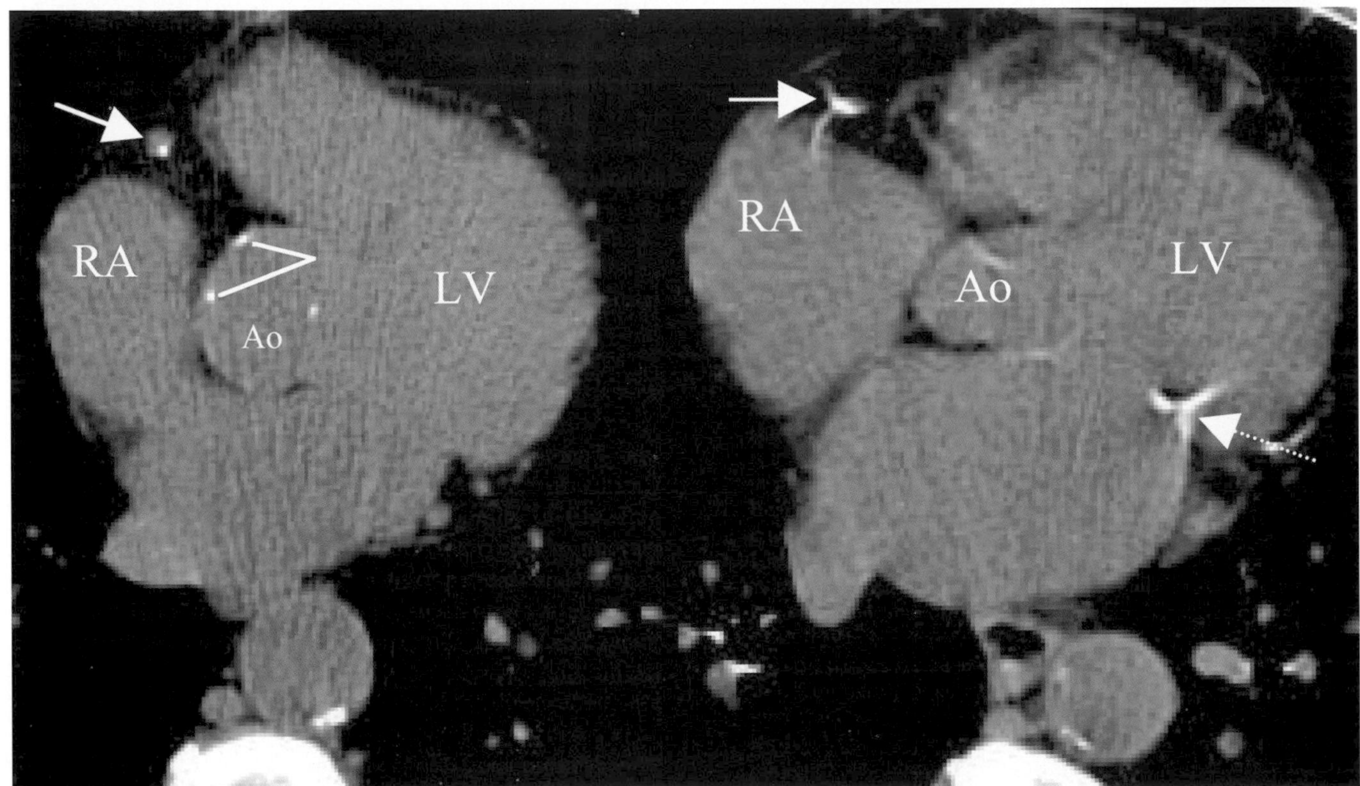

Fig. 3. A cross-sectional image through the aorta (Ao), the left ventricle (LV) and the right atrium (RA). Left image: high image quality, no image artifacts, aortic valve calcification. Right image: image artifacts in the right coronary artery (solid arrow) and mitral valve calcification (dashed arrow).

CAD. Consequently, the prevalence of disease (CAD) was very high in the study populations (with one exception >50%, in about a third of the studies 70–95%), and the clinically important question "What is the probability of having/not having significant CAD given a positive/negative test?" (positive predictive value/negative predictive value) is difficult to answer. In addition, most studies were designed only as observational studies, and blinding was not mentioned as a quality criterion in all but two of the analyzed studies. In summary, the available information is still limited, and the results cannot be general-

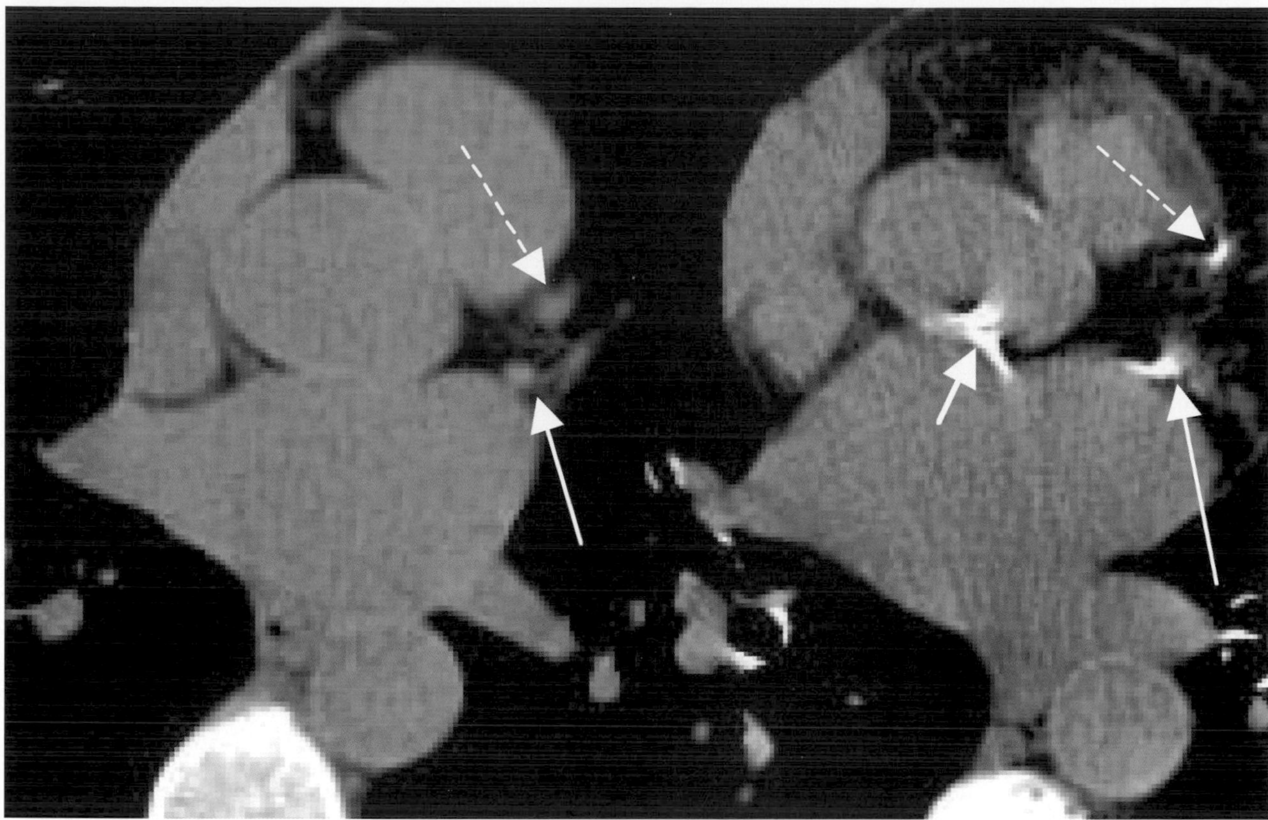

Fig. 4. A cross-sectional image through the aorta and the left atrium. Left image: high image quality, no image artifacts, arrow pointing at the circumflex and the left coronary artery. Right image: image artifacts in the circumflex, the left coronary artery, and the aortic valve (arrows).

ized. As a consequence, the use of CAC for the accurate prediction of prevalent significant CAD has not been implemented into clinical guidelines.

PREDICTIVE VALUE OF CORONARY CALCIFICATION FOR CARDIOVASCULAR EVENTS

Clinicians are currently interested in the role of CAC in prediction of cardiovascular events. Since a large proportion of all cardiovascular events occur in asymptomatic patients, it is justified to differentiate asymptomatic persons from symptomatic patients with known CAD.

CORONARY CALCIFICATION IN ASYMPTOMATIC PERSONS

A small number of prospective studies have evaluated the prediction of cardiac events by coronary calcification. In a recent meta-analysis of prospective studies, there was an increased risk for a combined outcome (nonfatal myocardial infarction [MI], congenital heart disease [CHD], death, or revascularization) associated with a calcium score elevated above a median value (risk ratio 8.7 [95% CI, 2.7–28.1]). The relative risk of hard endpoints (MI or death) was also increased (risk ratio 4.2 [95% CI 1.6–11.3]) *(9)*. Three more recent prospective studies have added data from more than 20,000 patients to the meta-analysis. In 5635 asymptomatic, low-to-medium-risk men and women self-referred for EBCT, there were 224 events, of which only 61 were "hard" endpoints (MI or death) after 37 ± 12 mo of follow-up. After adjustment for risk factors ascertained by questionnaire, there were statistically increased risks associated with the presence of CAC for hard events in men (95% CI, 3.9 [1.2–13]) and no significantly increased risks in women (95% CI, 1.5 [0.2 10]) *(10)*. In a second prospective study of all-cause mortality in 10,377 self-referred men and women, there were 249 deaths in approx 60 mo of follow-up. Increasing CAC scores were associated with significantly increased relative risks for death, and receiver operating characteristics (ROC) curves were significantly greater for CAC score added to risk factors compared with risk factors alone ($p < 0.001$) *(11)*. In a third prospective study of 5585 men and women recruits in whom an EBCT test was obtained to decide upon eligibility for inclusion in a randomized controlled lipid lowering trial, there were 122 events, of which 43 were hard events after over 50 mo of follow-up. Overall, there were statistically increased risks for hard events (9.9 [5.2–18.9]) as well as all endpoints associated with a high CAC score. In an analysis of the incremental predictive ability of CAC over Framingham risk score in a subset of 1817 subjects in whom risk factors was measured, there was a several-fold increase in risk for cardiovascular endpoints in the highest compared with the lowest tertile of CAC score *(12)*.

LIMITATIONS OF THE AVAILABLE DATA

While there is consistency across the available studies for an association of CAC scores with the presence of significant CAD and the risk of cardiovascular events, a number of methodological concerns make it difficult to interpret study results and apply them to clinical practice. Importantly, there are concerns regarding study generalizability/external validity, validity of the risk factor measures, and resultant multivariable models used in the studies. In addition, the conclusions are drawn from relatively small numbers of hard cardiovascular outcomes (all together numbering only several hundred).

A major limiting factor of most studies has been the inclusion of self-referred patients. None of the available evidence for CAC screening has been drawn from community-based cohorts representative of typical populations which might be considered for screening. Subjects studied to date have a high prevalence of subclinical CAD and CAD risk factors, often making them different from persons in the community of a similar age and sex. The baseline characteristics of many of these cohorts suggest that patient populations already at substantially elevated risk have been studied. Thus, data from these studies may not be representative of apparently healthy low- and medium-risk groups for whom screening may be more relevant. Moreover, the self-referred subjects to date may differ significantly in other unmeasured characteristics that accompany health-seeking behaviors.

In the available studies, data are limited for young persons, women, and non-Caucasians. Much of the data to date have been derived largely from middle-aged Caucasian men. As a consequence of this selection bias, age- and gender-specific CAC thresholds for younger individuals for subjects below 40 yr of age, women, and non-Caucasian populations may be relatively unreliable due to lack of statistical power (small sample sizes, insufficient numbers of events) or wholly unavailable. Potentially important racial differences in prevalence of CAC have been noted in the Multiethnic Study of Atherosclerosis (MESA) *(13)*; in particular, the prevalence of CAC appears to be lower in African Americans and other major ethnic groups in the United States *(14–16)*.

Another significant concern pertains to the method of ascertainment of risk factor data. It has been suggested that a high CAC score predicts coronary risk independently and probably incrementally to traditional coronary risk factors and coronary risk scores. ROC curve analyses are often provided to bolster the case for CAC screening over and above risk factors. However, in virtually every available study, blood pressure determinations, lipid levels, and other risk factors are obtained retrospectively by questionnaire, self-report from the study patient, and/or review of the medical record. There is a substantial risk of misclassification in self-reported risk-factor data. Therefore, calculations of Framingham coronary risk or other multivariable risk models using self-reported risk factors algorithms would tend to underestimate the risk conferred by risk factors (bias towards the null) and lead to a more favorable comparison of CAC scores with risk factors. Standardized research methods that mirror office-based methods for measurement of blood pressure, lipid levels, and diabetes have not been employed in the available studies. By way of contrast, prospective epidemiologic cohort studies such as the Framingham Heart Study and the Multiethnic Study of Atherosclerosis are recording risk factor data prospectively. A final set of concerns pertains to study follow-up and outcomes. First, the level of completion of follow-up is inconsistent across studies, with some studies having less than 90% follow-up. For example, in one of the largest recent studies, only a 64% follow-up was achieved *(10)*. Losses to follow-up can raise questions about the validity of study findings. A second concern is the focus of the available studies on either combined hard (i.e., MI and death) and/or soft (i.e., revascularization using percutaneous coronary interventions or coronary artery bypass surgery) outcomes. Soft intervention outcomes are often used, but may not be appropriate because neither the study patients nor their physicians were blinded to the CAC score. Thus, given the fact that many patients were self-referred and not part of a blinded study, there is a substantial risk that soft outcomes may be contaminated by intervention bias introduced by knowledge of the CAC test results. No study with cardiovascular mortality as a primary outcome has been reported to date, and in virtually all available studies, there have been too few cardiovascular deaths to reliably examine the association of CAC. The recent study of Shaw et al. shares many of the limitations of the other self-referral studies, but it did report a positive association of CAC score with all-cause mortality *(11)*. One strength of the Shaw study was its demonstration of consistent, statistically significant increases in mortality across increasing CAC scores in a large cohort. Nevertheless, mortality data were drawn from the National Death Index, and no further data on cause of death or on non-fatal outcomes were ascertained *(11)*.

Interestingly, there is a small and growing body of evidence in population-based cohorts that calcification of the aorta predicts risk for CAD and other cardiovascular diseases independent of measured risk factors. The prevalence of calcified lesions detected on thoracic and abdominal radiographs like that of coronary calcium, increases steeply with age *(17)*. A number of recent studies have demonstrated that thoracic and abdominal aortic calcifications are independent, prospective predictors of CVD. Calcification of the aortic arch detected by plain antero-posterior radiographs predicts an increased risk of cardiovascular diseases in men and women *(18)*. In the Framingham Heart Study, the presence and extent of abdominal aortic calcification detected by lateral lumbar radiographs is a predictor of CVD, CVD mortality, and CHD in middle-aged men and women (mean age 60 yr), independent of age and actually measured cardiovascular risk factors *(17)*. Abdominal aortic calcification would likely be detected quite reliably and accurately by CT imaging, and further study of the prognostic value of such CT findings in addition to or instead of coronary calcium is clearly warranted.

ADDITIONAL QUESTIONS SURROUNDING CAC SCREENING

A number of additional concerns have arisen surrounding CAC screening and are summarized in Table 1. First, the CT test does lead to significant exposure to radiation. The test exposes the patient to a limited amount of ionizing radiation (0.7 to 3 mSv) that is equivalent to 25–100% of the natural background radiation exposure that an individual in the United

Table 1
Suggested Guidelines and Implications for Coronary Artery Calcium Scoring (Adapted From Partner's HealthCare System 2002 Guidelines)

Guidelines for ordering a CT test for coronary calcium

Coronary calcium screening is not recommended for asymptomatic individuals at low risk.
Coronary calcium screening will be performed only upon a physician's request.
Patients should be informed that most insurers do not reimburse for coronary screening. The out-of-pocket expense for a multidetector-row CT test for coronary calcium is $350–$450.
A positive calcium score *might* be valuable in determining whether a patient who appears to be at intermediate congenital heard disease (CHD) risk is actually at high risk. However, we do not currently recommend coronary calcium scoring for this group.
Ongoing research will better define the clinical subgroups, such as elderly asymptomatic persons or those with a strong family history, in whom the management of other risk factors might be modified according to the calcium score.

Guidelines for Interpreting a CT Test for Coronary Calcium

Some patients and physicians will choose to obtain coronary calcium studies despite the lack of consensus for these studies. We recognize that clinicians who might not have ordered the test themselves are increasingly faced with the test "results" and asked for their advice. Therefore the following comments are provided from the recent ACC/AHA consensus document:
In the absence of coronary calcium (i.e., a "negative" CT test)
Atherosclerotic plaque, including unstable plaque, is very unlikely, although it is possible that significant coronary atherosclerosis may not be detected.
Significant luminal obstructive disease is highly unlikely.
Angiographically normal coronary arteries occur in the majority of such patients.
The absence of calcium may be consistent with a low risk of CHD events over the next 2 to 5 yr.

For a test that is positive for coronary calcium:

The presence of calcium confirms the presence of a coronary atherosclerotic plaque.
The greater the amount of calcium, the greater the likelihood of occlusive coronary artery disease, although there is not a one-to-one relationship, and findings may not be site specific.
The total amount of calcium correlates best with the total amount of atherosclerotic plaque, although the true "plaque burden" is underestimated.
A high calcium score (e.g., Agatston score > 400) *may* be consistent with moderate–high risk of CHD events over the next 2–5 yr.

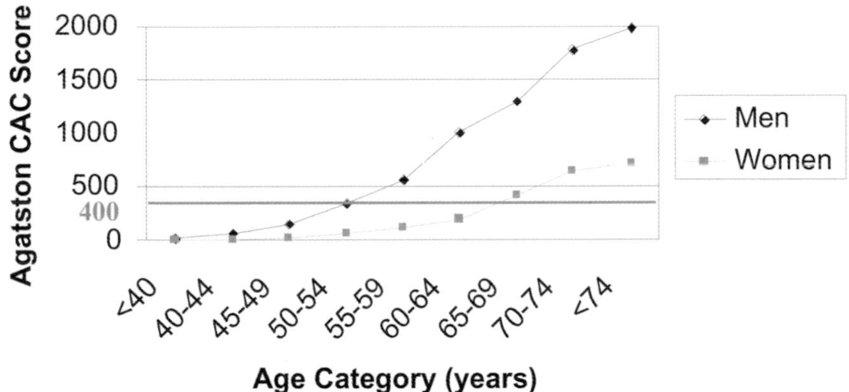

Fig. 5. 90th Percentile Agatston scores derived from large numbers of men and women screened with electron beam CT. Data from ref. *22*.

States receives per year (2.5 to 3 mSv). This is less than the dose received during a diagnostic cardiac catheterization (approx 4.5 mSv) and only a fraction of the occupational exposure limit for a radiation worker in the United States (50 mSv/y). Although the available data suggest that these risks are extremely low from such exposure *(19)*, for some individuals even this low risk may be considered unacceptably high. Second, several recent studies have demonstrated that there is a high prevalence of potentially clinically important findings that are incidentally detected on CT scans *(20,21)*. Such incidental findings may provoke significant anxiety in the patient and may require additional exposure to radiation or even invasive testing in order to confirm or exclude a potentially serious diagnosis such as an aortic aneurysm or malignancy. Third, as mentioned above, unbiased data on age-adjusted coronary calcium thresholds are not yet available, because the available data are derived from cohorts that may or may not be representative of general screening subjects. Moreover, simple thresholds (such as an Agatston score of 400) that do not adjust for age may overestimate risk in older persons and underestimate risk in younger persons (Fig. 5) *(22)*. A fourth and related concern is the fact that many different CT scan machines are now available (including both

EBCT and MDCT machines) and standardized scanning and scoring algorithms have not been implemented across machine types. Moreover, there is a small but significant level of measurement variability consistently seen across all scanner types, and the degree of variability may differ. Fifth, all CAC scoring to date has been conducted using the Agatston score. While the Agatston score has provided an invaluable reference score for research to date, newer mass-based scoring techniques may substantially reduced the misclassification introduced by image noise. A final concern regarding CT scanning is its currently high cost. The cost for the test ranges from \$375–\$450, and the test is not currently covered by most health insurance providers.

CRITICAL EVIDENCE NEEDED FOR CLINICAL GUIDELINES

Both risks and benefits must be considered for any potential screening test. The benefits would include potential for reduction of risk provided by an accurate diagnosis of increased risk and the potential benefits from early detection of incidental findings (e.g., small lung cancers). The risks include the morbidity and mortality risk of an incorrect diagnosis (negative or positive), risks of radiation exposure, morbidity and mortality from detection of benign incidental findings, and high costs of potentially unnecessary testing. The current body of studies suggests that there may be a role for CAC screening, but to date there are no strong unbiased data for or against CAC screening over and above traditional risk-factor assessments in the general population. The limitations of existing studies can be addressed only by prospective, observational studies conducted in unbiased, population-based cohorts of both Caucasian and non-Caucasian men and women. It has been suggested that coronary calcium screening may be most beneficial in persons at intermediate coronary risk *(5,6)*. At least 40% of the population of middle-aged men and women may fall into this category *(5)*. In the proposed studies, risk-factor measurements should be office-based rather than self-reported. Ideally, measures of risk factors as well as coronary calcification would be conducted in as blinded a manner as possible. Several such population-based studies are currently underway. These studies include the Framingham Heart Study and the Multiethnic Study of Atherosclerosis. Final recommendations regarding use of CT calcium awaits the completion of these studies.

CONCLUSION

Coronary atherosclerosis underlies CHD and is influenced by the interaction of multiple risk factors over time in a susceptible host. Traditional risk-prediction models, such as the Framingham risk score, are reasonable predictors of CHD risk. Interest in CAC screening is aimed at improving the prediction of risk for future clinical events. Future studies will need to ascertain the incremental benefit of CAC measures over traditional risk factors and the cost effectiveness of incorporating such measures into global risk-assessment algorithms.

In the future, CAC tests may play an important role in assessment of patients at intermediate risk for CHD events. Higher-risk individuals may be candidates for more aggressive pharmacological risk-factor modification using combinations of lipid-lowering agents, anti-platelet therapies, and angiotensin-converting enzyme inhibitors. While the optimal indications for the use of noninvasive tests for clinical monitoring of the response to therapy remain to be determined, existing expert consensus statements such as that provided by the ACC/AHA in 2000 provide cogent standards for the present time. CAC testing has not yet been reliably shown to add incremental information for risk stratification in generalizable patient cohorts, and ongoing studies should address the important outstanding questions regarding the appropriate types of men and women in whom to consider coronary calcium screening.

REFERENCES

1. American Heart Association. 2000 Heart and Stroke Statistical Update. 2000. Dallas, Texas, American Heart Association.
2. Wilson PW, D'Agostino RB, Levy D, et al. Prediction of coronary heart disease using risk factor categories. Circulation 1998;97: 1837–1847.
3. Third Report of the National Cholesterol Education Program (NCEP) Expert Panel on Detection, Evaluation, and Treatment of High Blood Cholesterol in Adults (Adult Treatment Panel III) final report. Circulation 2002;106:3143–3421.
4. Chobanian AV, Bakris GL, Black HR, et al. The Seventh Report of the Joint National Committee on Prevention, Detection, Evaluation, and Treatment of High Blood Pressure: the JNC 7 report. JAMA 2003;289:2560–2572.
5. Greenland P, Smith JS, Jr., Grundy SM. Improving coronary heart disease risk assessment in asymptomatic people: role of traditional risk factors and noninvasive cardiovascular tests. Circulation 2001;104:1863–1867.
6. Wilson PW, Smith SC, Blumenthal RS, et al. Task force #4—how do we select patients for atherosclerosis imaging? J Am Coll Cardiol 2003;41:1898–1906.

6a. Rumberger JA, Simons DB, Fitzpatrick LA, Sheedy PF, Schwartz RS. Coronary artery calcium area by electron-beam computed tomography and coronary atherosclerotic plaque area. A histopathologic correlative study. Circulation 1995;92:2157–2162.

7. Nallamothu BK, Saint S, Bielak LF, et al. Electron-beam computed tomography in the diagnosis of coronary artery disease: a meta-analysis. Arch Intern Med 2001;161:833–838.
8. O'Rourke RA, Brundage BH, Froelicher VF, et al. American College of Cardiology/American Heart Association expert consensus document on electron-beam computed tomography for the diagnosis and prognosis of coronary artery disease. J Am Coll Cardiol 2000;36: 326–340.
9. O'Malley PG, Taylor AJ, Jackson JL, et al. Prognostic value of coronary electron-beam computed tomography for coronary heart disease events in asymptomatic populations. Am J Cardiol 2000;85: 945–948.
10. Kondos GT, Hoff JA, Serukov A, et al. Electron-beam tomography coronary artery calcium and cardiac events: a 37-month follow-up of 5635 initially asymptomatic low- to intermediate-risk adults. Circulation 2003;107:2571–2576.
11. Shaw LJ, Raggi P, Schisterman E, Berman DS, Callister TQ. Prognostic value of cadiac risk factors and coronary artery calcium screening for all-cause mortality. Radiology 2003;228:826–833.
12. Arad Y, Roth M, Newstein D, Guerci AD. Coronary calcification, coronary disease risk factors, and atherosclerotic cardiovascular disease events: the St. Francis Heart Study. J Am Coll Cardiol Abstract 2003.
13. Bild DE, Bluemke DA, Burke GL, et al. Multi-ethnic study of atherosclerosis: objectives and design. Am J Epidemiol 2002; 156:871–881.
14. Hatwalkar A, Agrawal N, Reiss DS, et al. Comparison of prevalence and severity of coronary calcium determined by electron beam

tomography among various ethnic groups. Am J Cardiol 2003; 91:1225–1227.
15. Budoff MJ, Yang TP, Shavelle RM, et al. Ethnic differences in coronary atherosclerosis. J Am Coll Cardiol 2002;39:408–412.
16. Lee TC, O'Malley PG, Feuerstein I, et al. The prevalence and severity of coronary artery calcification on coronary artery computed tomography in black and white subjects. J Am Coll Cardiol 2003; 41:39–44.
17. Wilson PW, Kauppila LI, O'Donnell CJ, et al. Lumbar aortic calcification is an important predictor of vascular morbidity and mortality. Circulation 2001;103:1529–1534.
18. Witteman JC, Kannel WB, Wolf PA, et al. Aortic calcified plaques and cardiovascular disease (the Framingham Study). Am J Cardiol 1990;66(15):1060–1064.
19. Morin RL, Gerber TC, McCollough CH. Radiation dose in computed tomography of the heart. Circulation 2003;107:917–922.
20. Horton KM, Post WS, Blumenthal RS, et al. Prevalence of significant noncardiac findings on electron-beam computed tomography coronary artery calcium screening examinations. Circulation 2002;106:532–534.
21. Hunold P, Schmermund A, Seibel RM, et al. Prevalence and clinical significance of accidental findings in electron-beam tomographic scans for coronary artery calcification. Eur Heart J 2001;22: 1748–1758.
22. Hoff JA, Chomka EV, Krainik AJ, Daviglus M, Rich S, Kondos GT. Age and gender distributions of coronary artery calcium detected by electron beam tomography in 35,246 adults. Am J Cardiol 2001;87(12):1335–1339.

8 Coronary Calcium Scanning

Why We Should Perform It

Axel Schmermund, MD, Stefan Möhlenkamp, MD,
and Raimund Erbel, MD

It is increasingly recognized that only by preventing ischemic heart disease can morbidity and mortality associated with cardiovascular diseases be substantially reduced. There are two main preventive strategies: one that focuses on community-wide measures ("population approach") and one that focuses on high-risk individuals ("high-risk approach") *(1)*. Certainly, both approaches have strengths and limitations, and should work best if applied in a complementary fashion. Although clear goals can be set for community-wide measures (such as promoting healthy diet, increasing physical activity, and marginalizing smoking), strategies for successful implementation depend on political, cultural, and economic surroundings. Trials in Central and Western Europe have failed to fulfil the expectations *(2,3)*. By contrast, the high-risk approach has been demonstrated to be effective regarding both lifestyle and pharmacological interventions *(1)*. The problem with this approach is the need to reliably identify high-risk subjects.

Risk prediction algorithms derived from large epidemiological studies—in particular the Framingham study and the Münster (Germany) Procam study *(4,5)*—serve as the cornerstone of office-based risk assessment. Absolute 10-yr risk of myocardial infarction or cardiac death is calculated. However, risk factors identify adverse outcomes in a population. Because of the wide variability of atherosclerosis in subjects with formally identical risk-factor exposure *(6)*, individual discrimination is often unsatisfactory *(7)*. Further, there is considerable uncertainty as to the application in external populations with different characteristics *(8–11)*. The Framingham algorithm appears to overestimate absolute risk in a German population by approx 50% *(11)*.

To estimate the risk of a coronary event, risk-factor assessment is the most common procedure, and this is justified by overwhelming evidence. Risk factors lead to events by the patho-physiological intermediary of atherosclerotic plaque disease. In this sense, risk factors yield a statistical probability that coronary plaques have developed. Coronary calcium scanning allows for direct visualization of coronary atherosclerotic plaque disease. It can answer the question of whether risk-factor exposure in the actual individual has really led to the development of coronary atherosclerosis. The cumulative effect of risk-factor exposure over many years can be assessed by its impact on coronary plaque development *(12)*.

There is a relationship between the extent of calcified plaque burden and that of total plaque burden *(13,14)*. Thus, the primary aim is not to diagnose coronary stenoses, but rather to detect and quantify coronary plaque burden. Importantly, coronary calcium in many instances seems to indicate coronary disease activity. Calcium is a frequent feature of plaque rupture (found in 70–80% of cases) *(15–17)*. Among all types of plaques that can be defined histologically, the extent of calcium is greatest in healed plaque rupture, which is frequently observed in sudden coronary death *(16,18)*. Further, calcium is associated with positive arterial remodeling *(19)*. The mechanisms leading to positive arterial remodeling appear to share common aspects with those ultimately leading to plaque rupture, and plaques displaying positive remodeling of the arterial segment are prone to rupture.

All prospective studies in seemingly healthy older adults have found substantial increases in relative risk of a cardiovascular hard event in the presence of increased amounts of coronary calcium *(20–25)*. Consistently, a very high negative predictive value (99%) regarding cardiovascular hard endpoints has been reported. Conversely, high-risk persons were identified whose risk exceeded an event rate of 2% per year *(20–25)*. These studies have prompted the authors of the *American Heart Association Prevention Conference V* and the *National Cholesterol Education Program Adult Treatment Panel III* to list electron beam computed tomography coronary calcium scanning as a possible diagnostic modality in adults with several risk factors, in particular older adults *(26,27)*. The actual guidelines for the prevention of CAD issued by the European Society of Cardiology and other leading European societies (European Heart Journal) expand on this. It is stated that the calcium score "is an important parameter to detect asymptomatic individuals at high risk for future CVD events, independent of the traditional risk factors" *(28)*.

The favorable data from the above-mentioned trials were all obtained in selected cohorts, which has been criticized. Recently, however, results from population-based studies with unselected participants have confirmed these results. The

From: *Contemporary Cardiology: CT of the Heart: Principles and Applications*
Edited by: U. Joseph Schoepf © Humana Press, Inc., Totowa, NJ

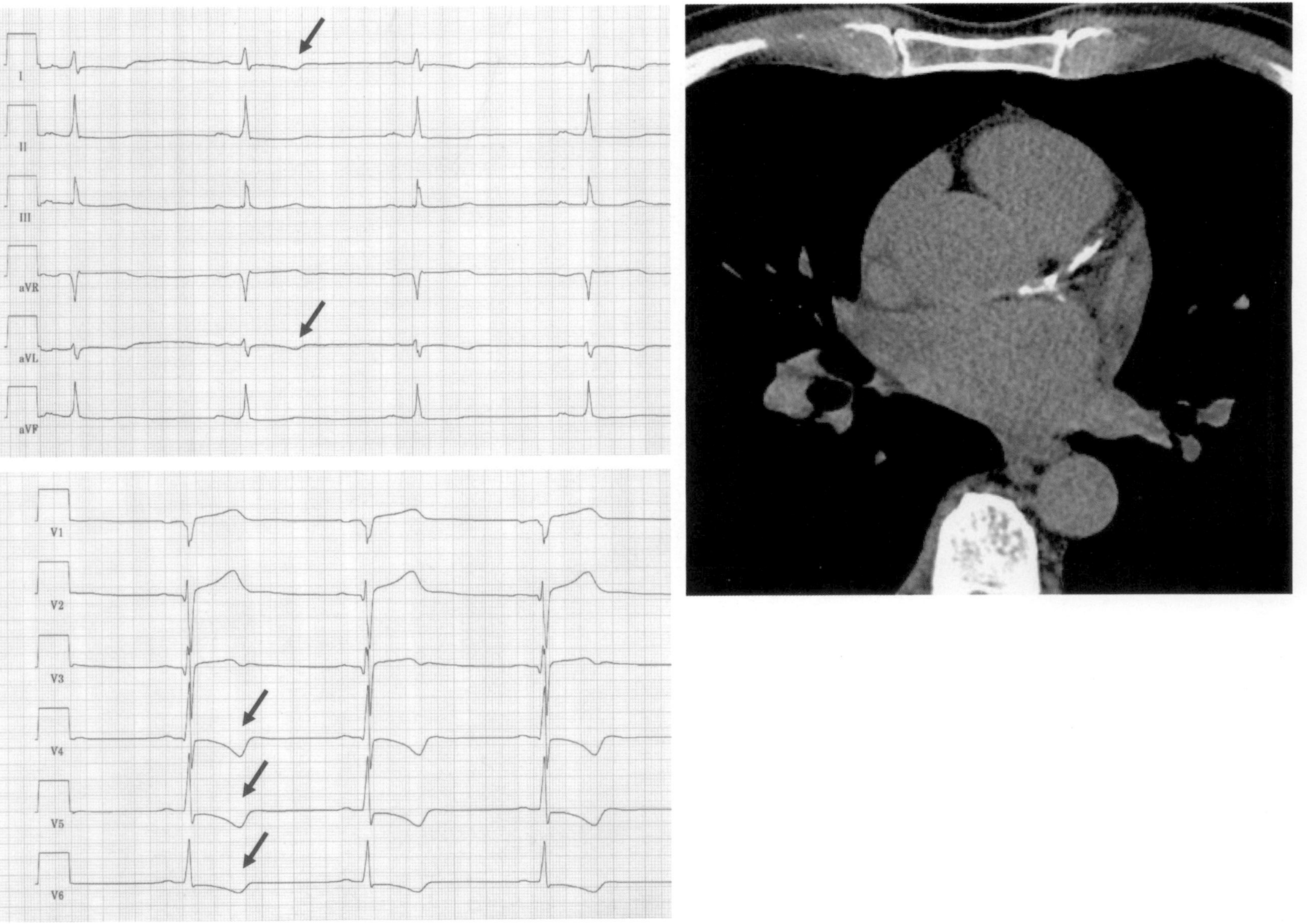

Fig. 1. Sixty-one-year-old male who agreed to participate in the Heinz Nixdorf Recall Study, an epidemiological project in the general population, 3 d after having run the Cologne marathon in 4:28 h. The man was in very good health and feeling well. His only cardiovascular risk factor was systemic hypertension, yielding a Framingham risk of 12% (intermediate risk category) and a Procam risk of 5.7% (low risk category). The electrocardiograph recording in the setting of the Heinz Nixdorf Recall Study and further laboratory analyses revealed subacute anterior myocardial infarction. The left panel shows his electrocardiogram with T inversion in I, aVL and V4-V6 (arrows) and slow R progression. His total coronary calcium score determined by electron-beam CT was 1105 (right panel). The figure shows a section at the base of the heart with massive calcification of the left main stem and proximal portion of the left anterior descending coronary artery. He had more coronary calcium than approx 94% of males his age (94th percentile). Coronary angiography showed severe three-vessel disease with left main stem involvement. He underwent successful aorto-coronary bypass surgery with complete revascularization and had an uneventful course.

Rotterdam Coronary Calcification Study and the St. Francis Heart Study, with a total of almost 7600 healthy subjects, have consistently observed relative risks associated with elevated coronary calcium scores on the order of 8–11 *(29–31)*. In both population-based studies, the predictive power of coronary calcium was independent of and additive to risk-factor information. In the Rotterdam study, subjects with a Framingham risk score below the median who had a calcium score in the upper tertile had a relative risk of 8.9 compared with subjects with the same Framingham risk score whose calcium score was in the lower tertile *(30)*.

Imaging of coronary calcium allows direct detection of coronary atherosclerotic plaques and estimation of the extent of disease and its distribution in the coronary tree *(32)*. As opposed to other methods of direct vessel wall diagnostics such as B-mode ultrasound analysis of carotid artery intima-media thickness and plaques, coronary atherosclerosis can be directly assessed. As opposed to noninvasive exercise tests such as exercise stress testing or stress echocardiography, actual coronary plaques are detected, with all the consequences regarding comparative predictive abilities. Coronary calcium scanning adds previously unachievable prognostic power to the information derived from risk-factor analysis. An example is shown in Fig. 1.

Coronary calcium scanning is helpful in particular in healthy subjects with an undetermined cardiovascular risk whose management is unclear. In these subjects, the coronary calcium score can direct the treating physician towards general advice in the case of a low or negative score, or towards intensive treatment in the case of a high score. If the score is intermediate, this is also helpful. The physician has much more security that indeed, an intermediate risk is present and the patient can be treated accordingly. Finally, selected symptomatic patients with known coronary artery disease can benefit from coronary calcium scanning if detailed information on the extent of atherosclerotic plaque disease is needed and prognostication is especially important.

REFERENCES

1. Yusuf S, Reddy S, Ôunpuu S, Anand S. Global burden of cardiovascular disease. Part II: variations in cardiovascular disease by specific ethnic groups and geographic regions and prevention strategies. Circulation 2001;104:2855–2864.
2. World Health Organization European Collaborative Group. European Collaborative Trial of Multifactorial Prevention of Coronary Heart Disease. Final report on the 6-year results. Lancet 1986;1: 869–872.
3. Thelle D. Prevention of cardiovascular diseases: a scientific dilemma. Scand Cardiovasc J 2000;34:103–105.
4. Wilson PWF, D'Agostino RB, Levy D, Belanger AM, Silbershatz H, Kannel WB. Prediction of coronary heart disease using risk factor categories. Circulation 1998;97:1837–1847.
5. Assmann G, Cullen P, Schulte H. Simple scoring scheme for calculating the risk of acute coronary events based on the 10-year follow-up of the prospective cardiovascular Munster (PROCAM) study [erratum: Circulation 2002;105:900]. Circulation. 2002;105: 310–315.
6. Greenland P, Abrams J, Aurigemma GP, et al. Prevention Conference V. Beyond secondary prevention: identifying the high-risk patient for primary prevention. Noninvasive tests of atherosclerotic burden. Writing Group III. Circulation 2000;101:e16–e22.
7. Wald NJ, Law M, Watt HC, et al. Apolipoproteins and ischaemic heart disease: implications for screening. Lancet 1994;343:75–79.
8. D'Agostino RB Sr, Grundy S, Sullivan LM, Wilson P. CHD Risk Prediction Group. Validation of the Framingham coronary heart disease prediction scores: results of a multiple ethnic groups investigation. JAMA 2001;286:180–187.
9. Laurier D, Chau NP, Cazelles B, Segond P. PCV METRA Group. Estimation of CHD risk in a French working population using a modified Framingham model. J Clin Epidemiol 1994;47:1353–1364.
10. Menotti A, Puddu PE, Lanti M. Comparison of the Framingham risk function-based coronary chart with risk function from an Italian population study. Eur Heart J 2000;21:365–370.
11. Hense HW, Schulte H, Lowel H, Assmann G, Keil U. Framingham risk function overestimates risk of coronary heart disease in men and women from Germany—results from the MONICA Augsburg and the PROCAM cohorts. Eur Heart J 2003;24:937–945.
12. Hoeg JM, Feuerstein IM, Tucker EE. Detection and quantitation of calcific atherosclerosis by ultrafast computed tomography in children and young adults with homozygous familial hypercholesterolemia. Arterioscler Thromb 1994;14:1066–1074.
13. Rumberger JA, Simons DB, Fitzpatrick LA, Sheedy PF, Schwartz RS. Coronary artery calcium area by electron-beam computed tomography and coronary atherosclerotic plaque area. A histopathologic correlative study. Circulation 1995;92:2157–2162.
14. Schmermund A, Denktas AE, Rumberger JA, et al. Independent and incremental value of coronary artery calcium for predicting the extent of angiographic coronary artery disease: comparison with cardiac risk factors and radionuclide perfusion imaging. J Am Coll Cardiol 1999;34:777–786.
15. Farb A, Burke AP, Tang AL, et al. Coronary plaque erosion without rupture into a lipid core. A frequent cause of coronary thrombosis in sudden coronary death. Circulation 1996;93:1354–1364.
16. Burke AP, Taylor A, Farb A, Malcom GT, Virmani R. Coronary calcification: insights from sudden coronary death victims. Z Kardiol 2000;89 Suppl 2:49–53.
17. Schmermund A, Erbel R. Current perspective: unstable coronary plaque and its relation to coronary calcium. Circulation 2001; 104: 1682–1687.
18. Burke AP, Kolodgie FD, Farb A, et al. Healed plaque ruptures and sudden coronary death: evidence that subclinical rupture has a role in plaque progression. Circulation 2001;103:934–940.
19. Burke AP, Kolodgie FD, Farb A, et al. Morphological predictors of arterial remodeling in coronary atherosclerosis. Circulation 2002; 105:297–303.
20. Raggi P, Callister TQ, Cooil B, et al. Identification of patients at increased risk of first unheralded acute myocardial infarction by electron-beam computed tomography. Circulation 2000;101:850–855.
21. Arad Y, Spadaro LA, Goodman K, Newstein D, Guerci AD. Prediction of coronary events with electron beam computed tomography. J Am Coll Cardiol 2000;36:1253–1260.
22. Wong ND, Hsu JC, Detrano RC, Diamond G, Eisenberg H, Gardin JM. Coronary artery calcium evaluation by electron beam computed tomography and its relation to new cardiovascular events. Am J Cardiol 2000;86:495–498.
23. Park R, Detrano R, Xiang M, et al. Combined use of computed tomography coronary calcium scores and C-reactive protein levels in predicting cardiovascular events in nondiabetic individuals. Circulation 2002;106:2073–2077.
24. Kondos GT, Hoff JA, Sevrukov A, et al. Electron-beam tomography coronary artery calcium and cardiac events: a 37-month follow-up of 5635 initially asymptomatic low- to intermediate-risk adults. Circulation 2003;107:2571–2576.
25. Shaw LJ, Raggi P, Schisterman E, Berman DS, Callister TQ. Prognostic value of cardiac risk factors and coronary artery calcium screening for all-cause mortality. Radiology 2003;228:826–833.
26. Greenland P, Smith SC, Grundy SN. Current perspective: improving coronary heart disease risk assessment in asymptomatic people. Role of traditional risk factors and noninvasive cardiovascular tests. Circulation 2001;104:1863–1867.

27. Third Report of the National Cholesterol Education Program (NCEP) Expert Panel on Detection, Evaluation, and Treatment of High Blood Cholesterol in Adults (Adult Treatment Panel III) Final Report. Circulation 2002;106:3143–3421.
28. De Backer G, Ambrosioni E, Borch-Johnsen K, et al. Executive Summary. European guidelines on cardiovascular disease prevention in clinical practice. Third Joint Task Force of European and Other Societies on Cardiovascular Disease Prevention in Clinical Practice. Eur Heart J 2003;24:1601–1610.
29. Vliegenthart R, Oei HH, Breteler MM, et al. Coronary calcification is a strong predictor of all-cause and cardiovascular mortality in elderly. Circulation 2002;106(Suppl):II–743.
30. Vliegenthart R. Coronary calcification and the risk of cardiovascular disease. An epidemiologic study. PhD Thesis. Thoraxcentre Rotterdam, Netherlands, March 19, 2003.
31. Arad Y, Roth M, Newstein D, Guerci A. Coronary calcification, coronary disease risk factors, and atherosclerotic cardiovascular disease events: the St. Francis Heart Study. Hotline Session, ACC 2003.
32. Schmermund A, Baumgart D, Möhlenkamp S, et al. Natural history and topographic pattern of progression of coronary calcification in symptomatic patients: an electron-beam CT study. Arterioscler Thromb Vasc Biol 2001;21:421–426.

9 Detection and Quantification of Coronary Calcium With Electron Beam CT

Axel Schmermund, md, Stefan Möhlenkamp, md, and Raimund Erbel, md

TECHNIQUE

Electron beam computed tomography (EBCT) employs well-known computed tomography technology. However, in distinction to other CT machines, no mechanical parts are moved. Whereas in usual CT machines, the distance between cathode and anode is very short, it measures approx 9 ft in EBCT. The electron beam, which produces the X-rays by striking the anode, is steered over this distance by an electromagnetic deflection system. The latest generation of EBCT machines (e-Speed™, GE Imatron) achieves an image acquisition time of only 30 ms, which is sufficient to freeze the motion of the heart.

Standardized methods for imaging, identification, and quantification of coronary calcium using EBCT have been established *(1,2)*. The current generation of EBCT scanners is usually operated in the high-resolution mode with continuous, nonoverlapping slices of 3-mm thickness and an acquisition time of 100 ms. Patients are positioned supine, and a sufficient number of slices is obtained to cover the complete heart through the apex (usually 36–40 slices). Electrocardiographic triggering is performed at a fixed point within the RR interval, generally 40% or 80%. Coronary calcium is defined as a hyperattenuating lesion above the threshold of a CT density of 130 Hounsfield units (HU) in an area of two or more adjacent pixels. The *calcium score* is a product of the area of calcium and a factor rated 1–4, dictated by the maximum CT density *(1)*. The calcium score can be calculated for a given coronary segment, a specific coronary artery, or for the entire coronary system (Fig. 1).

More recently, a volumetric score has been introduced, which uses isotropic interpolation and may thus be more reproducible *(3)*. Further, calcium mass measurements have been suggested, which would render measurements obtained with various CT technologies (EBCT or spiral CT with different slice thickness) comparable *(4)*. Such measurements require simultaneous phantom calibration and are currently not widely available. Because the above-mentioned calcium score has been employed since 1990, and all long-term data are based on this scoring algorithm, it should not be completely abandoned in favor of more recent algorithms.

CORONARY CALCIUM—WHAT DOES IT MEAN?

Non-contrast-enhanced cardiac EBCT allows for direct, noninvasive visualization of calcified coronary plaques (Fig. 1). The primary aim is not to diagnose coronary stenoses, but rather to detect and quantify coronary plaque burden. Coronary plaques, usually not highly stenotic, are the underlying substrate of the acute coronary syndromes *(5)*. Coronary calcium is a specific expression of coronary atherosclerotic plaque disease *(6,7)*. There is a relationship between the extent of calcified plaque burden and that of total plaque burden *(6–9)*. Total plaque burden is one of the most important predictors of coronary risk *(10,11)*. The more calcium detected, the more plaque there is. This carries direct implications for an individual's coronary risk *(5)*.

It may be argued that calcium is associated with an overall increased activity of coronary atherosclerotic disease. Histopathologic studies have demonstrated that coronary calcium is a frequent feature of plaque rupture *(5,12,13)* and is found even in subjects who die of sudden coronary death as the first manifestation of ischemic heart disease under the age of 50 yr *(14)*. Among all types of histologically defined types of plaques detected in young victims of sudden coronary death, acute ruptures contain calcium most frequently (80%), while healed ruptures contain the greatest amount of calcium *(13,15)*. Plaque erosions, on the other hand, are associated with little calcium *(12,13)*. Calcium is found preferentially in plaques with expansive ("positive") arterial remodeling *(16)*. The mechanisms leading to expansive arterial remodeling appear to share common aspects with those ultimately leading to plaque rupture, and plaques displaying positive remodeling of the arterial segment are prone to rupture *(17)*. Finally, lesions characterized by ultrasound radiofrequency analysis as unstable frequently contain calcium *(18)*.

The findings in studies using conventional intravascular ultrasound have been less unequivocal, perhaps as a result of differences in the ability to define calcium and lesion characteristics *(19–23)*. Whereas some studies have detected less calcium in the culprit lesion in patients with unstable angina

From: *Contemporary Cardiology: CT of the Heart: Principles and Applications*
Edited by: U. Joseph Schoepf © Humana Press, Inc., Totowa, NJ

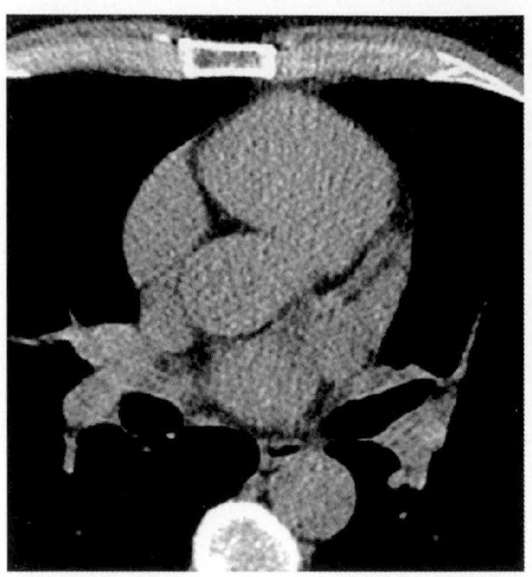
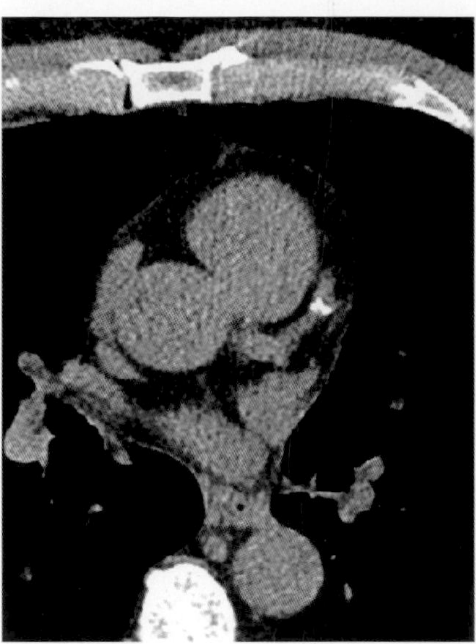
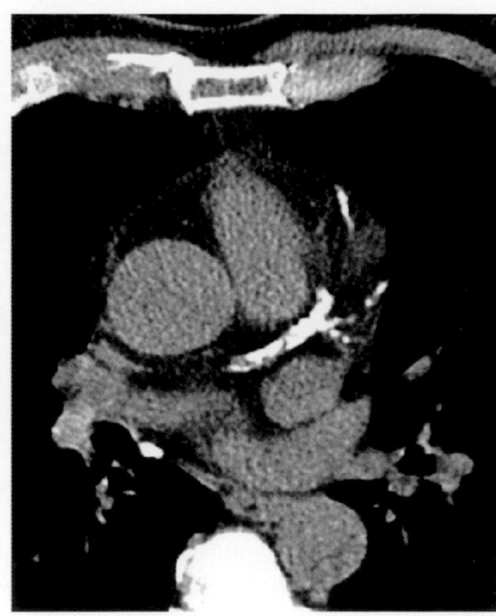

Fig. 1. Coronary calcium scans at the level of the left anterior descending coronary artery. Left panel: No coronary calcium. Mid panel: Moderate coronary calcium with typical localization in the area of bifurcation with first diagonal branch, total calcium score 108. Right panel: Extensive coronary calcium, total calcium score 3.532.

pectoris or acute myocardial infarction than in patients with stable symptoms *(19–21)*, others did not find a difference *(22,23)*, or, in a prospective study, detected more calcium in patients who later sustained an event *(24)*. In summary, coronary calcium indicates the presence and extent of coronary atherosclerotic plaque disease. The weight of evidence suggests that coronary calcium indicates atherosclerotic disease activity and is associated with healed or acute plaque rupture and positive arterial remodeling.

CORONARY CALCIUM—WHAT DOES IT PREDICT?

In patients presenting to the emergency room with chest pain and no initial objective signs of myocardial ischemia, a negative EBCT indicated an excellent prognosis with regard to major cardiac events over the subsequent 1–4 mo *(25–27)*. EBCT yielded negative predictive values in the range of 98–100%. In symptomatic patients undergoing coronary angiography, increased amounts of coronary calcium detected by EBCT were highly predictive of subsequent events over 30 mo *(28–30)*. In direct comparison, EBCT performed better than coronary angiography (that is, number of stenotic major coronary arteries) in this respect *(28–30)*.

A number of studies have examined the predictive value of EBCT coronary calcium quantification in selected asymptomatic populations. All of these studies have demonstrated that the coronary calcium score predicts coronary events, defined as an aggregate of coronary death, nonfatal myocardial infarction, and revascularization (Table 1). Arad et al. observed that the prespecified calcium score cutpoints of 80 and 160 both were associated with odds ratios of approx 22 for suffering coronary death or acute myocardial infarction, with wide confidence intervals (CIs) (95% CI, 5.1–97.4 and 6.4–77.4, respectively) *(31)*. There was a tendency for higher scores in subjects with hard events compared to subjects who underwent revascularization. In this study, the status of established risk factors was determined by questionnaire. In a multivariate analysis in a subgroup of patients with all information available ($n = 787$), the calcium score cutpoints were associated with odds ratios for suffering any event in the range of 14–20 and the risk factors, including age, with odds ratios in the range of 3–6 *(31)*.

Raggi et al. found that subjects with calcium scores in the highest quartile had an odds ratio of 21.5 (95% CI, 2.8–162.4) for suffering acute myocardial infarction or cardiac death *(32)*. Risk factor data were obtained by questionnaire. Subjects in the highest quartile of cardiovascular risk factor distribution had an odds ratio of 7.0 (95% CI, 1.6–31.5).

Wong et al. assessed risk factors (by questionnaire) and coronary calcium scores in 881 subjects. After adjustment for risk factors, coronary calcium scores in the third or fourth quartile were associated with a relative risk of 4.5 or 8.8 *(33)*. Accordingly, these three studies suggest that EBCT was independent of risk-factor information for predicting events and was clearly superior compared with risk-factor analysis alone. However, risk factors were determined only by questionnaire.

Detrano et al. reported an odds ratio of 2.7 associated with a calcium score above the median *(34)*. Receiver operating curve analysis of calcium scores for separating subjects with vs without acute myocardial infarction or coronary death yielded an area under curve (± SE) of 0.64 ± 0.05. For comparison, this value was 0.86 ± 0.07 in the study by Arad et al. *(31)*. Risk factors were assessed by questionnaire and direct measurements of laboratory values. An ECG was recorded in all subjects. The combined analysis of risk factors and ECG yielded an area under the curve of 0.69 ± 0.05, so that for predicting hard events, EBCT was not superior in this report. However, in a later analysis of the same data set, but excluding diabetic subjects, coronary calcium was a strong and independent predictor of coronary death and nonfatal myocardial infarction as well as revascularization *(35)*. After adjustment for risk factors, the relative risk of sustaining a hard event was 4.9–6.1

Table 1
Prognostic Studies in Selected Patient Populations

Author (reference)	*No. of patients*	*Mean age*	*Women (%)*	*Mean calcium score*	*Median calcium score*	*Follow-up (mo)*	*No. of events (%)*	*Patients with event: calcium score (mean ± SD, median)*	*Patients without event: calcium score (mean ± SD, median)*	*RR*	*Definition of events*
Arad *(31)*	1177	53 ± 11	29	~ 156	4	43	39 (3.3)	764 ± 935 (511)	135 ± 432 (3)	14.3	Coronary death, nonfatal MI, revasc.
Raggi *(32)*	632	52 ± 9	50	101 ± 254	3.1	32	27 (4.3)	303 ± 441 (141)	92 ± 240 (2.4)	12.5	Coronary death, nonfatal MI
Wong *(33)*	926	54 ± 10	21	143	5	40	28 (3.0)	n/a	n/a	4.5[a]	MI, revasc., cerebrovasc. event
Detrano *(34)*	1196	66 ± 8	11	452 ± 457	44	41	46 (3.8)	n/a	n/a	2.3	Coronary death, nonfatal MI, revasc.
Park *(35)*	967	66 ± 8	10	n/a	n/a	77	104	395 ± 571 (203)	195 ± 378 (37)	4.4–7.5[a]	Coronary death, nonfatal MI, revasc.

[a]Adjusted for risk factors. SD, standard deviation; MI, myocardial infarction.

in the highest vs the lowest tertile of calcium scores (depending on the level of C-reactive protein), and the risk for all endpoints (including revascularization) was 4.4–7.5. In this analysis, coronary calcium was superior to combined risk-factor analysis (on the basis of actual laboratory data) and ECG and also to C-reacting protein *(35)*.

These findings were corroborated by the analysis of large databases with a total of >15,000 patients *(36,37)*. Kondos et al. examined subjects who were all self-referred and who were followed over a mean of 3.1 yr. They observed a relative risk of myocardial infarction or cardiac death of 7.2 in men with a coronary calcium score in the upper quartile *(36)*. In women, the event rate was only 0.4%, so that no meaningful analysis was possible. Shaw et al. documented only total mortality *(37)*. A calcium score in the range between 400 and 1000 was associated with a 6.2-fold increase in death rate. A calcium score >1000 was associated with a 12.3-fold increase in death rate. Perhaps the most important aspect of these studies was that high-risk persons could be identified whose risk exceeded a rate of 2% per year (hard events) *(36,37)* or 1% per year for overall mortality.

Along the same lines, Wahys et al. reported retrospective data *(38)*. In analogy with a study in symptomatic patients *(30)*, asymptomatic patients with very high calcium scores (>1000) had a greatly elevated risk of sustaining an event *(38)*.

The Rotterdam Coronary Calcification Study was the first population-based study to have yielded data in unselected participants *(39,40)*. In this project, 2013 persons from a suburb of Rotterdam, the Netherlands, were recruited. After a mean follow-up time of 2.7 yr, 116 cardiovascular events occurred, including 73 coronary heart disease deaths. There was a strong and graded relationship between the EBCT-derived calcium score and cardiovascular disease events *(39)*. The 15% of participants with the highest scores had a relative risk of 11 of dying from ischemic heart disease. The yearly death rate regarding only ischemic heart disease was almost 2% (Fig. 2). In the approx 50% of participants with low or negative calcium scores, this rate was only 0.07% *(39)*. After adjustment for risk factors, the association between coronary calcium scores and cardiovascular as well as coronary morbidity and mortality

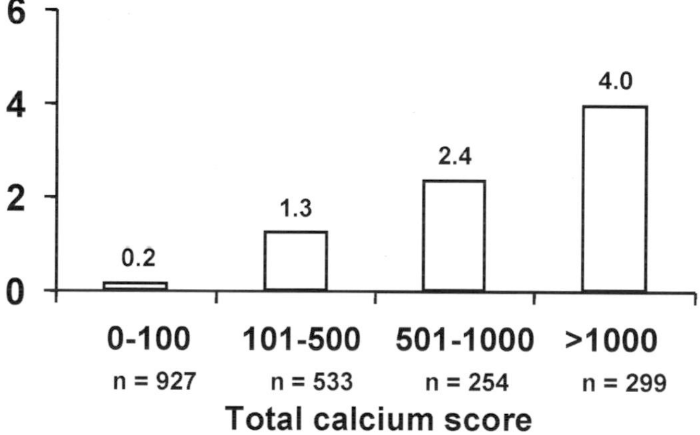

Fig. 2. Rate of coronary artery disease (CAD)-related deaths associated with different coronary calcium scores in the Rotterdam Coronary Calcification Study, a population-based study. Mean follow-up was 2.7 yr *(38)*.

Table 2
Indications for the Use of CT Coronary Calcium Scanning

Asymptomatic persons:
1. Persons with risk factors who cannot be determined by office-based risk assessment to have either a low or a high cardiovascular risk
2. Older persons in whom the established risk factors lose some of their predictive value and whose risk remains indeterminate

Symptomatic persons:
3. Patients in whom advanced risk stratification is useful, for example if extensive coronary plaque disease is suspected
4. Patients presenting to the emergency room with nonspecific chest pain ("rule out myocardial infarction")

remained strong *(40)*. The relative risk of coronary heart disease increased gradually in patients with higher coronary calcium scores compared with those in the reference category with calcium scores of 0–100, which comprised 50% of all participants *(40)*. It was 3.2 in subjects with scores of 101–500, 5.1 in subjects with 501–1000, and 8.3 in subjects with scores >1000. The coronary event rates in 2.7 yr were 0.8% in the lowest score group and increased to 3.3%, 5.0%, and 8.7% in the other calcium score groups.

In summary, the EBCT-derived coronary calcium score has demonstrated its ability to identify subjects with a very low risk of cardiovascular and coronary disease as well as subjects with a very high rate of events (>2% per year). This ability goes beyond that of conventional risk-factor analysis, is independent of it, and adds incremental predictive value.

PROGRESSION OF CORONARY CALCIUM

Follow-up coronary calcium scans appear to be useful, as the progression of calcification is influenced by low-density lipoprotein values and can be attenuated or even stopped by lipid-lowering ("statin") medication *(3,41)*. In patients followed in an outpatient setting, the progression of coronary calcium burden is approx 25% per year *(42)*. However, there is great inter-individual variability, probably as a result of the interplay of numerous factors which influence the process. Also, baseline plaque burden determines the rate of progression *(42)*. Progression is observed at typical predilection sites of atherosclerosis in the coronary tree. Changes in overall coronary calcium result from uniform changes at these sites. This uniform pattern of change suggests that the development of calcified plaque disease is a coronary systemic process *(42)*.

In patients with elevated cholesterol values, progression of coronary calcium appears to be accelerated and on the order of 50% per yr *(3)*. In patients treated with statin therapy, the annual progression is substantially reduced. Values between 10 and 20% per year have been reported *(3,41)*. If low-density lipoprotein (LDL)-cholesterol can be reduced to levels <100 mg/dL, it appears possible to stop the progression of coronary calcium *(41)*. The value of coronary calcium scanning for assessing the treatment effect in individual patients remains to be clarified.

CORONARY CALCIUM—HOW CAN IT BE USED?

There are four major areas where EBCT scanning for coronary calcium can offer clinical value (Table 2).

1. Application of coronary calcium scoring to define the extent of coronary atherosclerosis in asymptomatic individuals at risk for coronary disease is of great interest. The magnitude of the problem warrants tools for improved risk prediction, and published data suggest a prominent role for EBCT. However, it is currently unresolved who benefits from an EBCT scan in terms of future coronary events which can be prevented on the basis of the calcium study. Clearly, the indications for a scan need to be strictly defined to avoid "overdiagnosis" and disproportionate increases in health care expenditure.

Indeed, the authors of the American Heart Association Prevention Conference V and the National Cholesterol Education Program Adult Treatment Panel III list coronary calcium scanning as a useful diagnostic modality in adults with several risk factors, in particular older adults *(43,44)*. Fig. 3 shows how coronary calcium scoring might be used to improve individual risk stratification.

The most recent statement is provided in the actual guidelines for the prevention of CAD issued by the European Society of Cardiology and other leading European societies *(45)*. The European guidelines state that the calcium score "is an important parameter to detect asymptomatic individuals at high risk for future CVD events, independent of the traditional risk factors." This statement expands on the previous statements *(43,44)*.

The interpretation of the EBCT scan is straightforward with regard to prognostication, and it indeed applies to any person regardless of symptomatic status. Because it is internationally comparable, the Agatston calcium score remains the standard algorithm, but an increasing role of calcium area and/or volume-scoring algorithms can be expected. The absence of identifiable coronary calcium is consistent with no or at most minimal coronary atherosclerosis. Individuals in this group fall into a favorable prognostic group. On the other hand, Agatston calcium scores exceeding 80–100 are highly consistent with at least nonobstructive CAD *(46,47)*. The presence of moderate calcium scores in an otherwise asymptomatic individual suggests that further evaluations may be prudent, including careful identification and aggressive treatment of modifiable risk factors. It cannot be overemphasized that calcium scores need to be interpreted with regard to age and sex distribution. According to the natural history of coronary atherosclerosis, calcium scores increase in higher age groups. At the same time, the prognostic significance is shifted, because clinically overt coronary artery disease occurs in some patients with increasing age, but not in others. With this in mind, individuals with significant coronary calcium (calcium score >400–500) clearly have advanced coronary atherosclerosis and require strict measures regarding modifiable risk factors. Additionally,

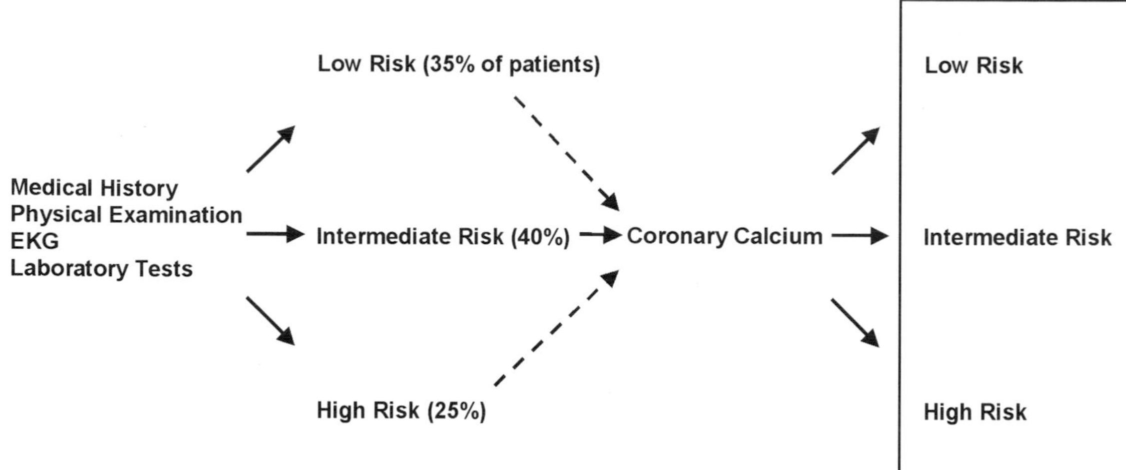

Fig. 3. Algorithm for the use of electron beam CT coronary calcium scanning for advanced risk stratification *(41,42)*. In patients in whom office-based risk assessment determines an intermediate risk level (approx 40% of patients), calcium scanning can be used for further—advanced—risk stratification (box). Even in the presence of a rather intermediate calcium score, the scan is useful. In this case, the probability of a truly intermediate risk is much greater than if determined by office-based risk assessment alone. Of note, the initial office-based risk estimate might be less accurate than the aggregate risk estimate including coronary calcium scanning. It is open to question whether one should concentrate on examining intermediate-risk patients in order to define their management more precisely or whether some patients with a presumably low or high risk on the basis of office-based risk assessment may also profit from undergoing a coronary calcium scan.

Step I		Step II	
EBCT-Score (Agatston method)	Interpretation	Age- and sex-specific interpretation (EBCT-Score percentiles)	Risk assessment
0 - 10	No/minimal plaque	0 - 25	Small risk
11 - 100	Some plaque present	26 - 50	Moderate risk
111 - 400	Moderate plaque burden	51 - 75	Increased risk
401-1000	Severe plaque burden	76 - 90	High risk
> 1000	Very severe plaque burden	> 90	Very high risk

Fig. 4. Algorithm used by the authors for interpreting electron-beam computed tomography coronary calcium scans *(2)*. In a first step, the total calcium score is considered. Because of the relationship between coronary calcified and coronary total plaque burden, a high calcium score indicates a high coronary plaque burden. In a second step, the total calcium score is put in perspective regarding age and sex of the individual person. If the calcium score is greater than expected (above the median value), cardiovascular risk is increasingly elevated.

depending on all available clinical information, further evaluations should probably be considered to determine the potential for myocardial ischemia *(47)*.

Apart from the calcium score, age and sex of the patient should be considered by using specific percentile values ("normogram") such as those provided for >35,000 adults in ref. *48*. These percentile values were calculated on the basis of EBCT studies. They appear to be very similar to values derived with four-slice spiral CT *(49)*. But, dynamic changes in imaging parameters need to be considered that may pose problems regarding the comparability and application of data from one system to another. On the basis of these considerations, the German Working Group on Cardio-CT has suggested a scheme for interpretation of EBCT coronary calcium scans (Fig. 4) *(2)*.

2. The issues explained above also pertain to symptomatic patients with known coronary artery disease in that the extent of coronary arteriosclerosis represents an important predictor of events *(28–30)*. Therefore, coronary calcium scanning may be helpful in selected individuals with coronary artery disease where it appears particularly important to obtain complete prognostic information.

10 Detection and Quantification of Coronary Calcium With Dual-Slice CT

Joseph Shemesh, MD

INTRODUCTION

The introduction of dual-slice spiral technique by Elscint in 1992 allowed the imaging of the heart with 3-mm slices within 30 s (a breath-hold). The advantage of double-helical computed tomography (DHCT) over single-slice helical CT is its ability to acquire data twice as fast as single-slice helical CT owing to its two parallel arcs of detectors that are simultaneously irradiated by a single node. Both single- and dual-slice techniques acquire a volume of spatial information over several seconds without electrocardiographic gating. These data can be reconstructed into thin overlapping axial images, with an acquisition time for each image of approx 0.6–1.0 s. The use of overlapping methods compensates for the absence of electrocardiogram (ECG) triggering, enabling the detection of minimal spotty calcific lesions with an area threshold of 0.5 mm^2. This technique was further improved by the 4- and 16-slice multidetector spiral techniques, which enable the use of ECG triggering with subsecond slice time. The dual-slice technique of the Twin system (Philips LTD) is a contribution to practical cardiology. The noninvasive detection and measurement of the early stages of atherosclerosis within the wall of the coronary arteries provides the clinician with a new perspective on coronary artery disease (CAD) and adds important information to the current noninvasive methods. This chapter will summarize our experience of using the coronary calcium score in clinical practice.

CORONARY CALCIUM AND ATHEROSCLEROSIS

In order to recommend the most appropriate diagnostic test for each individual, it is essential to recognize the underlying process of the disease. For CAD, it is atherosclerosis, which starts early in life. Atherosclerotic lesions (types I and II) are found in 69% of children by the time of puberty *(1)*. The changes are minimal in such lesions—lipids have not yet accumulated exracellularly, the matrix between cells remains unchanged, and they are not associated with the emergence of calcium deposits. Type III lesions are the link between the minimal changes of children and the atheroma of adults, and rarely contain a few calcium granules. Atheroma, type IV lesions, emerge primarily in the decade after puberty at the highly susceptible artery sites, and immediately contain calcium granules within some smooth muscle cells and extracellularly among the vast mass of lipidic particles (the lipid core) that now forms, replaces, and expands an extensive region in the deep intima. According to Stary *(1)*, cell organelles were damaged and sequestered calcium. Intracellular calcium granules become extracellular when dead cells break up, but calcification of cell components apparently also occurs only after their release into the extracellular space after cell disintegration. Lipidic cell remnants can calcify, including matrix vesicles, cell membranes, secondary and tertiary lysosomes, macrophage foam cells, and smooth muscle cells. The atheromas of people up to early middle age do not often obstruct the arterial lumen much, but are vulnerable to rupture or fissuring, leading to acute coronary syndrome *(2)*. These potentially dangerous lesions cannot be detected by the current noninvasive diagnostic methods, which are all based on flow-limiting protruding lesions that obstruct at least 50% of the vessel lumen. This preclinical stage of CAD can be detected by the high resolution of the spiral technique, providing a potential means for population screening and an anatomical basis for primary prevention measures.

The proportion of lipid-to-calcium deposit is much higher in young than old people. From about the fifth decade of life, advanced lesions contain lumps and plates of calcium rather than, or in addition to, the much smaller granules. Granules increase in size by encrustation, and adjacent granules fuse to form the larger structures. Type V and VI lesions contain large-sized deposits but continue to have a core of extracellular lipid. In high-grade calcifications, designated as type VII lesions, mineral dominates over all other lesion components. Lamellar bone (osseous metaplasia) may be present in such lesions. Type V–VII lesions are more often associated with lumen obstruction, forming the basis of the chronic manifestations of CAD, stable angina pectoris (SAP) with generally ischemic changes upon stress tests diagnostic modalities. These symptomatic obstructive lesions require revascularization by angioplasty or bypass operation—the "chronic," "soft," or "interventional" events.

From: *Contemporary Cardiology: CT of the Heart: Principles and Applications*
Edited by: U. Joseph Schoepf © Humana Press, Inc., Totowa, NJ

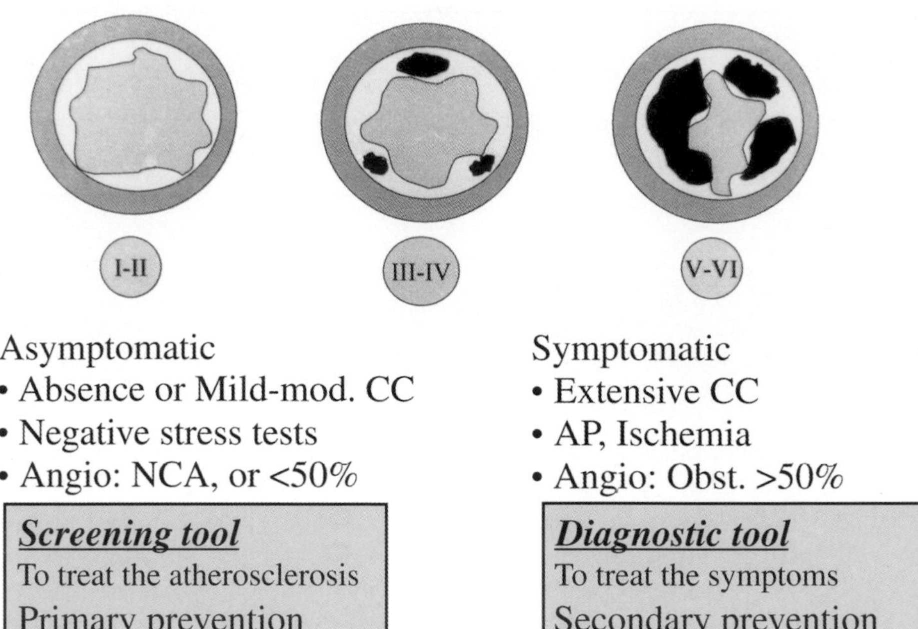

Fig. 1. The main indications for coronary calcium screening are summarized in relation to stages of the atherosclerotic process.
Screening: asymptomatic individuals may have mild to moderate amounts of coronary calcifications (CC) (Stary stages III–IV), or may have earlier noncalcific plaques (Stary I–II). At these stages the current noninvasive tests are normal, as well as the coronary angiogram. The goal of the coronary scan is to provide a more sensitive screening tool, in order to introduce early primary preventive measures to treat the atherosclerosis systematically.
Diagnostic: the diagnosis of heavy calcifications (Stary V–VII) helps to confirm the presence of obstructive disease in clinically equivocal patients. The goal is to identify obstructive vessels for revascularization in order to treat ischemia and anginal symptoms. Coronary CT for this indication should not be confused with its use as a screening tool.

CLINICAL MANIFESTATION OF CAD: CHRONIC VS ACUTE

CAD is clinically manifested by two different main syndromes. The acute syndrome strikes suddenly as sudden death, acute myocardial infarction (AMI), or unstable angina. This syndrome is related to fissure or rupture of one or more vulnerable plaques, generally characterized by a lipid-rich core and thin, fibrous cap. The chronic CAD syndrome manifests when obstructive lesions develop over many years, resulting in ischemic changes upon stress tests, with angina pectoris (AP), or without pain (silent ischemia) (Fig. 1). Pathologic, angiographic, and intracoronary ultrasound studies reveal sharp differences in the distribution of coronary atherosclerosis and plaque morphology between these two coronary syndromes.

Utilizing DHCT, we evaluated the coronary calcium patterns in 149 patients: 47 with chronic SAP and 102 patients surviving a first AMI *(3)*. Prevalence of coronary calcium was 81% among the AMI patients and 100% in the SAP patients. The 547 calcific lesions identified in the AMI patients and the 1242 lesions in the SAP patients were categorized into three groups according to their extent: mild, intermediate, and extensive. The age-adjusted percentages of the highest level of calcification, among AMI vs SAP patients, were as follows: mild 18 vs 3%, intermediate 49 vs 18%, and extensive lesions 33 vs 79% respectively ($p < 0.01$). In the AMI group, 73 culprit arteries were identified; 16 (22%) had no calcium detected, while 30 (41%) showed mild lesions, 20 (27%) had intermediate forms, and only 7 (10%) had extensive lesions. We demonstrated in this study that extensive calcium characterizes the coronary arteries of patients with chronic SAP, whereas first AMI most frequently occurs in mildly calcified or noncalcified culprit arteries. We recently confirmed this observation in a prospective study *(4)*, which investigated the underlying calcific atherosclerotic lesions in a cohort of 50 hypertensive patients who sustained acute vs chronic coronary events. Their mean age was 66 ± 6 yr, and 78% were male. They were all participants in the INSIGHT calcification study and sustained a coronary event during a 3-yr follow-up. Twenty-nine patients had an acute and 21 had a chronic event. High prevalence of coronary artery calcification (CAC) (total calcium score [TCS] >0) was observed in both groups: 93% in the acute and 96% in the chronic group. Three-vessel calcification was found in 82% of the chronic as compared to only 31% in the acute group. Median TCS was 906 in the chronic and 63 in the acute group. The main clinical application of these two studies *(3,4)* is the contribution of DHCT to the better understanding of the CAC characteristics and their potential as predictor of ischemic coronary events. While interventional procedures are related to higher amounts of CAC, many of the acute events occur against a background of minor or mild calcifications. This should draw attention to the malignant potential of the underlying atheromas presented by minor CAC. Furthermore it is essential to distinguish between acute and interventional events when the prognostic significance of CAC is assessed.

PREDICTION OF ANGIOGRAPHIC OBSTRUCTIVE CAD

When compared to coronary angiography, the presence of CAC determined by DHCT (measured as total coronary score >0) indicates the presence of obstructive CAD with a sensitivity of 91% and specificity of 52% in one study *(5)* and 88 and 52% respectively in another study *(6)*. The relatively low specificity reflects the presence of CAC in non- or mildly protruding atheromas within the vessel wall. In fact, the specificity of CT is low only when angiography is considered the gold standard. The truth is that patients who have CAC detected by CT and normal angiograms have false-negative angiograms rather than false-positive CT scans. Sekiya and colleagues showed that these patients have coronary atherosclerosis with reduced ventricular function and coronary reserve *(7)*. The accuracy of DHCT for the diagnosis of angiographically obstructive CAD is similar to that obtained by electron beam CT (EBCT), as indicated in a meta-analysis by Brahmajee and colleagues *(8)*. These authors pooled 1662 patients from nine studies and found a pooled sensitivity of 92.3% and pooled specificity of 51.2%.

CONTRIBUTION OF DHCT IN CHEST PAIN EVALUATION

Chest pain is one of the most frequent reasons for referring patients to cardiac evaluation. The diagnostic procedures in many of these patients are directed at excluding the presence of obstructive CAD. We found that for this indication, DHCT is particularly helpful as a first-line diagnostic procedure in equivocal clinical situations. However, in order to maximize the clinical benefits of this diagnostic tool and to avoid unnecessary costs and irradiation, it is essential to define the proper criteria for referring patients for coronary calcium CT. Our experience in this field can be summarized as follows:

CT for Chest Pain Evaluation Highly Recommended:

- When CAD is not yet diagnosed
- Chronic chest pain
- Atypical chest pain
- Equivocal results of stress tests, thallium, or echo stress
- In patients unable to undergo stress test
- In patients older than 50 yr, particularly women

Less Useful in Patients With:

- Known CAD
- Acute chest pain syndrome
- Typical AP in men
- Unequivocal positive stress test or thallium scintigraphy results

We evaluated the prevalence and score of CAC in patients categorized by chest pain type and by gender, and their value in determining which patients with chronic chest pain are optimal candidates for coronary artery calcification scoring with DHCT *(9)*. We found CAC in 87% of men with typical AP compared to only 52% of those with atypical chest pain. This difference was less pronounced in women—54% in women with typical AP vs 44% in those with atypical chest pain. This prevalence of CAC is in accordance with the estimated prevalence of angiographic CAD in patients with AP and atypical chest pain: 90% of the men and 60% of the women with typical AP had angiographically obstructive CAD, compared to 70% in men and 40% in women with atypical chest pain *(10)*. We could conclude that using DHCT for excluding coronary calcium yields the best results in middle-aged and elderly patients with chronic atypical chest pain.

CHEST PAIN IN WOMEN

Women have higher rates of false-positive ECG and thallium stress tests. They also show poor predictive value of anginal pains for the prediction of angiographically obstructive coronary disease. Moreover, women have a higher likelihood of alternative mechanisms of chest pain, making the diagnosis of CAD even more difficult than in men. Therefore, chest pain in women still poses a diagnostic challenge. The value of exercise electrocardiography as well as thallium scintigraphy have been questioned in women as a result of the higher frequency of false-positive results *(11)*. The demonstration of normal perfusion by radionuclide test, however, is not always predictive of the absence of CAD or future coronary events *(12)*. We studied 48 symptomatic women (mean age 65 ± 5 yr) referred for coronary angiography because of typical angina, or atypical chest pain with a positive exercise or thalium scintigraphy test *(13)*. Women with angiographically normal coronary arteries had lower TCS than those with CAD, 5.7 ± 11 vs 580 ± 634, respectively. Seven women with angiographically normal CAD demonstrated mild coronary calcification (TCS <50). Of the 11 women without CAC, none had CAD. The absence of CAC on DHCT scans in women >60 yr is highly predictive of normal coronary arteries with 61% sensitivity, 100% specificity, and 85% accuracy. DHCT provides a rapid and reliable noninvasive tool for the diagnosis of normal coronary arteries and may spare unnecessary invasive intervention in a great number of elderly female patients, as well as significant cost savings.

In another study we further evaluated the contribution of DHCT for the detection of diseased coronary arteries in women with anginal pain, positive exercise test, and angiographically normal coronary arteries—"Syndrome X" *(14)*. Eighty-one consecutive women (mean age 64 yr) referred to coronary angiography for chest pain evaluation underwent DHCT. They were divided into three groups according to stress test and angiographic results: Group 1, the "Normal," had a normal exercise test and angiographically normal coronary arteries; Group 2, "Syndrome X," were those with abnormal exercise test and normal coronary arteries; Group 3, the CAD group, comprised women with at least one angiographically diseased vessel. The prevalence of coronary calcification among Syndrome X patients was 63% compared to 96% in women with CAD and 22% in the normal group. The lowest values of TCS were obtained for the normal group. Significantly higher values were found for Syndrome X group, and the highest for the CAD group. This study demonstrates that the majority of women over 50 yr with Syndrome X exhibit calcific coronary atherosclerosis on DHCT. These changes of the coronary artery wall may lead to altered endothelial-dependent vasomotion and reduced coronary flow reserve *(15)*. We believe, therefore, that women with Syndrome X having CAC at DHCT should receive anti-atherosclerotic and probably anti-ischemic therapy.

In many of our patients, DHCT helped the clinician to achieve the accurate diagnosis, as in the following examples:

Case 1—A 58-yr-old asymptomatic subject. He used to perform an ECG stress test each year as a part of an annual check-up program. He has no other risk factors. During the last 6 yr his stress test revealed ST changes, which were interpreted by the cardiologists who performed the tests as false positive. The patient was referred for coronary scan, revealing extensive calcification of the left circumflex artery (Fig. 2). A thallium stress test was than performed, revealing ischemic perfusion defect at the corresponding site. Coronary angiography was recommended. A 90% obstruction of proximal left circumflex was found, which has been successfully opened (Fig. 3A,B).

Comments: This case demonstrates the potential of DHCT in the differentiation between false-positive ECG stress test and true silent ischemia: The target patients are those with or without chest pain who have a positive stress test but a normal thallium scan, or inconclusive tests. The differential diagnosis between false and true ischemia is easier if the clinician knows the coronary calcium score of the patient. The presence of extensive calcification, as shown in this case, favors the presence of obstructive CAD and strengthens the indication for coronary angiography.

Case 2—A 63-yr-old woman. She has hypercholesterolemia and positive family history for CAD. The patient complained of retrosternal chest burning pain and discomfort for 6 yr. She has diaphragmatic hernia. The clinical manifestations raise two main possible origins for her pains: gastric and coronary. She was referred for stress ECG, revealing unequivocal results with 1.5-mm ST depression at high rate. At this point the patient was referred for coronary scanning, upon which no calcium was detected (TCS = 0, Fig. 4A–C). No further cardiac test was done, and no cardiac events were recorded during 5 yr of follow-up.

Comments: Accurate diagnosis of angiographically normal coronary arteries in women over 60 yr old can be achieved by DHCT. This clinical application of the test is based on the well-accepted concept that angiographically obstructive disease is very unlikely in the absence of CAC. Absence of CAC indicates a false-positive ECG stress test and saves the patient from having to undergo coronary angiography.

Case 3—62-yr-old male, asymptomatic, without any other risk factors. He underwent a stress test during his routine annual check-up. (Bruce protocol, 10 min, maximal heart rate 156/min, 12.9 METS). Up-sloping ST depression of 2.5 mm was observed in leads II, III, aVF, V4–V6 without pain. The patient was referred for thallium single photon emission CT (SPECT) by his cardiologist, revealing a suspected small, mild, reversible defect at the distribution of marginal left circumflex. At this point, the cardiologist decided not to order coronary angiography. The patient then consented to undergo DHCT for one of our investigational protocols, revealing very high TCS of 1725 (>95th percentile) with four-vessel calcification, suggesting the presence of obstructive CAD (Fig. 5). Consequently, he was referred for coronary angiography, revealing severe multiple-vessel obstructions with main Lt obstruction of 65%, proximal LAD of 70%, and mid RCA with 85%, leading to a coronary bypass operation.

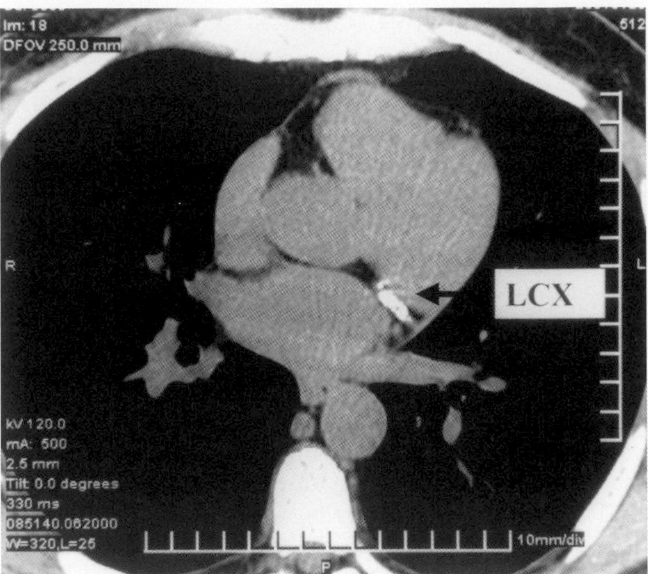

Fig. 2. Heavily calcific left circumflex (LCX) coronary artery.

Comments: This case demonstrates a failure of the stress ECG and thallium SPECT to correctly estimate the severity of CAD. The role of a high coronary calcium score as an indicator of obstructive CAD is emphasized: the DHCT results prompted the cardiologist in this case to perform coronary angiography, which led to the diagnosis of multiple obstructive lesions and resulted in a coronary bypass operation.

It should be remembered, however, that most of the patients with obstructive plaques are symptomatic. According to our experience, the estimated prevalence of extensive CAC in asymptomatic subjects ages 40–60 yr is approx 5%.

Case 4—A 55-yr-old male. Asymptomatic, current smoker. He walks 10 km daily. He performs an annual stress ECG test during a routine check-up. He completed 17 min of the Bruce protocol up to the maximal predictive heart rate without any limiting symptoms or ECG ischemic changes. He consented to undergo DHCT for one of our investigational protocols. Extensive calcification was found, with TCS = 1350 (Fig. 6A–C). Consequently, he was referred for thallium SPECT, which was completely normal; further diagnostic procedures were not recommended. During 2 yr of follow-up, the patient remained asymptomatic and has not sustained a coronary event.

Comments: This case demonstrates that extensive CAC may be present without any clinical signs of obstructive CAD. An angiographically patent lumen may be observed despite the presence of extensive CAC within the vessel wall. This can be explained by the Glagov remodeling phenomenon *(16)*.

The presence of extensive calcification (above the 90th percentile) in asymptomatic subjects requires thallium stress test. If thallium is normal, coronary angiography is not recommended.

Case 5—A 75-yr-old woman, hypertensive and hypercholesterolemic. She complained of chest pain for 15 yr and has deep negative T waves in the precordial leads of her ECG. Echocardiography revealed concentric LVH. Her cardiologist

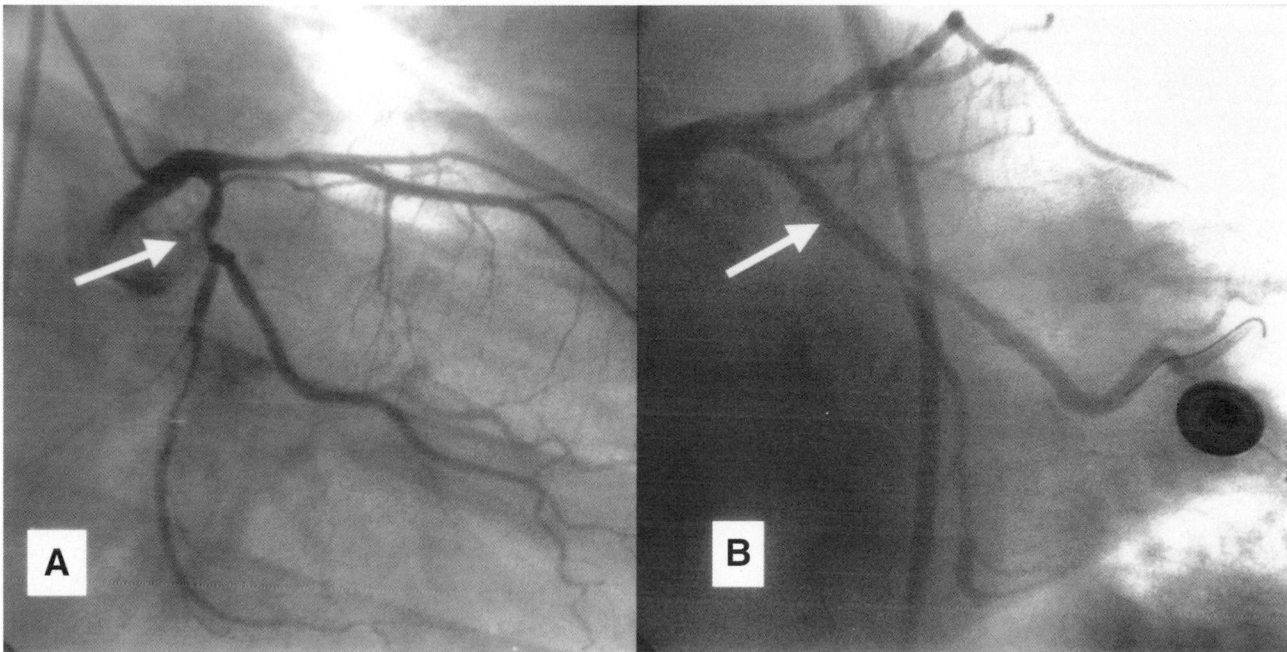

Fig. 3. Heavily calcific left circumflex coronary artery (*see* Fig. 2) led to angiography, which revealed >90% obstruction at the corresponding portion of the vessel (**A**). Successful angioplasty was performed (**B**).

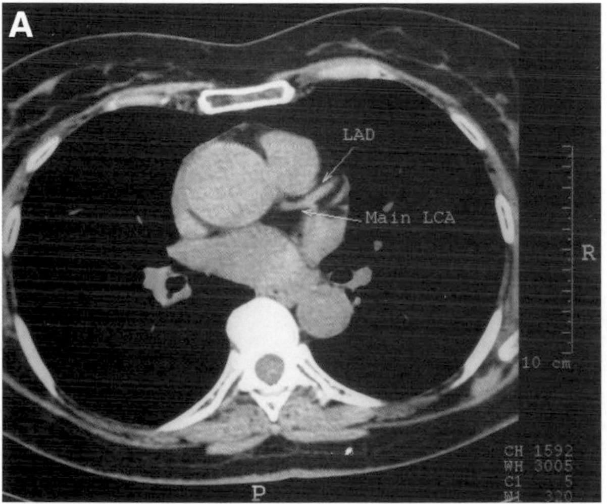

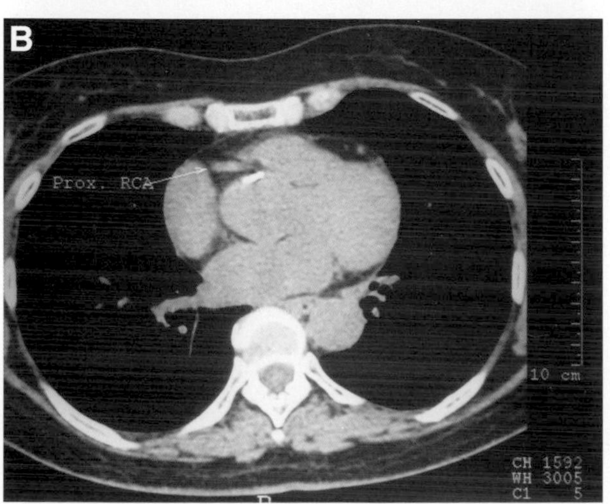

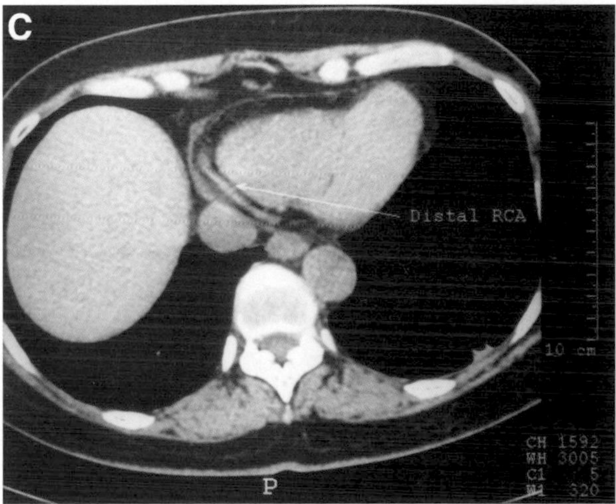

Fig. 4. Coronary vessel without calcifications. (**A**) Main left coronary (main LCA) and left anterior descending (LAD) arteries. (**B**) Proximal right coronary artery (RCA). (**C**) Distal RCA.

suspected a concomitant obstructive CAD with previous silent non-q-wave MI. He recommended thallium SPECT, which was nonconclusive with a small perfusion defect, interpreted as breast attenuation artifact. At this point the cardiologist considered coronary angiography. We suggested performing a DHCT. The scan was done and revealed no CAC (Fig. 7); further diagnostic tests were not recommended. The patient has now completed 6 yr of follow-up and has not sustained a coronary event.

Comments: This case emphasizes the negative predictive value of DHCT. The absence of CAC in a 75-yr-old woman made the diagnosis of angiographically obstructive CAD very

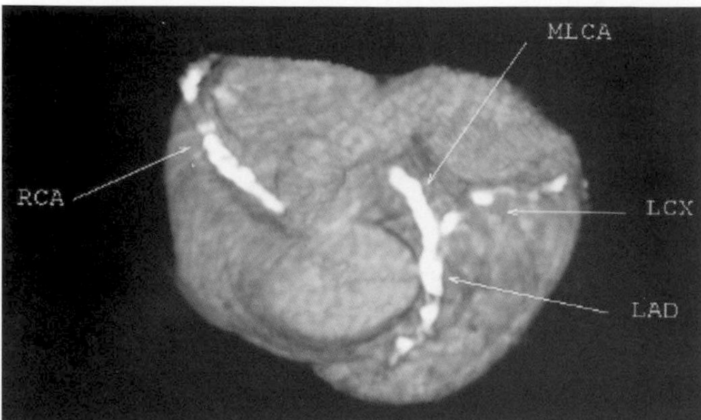

Fig. 5. Three-dimensional reconstruction of the heart with extensive coronary calcification. MLCA, main left coronary artery; LAD, left anterior descending artery; LCX, left circumflex artery; RCA, right coronary artery.

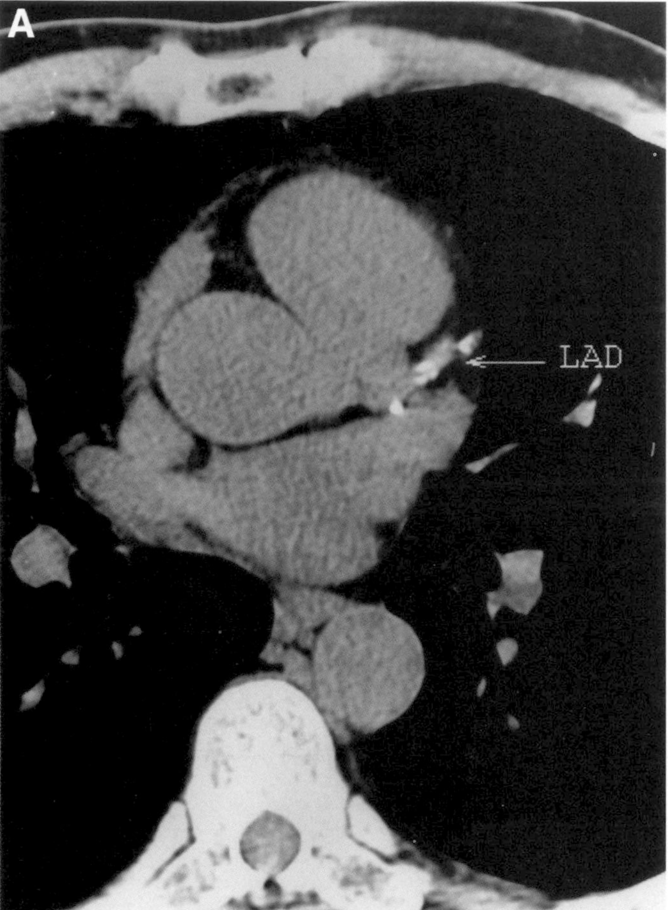

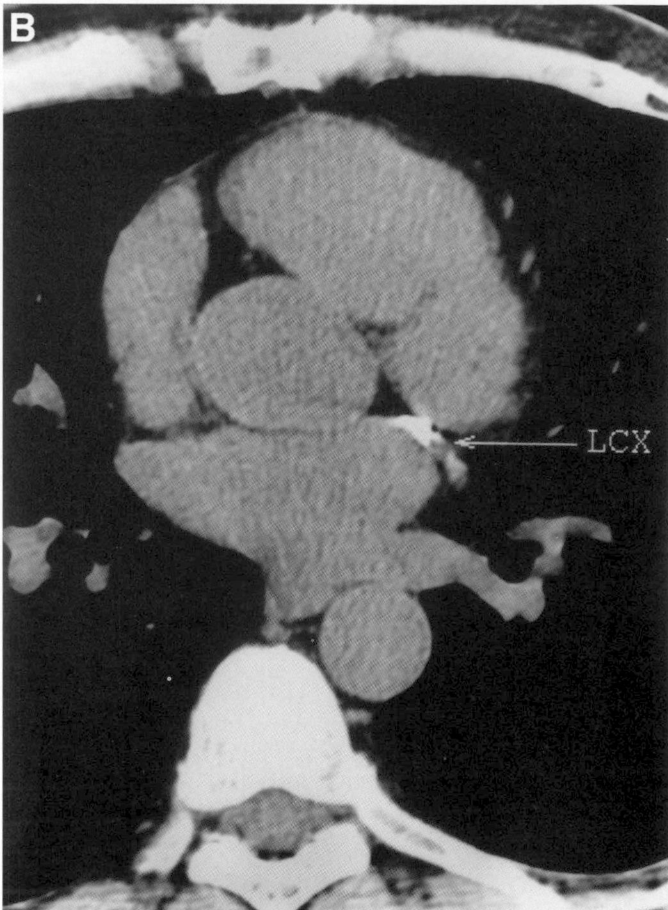

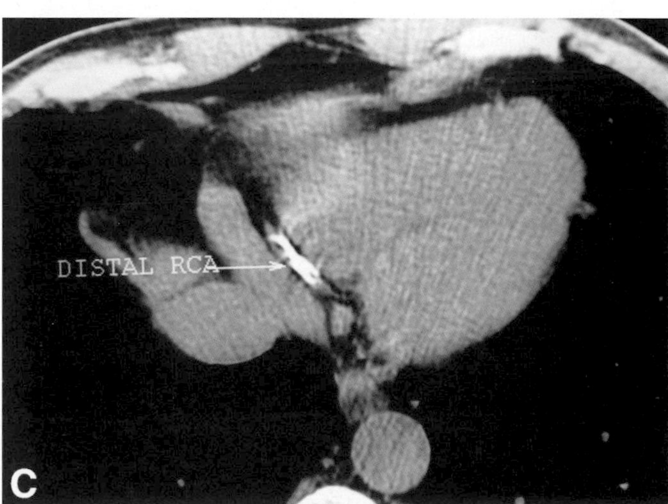

Fig. 6. Extensive coronary calcifications may be present without symptoms, as in this 55-yr-old male patient. **(A)** Left anterior descending (LAD). **(B)** Left circumflex coronary artery (LCX). **(C)** Distal right coronary artery (RCA).

unlikely. The deep negative T waves of the woman reflects her left-ventricular hypertrophy.

Coronary CT may also help the diagnosis of co-existing CAD in patients with atrial fibrillation *(17)* or CLBBB. The main limitations of the use of DHCT for chest-pain evaluation are in patients younger than 50 yr who might have noncalcific CAD, and in cases of acute chest pain, which may be the consequence of soft-plaque rupture. (In our studies, up to 19% of patients with first AMI had no CAC on DHCT; the younger the patient, the higher this percentage may be.)

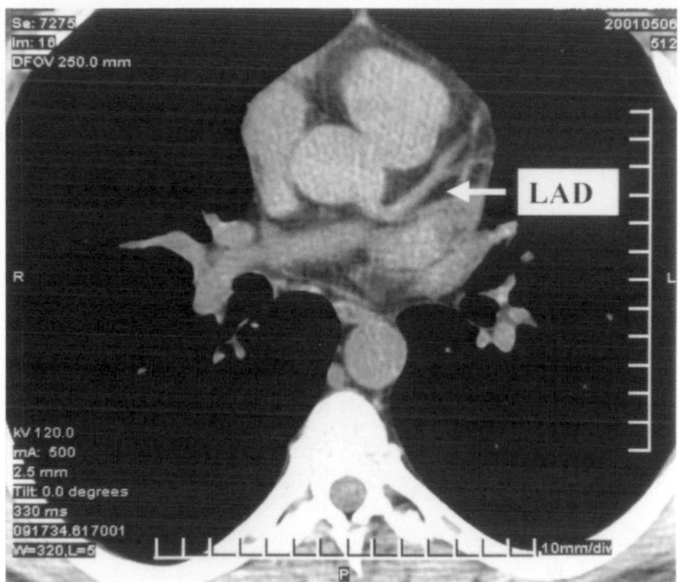

Fig. 7. Absence of calcium excludes the presence of concomitant obstructive coronary artery disease in a 75-yr-old female with hypertrophic cardiomyopathy. LAD, left anterior descending artery.

In summary: Coronary calcium scoring can help the clinician to confirm the presence of CAD and to inform him about its extent. Further diagnostic procedures can be used more efficiently, reducing costs by saving unnecessary procedures.

The test is useful to exclude obstructive CAD in patients older than 50 yr with chronic atypical chest pain, particularly in women, due to their higher prevalence of false-positive stress tests.

DIAGNOSIS OF ISCHEMIC ETIOLOGY OF DILATIVE CARDIOMYOPATHY OF UNKNOWN ORIGIN

The etiology of dilative cardiomyopathy (DCMP) is important for both therapeutic and prognostic implications, but the differential diagnosis may still be difficult after evaluation of the clinical data and generally requires coronary angiography. We have demonstrated that the presence or absence of CAC on DHCT provides a useful tool in differentiating between ischemic and nonischemic DCMP in middle-aged patients *(18)*. Thirty-two consecutive patients with DCMP who underwent coronary angiography were scanned. Thirteen patients (mean age 60 ± 8) had nonischemic DCMP with normal coronary arteries, whereas 19 (mean age 60 ± 6) exhibited ischemic DCMP with at least two obstructed vessels. CAC was found in all patients with ischemic DCMP and was absent in 12 of the 13 with nonischemic DCMP. The presence of CAC on DHCT can thus identify ischemic DCMP with a sensitivity of 100%, specificity of 92%, and total accuracy of 97%, providing a reliable noninvasive tool for the differential diagnosis of ischemic from nonischemic DCMP. The results of this study were reproduced by Budoff et al. on EBCT *(19)*.

TRACKING THE PROGRESSION OF THE CORONARY ATHEROSCLEROTIC PROCESS

DHCT CAN ACCURATELY TRACK THE CALCIUM PROGRESSION

Studies of the progression of coronary atherosclerosis have hitherto been limited to invasive angiographic techniques among symptomatic patients. The ability to quantify coronary atherosclerosis by a simple noninvasive technique provides clinicians and researchers with a simple method to monitor the effect of anti-atherosclerotic treatment. We have demonstrated the accuracy of DHCT in tracking the progression of CC as measured during a 3-yr follow-up *(20)* (Fig. 8). Ninety-four of the 246 patients who entered the study had no calcium (TCS = 0). Among the 152 with calcium (TCS >0), 33 had minimal amounts of calcium (TCS 1–9), and 119 had a total score >9; 60 of them (50%) had baseline TCS <100 and 75% had TCS <250. The mean TCS of the patients with calcium increased significantly each year from 245 at baseline to 288, 322, and 349 at the end of the first, second, and third year of follow-up (p for trend <0.01). This corresponds to a percent change from baseline TCS of 33, 71, and 117% respectively. This progression of calcium was not related to age, sex, or any other risk factor by univariant analysis. The incidence of 3 yr progression of calcium was almost three times higher among the patients with calcium at baseline compared to those without calcium: 70% (106/152) compared to 28% (26/94). All the 33 patients with baseline minimal amounts of calcium (TCS <9) had detectable calcium at follow-up, with increasing mean TCS from 3.8 ± 0.45 to 14.9 ± 2.7. We found that baseline TCS is a very strong predictor of the follow-up TCS. This was found by other researchers who used EBCT *(21)* and described by Yoon and colleagues *(22)* as "calcium begets calcium."

CLINICAL SIGNIFICANCE OF CAC PROGRESSION

We investigated the hypothesis that a higher progression rate of CAC is related to cardiac events, in a cohort of hypertensive patients who were followed during a period of 3 yr *(23)*. One hundred sixty-eight consecutive hypertensive patients who underwent annual CT scans over a 3-yr period were selected among the 547 participants of the INSIGHT calcification side arm study *(24)*. Patients were divided into three groups:

1. Asymptomatic with prominent atherosclerotic risk factors (n = 116).
2. Patients with clinical CAD at baseline (n = 28) ("Stable CAD").
3. Patients who sustained a coronary event (n = 24) during follow-up ("Event").

Clinical CAD was defined as previous myocardial infarction, typical AP with positive stress test, or positive coronary angiography (>50% lumen obstruction in at least one epicardial vessel). Coronary events were AMI, unstable AP, sudden death, hospitalization for increased preexisting angina, coronary angiography, coronary angioplasty, or coronary bypass operation. The progression of CAC was calculated as percent increase from baseline total coronary calcium score. A significant annual progression of total coronary calcium score was

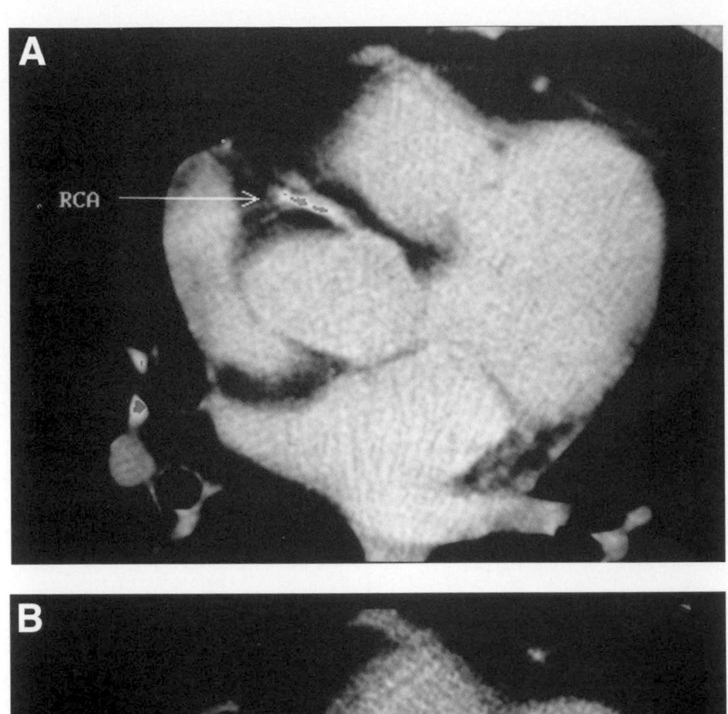

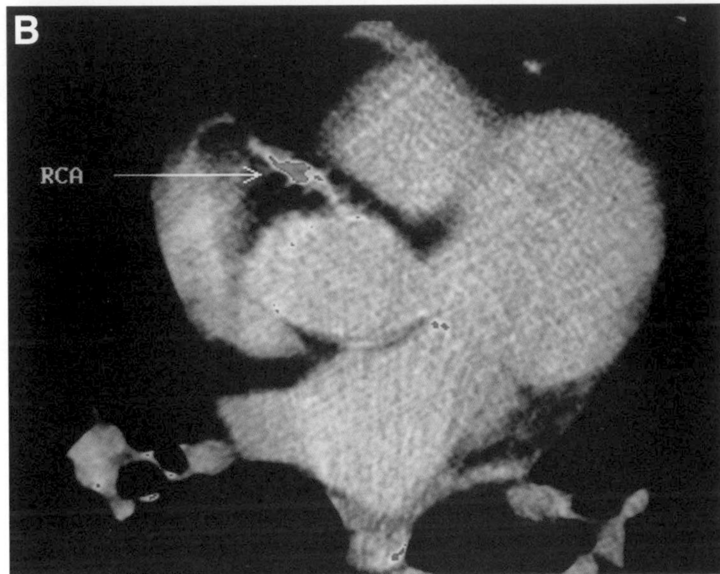

Fig. 8. Progression of coronary calcium. Two spotty lesions at baseline in the proximal right coronary artery (RCA) (**A**), with significant increase after 3 yr (**B**).

observed within each of the three study groups ($p < 0.01$). Both patients with stable CAD and asymptomatic patients with a stable rate of CAC developed a coronary event. There was a higher progression rate at the end of follow-up of patients who sustained a coronary event compared to those who did not: 180% vs 124 in asymptomatic and 118% in the group of stable CAD ($p < 0.05$).

Prevalence, extent and annual progression of CAC in patients with documented CAD are significantly higher than in asymptomatic subjects. The mean annualized percent of progression in asymptomatics is 15%, and three times higher (47%) in patients with CAD. These results sharpen the importance of excluding patients with documented CAD from studies designed to evaluate interventional effects and prognostic value of CAC in asymptomatic populations.

PROGRESSION UNDER INTERVENTION

Using DHCT we have been able to demonstrate different progression rates of CAC over a 3-yr period, in hypertensive patients treated by nifedipine once daily vs co-amilozide following the protocol of the INSIGHT study *(24)*. A total of 201 patients with a TCS > 9 at the onset of the study underwent an annual DSCT for 3 yr. Coronary calcium progression was significantly lower in the group treated by nifedipine as compared to the co-amilozide group, 40% vs 78% at the third year.

PROGRESSION IN TRANSPLANTED HEARTS

Tracking the progression of allograft atherosclerosis in heart transplant recipients is currently accomplished using invasive techniques. We used DHCT to track CAC progression in 24 consecutive heart transplant patients *(25)*. The first scan was performed 1.9 ± 1.3 yr after transplantation. After 2 yr of follow-up, 4 died and the remaining 20 patients underwent a second scan. The incidence of CAC at the first scan was 4.2% and increased to 40% at the second scan. We could identify very mild new spotty lesions with a mean TCS of 6.7. Our findings confirm the results of previous studies done by Barbir and colleagues using EBCT on 102 heart transplant recipients. They found calcific lesions in 45% of the patients with a similar minimal amount of CAC *(26)*.

Spiral CT can be a noninvasive alternative for the detection of newly developed atherosclerotic changes in heart transplant recipients. The delayed appearance of CAC in heart transplants suggests that CT should be done no less than 2 yr after transplantation.

SUMMARY

Evaluation of chest pain, diagnosis of false-positive ST changes upon stress test, diagnosis of obstructive CAD, and evaluation of the effect of anti-atherosclerotic treatment constitute a major part of the daily clinical practice. We have demonstrated that a comprehensive use of DHCT substantially contributes to these topics. The accordance between data obtained from DHCT and EBCT devices in many of these subjects indicates that for clinical practice, coronary calcium detection and measurement is relevant regardless of the device or the technique used. We strongly believe that our and others' results demonstrate the usefulness of the new multislice spiral CT devices. The differentiation between minimal, mild, moderate, and extensive CAC is universal. The numerical scale of each category should be individualized to each specific device after the most accurate and reproducible protocol has been defined.

Essential questions such as whom to refer for this test, for which diagnostic question, how to interpret the results, and the contribution of the test for better treatment of the patients should be further discussed.

REFERENCES

1. Stary HC. The development of calcium deposits in atherosclerotic lesions and their persistence after lipid regression. Am J Cardiol 2001;88:16–19
2. Fuster V. Mechanisms leading to myocardial infarction: insights from studies of vascular biology. Circulation 1994;90:2126–2146.
3. Shemesh J, Stroh CI, Tenenbaum A, et al. Comparison of coronary calcium in stable angina pectoris and in first acute myocardial infarction utilizing double helical computerized tomography. Am J Cardiol 1998;81:271–275.
4. Shemesh J, Apter S, Itzchak Y, Motro M. Coronary calcification compared in patients with acute versus in those with chronic coronary events using dual-sector spiral CT. Radiology 2003;226:483–488.
5. Shemesh J, Apter S, Rozenman J, et al. Calcification of coronary arteries: detection and quantification with double helix CT. Radiology 1995;197:779–783.
6. Broderick LS, Shemesh J, Wilensky RL, et al. Measurement of coronary artery calcium with double helical CT compared to coronary angiography: evaluation of CT scoring methods, interobserver variation, and reproducibility. AJR Am J Roentgenol 1996;167: 439–444.
7. Sekiya M, Mukai M, Suzuke M, et al. Clinical significance of the calcification of coronary arteries in patients with angiographically normal coronary arteries. Angiology 1992;43:401–407.
8. Brahmajee KN, Saint S, Bielak LF, Sonnad SS, Peyser PA, Rubenfire M, Fendrick M. Electron-beam computed tomography in the diagnosis of coronary artery disease: a meta-analysis. Arch Intern Med 2001;161:833–838.
9. Shemesh J, Weg N, Tenenbaum A et al. Usefulness of spiral computed tomography (dual-slice mode) for the detection of coronary artery calcium in patient with chronic atypical chest pain, in typical angina pectoris, and in asymptomatic subjects with prominent atherosclerotic risk factors. Am J Cardiol 2001;87:226–228.
10. DeSanctis RW. Clinical manifestations of coronary artery disease: chest pain in women. In: Wenger NK, Speroff L, and Packard B (eds), Cardiovascular Health and Disease in Women. Le Jack Communications, Greenwich, CT: 1993;67.
11. Hung J, Chaitman BR, Lam J, et al. Non-invasive diagnostic test choices for the evaluation of coronary artery disease in women: a multivariate comparison of cardiac fluoroscopy, exercise electrocardiography, and exercise thallium myocardial scintigraphy. J Am Coll Cardiol 1984;4:8–16.
12. Niemeyer MG, Van Der Wall EE, Kuyper AF, et al. Discordance of visual and quantitative analysis regarding false negative and false positive test results in thallium-201 myocardial perfusion scintigraphy. Am J Physiol Imaging 1991;6:34–43.
13. Shemesh J, Tenenbaum A, Fisman EZ, et al. Absence of coronary calcification on double helical CT scans: predictor of angiographic normal coronary arteries in elderly women? Radiology 1996;199: 665–668.
14. Shemesh J, Fisman EZ, Tenenbaum A, et al. Coronary artery calcification in women with syndrome X: usefulness of double helical CT for detection. Radiology 1997;205:697–700.
15. Gage JE, Hess OM, Murakami T, et al. Vasoconstriction of stenotic coronary arteries during dynamic exercise in patients with classic angina pectoris: reversibility by nitroglycerin. Circulation 1986;73: 865–876.
16. Glagov S, Weisenberg E, Zarins CK, Stankunavicius R, Kolettis GJ. Compensatory enlargement of human atherosclerotic coronary arteries. New Engl J Med 1996:316:1371–1375
17. Stroh CI, Shemesh J, Motro M. Using fast CT to exclude CAD in elderly women (60 and above). N Engl J Med 1996;335 (8):595.
18. Shemesh J, Tenenbaum A, Fisman EZ, et al. Coronary calcium as a reliable tool for differentiating ischemic from nonischemic cardiomyopathy. Am J Cardiol 1995;77:191–194.
19. Budoff MJ, Shavelle DM, Lamont DH, Kim HT, Akinwale P, Kennedy JM, Brundage BH.Usefulness of electron beam computed tomography scanning for distinguishing ischemic from nonischemic cardiomyopathy. J Am Coll Cardiol 1998;32(5):1173–1178.
20. Shemesh J, Apter S, Stroh CI, Itzchak Y, Motro M. Tracking coronary calcification by using dual-section spiral CT: a 3-year follow-up. Radiology 2000;217:461–465.
21. Schmermund A, Baumgart D, Möhlenkamp S, et al. Natural history and topographic pattern of progression of coronary calcification in symptomatic patients: an electron beam CT study. Arterioscler Thromb Vasc Biol 2001;3:421–426.
22. Yoon HC, Emerick AM, Hill JA, Gjertson DW, Goldin JG. Calcium begets calcium: progression of coronary artery calcification in asymptomatic subjects. Radiology 2002;224:236–241.
23. Shemesh J, Apter S, Stolero D, Itzchak Y, Motro M. Annual progression of coronary artery calcium by spiral computed tomography in hypertensive patients without myocardial ischemia but with prominent atherosclerotic risk facors, in patients with previous angina pectoris or acute myocardial infarction which healed, and in patients with coronary events during follow-up. Am J Cardiol 2001; 87:1935–1937.
24. Motro M, Shemesh J. Calcium channel blocker nifedipine slows down progression of coronary calcification in hypertensive patients compared with diuretics. Hyprtension 2001;37:1410–1413.
25. Shemesh J, Tenenbaum A, Stroh CI, et al. Double helical CT as a new tool for tracking of allograft atherosclerosis in heart transplant recipients. Invest Radiol 1999;32:503–506.
26. Barbir M, Lazem F, Bowker T et al. Determinant of transplanted coronary calcium detected by ultrafast computed tomography scanning. Am J Cardiol 1997;79:1606–1609.

11 Detection and Quantification of Calcified Coronary Plaque With Multidetector-Row CT

J. Jeffrey Carr, MD, MSCE

INTRODUCTION

Multidetector-row computed tomography (MDCT) has rapidly developed into a powerful tool for noninvasive measurement of calcified plaque in the coronary arteries over the past decade. Identification and quantification of coronary artery calcifications (CAC) with X-ray devices is well established in the literature with chest radiographs, fluoroscopy, computed tomography (CT without electrocardiogram [ECG] gating) and cardiac CT (electron beam CT [EBCT], helical CT, and MDCT with cardiac gating) *(1–6)*. Calcified plaque is an established component of coronary atherosclerosis, and radiographic techniques are highly sensitive to calcified atherosclerotic plaque *(1,7)*. The presence of calcified plaque documents the presence of subclinical atherosclerosis in the coronary artery. Calcified plaque is an active and regulated process occurring in the vessel wall, with pathways similar to those of bone metabolism *(8,9)*. As of 2003, two consensus documents *(1,10)* concerning cardiac CT and the recommendations of the Prevention V Conference *(11)* are available to guide clinical application. The results of several large epidemiological studies, as well as pharmaceutical trials, will become available during the next five years and will provide new information to guide the medical community and society at large as to the appropriate utilization of CAC screening in the population.

Cardiac CT is rapidly transitioning from a research tool with modest clinical application to a diagnostic test integral in our management of cardiovascular disease. There is increasing evidence that cardiac CT applied to measuring CAC will be effective in the risk stratification of individuals asymptomatic for cardiovascular disease (CVD), as will be discussed later in this chapter. The rapid development of the cardiac-gated MDCT techniques was made possible through the pioneering work performed with EBCT in the 1980s and 1990s. Technological advances in engineering, manufacturing, and computer sciences made possible the current-generation MDCT systems. The strengths of cardiac CT and, specifically, MDCT, are detailed in the technical chapters, but are based on high spatial resolution, volumetric coverage, high temporal resolution, rapid scan times, high patient productivity, robust protocols, consistent results, and high patient acceptance. In this chapter we will review the history of MDCT for the measurement of CAC, discuss the technical aspects and various implementations of MDCT protocols for measuring CAC, and review scientific results published and in-progress with cardiac CT and MDCT specifically.

EVOLUTION OF HELICAL CT TO CARDIAC-GATED MDCT

The ability to identify the heart and calcifications related to the coronary arteries was noted even with early-generation CT scanners, despite insufficient temporal resolution to stop cardiac motion *(12,13)*. The motion of the heart blurred anatomic detail related to the coronary arteries and cardiac chambers. The development of slip-ring CT technology, which enabled spiral or helical CT scanning, dramatically improved the temporal resolution of mechanical CT systems. Increased gantry speed provided improved temporal resolution and greater scan coverage per unit time, which facilitated protocols incorporating suspended respiration *(14)*. When CT gantries capable of 1 s were possible, the nongated ECG scans through the chest clearly demonstrated improved cardiac and coronary morphology, and strategies for quantifying CAC were developed *(2,15,16)*. Cardiac gating of helical CT exams using a helical acquisition was first coupled with low-pitch overlapping reconstruction algorithms designed to maximize temporal resolution and create multilevel, multiphase images of the entire coronary circulation. *(17)*. Synchronized recording of the ECG tracing during the scan acquisition allowed the images to be aligned with the ECG tracing of cardiac activity. This retrospective ECG gating was performed after the scan was acquired (i.e., postexam processing) on a computer workstation, and allowed the user or computer algorithm to select the appropriate diastolic phase image for measuring CAC (Fig. 1). The introduction of the 0.8-s gantry rotation and higher heat unit X-ray tubes made possible a more clinically feasible study with further improved image quality. The 0.8-s gantry rotation resulted in cardiac imaging with a temporal resolution of 520 ms per image, and the high heat unit tube meant that the scans could be obtained in clinical practice without extended wait periods for tube cooling. This first-generation cardiac-gated helical CT technique allowed scanning the entire heart in a single breath-hold ranging from 30 to 50 s, depending on heart rate, which determined the helical pitch *(4)*.

From: *Contemporary Cardiology: CT of the Heart: Principles and Applications*
Edited by: U. Joseph Schoepf © Humana Press, Inc., Totowa, NJ

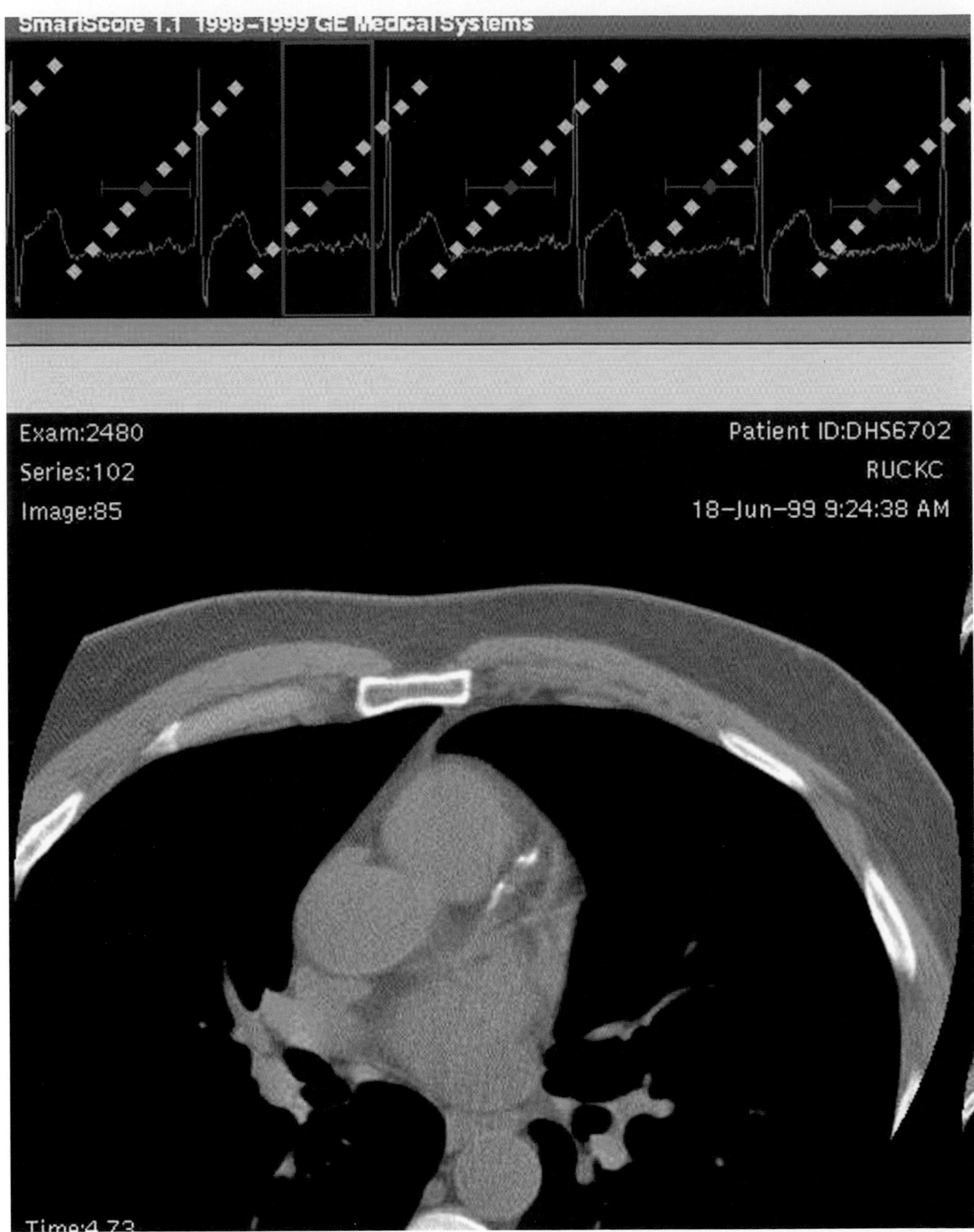

Fig. 1. Retrospective gating with a single-slice helical CT system. The image is from a retrospectively gated helical scan performed in June of 1999 (General Electric Medical Systems)—CTi, with 0.8-s gantry, SmartScore calcium scoring package on the Advantage Windows workstation). Overlapping images are reconstructed throughout each cardiac cycle, represented by the gray diamonds. An automated selection algorithm picks the diastolic phase image at a preprogrammed percentage of the cardiac cycle (red diamond) and is displayed in the image window below the electrocardiogram (ECG) tracing. As discussed in the text, images are obtained throughout the cardiac cycle, resulting in significantly higher exposure than in a prospectively triggered sequential protocol. Modern multidetector-row CT systems obtain multiple channels of data simultaneously (4, 8, 12, or 16, depending on model). However, like the single-slice helical CT system, the helical reconstruction algorithm requires data throughout the scan, and thus the X-ray tube is on continuously. ECG dose modulation is available and reduces tube current during systole to improve the dose profile of the study. However, even with tube modulation, prospective triggering results in the lowest dose profile while maintaining comparable image-quality factors. Calcified plaques are demonstrated in the left anterior descending coronary artery.

The studies comparing the single-slice scanners with ECG gating demonstrated high correlation and good agreement between calcium scores obtained with that generation of EBCT systems (C150) and the single-slice helical CT systems *(3,4,18–20)*. This new capability for helical CT came with limitations. First, the overlapping reconstructions resulted in a large number of images—typically 450–600 images per scan series. The large number of images required significant computational resources to reconstruct the images, and this process would often have to be completed offline to reduce impact on patient throughput on the CT scanner. The scans also tended to result in relatively long breath-holds, ranging from 35 to 50 s. With the single-slice helical CT, the breath-hold time was dependent upon the patient's heart rate, which was used to set the speed of the CT couch as it moved the patient through the scanner. The single-slice helical CT exam was dose-inefficient in that the patient was irradiated for the entire cardiac cycle, but only a few cardiac phases at most were utilized for calcium scoring. Prospective ECG triggering was developed and tested on these systems, but the application was limited by long scan times, which required multiple breath-holds to image the entire heart *(3)*. Nonetheless, single-slice helical CT systems operating with effective temporal resolutions of 520 ms demonstrated the capability of mechanical CT scanners to accurately and reproducibly measure CAC with comparable measurement error to EBCT. Direct comparison of helical CT and EBCT with individuals receiving paired scans on each system demonstrated no statistically significant difference in the interexam or intraobserver variability when using the standard 130-Hounsfield unit (HU) threshold *(21)*. The foundation developed for single-slice helical CT was critical for developing cardiac applications, reconstruction algorithms, ECG and non-ECG gating strategies, and postprocessing for the revolution in CT—the introduction of multislice scanners.

MDCT SYSTEMS—APPLICATION TO CORONARY CALCIUM MEASUREMENT

The introduction of the four-channel MDCT systems created new possibilities for cardiac imaging. The ability to acquire four 2.5-mm slices results in covering 10 mm along the z axis with each heart beat. The entire heart, typically 120 mm in z axis length, could be imaged with only 12 movements of the CT couch. For the first time the entire heart could be covered with prospective ECG gating in a clinically acceptable breath-hold time. The initial release of the four-channel MDCT systems had gantry rotations of 0.8 s, although this was followed by systems with gantry rotation speeds of 0.5, 0.42, and 0.4 s, resulting in temporal resolutions ranging from 520 to 240 ms when scanning in the cardiac mode (i.e., partial scan reconstruction). The MDCT scanner is operated in the sequential scan mode (on some systems this is called axial or cine scan mode), resulting in significantly less radiation exposure than the helical approach utilizing retrospective ECG gating. This approach is fundamentally identical to calcium screening protocols implemented with EBCT systems that also utilize a "step-and-shoot" sequential scan technique.

The basic operation of a MDCT system for sequential CAC study with prospective ECG gating is the same whether it is 4, 8, or 16 slices. The operator prescribes the start and end locations based on the scout image of the thorax. The MDCT scanner moves the CT couch so that the first block of 4, 8, or 16 images is appropriately positioned inside the gantry. The scan sequence is started by the breathing instructions, and the first block of images is obtained at the prescribed offset from the R wave on the ECG. In the sequential mode, the X-ray beam is on for only a very brief exposure at each level. For a 0.5-s gantry system this time is slightly more than the number of views required to reconstruct an image, and is typically in the range of 330–360 ms, depending upon manufacturer. For a General Electric LightSpeed™ 8 or 16 MDCT with a 0.5-s gantry, the X-ray exposure time is only 2 s for the entire scan. During the majority of the 10–20-s scan time, the X-ray tube is off because the CT couch is moving to the next location or the CT is waiting for the appropriate cardiac phase. Upon completion of the first set of images, the CT couch then moves the patient to the next block of scans along the z axis. This movement occurs during the second cardiac cycle, which then allows the second block of slices to be obtained during the third cardiac cycle of the breath hold. This sequence of acquiring and skipping a heartbeat continues until all the prescribed scan locations have been completed.

As of 2003, MDCT systems use various detector arrays with a length along the z axis of 20 mm. For the MDCT(4) systems, a 4 × 2.5-mm slice protocol uses the center 10 mm of the detector. The introduction of the MDCT(8) and MDCT(16) systems allowed scans for coronary calcium using an 8 × 2.5-mm configuration, thus utilizing the entire 20-mm width of the detector array. A comparison of MDCT systems is presented in Table 1. The direct benefits of this for coronary calcium scanning are the reduction in reduced breath-hold time to 10–20 s as opposed to 20–40 with MDCT(4). Only six CT couch translations and thus only 6 cardiac cycles—as opposed to 12 with MDCT(4)—are needed to image the entire heart, which improves the image quality by reduced variability related to cardiac beat-to-beat variations, improved slice registration along the z axis, and reduced patient dose through improved dose efficiency.

One way to conceptualize prospective ECG gating with MDCT is to mentally construct the "ideal" CT device, in which a detector covers the entire heart. This system might have 48 channels or rows (i.e., capable of 2.5-mm slices × 48 levels = 128-mm detector) through the use of either a panel or dramatically expanded matrix array detector *(22,23)*. To measure coronary calcium with a similar protocol to today's CT systems, the hypothetical "MDCT(48)" scanner would operate in the sequential mode and acquire 48 slices, each 2.5 mm thick, within a single heart beat. If we assume no further improvement in gantry rotation speeds beyond 0.4 s and utilize the current partial scan reconstruction algorithm, then scan acquisition and breath-hold time would be 250 ms! The entire coronary arterial tree would be acquired within a 250-ms phase of a single cardiac cycle, and no movement of the patient by the CT couch

Table 1
Comparison of MDCT Multislice Capability on Scan Time—Sequential Scan Mode With Prospective ECG Gating

Multislice capability	*Slice thickness (mm)*	*Slab thickness (mm)*	*Slabs per 120 mm coverage*	*Scan time (s)*
1	2.5	2.5	48	80–160
4	2.5	10	12	20–40
8	2.5	20	6	10–20
8 or 16	2.5 or 1.25	20		
20	6	10–20		
48	*2.5*	*120*	*1*	*0.24*

Slab thickness roughly corresponds to beam collimation; however, the beam must be slightly wider than the nominal detector configuration. Current 16-channel systems are limited in their z axis coverage by the 20-mm width of the detector. These systems can typically acquire in either an 8-slice mode (8 × 2.5 mm) or 16-slice (16 × 1.25 mm) with increased spatial resolution in the slice direction (z axis). The hypothetical 48-slice MDCT system is provided as an example of how the increasing size of the detector along the z axis will impact future cardiac CT protocols. Numerous technical challenges remain to be solved before this type of system or some variant is ready for clinical applications.

would be required. "Sequential" would be a misnomer, since only one block or set of 48 images would be obtained. By acquiring all levels or slices of the coronary tree in a single heartbeat, slice misregistration related to beat-to-beat coronary motion, breath-holding, and voluntary patient motion would be eliminated. A more likely scenario is that this enhanced imaging capability would be coupled with more sophisticated reconstruction algorithms, providing either enhanced temporal resolution or increased coverage of cardiac motion (multiphase imaging) or both to varying degrees.

MDCT systems will continue to rapidly develop new capabilities focused on cardiac imaging, based in large part on the intense global competition between CT manufacturers. Based on the rapid developments with CT of the past decade, it is foolhardy to speculate what capabilities may be available to cardiac imagers even in the near future from the descendents of today's MDCT systems. It is clear that future MDCT systems will incorporate enhanced resolution both temporal and spatial, greater coverage of the heart, new methods for cardiac motion compensation, dose reduction techniques, scan reconstruction and postprocessing applications specifically designed for cardiac imaging. What remains unknown is when, and what impact these advances in cardiac imaging with CT will have on clinical management.

MEASURING CALCIFIED CORONARY PLAQUE WITH CARDIAC CT

In quantifying the amount of calcified plaque in the coronary arteries, the CT system is acting as a measurement device. Something common to all measurement techniques is the presence of measurement error. Comparison of two measurements will by definition incorporate the combined errors of the two measurements. The problems associated with comparing a new technique to an established technique are well documented in medical and statistical literature *(24,25)*. Accuracy is defined as how well the instrument is calibrated to the true value of the object being measured. Precision indicates the degree of refinement of the reported value. Thus a measurement can have high precision (alternatively, highly reproducible or refined), providing nearly the same value on multiple measurements but biased from the true value. Likewise a device can be well calibrated but have significant variability, resulting in decreased precision. Most importantly, the degree of accuracy and precision must be appropriate for the desired task. Fortunately, cardiac CT can measure plaque burden with high accuracy and good precision in the range of values for which clinical decisions are likely to be made, based on existing outcomes data. Specifically, EBCT and MDCT have extremely good measurement characteristics for plaque burden above Agatston scores of 50. More problematic, as will be discussed later, are the low scores, where detection and image noise issues have been shown to negatively impact the ability to measure calcified plaques. Likewise, changes in calcium scores over short time intervals can easily be shown in groups of patients, with reasonable statistical power; however, tracking change in CAC in an individual over a year requires significantly greater precision and accuracy.

CT was developed as a medical imaging device, with less emphasis on quantification of the X-ray attenuation values (a.k.a. CT numbers or HU). The CT attenuation values extend from –1000 to +4000. CT number 0 is calibrated to water, –1000 to air, +1000 to dense bone, and >1000 to metal objects. Limitations in the CT scanners' ability to measure small calcified objects were established early in the history of CT, during attempts to quantify calcification in pulmonary nodules. Since this effort, there has been significant improvement in the CT system stability and quality control over the past decade *(26)*.

When comparing CT devices (EBCT vs EBCT, MDCT vs MDCT, or EBCT vs MDCT) an understanding of the influences of accuracy and precision are important to understand any observed differences. Significant variability in the measurement of coronary calcium between EBCT systems at the same site maintained and calibrated by the same engineers has been reported with the 130 HU threshold varying between 77.1

and 136.4 mg/cm^3 of calcium hydroxyapatite *(27)*. Likewise, when replicate calcium determinations are performed using EBCT, significant measurement error has been documented. Mean interscan variability using the Agatston scoring method has ranged from 18 to 43%, and there remains debate about the impact of a 40% vs 80% phase for image acquisition *(28–32)*. The nature of the calcium score and the range of values from 0 to greater than 10,000 requires an understanding that the measurement error changes based on the amount of calcified plaque; a more detailed analysis using methods proposed by Bland to determine limits of agreement is indicated and has been performed by some researchers *(24,33)*. Comparable degrees of measurement error, as will be discussed later, have been documented for MDCT. It must be remembered that if one measurement device is labeled the "gold standard," all comparison instruments will have the error inherent in the gold standard included and in some cases erroneously attributed as error related to the comparison device. The measurement error is related to the physiology of the heart and the size of the calcified plaques we are measuring with the CT systems. Specifically, we are asking the CT system to measure relatively small calcified plaques located on 3-mm or smaller coronary arteries using a slice collimation of 2.5–3 mm, depending on CT system. This results in partial volume averaging of the plaque within or between two slices, which can dramatically alter the CT numbers of the plaque. In addition, motion blurring is present with EBCT and to a greater extent with MDCT. Blurring of the plaque secondary to coronary motion is most common in the right coronary artery, and alters the values of the picture elements (pixels) within a given image. Lastly, detection of calcified plaques is determined by the presence of more signal (information about the plaque and surrounding structures) than noise. Image noise is random by definition and obscures information or signal. The noise in the CT images creates false-positive plaques that cannot be differentiated from true calcified plaques. The impact of image noise on small-lesion detection has been documented with EBCT *(34)*. A limitation of EBCT is the fixed mAs (approx 60). With mAs fixed, image noise increases with thoracic size and degrades image quality in larger patients. The established relation between body size and image noise will creates an erroneous relationship between obesity and CAC *(35,36)*. Since both obesity and CAC are associated with CVD, this results in confounding the true relationship. The ability to alter technique and maintain a constant image quality (i.e., an acceptable level of image noise) is a critical benefit of MDCT techniques for CAC *(37,38)*. There is by definition a trade-off between improved image quality (i.e., less image noise means more signal and more X-ray photons) and increased dose. Thus, image quality should be selected based on the clinical application of the results. Current and likely future clinical recommendations indicate changes in management using significant levels of plaque burden corresponding to Agatston scores ranging from 100 to 400. However, if a percentile approach or progression rates are to be utilized in clinical practice, then these issues become critical and further research into the optimal level of image quality is required.

STUDIES EVALUATING CALCIFIED PLAQUE MEASUREMENT WITH CARDIAC CT

In the studies to date, extremely high correlations have been seen between CT devices for both the amount of calcified plaque and the rank ordering of patients' calcium burdens. In the initial comparisons of EBCT to single-slice helical CT with ECG gating, the correlation between scores performed on the same individuals was near perfect ($R > 0.97$), and mean interscan variability was 25% *(3,4)*. In addition, the more conservative nonparametric Spearman's test of rank order was shown to be extremely high (0.96), and agreement at grouping patients based on Agatston scores of 100, 200, and 400 was 97%, 92%, and 94% respectively. The study by Goldin et al. is the only study to date in which a direct comparison of interscan variability between EBCT and helical CT/MDCT has been performed. In this study, participants had paired scans and calcium measurements on an EBCT (C150) and a GE helical CT system with cardiac gating (0.8-s gantry), and no statistically significant difference in interscan or interobserver variability was found when using the 130 CT threshold and Agatston scoring method. Differences in risk stratification were observed between the two methods. The documented high correlations for both amount of calcium and ordering of calcified plaque burden in these studies indicates that differences in agreement could be improved through calibration of calcium plaque measured by CT to an external standard *(4,27)*. This calibration would reduce systematic bias related to the CT system and further improve agreement.

The National Heart, Lung and Blood Institute of the National Institutes of Health is funding the Multi-Ethnic Study of Atherosclerosis (MESA), in which 6800 individuals asymptomatic for CVD have received an extensive CVD exam, including cardiac CT measurement of CAC. MESA exams are performed at six field centers across the United States *(39)*. The participants had replicated measures of coronary calcium made during the baseline CT visit in order to measure interscan variability and to improve the ability to track progression of calcified plaque in subsequent planned exams of the cohort. In MESA, three field centers utilized EBCT (C150) and three MDCT (4-slice). Findings from the baseline exam on cardiac CT interscan variability were presented at the American Heart Association Scientific Session in 2002 *(40)*. After adjusting for mean calcium score and body mass index, there was no significant difference between median interscan variability using the Agatston score (EBCT 22.7 vs MDCT 24.7, $p = 0.15$) or volume score (EBCT 11.0 vs MDCT 11.9, $p = 0.84$). The median interscan percentage differences using the Agatston score were 18.1 % (EBCT) and 18.7% (MDCT), and are consistent with the range of interscan variability published for EBCT of 18–43% as well as the result published with MDCT(4) demonstrating interscan variability of 20.4%, 13.9%, and 9.3% for Agatston score, volume, and mass respectively *(41)*. The conclusions we can draw from these data is that the measurement precision of EBCT and MDCT(4) are very similar. The component of the overall observed variability attributable to the CT systems (EBCT vs EBCT, MDCT vs MDCT, EBCT vs MDCT) is small relative to the intrinsic variability present in measuring CAC with existing cardiac CT technology.

MDCT—CARDIAC-GATED HELICAL ACQUISITIONS FOR CAC

MDCT systems can scan in a helical mode and can reconstruct images compensated for cardiac motion using either ECG waveform or the inherent motion of the heart *(42–44)*. These techniques are detailed in other chapters, but evolved directly from the single-slice helical CT retrospective gating described previously (Fig. 1). Although currently used and developed for MDCT coronary angiography, it is clear that these advances in coronary imaging can be applied to measuring calcified plaque in the coronary arteries during a non-contrast-enhanced study. Specifically, the improved spatial and temporal resolution possible with these techniques has already been shown to reduce inter-exam variability from 35% with EBCT using the standard sequential technique and 3-mm slices to 4% with volumetric MDCT using a helical scan with overlapping 2.5-mm slices in controlled testing with a motion phantom of the coronary arteries *(45,46)*. These methods hold significant potential. The increased radiation exposure and limited clinical experience has limited their application to date. Lower-dose methods incorporating mA modulation and low-kV imaging are available, and initial reports have demonstrated promising results *(47–49)*. At this time, prospective ECG gating with a sequential scan acquisition is the preferred standard for clinical use, based on the lower radiation exposure and more extensive clinical and research experience to date. The future application of the helical technique to coronary calcium imaging, although promising, remains to be fully defined and validated for clinical practice.

IMAGE NOISE AND CARDIAC CT

Atherosclerosis begins as early as the second decade of life, and includes the formation of small calcified lesions *(50)*. Detection of calcified plaques in the walls of the coronary arteries requires increasing image quality as the size of the plaque becomes smaller. In essence, with CT (EBCT or MDCT) the device is measuring those calcified plaques above the predefined threshold and size criteria configured in the scoring software. These factors are determined not by the pathobiology of atherosclerosis but by the imaging specifications of the CT devices. Individuals with a calcium score of zero represent a range of calcified coronary plaque not measurable by existing CT technologies. Previous authors have suggested lowering the threshold for CT-measurable calcified plaque from 130 to 90 CT units *(16)*. This effectively increases the sensitivity of the CT test for earlier plaque. For helical CT and MDCT systems, this is possible through the ability to maintain sufficient image quality by adjusting the mA or tube current to maintain the signal-to-noise ratio (SNR) at an acceptable level. Without maintaining the SNR, the image quality is degraded to the point that image noise obscures the small, calcified plaques. With EBCT, mAs is fixed. Individuals with increasing thoracic girth have increasing image noise. Image noise can vary on MDCT systems depending upon the technique employed, but typically range between 8 and 16 noise/HU, compared to 24 noise/HU for EBCT. Image noise can be scored as CAC resulting in false-positive results and inflate the size of true lesions. This relation between patient size and image noise with EBCT has been demonstrated to confound the true relation between CAC and obesity *(35)*. Cardiac imaging requires all aspects of image quality (SNR, temporal resolution, contrast-to-noise, and spatial resolution) to be balanced appropriately for the desired task. In the specific case of detecting and quantifying small calcified plaques in the coronary arteries, the critical influence of image noise was established early in the literature with EBCT *(34)*. The epidemic of obesity in industrialized societies and the elevated risk of CVD seen in individuals with the metabolic syndrome (which includes obesity) means that any device that will be used for screening the general population for CVD must be able to handle individuals weighing greater than 100 kg (220 lb) without creating false-positive calcium scores. Maintaining a consistent level of image quality across various patient sizes will significantly improve image quality and the measurement of CAC.

IMPROVED SPATIAL RESOLUTION

The continued technological advancement of MDCT systems will allow imaging with increasing spatial resolution in the slice or z direction. Current MDCT-16 systems can provide 1.25-mm slices by 16 levels simultaneously with protocols reconstructing 2.5 mm × 8 levels at no increased dose or exposure to patient. With increasing spatial resolution, issues related to dose and SNR become increasingly important. Fundamentally, improved spatial resolution will allow more accurate measurement of small coronary plaques (Fig. 2). If the CT technique and radiation exposure is held constant, by definition greater image noise will be present on the thinner 1.25-mm images, when compared to the 2.5-mm images reconstructed from the same scan data. These improvements in measurement capability may be particularly important in measuring the change in plaque burden over time, and this is an area of extremely active research. Rapid progression of coronary atherosclerosis and thus potentially calcified plaque may be a key predictor of future clinical events.

STANDARDIZED SCANNING PROTOCOL FOR MDCT

The continued technological change in MDCT makes standardization problematic. For measuring CAC, by far the greatest experience is using prospective ECG gating (also called triggering) and scanning in a sequential scan mode. Gantry speeds of 0.5 s or greater should be used for cardiac applications. 120 kVp with mAs ranging from 50 to 100 are consistently used in research and clinical applications. The tradeoff between 50 and 100 mAs is between dose (effective dose ranges between 1 and 2 mSv, respectively) and image noise. Note that increasing mAs with patient size is desirable to maintain image quality. In the MESA CT protocol, mA was increased by 25% for those individuals weighing greater than 100 kg (220 lb). Slice collimation is relatively standardized at 2.5 mm for MDCT systems when operating in the sequential mode. MDCT scans should be performed at the maximum multislice capability (i.e., widest nominal beam width) possible in order to reduce variability related to coronary and

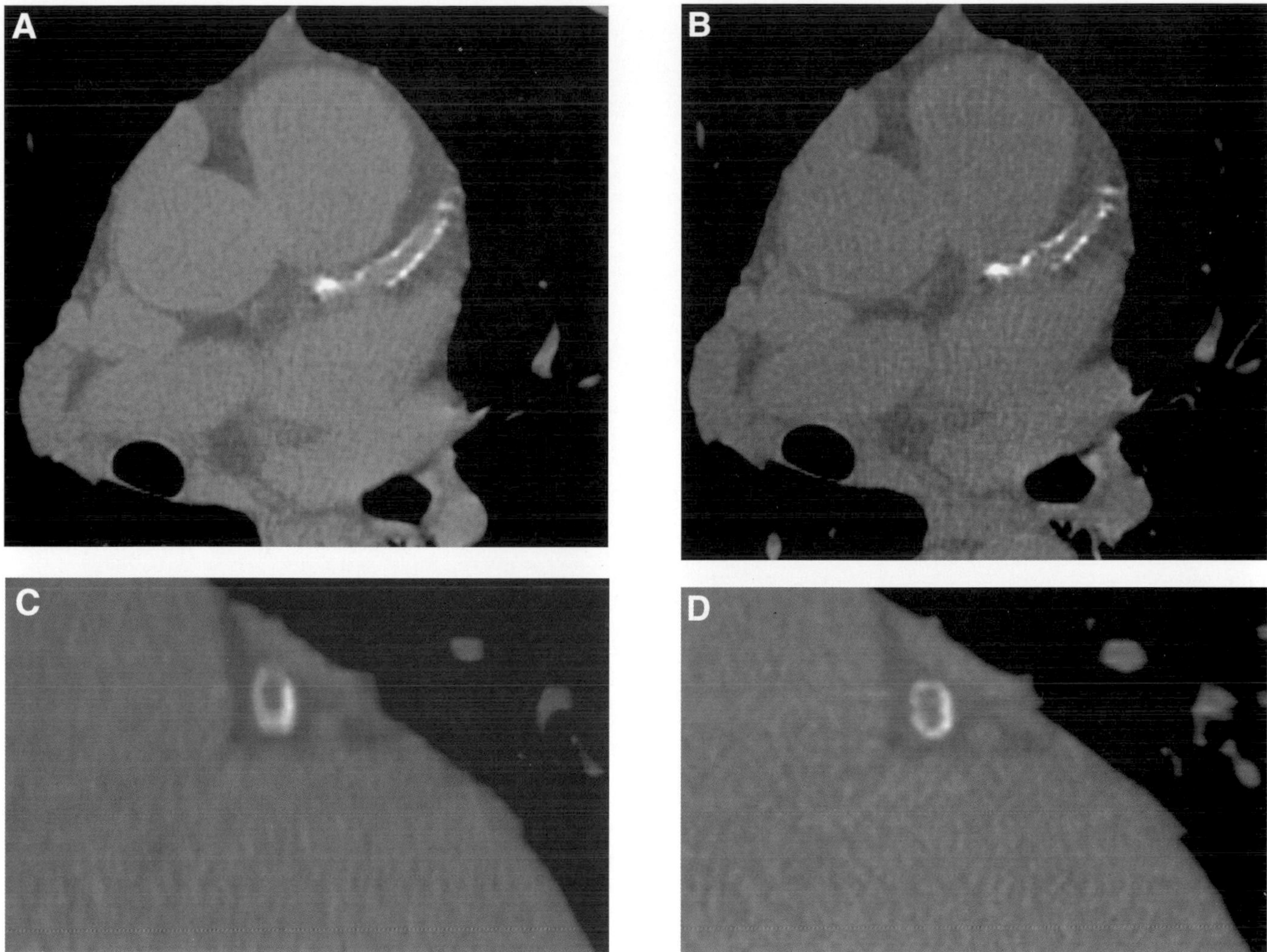

Fig. 2. Improvement in spatial resolution using 1.25-mm slice collimation. Images **A** and **B** are from the same cardiac-gated scan through the heart performed on a multidetector-row CT(16) system (General Electric LightSpeed Pro) using 0.4-s gantry rotation and segmented reconstruction algorithm. (**A**) The direct axial slice reconstructed with 2.5-mm slice thickness; (**B**) the same data reconstructed at 1.25-mm slice thickness. Note how there is increased image noise apparent in the 1.25 slice by the more "textured" appearance of the homogenous blood in the ascending aorta and main pulmonary artery. (**C,D**) Oblique reconstructions positioned to create a cross-section through the left anterior descending coronary artery using the 2.5-mm and 1.25-mm data respectively. Note how the calcifications in the wall of the left anterior descending artery demonstrate more detail secondary to the improved spatial resolution with the 1.25-mm dataset. These sets of images demonstrate how improved technique will be required as slice thickness is reduced if the level of noise is to remain constant.

patient motion. The wider beam will also reduce extraneous scatter radiation and increase dose efficiency while reducing patient exposure.

CALIBRATED CALCIUM MASS

Calibration of any measurement device is central to improving accuracy. The Agatston score is a quantitative scoring system with limitations related to the discrete weighting factors that increase variability, and it has no straightforward means of calibration *(41,51,52)*. The various volume-scoring methods allow calculation of the volume of calcified plaque in S.I. units such as milliliters. Volume methods are strongly influenced by the threshold of "CT measurable calcium," typically set at 130 HU. It has already been demonstrated that there is variability between patient and CT system in the determination of this threshold *(27)*. Plaque volume does not account for plaque density, which may provide important information in relationship to CVD risk assessment. There are several methods of determining a calibrated mass, which include calibrating the CT scanner to an external standard as well as including a calibration phantom within the scan field of view for each scan (Fig. 3). The calibrated calcium mass in milligrams has several advantages. Based on imaging principles, it is more robust to the effect of partial volume averaging than either a volume score or Agatston score. Data with MDCT in both phantom studies and with human research participants have demonstrated less variability with a calibrated mass measurement than either volume or Agatston methods *(41,52)*. Lastly, the calibrated mass can be reported in milligrams of calcium and will allow for standardization of measurements across CT systems and techniques as well as for currently undiscovered future techniques.

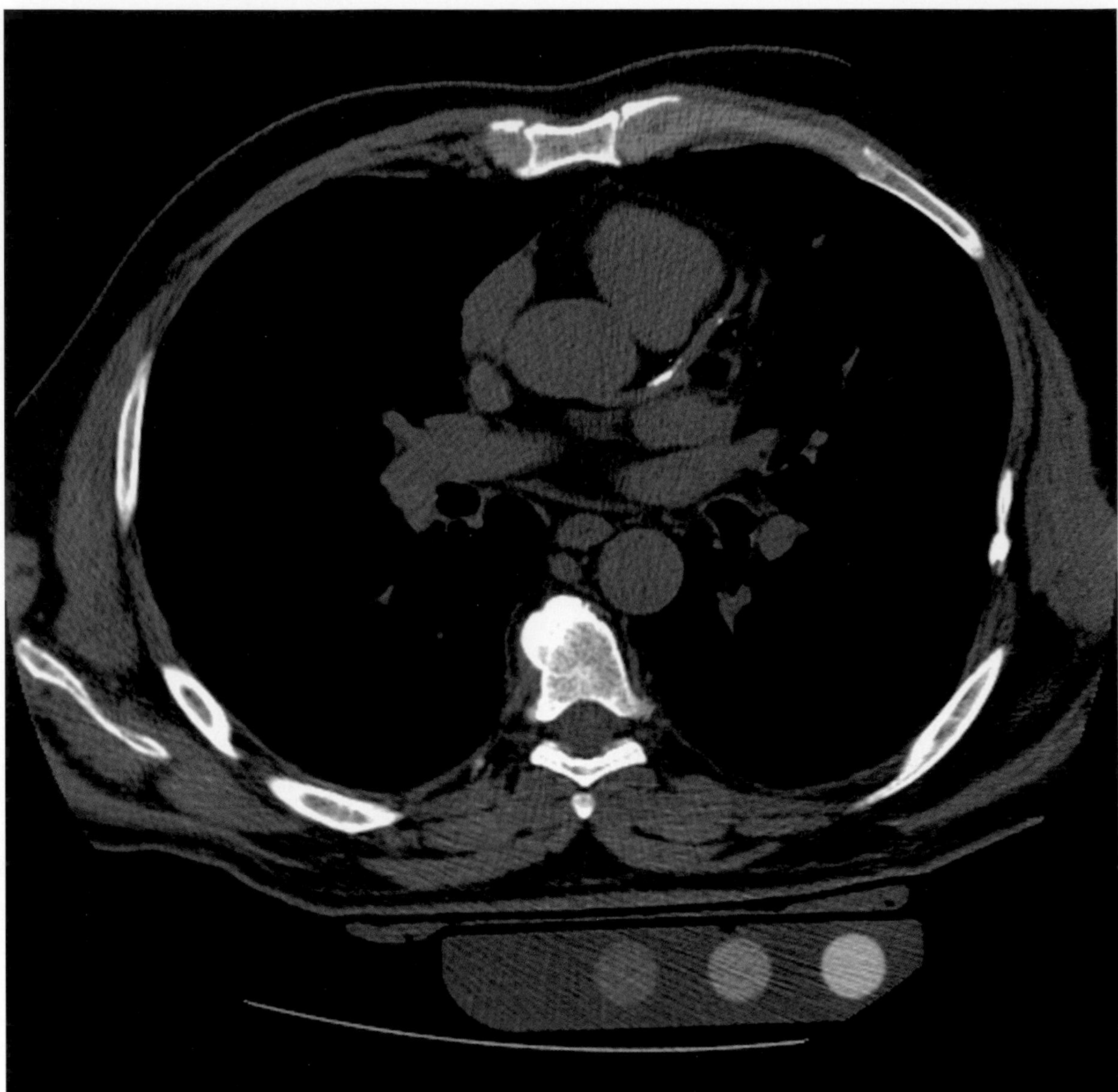

Fig. 3. Calibration phantom for calcium mass. One slice from a research study in which a calcium calibration phantom is used. These phantoms were originally designed for measurement of trabecular bone mineral density with CT, also known as quantitative computed tomography (QCT). The phantom is positioned underneath the participant during the scan and contains four cylinders with the following concentrations of calcium hydroxyapatite: 0 mg/mL, 50 mg/mL, 100 mg/mL, and 200 mg/mL. These known quantities of calcium are then used to calibrate the CT numbers such that the resulting mass determination is reported in mg of calcium hydoxyapatite. Calibration of each patient's scan provides the greatest gain in accuracy.

STUDIES IMPACTING THE CLINICAL APPLICATION OF CAC

Increasing evidence supports the use of CAC as a tool for better quantifying coronary heart disease risk among asymptomatic individuals. The Saint Francis Heart Study has recently reported data with 4.3 yr on average of follow-up of asymptomatic individuals aged 50–70 yr using EBCT *(53)*. In this study, participants with CAC scores >100 had a 10-fold increase in relative risk for CVD events. The calcium score had significantly better prognostic ability for coronary events than the Framingham Risk Index. The National Heart, Lung and Blood Institute's MESA is following an asymptomatic cohort of 6800 individuals whose coronary calcium was measured by either EBCT or MDCT between 2000 and 2002 *(39)*. The results from MESA will provide data on both prevalence and the predictive ability of CAC for CVD events in men and women as well as four ethnic groups.

CONCLUSION

Accumulating evidence supports the use of the calcified plaque as measured by cardiac CT (EBCT or MDCT) as a valuable predictor of future CVD risk. Ongoing population-based research and clinical trials will provide additional information to determine the appropriate clinical role. Calibration of cardiac CT measurements of coronary calcified plaque burden to mass of calcium will improve accuracy and reduce variability. As both EBCT and MDCT systems continue to improve in terms of image quality, tracking the progression of plaque burden and greater understanding of calcified plaque morphology will provide important new information on coronary heart disease. Based on preliminary data, it is likely that coronary calcium provides additive information to traditional CVD risk factors. The specific results of ongoing epidemiological studies will help determine the appropriate at-risk population for CVD screening with cardiac CT for coronary calcium. Cardiac CT with MDCT is well positioned to make screening for subclinical coronary atherosclerosis a viable and cost-effective option for identifying the individual at elevated CVD risk. Once these individuals are identified, proven interventions for CVD prevention are currently available and can be employed to reduce the tremendous burden of CVD on the population.

REFERENCES

1. Wexler L, Brundage B, Crouse J, et al. Coronary artery calcification: pathophysiology, epidemiology, imaging methods, and clinical implications. A statement for health professionals from the American Heart Association. Writing Group. Circulation 1996;94: 1175–1192.
2. Shemesh J, Apter S, Rozenman J, et al. Calcification of coronary arteries: detection and quantification with double-helix CT. Radiology 1995;197:779–783.
3. Becker CR, Jakobs TF, Aydemir S, et al. Helical and single-slice conventional CT versus electron beam CT for quantification of coronary artery calcification. AJR Am J Roentgenol 2000;174:543–547.
4. Carr JJ, Crouse JR, 3rd, Goff DC, Jr., D'Agostino RB, Jr., Peterson NP, Burke GL. Evaluation of subsecond gated helical CT for quantification of coronary artery calcium and comparison with electron beam CT. AJR Am J Roentgenol 2000;174:915–921.
5. Becker CR, Schoepf UJ, Reiser MF. Methods for quantification of coronary artery calcifications with electron beam and conventional CT and pushing the spiral CT envelope: new cardiac applications. Int J Cardiovasc Imaging 2001;17:203–211.
6. Agatston AS, Janowitz WR, Hildner FJ, Zusmer NR, Viamonte M, Jr., Detrano R. Quantification of coronary artery calcium using ultrafast computed tomography. JACC 1990;15:827–832.
7. Rumberger JA, Simons DB, Fitzpatrick LA, Sheedy PF, Schwartz RS. Coronary artery calcium area by electron-beam computed tomography and coronary atherosclerotic plaque area. A histopathologic correlative study. Circulation 1995;92:2157–2162.
8. Doherty TM, Detrano RC. Coronary arterial calcification as an active process: a new perspective on an old idea. Calcif Tissue Int 1994;54: 224–230.
9. Wallin R, Wajih N, Greenwood GT, Sane DC. Arterial calcification: a review of mechanisms, animal modes, and the prospects for therapy. Med Res Rev 2001;21:274–301.
10. O'Rourke RA, Brundage BH, Froelicher VF, et al. American College of Cardiology/American Heart Association Expert Consensus Document on Electron-Beam Computed Tomography for the Diagnosis and Prognosis of Coronary Artery Disease. JACC 2000:236–240.
11. Smith SC, Jr., Amsterdam E, Balady GJ, et al. Prevention Conference V: Beyond secondary prevention: identifying the high-risk patient for primary prevention: tests for silent and inducible ischemia: Writing Group II. Circulation 2000;101:E12–6.
12. Sasaki F, Koga S, Takeuchi A. [Computed tomographic detection of calcification within the heart and the thoracic aorta (author's transl)]. Nippon Igaku Hoshasen Gakkai Zasshi—Nippon Acta Radiologica 1982;42:123–129.
13. Reinmuller R, Lipton MJ. Detection of coronary artery calcifications by computed tomography. Cardiovascular Imaging 1987;1:139–145.
14. Kalender WA, Seissler W, Klotz E, Vock P. Spiral volumetric CT with single-breath-hold technique, continuous transport, and continuous scanner rotation. Radiology 1990;176:181–183.
15. Callaway MP, Richards P, Goddard P, Rees M. The incidence of coronary artery calcification on standard thoracic CT scans. Brit J Radiol 1997;70:572–574.
16. Broderick LS, Shemesh J, Wilensky RL, et al. Measurement of coronary artery calcium with dual-slice helical CT compared with coronary angiography: evaluation of CT scoring methods, interobserver variations, and reproducibility. Am J Roentgenol 1996;167: 439–444.
17. Woodhouse CE, Janowitz WR, Viamonte M, Jr. Coronary arteries: retrospective cardiac gating technique to reduce cardiac motion artifact at spiral CT. Radiology 1997;204:566–569.
18. Becker CR, Knez A, Jakobs TF, et al. Detection and quantification of coronary artery calcification with electron-beam and conventional CT. Eur Radiol 1999;9:620–624.
19. Knez A, Becker C, Becker A, et al. New generation computed tomography scanners are equally effective in determining coronary calcium compared to electron beam CT in patients with suspected CAD. Circulation 1998;Suppl I:I-655.
20. Carr JJ, Burke GL, Goff DC, Crouse JR, D'Agostino RA. Coronary artery calcium scores correlate strongly between fast gated helical and electron beam computed tomography. Circulation 1999;99: 1106.
21. Goldin JG, Yoon HC, Greaser LE, 3rd, et al. Spiral versus electron-beam CT for coronary artery calcium scoring. Radiology 2001; 221:213–221.
22. Carr JJ. Coronary calcium: the case for helical computed tomography. J Thorac Imaging 2001;16:16–24.
23. Ning R, Chen B, Yu R, Conover D, Tang X, Ning Y. Flat panel detector-based cone-beam volume CT angiography imaging: system evaluation. IEEE Trans Med Imaging 2000;19:949–963.
24. Bland MJ, Altman DG. Statistical methods for assessing agreement between two methods of clinical measurement. Lancet 1986;1 (8476):307–310.
25. Carr JJ, Reed JC, Choplin RH, Case LD. Pneumothorax detection: a problem in experimental design. Radiology 1993;186:23–25; discussion 25–26.
26. Zerhouni EA, Spivey JF, Morgan RH, Leo FP, Stitik FP, Siegelman SS. Factors influencing quantitative CT measurements of solitary pulmonary nodules. J Comput Assist Tomo 1982;6:1075–1087.
27. McCollough CH, Kaufmann RB, Cameron BM, Katz DJ, Sheedy PF, 2nd, Peyser PA. Electron-beam CT: use of a calibration phantom to reduce variability in calcium quantitation. Radiology 1995;196: 159–165.
28. Mao S, Budoff M, Bakhsheshi H, Liu SCK. Improved reproducibility of coronary artery calcium scoring by electron beam tomography with a new electrocardiographic trigger method. Invest Radiol 2001;36:363–367.
29. Achenbach S, Ropers D, Mohlenkamp S, et al. Variability of repeated coronary artery calcium measurements by electron beam tomography. Am J Cardiol 2001;87:210–213, A8.
30. Becker CR, Jakobs TF, Aydemir S, et al. Helical and single-slice conventional CT versus electron beam CT for the quantification of coronary artery calcification. Am J Roentgenol 2000;174:543–547.
31. Yoon HC, Goldin JG, Greaser LE, 3rd, Sayre J, Fonarow GC. Interscan variation in coronary artery calcium quantification in a large asymptomatic patient population. Am J Roentgenol 2000;174: 803–809.
32. Greaser LE, 3rd, Yoon HC, Mather RT, McNitt-Gray M, Goldin JG. Electron-beam CT: the effect of using a correction function on coronary artery calcium quantitation. Acad Radiol 1999;6:40–48.
33. Bielak LF, Sheedy PF, 2nd, Peyser PA. Coronary artery calcification measured at electron-beam CT: agreement in dual scan runs and change over time. Radiology 2001;218:224–229.
34. Bielak LF, Kaufmann RB, Moll PP, McCollough CH, Schwartz RS, Sheedy PF, 2nd. Small lesions in the heart identified at electron beam CT: calcification or noise?. Radiology 1994;192:631–636.

35. Sevrukov A, Pratap A, Doss C, Jelnin V, Hoff JA, Kondos GT. Electron beam tomography imaging of coronary calcium: the effect of body mass index on radiologic noise. J Comput Assist Tomogr 2002;26:592–597.
36. Sevrukov A, Jelnin V, Hoff JA, Kondos G. Electron-beam tomography coronary artery calcium scanning: effect of image noise on calibration phantom computed tomography values. Am J Cardiol 2001; 88:85E.
37. Van Hoe LR, De Meerleer KG, Leyman PP, Vanhoenacker PK. Coronary artery calcium scoring using ECG-gated multidetector CT: effect of individually optimized image-reconstruction windows on image quality and measurement reproducibility. Am J Roentgenol 2003;181:1093–1100.
38. Mahnken AH, Wildberger JE, Simon J, et al. Detection of coronary calcifications: feasibility of dose reduction with a body weight-adapted examination protocol. Am J Roentgenol 2003; 181:533–538.
39. Bild DE, Bluemke DA, Burke GL, et al. Multi-ethnic study of atherosclerosis: objectives and design. Am J Epidemiol 2002;156: 871–881.
40. Detrano R, Anderson M, Nelson J, et al. Effect of scanner type and calcium measure on the re-scan variability of calcium quantity by computed tomography. Circulation 2002.
41. Hong C, Bae KT, Pilgram TK. Coronary artery calcium: accuracy and reproducibility of measurements with multi-detector row ct—assessment of effects of different thresholds and quantification methods. Radiology 2003;227:795–801.
42. Ohnesorge B, Flohr T, Becker C, et al. Cardiac imaging by means of electrocardiographically gated multisection spiral CT: initial experience. Radiology 2000;217:564–571.
43. Flohr T, Prokop M, Becker C, et al. A retrospectively ECG-gated multislice spiral CT scan and reconstruction technique with suppression of heart pulsation artifacts for cardio-thoracic imaging with extended volume coverage. Eur Radiol 2002;12:1497–1503.
44. Kachelriess M, Sennst DA, Maxlmoser W, Kalender WA. Kymogram detection and kymogram-correlated image reconstruction from subsecond spiral computed tomography scans of the heart. Med Phys 2002;29:1489–1503.
45. Kopp AF, Ohnesorge B, Becker C, et al. Reproducibility and accuracy of coronary calcium measurements with multi-detector row versus electron-beam CT. Radiology 2002; 225:113–119.
46. Hong C, Becker CR, Schoepf UJ, Ohnesorge B, Bruening R, Reiser MF. Coronary artery calcium: absolute quantification in nonenhanced and contrast-enhanced multi-detector row CT studies. Radiology 2002;223:474–480.
47. Ohnesorge B, Becker C, Flohr T, et al. Coronary calcium scoring with electrocardiographically pulsed multislice spiral computed tomography and reduced radiation exposure. Am J Cardiol 2001;88:82E.
48. Jakobs TF, Becker CR, Ohnesorge B, et al. Multislice helical CT of the heart with retrospective ECG gating: reduction of radiation exposure by ECG-controlled tube current modulation. Eur Radiol 2002;12:1081–1086.
49. Jakobs TF, Wintersperger BJ, Herzog P, et al. Ultra-low-dose coronary artery calcium screening using multislice CT with retrospective ECG gating. Eur Radiol 2003;13:1923–1930.
50. Strong JP. Natural history and risk factors for early human atherogenesis. Pathobiological Determinants of Atherosclerosis in Youth (PDAY) Research Group. Clin Chem 1995;41:134–138.
51. Callister TQ, Cooil B, Raya SP, Lippolis NJ, Russo DJ, Raggi P. Coronary artery disease: improved reproducibility of calcium scoring with an electron-beam CT volumetric method. Radiology 1998;208:807–814.
52. Ferencik M, Ferullo A, Achenbach S, et al. Coronary calcium quantification using various calibration phantoms and scoring thresholds. Invest Radiol 2003;38:559–566.
53. Arad Y, Roth M, Newstein D, Guerci AD. Heart Scan May Be Better Than Standard Risk Factors at Estimating Heart Disease Risk, American College of Cardiology 52nd Annual Scientific Session, Chicago, Ill, 2003.

12 Coronary Calcium Scoring With Multidetector-Row CT

Rationale and Scoring Techniques

ROMAN FISCHBACH, MD AND DAVID MAINTZ, MD

INTRODUCTION

Coronary heart disease is the leading cause of death, illness, and disability in populations worldwide. Strategies to reduce the risk of coronary heart disease include the early initiation of primary preventive measures including lifestyle changes and/ or medical therapy in patients with subclinical disease. The reliable identification of presymptomatic patients, however, is problematic by conventional risk assessment based on traditional risk factors. Direct visualization and quantification of the coronary atherosclerotic plaque burden would be desirable to more precisely determine a patient's coronary heart risk. In recent years, there has been an important increase of interest in the use of noninvasive measurement of coronary arterial calcification as a screening test for coronary atherosclerosis. Since coronary artery calcification is conceived as a manifestation of atherosclerosis in the arterial wall, the detection of coronary calcifications may serve as a marker for the presence of coronary artery disease. The most frequent application of coronary calcium scoring has thus become the assessment of an individual's future risk for a myocardial event. This indication and the predictive value of coronary artery calcium measurement and its role in the assessment of myocardial event risk has always been a matter of debate.

Until the introduction of subsecond mechanical computed tomography (CT) scanners, coronary calcium measurement remained a domain of electron beam CT (EBCT). Owing to the limited number of EBCT scanners available in dedicated imaging centers, access to coronary CT scanning has long been restricted. On the other hand, the scan protocol and the quantification method remained quite uniform for a decade. Many of the whole-body multidetector-row CT (MDCT) systems installed today are equipped with the necessary hard- and software to perform examinations of the heart using either prospective triggering of sequential scans or retrospective gating of spiral CT scans. This development opens CT scanning of the heart for a larger patient population. Parallel to the introduction of a growing range of MDCT systems capable of performing electrocardiogram (ECG)-synchronized cardiac scans, different scan protocols have been suggested and new approaches for the quantification of coronary artery calcifications have been introduced. Today no accepted standards exist for performing MDCT studies for quantification of coronary artery calcifications.

This chapter will give an overview of the basic concepts of imaging of coronary artery calcification and will review current techniques and indications for the "calcium scoring" examination, with special regard to MDCT technique.

CORONARY HEART DISEASE

Cardiovascular disease has been the leading cause of death in the United States ever since 1900, with the exception of the influenza epidemic in 1918. Although remarkable advances have been made in prevention and treatment of coronary heart disease, it remains the major cause of mortality and morbidity in the industrialized nations and accounts for 54% of all cardiovascular deaths and 22% of all deaths in the United States *(1)*. From 1990 to 2000, the death rate from coronary heart disease declined 25%, but the absolute number of deaths decreased only 7.6%. Coronary heart disease typically manifests in middle-aged and older, predominantly male, individuals. The average age of a person having a first myocardial infarction is 65 yr in males and 70 yr in women. In up to 50% of coronary heart disease victims, sudden coronary death or nonfatal myocardial infarction is the first manifestation of disease, and approx 50% of patients with acute myocardial infarction die within the first month of the event *(2,3)*. The identification of asymptomatic persons with subclinical disease who are at high risk of developing a future coronary event and who could potentially benefit from preventive efforts thus is of major economic and clinical importance. Coronary heart disease is the product and manifestation (myocardial infarction, stable and unstable angina, and myocardial dysfunction) of coronary artery disease (CAD), in the form of coronary atherosclerosis.

Traditionally, coronary heart disease risk stratification has been based on well-known clinical and biochemical factors. Moderately effective preventive treatment is available: lipid lowering with HMG-CoA reductase inhibitors (statins) or antiplatelet therapy (aspirin) have both resulted in decreased incidence rates of coronary events *(4,5)*. Coronary heart disease thus seems to be a suitable target for screening efforts. However, many myocardial events are not accounted for by these risk factors alone. Therefore efforts have been made

From: *Contemporary Cardiology: CT of the Heart: Principles and Applications*
Edited by: U. Joseph Schoepf © Humana Press, Inc., Totowa, NJ

to develop new diagnostic modalities that may provide an improved approach to coronary heart disease risk assessment.

CORONARY ARTERY CALCIFICATION

Autopsy studies have shown that coronary artery calcification is an excellent marker of CAD *(6,7)*. Histomorphological evaluation of coronary arteries at autopsy has produced good correlation between coronary artery calcification and overall plaque burden *(8–10)*, but it is not known whether the amount of calcium reflects the amount of total plaque over time or after therapeutic intervention. Calcification seems to be a better marker for overall coronary plaque burden than individual stenosis based on residual lumen size *(9)*. Calcifications are frequently present long before clinical manifestation of atherosclerotic disease. Although coronary artery calcification is found more frequently in advanced lesions, it may be histologically identified early in the disease process and has been detected in lesions that are seen as early as the second decade of life. On the other hand, atherosclerotic plaque can be present when coronary calcium is either absent or not detectable by CT, even though histopathologic studies confirmed an intimate relation between coronary atherosclerotic plaque area and coronary calcium area.

PATHOPHYSIOLOGY OF CORONARY ARTERY CALCIFICATION

The development of coronary atherosclerosis can be described as a sequence of changes in the arterial wall. An in-depth description of the pathophysiology would be beyond the scope of this work, and the interested reader is referred to the literature *(11–13)*. Initial lesions seem to occur secondary to an injury of the coronary artery endothelium. Circulating histiocytes traverse the injured vascular endothelium and gather in the arterial wall. These histiocytes transform into macrophages and can accumulate lipid. Lipid accumulation can be identified as fatty streaks, the initial and intermediate lesions in atherosclerotic plaque formation. Histologically, different types of atherosclerotic lesions can be distinguished, which has led to a classification system suggested by the American Heart Association. Lesions are designated by Roman numerals I through VI (*see* Fig. 1).

Initial and intermediate lesions are types I, II, and III. The advanced atherosclerotic lesions are subdivided into lesions type IV, V, and VI. The type IV lesion (atheroma) is characterized by extracellular intimal lipid accumulation, the lipid core. The type V lesion contains fibrous connective tissue formations. If parts of the lesion are calcified, it becomes a Vb lesion. If the lipid core is absent, the type Va or Vb lesion is classified as type Vc. Type IV and type V lesions may develop fissures, hematoma, and/or thrombus (type VI lesion). Although this classification system suggests a linear sequence of events, plaque development seems to be more complex *(13)*. This is suggested by angiographic studies, which have shown that rapid progression of minor lesions to high-grade stenosis may occur in only a few months *(14,15)*.

PLAQUE MORPHOLOGY AND DEGREE OF CALCIFICATION

Apatite in the form of $\{Ca\,[Ca_3\,(PO_4)_2]_3\}^{2+} \times 2\,OH^-$ (hydroxyapatite) and carbonate apatite is the predominant mineral

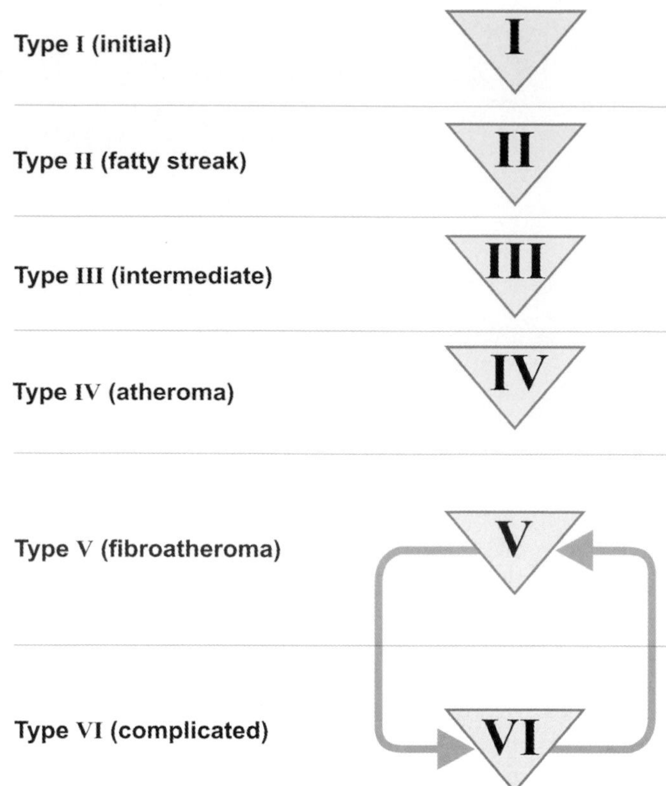

Fig. 1. Sequence of atherosclerotic lesions according to the classification system by the American Heart Association and the American College of Cardiology. The early lesion is characterized by isolated macrophage foam cells (type I lesion) or mainly intracellular lipid accumulation (type II). Type II changes and early extracellular lipid pools characterize the intermediate lesion. The more advanced lesions contain a core of extracellular lipids (atheroma, type IV), or multiple lipid cores and fibrotic layers or calcifications (type V). A lesion with a surface defect and associated thrombus or hematoma is the "complicated" type VI lesion. Diagram modified according to *(11)*.

form in calcified lesions. Atherosclerotic calcification is an organized, regulated process (similar to bone formation) that occurs only when other aspects of atherosclerosis are also present. Nonhepatic Gla-containing proteins like osteocalcin, which are actively involved in the transport of calcium out of vessel walls, are suspected to have key roles in the pathogenesis of coronary calcification. Osteopontin and its mRNA, known to be involved in bone mineralization, and mRNA for bone morphogenetic protein-2a, a potent factor for osteoblastic differentiation, have been identified in calcified atherosclerotic lesions. Although the process of calcium accumulation in atherosclerotic lesions is not fully understood, it seems to be an active process, which involves mechanisms similar to bone formation and resorption *(16–18)*. Regardless of the mechanisms involved, it is evident that calcium is very common in advanced atherosclerotic lesions.

Histologically, coronary artery plaque can be also classified as plaque rupture, plaque erosion, vulnerable plaque, fibroatheroma, fibrous plaque, plaque hemorrhage, and healed plaque rupture. Rupture is characterized by an acute luminal thrombus with connection to a plaque with a lipid-rich core. Plaque erosion represents a plaque with an intact fibrous cap

Table 1
Prevalence of Coronary Artery Calcification Detected by CT in Asymptomatic Men and Women (adapted from ref. *22*)

	Asymptomatic	
Age	*Men (%)*	*Women (%)*
–29	11	6
30–39	21	11
40–49	44	23
50–59	72	35
60–69	85	67
70–79	94	89
80–89	100	100

and acute luminal thrombus. The "vulnerable plaque" or thinned-cap fibroatheroma shows a plaque with a thin fibrous cap and infiltration of macrophages. The pattern of calcification was correlated with the plaque morphology in a histomorphologic study of patients dying suddenly with severe coronary disease *(19)*. The greatest amount of calcium was found in healed ruptures, followed by fibroatheroma. Acute plaque ruptures were most frequently seen in segments with speckled or no calcification, but did also occur in areas with diffuse calcifications. From these observations it can be assumed that calcification reflects healing of plaque rupture and intraplaque hemorrhage as well as a response to inflammation in the plaque. Calcification may thus be seen as an attempt of the arterial wall to stabilize itself, since calcified and fibrotic plaques are much stiffer than lipid-rich lesion. The earlier concepts suggesting that calcification is associated with plaque instability are not supported by recent data.

In a study of 40 patients with acute coronary syndromes and no or moderate angiographic coronary disease, 36% of culprit lesions were not calcified *(20)*. Because most acute ruptures seem to occur in areas with only little calcification, it is questionable whether coronary calcification could be a marker for plaque instability. Furthermore, we will have to accept that calcification pattern is not helpful in localizing potentially vulnerable lesions, as it has been shown that unstable plaque can be present in vessels with a wide range of calcification patterns as well as in vascular segments without detectable calcium deposits.

Even if the individual calcification or calcified plaque does not equal a possible future culprit lesion, the presence and extent of coronary artery calcifications reflect the total plaque burden, and as such the likelihood of the presence of potentially vulnerable lesions. Using this concept, the demonstration of coronary artery calcium accumulation identifies the patient with coronary artery disease, and the degree of calcification can be considered a potential risk factor *(21)*.

PREVALENCE OF CORONARY ARTERY CALCIFICATION

The prevalence of coronary artery calcification in asymptomatic as well as symptomatic persons is well studied. Table 1 shows data from an early study investigating the prevalence of coronary artery calcification in asymptomatic men and women of various ages *(22)*. The prevalence in men is evidently higher than the prevalence in women well into the postmenopausal period, and it is obvious that the prevalence is age dependent. Several investigators have since reported coronary calcium scores in large asymptomatic populations (*see* Fig. 2). The calcium score distributions published for these asymptomatic mainly white American populations can be used to classify patients compared with the expected norm. All investigators *(23–25)* report a steep increase in coronary calcium score with age: the 75th percentile ranges between 36 and 44 for males aged 45–50 yr, between 101 and 116 for males aged 50–55 yr, and between 410 and 434 for males aged 60–65 yr. Interestingly, the absolute calcium scores are quite similar in the different US populations studied.

Even though there is a positive association of the amount of coronary artery calcium and age, coronary artery calcification is not an inevitable aspect of aging. In older adults with minimal clinical cardiovascular disease, 16% of the individuals examined had no detectable coronary artery calcifications *(26)*.

IMAGING OF CORONARY ARTERY CALCIFICATION

Calcium strongly attenuates X-rays as a result of its relatively high atomic number; therefore, a variety of radiological imaging techniques, including chest X-ray, fluoroscopy, EBCT, conventional, spiral, and MDCT are suitable methods for detecting coronary calcifications.

CONVENTIONAL X-RAY TECHNIQUES

The chest film has the least sensitivity, and only extensive calcifications can be identified *(27)*. Fluoroscopy has a much higher sensitivity compared to plain chest radiography, but characterization, quantification, and documentation are problematic using a projection technique. Furthermore, fluoroscopy requires a skilled and experienced examiner. Nevertheless, fluoroscopically detected calcifications were shown to carry significant prognostic information. A prospective study using fluoroscopy in high-risk asymptomatic populations found that individuals with detectable coronary calcifications were three times as likely to develop angina or to experience myocardial infarction or death than persons without coronary calcifications *(28)*. Margolis et al. assessed the significance of coronary artery calcification in 800 symptomatic patients who underwent cardiac fluoroscopy. Calcification was shown by fluoroscopy in 250 patients, of whom 236 (94%) had greater than or equal to 75% stenosis of one or more major coronary arteries at angiography. The 5-yr survival for patients with coronary artery calcifications was 58%, compared with 87% in patients without coronary artery calcifications. The prognostic significance of coronary artery calcification was independent of sex, status of the coronary vessels at angiography, left-ventricular function, or results of exercise tests *(29)*.

CT IMAGING TECHNIQUES

Because of the high attenuation of calcium, CT is extremely sensitive in depicting vascular calcifications (Fig. 3). Conventional single-section imaging with acquisition times in the range of 2–5 s allowed identification of coronary artery calcifications, but calcifications are blurred because of cardiac motion, and small lesions may not be detected. Despite these drawbacks, conventional CT seems to be more sensitive in detecting calcifications than fluoroscopy *(30)*. Still, motion artifacts and

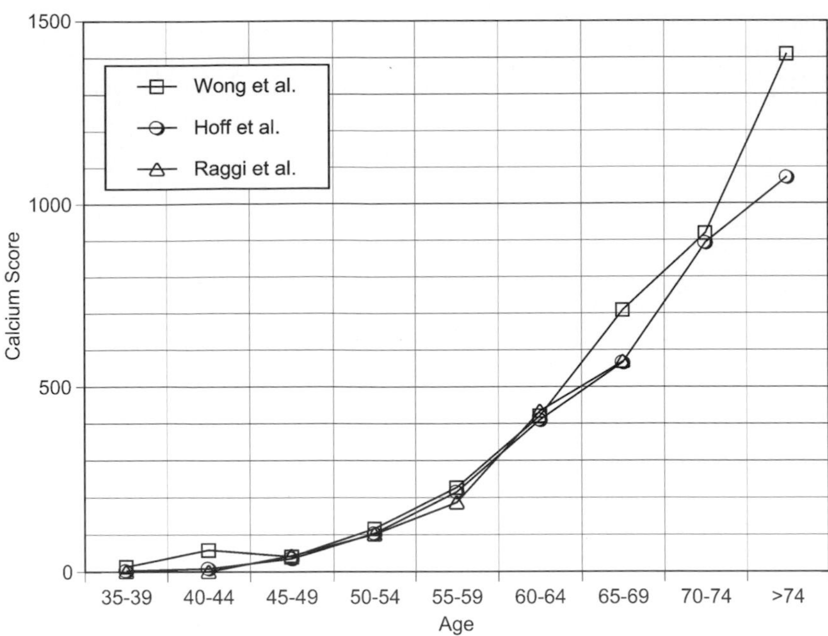

Fig. 2. Coronary artery calcium score in asymptomatic populations. Age- and gender-adjusted 75th percentile of coronary artery calcium in asymptomatic male patient populations reported by *(24)*, *(23)*, and *(25)*. All investigators found a remarkable increase of calcium scores with age. The reported 75th percentile calcium score is quite similar in the different groups.

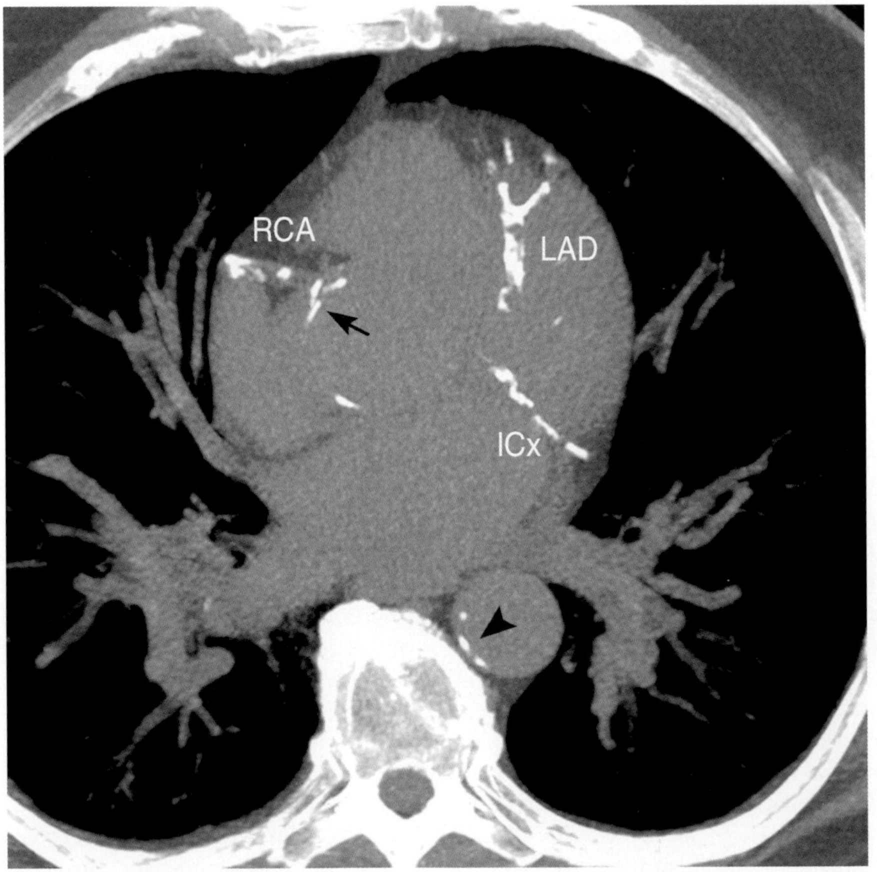

Fig. 3. Maximum-intensity projection image of a multidetector-row CT coronary scan depicting severely calcified coronary arteries. The right coronary artery (RCA), the left anterior descending artery (LAD), and the left circumflex (lCx) show diffuse calcifications. Small calcium accumulations are seen in the wall of the ascending (arrow) and descending aorta (arrow head).

Table 2
Results of Reproducibility Measurements Using Electron Beam CT

Author (reference)	*Patients*	*Calcium score variability (%)*	*Volume score variability (%)*
Kajinami et al., 1993 *(79)*	25	34	
Shields et al., 1995 *(80)*	50	38	
Wang et al., 1996 *(81)*	72	29	
Yoon et al., 1997 *(82)*	50	37	28.2
Callister et al., 1998 *(39)*	52	19	18
Devries et al., 1995 *(83)*	91	49	
Achenbach et al., 2001 *(47)*	120	19.9	16.2
Mao et al., 2001 *(43)*	60	24	
	57	15[a]	

[a] Triggering of the scan at 40% RR interval.

resulting volume averaging and breathing misregistration due to different inspiration depth precluded exact calcium quantification.

Electron Beam CT

The introduction of EBCT in the mid-1980s made quantification of coronary artery calcifications feasible. The first reports on EBCT to quantify coronary artery calcifications were published in the late 1980s *(31,32)*. EBCT was shown to be much more sensitive than fluoroscopy to detect small and less densely calcified plaque. Only 52% of calcifications detected by EBCT had been detected by fluoroscopy in the study by Agatston and coworkers.

EBCT uses an electron beam to sweep stationary tungsten target rings to generate images. A typical scan protocol for coronary calcium detection consists of contiguous 3-mm sections covering the heart with 100-ms exposure time per slice. The scans are prospectively triggered from the electrocardiogram (ECG) of the patient, usually at 80% of the RR interval. The examination is performed during one or two breath-holds. Using EBCT with ECG triggering allowed investigators for the first time to obtain cross-sectional images of the heart with high spatial and temporal resolution. The current is currently limited to 630 mAs, which results in image noise, especially in obese patients. Signal-to-noise ratio, however, is critical for distinguishing small calcifications from image noise.

EBCT-based calcium quantification has been criticized for its rather high variability in measurement results. Interscan variability may hamper accurate serial measurements in follow-up studies. The reported mean percentage variability for the calcium score in repeat examinations ranges between 15% and 49% (*see* Table 2). This variability is well within the reported annual calcium progression rate, rendering interpretation of yearly follow-up examinations difficult.

Major reasons for this variability are artifacts resulting from either cardiac motion in scan misregistration or patient motion occurring during the long breath-hold times. The most important factor, however, seems to be the quantification method (see below) and the rather thick section thickness, which renders the measurement susceptible to partial-volume effects.

Multidetector-Row CT

The development of subsecond rotation speeds in mechanical scanners in conjunction with the development of partial scan reconstruction algorithms provided a significant improvement in temporal resolution. Limited volume coverage and slow scan speed were major drawbacks of single-section CT. In comparisons of EBCT and ECG-controlled sequential CT scanning *(33,34)*, the variability between the two modalities was rather poor (42–84%). In combination with ECG-based synchronization of image reconstruction from subsecond single-section spiral CT, agreement in the classification of subjects as "healthy" or "diseased" based on calcium score categories was above 90% *(35)*.

The now widely available MDCT scanners offer the possibility of cardiac imaging with similar or even better image quality than EBCT. This is mainly a result of advantages of acquisition geometry, adjustable tube current, and the possibility of continuous spiral scanning. Four-slice CT systems were introduced in 1998. These systems achieved rotation times as fast as 500 ms, resulting in a temporal resolution of a partial scan of 250 ms for a prospective triggering technique. Latest generation systems offer rotation times of down to 370 ms and can acquire up to 16 slices with nearly isotropic resolution. Despite the fast technological development in MDCT systems, these systems still have a potential disadvantage of inferior temporal resolution compared to a 100-ms exposure time by EBCT. Motion artifacts, especially in the rapidly moving right coronary artery, become increasingly problematic with higher heart rates or cardiac contractility. However, the tube current can be adjusted to improve the signal to noise ratio considerably, which helps to distinguish small calcifications from image noise *(36)*.

Extensive validation studies to determine the equivalence of EBCT and MDCT have not been performed. Initial experiences show good correlation of EBCT measurement and prospectively triggered MDCT. A recent study compared different quantification methods and found volume and mass indexes to be superior to the traditional calcium score for comparing the results of EBCT and MDCT, and for determining significant coronary artery disease *(37)*.

QUANTIFICATION OF CORONARY ARTERY CALCIFICATION

CT allows for reliable measurements of lesion area and lesion attenuation. On the basis of these measurements quanti-

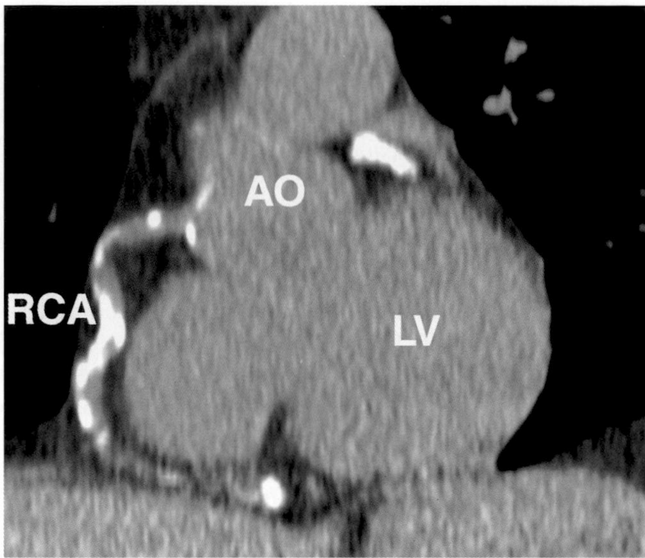

Fig. 5. Retrospective electrocardiogram gating and overlapping image reconstruction yields motion-free high-resolution images, which allow multiplanar reformation showing the heavily calcified right coronary artery (RCA). High-attenuation calcification, intermediate-attenuation vascular and cardiac structures, and the dark perivascular fat are well differentiated.

MDCT EXAMINATION TECHNIQUE

Imaging of coronary calcifications is typically performed using a low-dose technique without contrast enhancement. The scan time should be as short as possible to avoid patient motion and breathing artifacts. Synchronization of the image acquisition or image calculation with the cardiac motion is mandatory to scan the heart at reproducible positions to avoid gaps or overlaps, which would result in image misregistration. Therefore, continuous ECG recording is necessary to either trigger image acquisition in sequential scanning or to synchronize the image generation in spiral scans. The best possible temporal resolution is required for motion-free image acquisition.

The coronary arteries are easily recognized in their epimyocardial course surrounded by the low-attenuation periarterial fat. Owing to the high density of vascular calcifications, even small calcium deposits are detected with high sensitivity (Fig. 5).

The patient is positioned as in any other examination of the thorax. The scan extends form the midlevel of the left pulmonary artery down to the diaphragm, and is planned on a scout image. All MDCT scanners are able to cover this 10- to 15-cm range in one breath-hold. Continuous table feed as in spiral technique allows for somewhat faster volume coverage than sequential, stepwise scanning. In order to keep the scan protocols comparable with the increasing number of scanners and possible image-acquisition parameters, standard parameters for MDCT scanning should be developed. So far no official recommendations exist. A recommendation of image and acquisition and evaluation parameters is given in Table 3.

SEQUENTIAL SCANNING

In prospectively triggered sequential scanning, each scan is started at a predefined position in the cardiac cycle. In this approach, the next RR interval is estimated from the previous RR intervals. As long as the heart rate and rhythm remain constant, a prospective estimation of the duration of the next RR interval can be used to reliably position the scan in the mid to late diastole. In patients with change in heart rate during the necessary breath-hold or with arrhythmia, motion artifacts can impose a major problem for reliable calcium quantification *(42)*. In EBCT scanning, most groups use an 80% delay of the RR interval for the scan. Recently, a 40% delay has been recommended to increase the scan reproducibility *(43)*. For sequential MDCT scanning, no systematic evaluations have been performed to determine the optimal timing of scan triggering. As a result of the longer image exposure in MDCT, an earlier trigger time in the RR interval than the 80% commonly used in EBCT seems to be better. In coronary MDCT angiography, initial investigations based on spiral scanning and retrospectively gated image reconstruction have shown a wide variation of optimal reconstruction windows. A reconstruction window of 50–60% yielded the best results in terms of motion-free images *(44,45)*. Since motion-free images are crucial for reliable calcium quantification, a similar timing can be expected to yield favorable results in prospectively triggered MDCT scanning. In our experience, individual test scans at the mid-cardiac level with 50%, 60%, or 70% RR interval can be used to check for the optimal timing (Fig. 6). The best result can then be used for the entire cardiac scan.

SPIRAL SCANNING

Spiral image acquisition has several advantages over sequential scanning. The continuous data acquisition speeds up the scanning process, and images can be reconstructed at any position in the scanned volume. A slow table motion during the spiral data acquisition is necessary to allow for oversampling of spiral scan projections *(46)*. This is necessary to allow consistent retrospective ECG-synchronized selection of data for image reconstruction in a predefined phase of the cardiac cycle. As with prospectively ECG-triggered scanning, a specific

Table 3
Recommendations for Image Acquisition and Evaluation Parameters for Coronary Calcium Quantification With Multidetector-Row CT Scanners

Data acquisition	
Scan mode	Spiral
Tube voltage (kV)	120
Tube current	100
ECG gating	Retrospective gating in mid to late diastole, usually 50–60% RR interval; individual selection of reconstruction window with least motion artifacts is suggested
Breath hold	Inspiration
Field of view (cm)	22
Matrix	512
Scan range	Entire heart from 1 cm below tracheal bifurcation to diaphragm
Image reconstruction	
Section thickness (mm)	3
Reconstruction increment	1.5
Filter kernel	Medium smooth
Data evaluation	
Threshold (HU)	130
Minimal lesion size	1 pixel
Motion artifacts	Include in region of interest
Reporting	Number of calcified vessels, calcium mass and calcium volume score. The Agatston score cannot be recommended

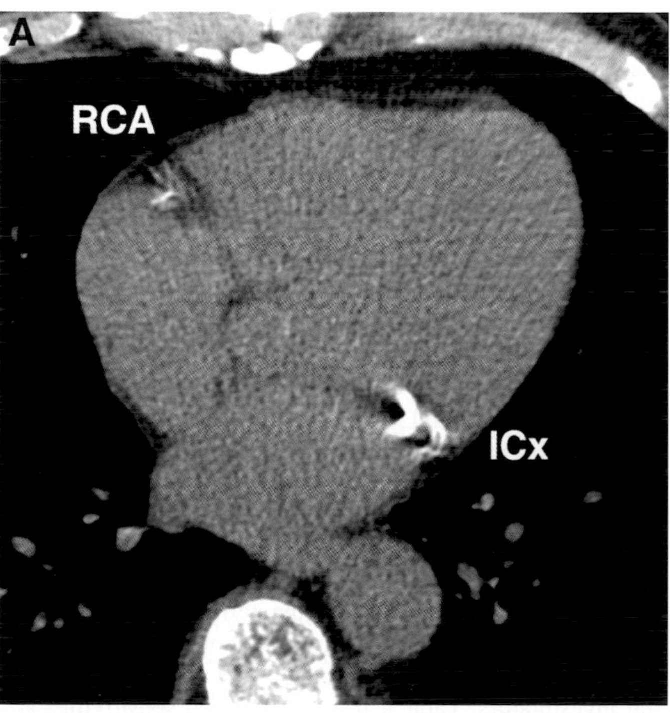

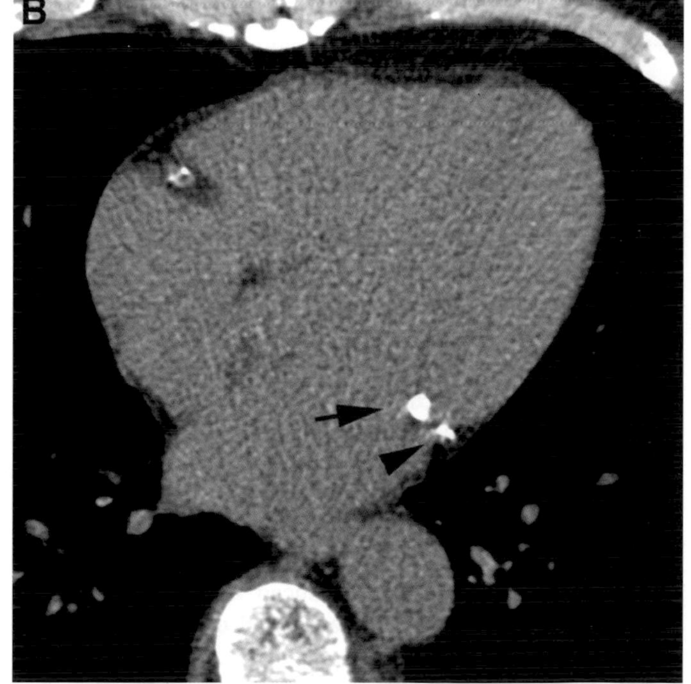

Fig. 6. Scan in the mid-cardiac level at 50% RR interval (**A**) and 60% RR interval. Motion artifacts affect the depiction of the right coronary artery (RCA) and the left circumflex (lCx). The LCx is not well delineated from calcifications of the mitral valve, which is better appreciated on the motion-free image obtained at 60% RR interval.

position of the reconstruction window in relation to the R peaks of the recorded ECG trace is chosen. Since image reconstruction is performed retrospectively after the data acquisition, an optimal agreement with the desired phase of cardiac cycle is assured. The user can perform additional reconstruction, if motion artifacts should occur. Thus misregistration because of changes in heart rate is minimal, and spiral scanning can improve the robustness of image reconstruction in arrhythmia,

Table 5
Risk Factors for Developing Coronary Heart Disease

Causal risk factors	*Predisposing risk factors*	*Conditional risk factors*
Hypercholesterolemia	BMI > 30 kg/m^3	Triglycerides
Arterial hypertension	Sedentary life style	Lipoprotein (a)
Cigarette smoking	Family history of premature myocardial infarction	Homocystein
Diabetes mellitus	Male gender	Fibrinogen
	Metabolic syndrome	Plasminogen acitvator inhibitor
	Social factors	C-reactive protein

plaque cannot be excluded. In this context, it has to be stressed that culprit plaque in sudden coronary death may contain only a little calcium and consequently is not reliably identified by CT.

CORONARY ARTERY CALCIFICATION AND DISEASE PROGRESSION

Coronary artery calcification constitutes a surrogate of total plaque burden, and plaque burden is closely related to the risk of future myocardial events. The possibility to observe changes in coronary atherosclerotic involvement noninvasively is an appealing concept for assessment of disease progression and efficacy of primary or secondary preventive measures in CAD.

Several studies have tracked changes of coronary calcium by EBCT. Score progression seems to be accelerated in patients with obstructive CAD compared with patients who have no clinically manifest disease (27% vs 18%) *(58)*. A mean annual rate of calcium score increase for untreated patients between 24% and 36% has been found. Recent studies have shown the ability of calcium quantification to monitor the progression of coronary calcification and to document the effect of risk-factor modification and medical treatment *(38,59,60,61)*. In 66 patients with coronary calcifications, the observed increase in coronary calcium volume score was 25% without treatment and decreased to 8.8% under treatment with statins *(59)*. It has not been shown whether a decrease in calcium progression also represents a decrease in future event risks. Because multiple trials on lowering cholesterol levels have shown a decrease in mortality, it is plausible that decrease in calcium score progression may be a valuable tool in monitoring and comparing such therapies.

If progression is to be assessed in an individual person, a high reliability of the calcium quantification is mandatory. Reported variability from many EBCT studies ranges between 14% and 38%, however, precluding a meaningful interpretation of calcium measurements in the individual patient. MDCT with spiral scanning, overlapping image reconstruction, and use of calcium mass measurement has resulted in a variability of 5% in a first study *(48)*. This study will need confirmation, but a significant improvement for follow-up or therapy control studies may be expected.

CORONARY ARTERY CALCIFICATION AND SCREENING FOR CAD

Conventional Identification of Subjects at Risk of CAD

According to the Air Force/Texas Coronary Atherosclerosis Prevention Study (AFCAPS/TexCAPS) only 37% of acute events can potentially be prevented using lipid-lowering therapy as primary prevention in individuals with average cholesterol levels *(62)*. Therefore, risk-assessment tools or screening tests are required that will reliably identify asymptomatic individuals at high risk of hard coronary events to efficiently target therapy.

The risk of developing CAD depends on a wide range of environmental and biochemical factors, many of which have been identified in prospective epidemiological studies. Among these well-recognized risk factors are tobacco smoking, high low-density lipoprotein cholesterol levels, low high-density lipoprotein cholesterol, diabetes mellitus, arterial hypertension, and family history of premature myocardial infarction (Table 5). These and other risk factors interact in a complex way, making risk assessment in the individual patient complicated. However, algorithms derived from large prospective epidemiological studies like the Framingham Study *(63,64)* in the United States and the Prospective Cardiovascular Münster (PROCAM) Study *(65)* in Germany can be used to calculate a person's risk of CAD. A person is said to be at increased risk if his or her absolute risk of suffering a future myocardial event within the next 10 yr exceeds 20%. Calculation of an individual's CAD risk is possible either by using scoring systems and risk charts or computer-assisted algorithms.

Subpopulations at a significantly increased global risk of CAD can be identified with a high level of exactness using scores or algorithms for risk assessment. Epidemiological studies have shown that in many individuals without clinically apparent symptoms, the risk of developing a future myocardial infarction may equal or even exceed that of persons with a history of coronary heart disease *(65)*. However, it remains questionable whether the presence of subclinical manifestations of atherosclerosis in these presymptomatic patients can be diagnosed with sufficient certainty based on traditional risk factors alone.

Even if standard or traditional risk-factor analysis is quite accurate in identifying populations at risk, exercise stress testing, which is also commonly used to screen for CAD, is characterized by a rather low accuracy in predicting events. The sensitivity of stress testing for identification of asymptomatic middle-aged males at risk for a future myocardial event is less than 40% *(66)*. This is not surprising, since more than two-thirds of acute coronary events in previously asymptomatic individuals are due to rupture or erosion of nonobstructive

Table 6
Coronary Calcium Thresholds and Test Performance for Identifying Subjects With Future Myocardial Infarction or Coronary Death (adapted from Guerci and coworkers *[78]*)

Score	*Sensitivity*	*Specificity*	*Positive predictive value*	*Negative predictive value*	*Overall accuracy*	*Odds ratio (95% CI)*
>80	0.89	0.74	0.05	0.99	0.74	22.3 (5.1–97.4)
>160	0.83	0.82	0.07	0.99	0.82	22.2 (6.4–77.4)
>600	0.55	0.94	0.13	0.98	0.94	20.3 (7.8–53.1)

CI, confidence interval.

coronary plaque *(67,13)*. Nonobstructive CAD seldom causes stress-induced myocardial ischemia, and thus perfusion imaging does not improve the detection rate of subclinical CAD.

Coronary Artery Calcification and Predicting Events

The use of noninvasive measurement of coronary artery calcification as a screening test for coronary atherosclerosis has received remarkable interest in recent years and has generated much controversy. Coronary calcium detection by CT makes the assumption that direct demonstration of atherosclerotic vessel-wall involvement in asymptomatic populations with increased coronary heart disease risk is helpful to identify as well as to stratify individuals at risk.

To evaluate a possible benefit from CT calcium screening, we first should realize that the main purpose of CAD screening is classification of asymptomatic persons as likely or not likely to have CAD. Early diagnosis of cases with subclinical CAD ought to reduce morbidity and mortality from the specific disease among the population screened, because screening leads to a course of action proven to save lives. If coronary CT screening cannot achieve a significant reduction of morbidity and mortality, it cannot be deemed effective. Therefore, we need to prove that calcium screening of the entire adult population, or even a subpopulation, leads to effective preventive therapy with a substantial benefit, before we can recommend this diagnostic test to healthy individuals and accept the involved expenditure of health care resources. Furthermore, calcium screening should identify high-risk individuals better then traditional risk-factor analysis.

In a comparison of persons dying of coronary heart disease and age- and sex-matched individuals dying of other causes, three times as much calcium was found in the coronary heart disease group *(68)*. Coronary calcium was even nine times as abundant in young persons under 50 yr of age dying suddenly, when compared to matched controls dying from accidents *(10)*.

Four prospective studies have addressed the prognostic information of coronary calcium scanning in asymptomatic individuals for predicting coronary events *(69,70,24,71)*. Results of these studies are not conclusive, since most of the studies report on a limited number of hard coronary events, the majority of endpoints being revascularizations (possibly triggered by the scan results). Furthermore, some of the studies enrolled self-referred subjects or subjects referred for scanning because of cardiovascular risk factors.

Arad et al. reported an odds ratio of 22 for the prediction of myocardial infarction or death in 1173 self-referred men and women, when comparing event rates in the group with calcium scores greater than 160 vs event rates among subjects with calcium scores less than 160 (*see* Table 6). The subjects were followed for 3.6 yr, and 18 myocardial infarctions and coronary deaths were registered. The positive predictive value increased as a function of the calcium score, indicating that calcium quantification may be a valid test for vulnerable atherosclerotic plaque.

Raggi et al. gave a relative risk of 21 for myocardial infarction or cardiovascular death in subjects with a calcium score greater than the 75th percentile when compared to individuals with a calcium score lower than the 25th percentile *(24)*. While the absolute calcium score had a wide variation in the asymptomatic individuals studied, a calcium score in the upper age- and gender-adjusted quartile seemed to identify subjects at risk better (*see* Table 7) than an increased absolute calcium score. Twenty-seven events were registered in the 632 subjects during a mean observation of 32 mo. Approximately two-thirds of the observed events occurred in patients with mild to moderate amounts of coronary artery calcium (calcium scores below 400). Subjects with massive calcifications (calcium scores >400) represented only 7% of the population scanned and accounted for 22% of all events. On the other hand, 70% of the events observed (19 of 27) occurred in 181 subjects with a calcium score above the 75th percentile adjusted for sex and age.

In a study of 926 subjects, who were either referred because of risk factors or self-referred, the highest calcium score quartile was associated with a relative risk of cardiovascular events of 9 compared to subjects without coronary calcification *(71)*. A limitation of this investigation is the high number of revascularizations (23 of 28 reported events) during a mean follow-up of 3.3 yr after scanning.

In the South Bay Heart Watch Study, 29 myocardial infarctions and 17 coronary deaths were reported during 44 mo of follow-up in 1196 asymptomatic high-risk subjects *(70)*. Calcium detection by CT failed to improve the identification of patients at risk compared to traditional risk-factor assessment in this study, which was carried out in a population originally screened by fluoroscopy.

O'Malley et al. performed a meta-analysis regarding the literature on using CT calcium to predict future events in asymptomatic adults *(72)*. Their results show that the relative risk of calcification for a myocardial infarct or CAD-related death varies from 1 to 22, with a weighted mean of 4.2. Thus, there is a strong indication that coronary calcium scanning may predict myocardial infarction in asymptomatic populations.

Table 7
Coronary Calcium Scores and Risk of Myocardial Events (according to Raggi et al. *[24]*)

In 632 asymptomatic persons, 8 fatal and 19 nonfatal myocardial infarcts were observed. The use of adjusted calcium quartiles discriminates better between risk statuses than the use of an absolute calcium score.

	Absolute calcium scores			
	0	1–99	100–400	>400
Patients	292	219	74	47
Annual event rate	0.11	2.1	4.1	4.8
	Age- and gender-adjusted calcium score quartile			
	1st	2nd	3rd	4th
Patients	351	351	100	181
Annual event rate	0.2	0.2	1.4	4.5

The question remains, whether calcium scanning performs better than conventional risk-factor analysis.

On the basis of the investigations in asymptomatic persons, some would argue that the demonstration of coronary artery calcium, which means the presence of subclinical CAD, should shift an asymptomatic patient from a primary to a secondary prevention category *(73)*. Even though this seems logical, it has not been proven that a positive or increased calcium score is equivalent to a prior myocardial infarction. Even if an increased calcium score puts a person at increased risk, as several investigations imply, one cannot be sure that any benefit would be reached by therapeutic intervention. It has been suggested that the coronary plaque burden should provide a better indicator of the probability of developing an acute coronary syndrome than a person's age and could replace age as a risk factor in the Framingham risk scores to improve risk assessment *(74)*.

Ongoing Trials

Three prospective epidemiological trials under way will examine this issue. One part of the Prospective Army Coronary Calcium (PACC) study *(75)* is a prospective cohort study of 2000 participants followed for at least 5 yr to establish the relation between coronary calcification and cardiovascular events in an unselected, "low-risk" Army population. The Multi-Ethnic Study of Atherosclerosis (MESA) will use a cohort of 6500 American adults who will undergo CT scanning and will be followed for coronary events for 7 yr.

Another population-based, prospective cohort study was begun in Germany in 2000. The RECALL (Risk Factors, Evaluation of Coronary Calcium and Lifestyle) study is designed to define the relative risk associated with EBCT-derived coronary calcium score for myocardial infarction and cardiac death in 4200 males and females aged 45 to 75 yr in an unselected urban population from the large, heavily industrialized Ruhr area *(76)*.

CONCLUSION

Risk-factor assessment and noninvasive imaging of atherosclerosis by CT calcium scanning aim at selecting subjects at a high risk for a future coronary event. While cardiovascular risk factors have been shown to increase CAD risk 1.5–5 times *(77,64)*, odds ratios for increased coronary calcium detected by CT of 22 are reported. This indicates a strong association between coronary calcification and CAD risk, even though formal proof in prospective population-based studies is still lacking.

Because atherogenesis is a dynamic process, which represents the result of a life-long exposure of an individual to a variety of predisposing factors, manifestations of subclinical coronary artery disease, as indicated by a positive CT calcium scan, may point to individuals with an increased future cardiac risk. In this respect, coronary calcium may outperform clinical risk-factor analysis in asymptomatic subjects, since the simple presence of even a combination of risk factors does not mean presence of subclinical CAD. Coronary plaque burden has been shown to be a good predictor for future coronary events in angiographic follow-up studies. Since coronary calcium is a reliable marker for CAD and since the amount of coronary calcium reflects total coronary plaque burden, demonstration of coronary artery calcification may thus be of value in improving risk stratification of asymptomatic populations with moderate to increased global coronary heart risk, or in assessing disease progression.

There is no formal proof that coronary heart disease risk can be reduced in patients with elevated coronary calcium scores. Neither is there a consensus in the professional societies on how to use the results of calcium scoring for risk-factor management or therapeutic decisions, or who should undergo CT scanning at all. In groups with intermediate or increased risk, calcium scanning may be of value, but long-term prospective studies will have to decide this issue.

MDCT scanning, especially using spiral technique with overlapping slice reconstruction and calcium quantification based on calibrated system and calcium mass measurement, holds promise to develop as the reference in the future.

REFERENCES

1. American Heart Association. Heart Disease and Stroke Statistics—2003 Update. 2002. Dallas, TX: American Heart Association.
2. Chambless L, Keil U, Dobson A, et al. Population versus clinical view of case fatality from acute coronary heart disease: results from the WHO MONICA Project 1985–1990. Multinational MONItoring of Trends and Determinants in CArdiovascular Disease. Circulation 1997;96:3849–3859.
3. Thaulow E, Erikssen J, Sandvik L, et al. Initial clinical presentation of cardiac disease in asymptomatic men with silent myocardial ischemia and angiographically documented coronary artery disease (the Oslo Ischemia Study). Am J Cardiol 1993;72:629–633.
4. Antiplatelet Trialists' Collaboration. Collaborative overview of randomized trials of antiplatelet therapy. I: Prevention of death, myocardial infarction, and stroke by prolonged antiplatelet therapy in various categories of patients. Br Med J 1994;308:81–106.
5. Shepherd J, Cobbe S, Ford I, et al. West of Scotland Coronary Prevention Study Group. Prevention of coronary heart diesease with pravastatin in men with hypercholesterolemia. N Engl J Med 1995; 333:1301–1307.
6. McCarthy J, Palmer F. Incidence and significance of coronary artery calcification. Br Heart J 1974;36:499–506.
7. Rifkin R, Parisi A, Folland E. Coronary calcification in the diagnosis of coronary artery disease. Am J Cardiol 1979;44:141–147
8. Rumberger JA, Simons DB, Fitzpatrick LA, et al. Coronary artery calcium area by electron-beam computed tomography and coronary atherosclerotic plaque area. A histopathologic correlative study. Circulation 1995;92:2157–2162
9. Sangiori G, Rumberger J, Severson A, et al. Arterial calcification and not lumen stenosis is correlated with atherosclerotic plaque burden in humans: a histologic study of 723 coronary artery segments using nondecalcifying methodology. J Am Coll Cardiol 1998; 31:126–133
10. Schmermund A, Schwartz RS, Adamzik M, et al. Coronary atherosclerosis in unheralded sudden coronary death under age 50: histopathologic comparison with healthy subjects dying out of hospital. Atherosclerosis 2001;155:499–508.
11. Stary HC, Chandler AB, Dinsmore RE, et al. A definition of advanced types of atherosclerotic lesions and a histological classification of atherosclerosis. A report from the Committee on Vascular Lesions of the Council on Arteriosclerosis, American Heart Association. Circulation 1995;92:1355–1374.
12. Stary HC, Chandler AB, Glagov S, et al. A definition of initial, fatty streak, and intermediate lesions of atherosclerosis. A report from the Committee on Vascular Lesions of the Council on Arteriosclerosis, American Heart Association. Arterioscler Thromb 1994;14:840–856.
13. Virmani R, Kolodgie FD, Burke AP, et al. Lessons from sudden coronary death: a comprehensive morphological classification scheme for atherosclerotic lesions. Arterioscler Thromb Vasc Biol 2000;20:1262–1275.
14. Ambrose JA, Tannenbaum MA, Alexopoulos D, et al. Angiographic progression of coronary artery disease and the development of myocardial infarction. J Am Coll Cardiol 1988;12:56–62.
15. Mancini GB, Pitt B. Coronary angiographic changes in patients with cardiac events in the Prospective Randomized Evaluation of the Vascular Effects of Norvasc Trial (PREVENT). Am J Cardiol 2002; 90:776–778.
16. Doherty T, Detrano R. Coronary arterial calcification as an active process: a new perspective on an old problem. Calcif. Tissue. Int. 1994;54:224–230.
17. Jeziorska M, McCollum C, Wooley D. Observations on bone formation and remodelling in advanced atherosclerotic lesions of human carotid arteries. Virchows Arch 1998;433:559–565.
18. Wexler L, Brundage B, Crouse J, et al. Coronary artery calcification: pathophysiology, epidemiology, imaging methods, and clinical implications. A statement for health professionals from the American Heart Association. Circulation 1996;94:1175–1192.
19. Burke AP, Weber D, Kolodgie F, et al. Pathophysiology of calcium deposition in coronary arteries. Herz 2001;26:239–244.
20. Schmermund A, Baumgart D, Adamzik M, et al. Comparison of electron-beam computed tomography and intracoronary ultrasound in detecting calcified and noncalcified plaques in patients with acute coronary syndromes and no or minimal to moderate angiographic coronary artery disease. Am J Cardiol 1998;81:141–146.
21. Schmermund A, Erbel R. Unstable coronary plaque and its relation to coronary calcium. Circulation 2001;104:1682–1687.
22. Janowitz WR, Agatston AS, Kaplan G, et al. Differences in prevalence and extent of coronary artery calcium detected by ultrafast computed tomography in asymptomatic men and women. Am J Cardiol 1993;72:247–254.
23. Hoff JA, Chomka EV, Krainik AJ, et al. Age and gender distributions of coronary artery calcium detected by electron beam tomography in 35,246 adults. Am J Cardiol 2001;87:1335–1339.
24. Raggi P, Callister TQ, Cooil B, et al. Identification of patients at increased risk of first unheralded acute myocardial infarction by electron-beam computed tomography. Circulation 2000;101:850–855.
25. Wong ND, Budoff MJ, Pio J, et al. Coronary calcium and cardiovascular event risk: evaluation by age- and sex-specific quartiles. Am Heart J 2002;143:456–459.
26. Newman A, Naydeck B, Sutton-Tyrell K, et al. Coronary artery calcification in older adults with minimal clinical or subclinical cardiovascular disease. J Am Geriatr Soc 2000;48:256–263.
27. Souza A, Bream P, Elliott L. Chest film detection of coronary artery calcification: the value of CAC triangle. Radiology 1978;129:7–10.
28. Detrano R, Wong N, Tang W. Prognostic significance of cardiac cinefluoroscopy for coronary calcifc deposits in asymptomatic high risk subjects. J Am Coll Cardiol 1994;24:354–358.
29. Margolis JR, Chen JT, Kong Y, et al. The diagnostic and prognostic significance of coronary artery calcification. A report of 800 cases. Radiology 1980;137:609–616.
30. Rienmüller R, Lipton M. Detection of coronary artery calcification by computed tomography. Dynam Cardiovasc Imag 1987;1:139–145.
31. Agatston A, Janowitz W, Hildner F, et al. Quantification of coronary artery calcium using ultrafast computed tomography. J Am Coll Cardiol 1990;15:827–832.
32. Tannenbaum S, Kondos G, Veselik K, et al. Detection of calcific deposits in coronary arteries by ultrafast computed tomography. J Am Coll Cardiol 1989;15:827–832.
33. Becker CR, Knez A, Jakobs TF, et al. Detection and quantification of coronary artery calcification with electron-beam and conventional CT. Eur Radiol 1999;9:620–624.
34. Budoff MJ, Mao S, Zalace CP, et al. Comparison of spiral and electron beam tomography in the evaluation of coronary calcification in asymptomatic persons. Int J Cardiol 2001;77:181–188.
35. Carr JJ, Crouse JR, 3rd, Goff DC, Jr., et al. Evaluation of subsecond gated helical CT for quantification of coronary artery calcium and comparison with electron beam CT. AJR Am J Roentgenol 2000; 174:915–921.
36. Bielak LF, Kaufmann RB, Moll PP, et al. Small lesions in the heart identified at electron beam CT: calcification or noise? Radiology 1994;192:631–636.
37. Becker CR, Kleffel T, Crispin A, et al. Coronary artery calcium measurement: agreement of multirow detector and electron beam CT. Am J Roentgenol 2001;176:1295–1298.
38. Callister T, Raggi P, Lippolis N, et al. Effect of HMG-CoA reductase inhibitors on coronary disease as assessed by electron-beam computed tomography. N Engl J Med 1998;339:1972–1978.
39. Callister TQ, Cooil B, Raya SP, et al. Coronary artery disease: improved reproducibility of calcium scoring with an electron-beam CT volumetric method. Radiology 1998;208:807–814.
40. Ulzheimer S, Kalender WA. Assessment of calcium scoring performance in cardiac computed tomography. Eur Radiol 2003;13:484–497.
41. Hong C, Becker CR, Schoepf UJ, et al. Coronary artery calcium: absolute quantification in nonenhanced and contrast-enhanced multi-detector row CT studies. Radiology 2002;223:474–480.
42. Mao SS, Oudiz RJ, Bakhshesh H, et al. Variation of heart rate and electrocardiograph trigger interval during ultrafast computed tomography. Am J Card Imaging 1996;10:239–243.

43. Mao S, Bakhsheshi H, Lu B, et al. Effect of electrocardiogram triggering on reproducibility of coronary artery calcium scoring. Radiology 2001;220:707–711.
44. Hong C, Becker CR, Huber A, et al. ECG-gated reconstructed multidetector row CT coronary angiography: effect of varying trigger delay on image quality. Radiology 2001;220:712–717.
45. Kopp AF, Schroeder S, Kuettner A, et al. Coronary arteries: retrospectively ECG-gated multi-detector row CT angiography with selective optimization of the image reconstruction window. Radiology 2001;221:683–688.
46. Ohnesorge B, Flohr T, Becker C, et al. Cardiac imaging by means of electrocardiographically gated multisection spiral CT: initial experience. Radiology 2000;217:564–571
47. Achenbach S, Meissner F, Ropers D, et al. Overlapping cross-sections significantly improve the reproducibility of coronary calcium measurements by electron beam tomography: a phantom study. J Comp Assist Tomogr 2001;25:569–573.
48. Ohnesorge B, Flohr T, Fischbach R, et al. Reproducibility of coronary calcium quantification in repeat examinations with retrospectively ECG-gated multisection spiral CT. Eur Radiol 2002;12: 1532–1540.
49. McCollough CH. Patient dose in cardiac computed tomography. Herz 2003;28:1–6.
50. Jakobs TF, Becker CR, Ohnesorge B, et al. Multislice helical CT of the heart with retrospective ECG gating: reduction of radiation exposure by ECG-controlled tube current modulation. Eur Radiol 2002;12:1081–1086.
51. Detrano R, Hsiai T, Wang S, et al. Prognostic value of coronary calcification and angiographic stenoses in patients undergoing coronary angiography. J Am Coll Cardiol 1996;27:285–290.
52. Glagov S, Weisenberg E, Zarins CK, et al. Compensatory enlargement of human atherosclerotic coronary arteries. N Engl J Med 1987; 316:1371–1375.
53. Friedrich G, Moes N, Muhlberger V, et al. Detection of intralesional calcium by intracoronary ultrasound depends on the histologic pattern. Am Heart J 1994;128:435–441.
54. Kajinami K, Seki H, Takekoshi N, et al. Noninvasive prediction of coronary atherosclerosis by quantification of coronary artery calcification using electron comuted tomography: comparison with electrocardiographic and thallium exercise stress results. J Am Coll Cardiol 1995;26:1209–1221.
55. Tuzcu E, Berkalp B, De Franco A, et al. The dilemma of diagnosing coronary calcification: angiography versus intravascular ultrasound. J Am Coll Cardiol 1996;27:832–838.
56. McLaughlin VV, Balogh T, Rich S. Utility of electron beam computed tomography to stratify patients presenting to the emergency room with chest pain. Am J Cardiol 1999;84:327–328, A328.
57. Georgiou D, Budoff MJ, Kaufer E, et al. Screening patients with chest pain in the emergency department using electron beam tomography: a follow-up study. J Am Coll Cardiol 2001;38:105–110.
58. Janowitz WR, Agatston AS, Viamonte M, Jr. Comparison of serial quantitative evaluation of calcified coronary artery plaque by ultrafast computed tomography in persons with and without obstructive coronary artery disease. Am J Cardiol 1991;68:1–6.
59. Achenbach S, Ropers D, Pohle K, et al. Influence of lipid-lowering therapy on the progression of coronary artery calcification: a prospective evaluation. Circulation 2002;106:1077–1082.
60. Budoff M, Lane K, Bakhsheshi H, et al. Rates of progression of coronary calcium by electron beam tomography. Am J Cardiol 2000;86:8–11.
61. Maher JE, Bielak LF, Raz JA, et al. Progression of coronary artery calcification: a pilot study. Mayo Clin Proc 1999;74:347–355.
62. Downs J, Clearfield M, Weis S, et al. Primary prevention of acute coronary events with lovastatin in men and women with average cholesterol levels: results of the AFCAPS/TexCAPS research. JAMA 1998;279:1615–1622.
63. Anderson K, Wilson P, Odell P, et al. An updated coronary risk profile—a statement for health professionals. Circulation 1991;83: 356–362.
64. Wilson PW, D'Agostino RB, Levy D, et al. Prediction of coronary heart disease using risk factor categories. Circulation 1998;97: 1837–1847.
65. Assmann G, Cullen P, Schulte H. Simple scoring scheme for calculating the risk of acute coronary events based on the 10-year follow-up of the prospective cardiovascular Munster (PROCAM) study. Circulation 2002;105:310–315.
66. Detrano RC, Froelicher VF. Exercise testing: uses and limitations considering recent studies. Prog Cardiovasc Dis 1988;31:837–845.
67. Petursson M, Jonmundsson E, Brekkan A, et al. Angiographic predictors of new coronary occlusions. Am Heart J 1995;129: 515–520.
68. Eggen DA, Strong JP, McGill HC. Coronary calcification: Relationship to clinically significant coronary lesions and race, sex and topographic distribution. Circulation 1965;32:948–955.
69. Arad Y, Spadaro LA, Goodman K, et al. Prediction of coronary events with electron beam computed tomography. J Am Coll Cardiol 2000;36:1253–1260.
70. Detrano RC, Wong ND, Doherty TM, et al. Coronary calcium does not accurately predict near-term future coronary events in high-risk adults. Circulation 1999;99:2633–2638.
71. Wong ND, Hsu JC, Detrano RC, et al. Coronary artery calcium evaluation by electron beam computed tomography and its relation to new cardiovascular events. Am J Cardiol 2000;86:495–498.
72. O'Malley PG, Taylor AJ, Jackson JL, et al. Prognostic value of coronary electron-beam computed tomography for coronary heart disease events in asymptomatic populations. Am J Cardiol 2000; 85:945–948.
73. Hecht HS. Impact of plaque imaging by electron beam tomography on the treatment of dyslipidemias. Am J Cardiol 2001;88:406–408.
74. Grundy SM. Coronary plaque as a replacement for age as a risk factor in global risk assessment. Am J Cardiol 2001;88:8E–11E.
75. O'Malley PG, Taylor AJ, Gibbons RV, et al. Rationale and design of the Prospective Army Coronary Calcium (PACC) Study: utility of electron beam computed tomography as a screening test for coronary artery disease and as an intervention for risk factor modification among young, asymptomatic, active-duty United States Army personnel. Am Heart J 1999;137:932–941.
76. Schmermund A, Möhlenkamp S, Stang A, et al. Assessment of clinically silent atherosclerotic disease and established and novel risk factors for predicting myocardial infarction and cardiac death in healthy middle-aged subjects: rationale and design of the Heinz Nixdorf RECALL Study. Risk Factors, Evaluation of Coronary Calcium and Lifestyle. Am Heart J 2002;144:212–218.
77. Chambless LE, Heiss G, Folsom AR, et al. Association of coronary heart disease incidence with carotid arterial wall thickness and major risk factors: the Atherosclerosis Risk in Communities (ARIC) Study, 1987–1993. Am J Epidemiol 1997;146:483–494.
78. Guerci AD, Arad Y. Potential use of Ca++ scanning to determine the need for and intensity of lipid-lowering therapy in asymptomatic adults. Curr Cardiol Rep 2001;3:408–415.
79. Kajinami K, Seki H, Takekoshi N, Mabuchi H. Quantification of coronary artery calcification using ultrafast computed tomography: reproducibility of measurements. Coron Artery Dis 1993;4(12): 1103–1108.
80. Shields JP, Mielke CH, Jr, Rockwood TH, Short RA, Viren FK. Reliability of electron beam computed tomography to detect coronary artery calcification. Am J Card Imaging 1995;9(2):62–66
81. Wang S, Detrano RC, Secci A, et al. Detection of coronary calcification with electron-beam computed tomography: evaluation of interexamination reproducibility and comparison of three image-acquisition protocols. Am Heart J 1996;132(3):550–558.
82. Yoon HC, Greaser LE, 3rd, Mather R, et al. Coronary artery calcium: alternate methods for accurate and reproducible quantitation. Acad Radiol 1997;4(10):666–673.
83. Devries S, Wolfkiel C, Shah V, Chomka E, Rich S. Reproducibility fo the measurement of coronary calcium with ultrafast computed tomography. Am J Cardiol 1995;75(14):973–975.
84. Breen JB, Sheedy PF, Schwartz RS, et al. Coronary artery calcification detected with ultrafast CT as an indication of coronary artery disease. Radiology 1992;185:435–439.

85. Fallavollita JA, Brody AS, Bunnell IL, Kumar K, Canty JM, Jr. Fast computed tomography detection of coronary calcification in the diagnosis of coronary artery disease. Comparison with angiography in patients <50 years old. Circulation 1994;89(1):285–290.

86. Rumberger JA, Sheedy PF, III, Breen JF. Coronary calcium, as determined by electron beam computed tomography, and coronary disease on arteriogram: Effect of patient's sex on diagnosis. Circulation 1995;91:1363–1367.

87. Budoff MJ, Georgiou D, Brody A, et al. Ultrafast computed tomography as a diagnostic modality in the detection of coronary artery disease: a multicenter study. Circulation 1996;93(5): 898–904.

88. Haberl R, Becker A, Leber A, et al. Correlation of coronary calcification and angiographically documented stenoses in patients with suspected coronary artery disease: results of 1,764 patients. J Am Coll Cardiol 2001;37(2):451–457.

13 Noninvasive Quantification of Coronary Calcium

Quantification Methods, Scanner Types, Scan Protocols, Accuracy, and Reproducibility

STEFAN ULZHEIMER, PhD, KAISS SHANNEIK, MSc,
AND WILLI A. KALENDER, PhD

INTRODUCTION

Calcium in the form of hydroxyapatite (HA) is regarded as a known marker for the presence of atherosclerotic lesions of the coronary arteries. Several studies have demonstrated that the risk for coronary events is associated and strongly correlated with the amount of coronary calcium *(1,2)*. The absence of coronary calcium does almost certainly imply the absence of coronary artery disease (CAD) *(3)*, which, according to a World Health Report by the World Health Organization (WHO), is the leading cause of mortality in the world, amounting to 13.7%.

Calcium strongly attenuates X-rays as a result of its relatively high atomic number. Therefore, X-ray techniques are quite suitable methods to detect and quantify coronary calcifications. In the past, plain chest radiographs and fluoroscopy were used to detect coronary calcifications, but they are both not sensitive enough and could not be used for the quantification of calcium *(4)*.

Since its introduction in the late 1980s, electron beam computed tomography (EBCT) has been well established as a noninvasive imaging modality for the quantification of coronary calcium *(5)* and the effective diagnosis of CAD. In addition, EBCT has offered the potential to image coronary arteries using CT angiography (CTA) for diagnostic and follow-up studies (e.g., detecting and tracking any changes in the observed parameters, such as the progress of the disease or the response to a certain medication). For the first time, these scanners allowed the tomographic depiction of the entire heart volume (about 120 mm) to be imaged during one breath-hold and with high temporal resolution (≥50 ms). For common protocols, the total acquisition time was 100 ms for single axial sections of 3 mm.

From: *Contemporary Cardiology: CT of the Heart: Principles and Applications*
Edited by: U. Joseph Schoepf © Humana Press, Inc., Totowa, NJ

Imaging of the heart has some very high demands to any imaging modality. For instance, it is of great importance to have a very high reproducibility when detecting coronary calcifications in order to be able to track the progress of the disease or the effectiveness of a certain medication. Despite its good temporal resolution, EBCT does suffer from a number of drawbacks, such as its restriction to cardiac applications as a result of limited performance in other fields compared to conventional CT scanners.

Therefore, conventional CT has tried to challenge EBCT in its domain of cardiac imaging since the first scanners became available. So, while conventional mechanical scanners without any special arrangements to reduce motion artifacts have been used for the quantification of coronary calcium *(6–11)*, much attention has been put to improve cardiac imaging by developing new reconstruction approaches in image acquisition *(12)*. However, owing to restrictions and limitations in image acquisition speed and low volume coverage (single-slice scanners with 0.75-s gantry rotation time), this early generation of scanners has not completely achieved this ambitious goal. It was not until the introduction of multislice computed tomography (MSCT) in 1998, with the acquisition of four slices simultaneously and an increase of the gantry rotation speed (0.5 ms), that several new clinical applications became much more feasible, such as motion artifact-free imaging of the human heart. The complex 3D motion of the heart can cause any single-slice CT scanner, and even the EBCT in a much higher probability, to miss certain calcifications or even to count them more than once. The new mechanical CT scanners do not suffer from this problem, as they offer continuous spiral image data acquisition. Electrocardiogram (ECG)-triggered and ECG-gated reconstruction techniques have helped with new dedicated reconstruction algorithms to obtain a much better temporal resolution of typically 100–250 ms. These scanners also allowed for thinner slices (4 × 1-mm collimation) to be applied,

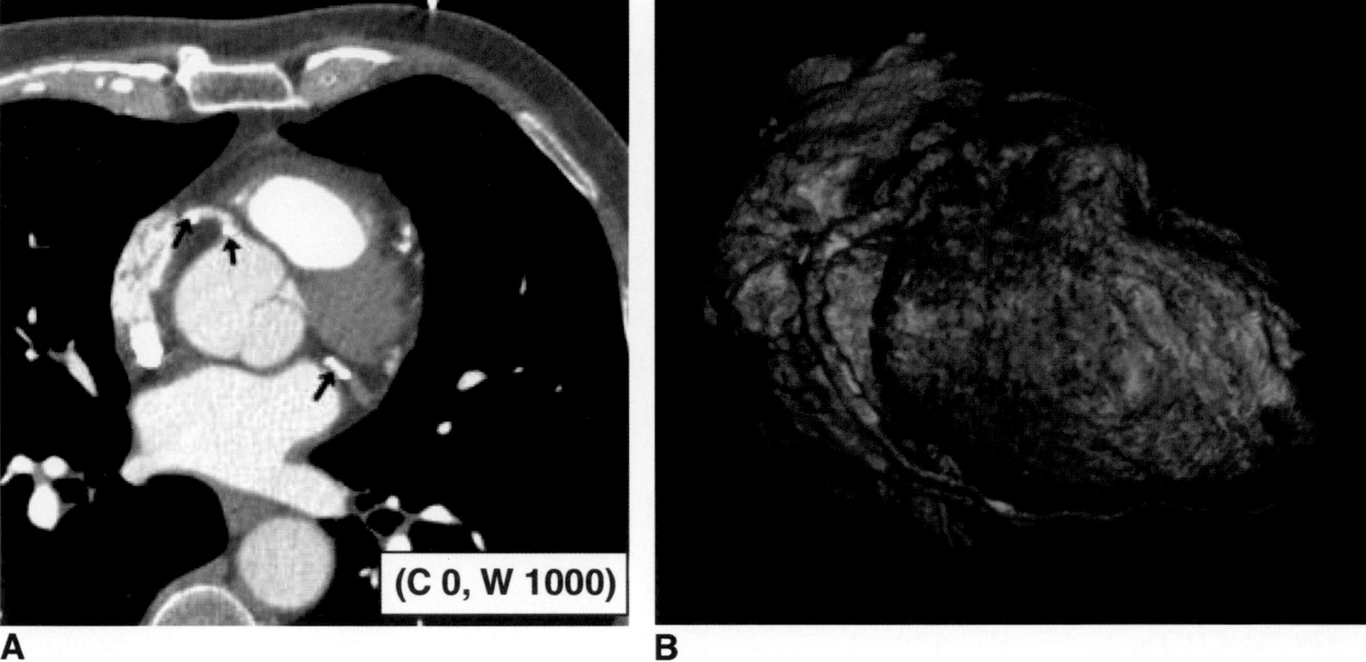

Fig. 1. (**A**) Severe calcifications of the coronary arteries are clearly depicted even in contrast enhanced CT images for CTA studies. Obviously contrast enhanced scan are not the method of choice to detect small amounts of calcium and for exact quantification of calcium. The scan was performed on a Siemens SOMATOM Sensation 16 scanner with a standard cardiac scan protocol with a slice collimation of 12 × 0.75 mm and a rotation time of 0.42 s. (**B**) shows a volume rendering of the showing the whole extent of the coronary arteries without any interruptions.

and offered excellent, almost isotropic resolution in the visualization of the coronary anatomy, thereby making it more than suitable in detecting CAD in an early stage of development (Fig. 1). In 2001, a new generation of scanners was introduced by various manufacturers *(13,14)*. These scanners offered further improved spatial and temporal resolution, a reduced scanning time because of the faster gantry rotation (down to 0.42 s), and an increased number of simultaneously acquired slices (up to 16 submillimeter slices). Rapid developments in computer and engineering technology have provided an opportunity to explore new clinical applications and to use cardiac CT imaging as a valuable quantification tool in clinical routine.

With the advent of these new MSCT scanners, it becomes even more important to develop and establish standardized concepts for quality assurance in order to determine the systems' performance characteristics. It clearly becomes mandatory to know the errors of the methods applied and to develop tools which allow for calibration and direct comparison of results obtained on arbitrary scanners. Unfortunately, in the case of the quantification of coronary calcium, this crucial task has been neglected. Moreover, as the quantification of coronary calcium with EBCT is still considered by many to be the "gold standard," the new methods have to be compared to EBCT. Therefore, a phantom that provides an anthropomorphic and reproducible environment has been designed and developed *(15,16)*.

The issue of calcium score reproducibility has been addressed by several clinical studies *(17–24)*. One paper determined the reproducibility to be around 30% *(25)*, while another judged the method as being ". . . not sufficiently reproducible to allow serial quantification of coronary calcium in individual patients over relatively short periods (<2 years)" *(24)*. In order to determine small changes with statistical significance, the standard deviation of the measurement has to be low.

In the following sections we will review scoring methods and concepts for quality assurance and standardization in this field.

QUANTIFYING CORONARY CALCIUM

THE AGATSTON SCORE

The first group that used EBCT images for the quantification of coronary calcium were Agatston et al. in 1990. They introduced a pseudo-quantitative scoring method—later called *Agatston score*—which became the traditional scoring method. The Agatston score in its original form *(5)* is determined from 20 contiguous EBCT slices of the heart (3-mm slice thickness, no interslice gaps, 100-ms data acquisition time per slice and breath-holding). The most cephalad slice is placed at the lower margin of the main pulmonary artery, and image acquisition is triggered at 80% of the simultaneously recorded ECG signal. Calcified lesions are identified by applying a segmentation threshold of 130 Hounsfield units (HU) on each of the 20 images and ignoring structures with sizes below 1 mm^2 to exclude noise from evaluation. For each coronary artery i a region of interest (ROI) is placed around each calcified lesion j in each of the 20 images. In a succeeding step, the area A_{ij} of the ROI in mm^2 and the maximum CT number $CT\#^{max}$ in HU are determined. The Agatston score, S_{ij} of lesion j in coronary artery i is calculated as the product of the area of the lesion A_{ij} with a weighting factor w_{ij} that depends on the maximum CT number $CT\#_{ij}^{max}$ in the lesions for each image:

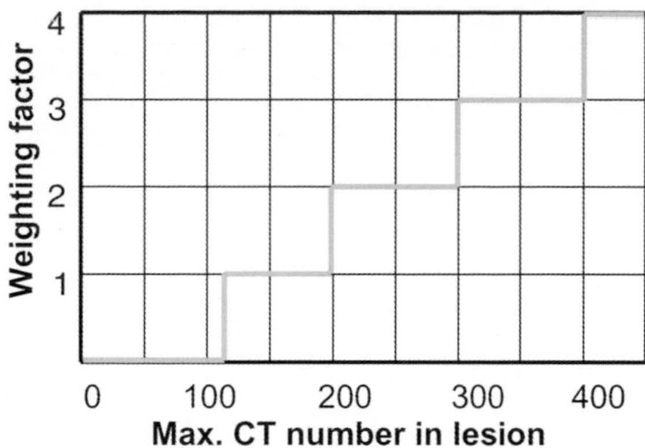

Fig. 2. Determination of the weighting factor for calculating the Agatston score.

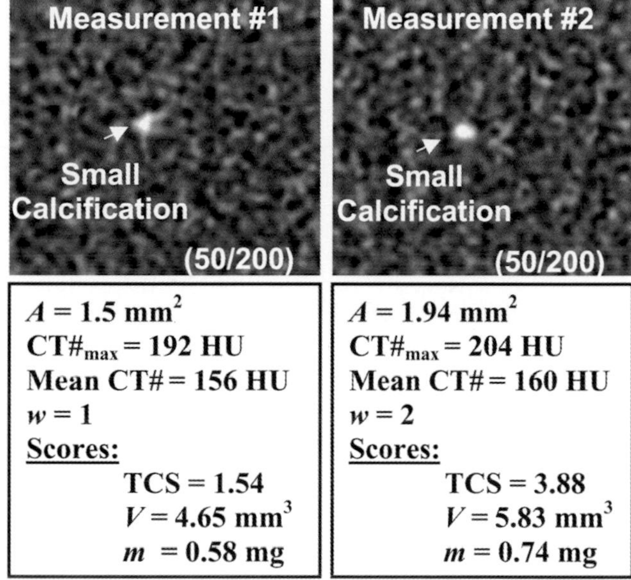

Fig. 3. Evaluation of two measurements of the same small calcification with EBCT. Agatston score TCS, volume score *V* and calcium mass *m* are calculated. The Agatston score shows a variability of 150%. For the volume score and the calcium mass the reproducibility errors are much smaller.

$$S_{ij} = w_{ij} \cdot A_{ij} \tag{1}$$

with

$$w_{ij} = \begin{cases} 1 \text{ if } 150\text{ HU} = CT\,\#_{ij}^{\max} < 200\text{HU} \\ 2 \text{ if } 200\text{ HU} = CT\,\#_{ij}^{\max} < 300\text{HU} \\ 3 \text{ if } 300\text{ HU} = CT\,\#_{ij}^{\max} < 400\text{HU} \\ 4 \text{ if } 400\text{ HU} = CT\,\#_{ij}^{\max} \end{cases} \tag{2}$$

The total calcium score (S_{tot} or TCS) for all lesions in all coronary arteries is determined by summing up the scores of the lesions for all arteries in all images:

$$S_{tot} = \Sigma_{ij} S_{ij} = \Sigma_{ij} w_{ij} \cdot A_{ij} \tag{3}$$

In later publications the score for each of the coronary arteries alone was given separately, e.g.,

$$S_{LAD} = \Sigma_{ij} S_{LAD,j} \tag{4}$$

for the left anterior descending artery (LAD).

Figure 2 illustrates the determination of the weighting factor *w* from the maximum CT number in the lesion, which is described mathematically in equation 2. However, it should be noted that there is not a linear relationship when considering the Agatston score because of the definitive weighting factors being used. Figure 3 demonstrates how the Agatston score is calculated for two EBCT scans of one and the same small artificial calcification with a diameter of 2 mm. By considering this example it becomes evident what the drawbacks of this score are (Table 1) and why the Agatston score can show a quite high variability, which in this case is 150%. Noise and motion are the cause for artifacts and result in small differences in images. The strong dependence of the Agatston score on noise results from the fact that it is based on the maximum CT number

Table 1
Pros and Cons of the Agatston Score

Pros	*Cons*
Has been used for >10 yr, which resulted in an accumulation of a large amount of data	Is unnecessarily complex
Has been shown to correlate with coronary events	Was created for a special modality and protocol
	Uses absolute CT numbers that depend upon reconstruction kernel, data corrections, etc.
	Does not correspond to any physical measure
	Is not a linear measure—weighting factors are used
	Because its definition is based on contiguous, nonoverlapping 3-mm slices, an adaptation of the equations must be undertaken for scanners other than electron beam CT
	Uses maximum CT numbers and is therefore prone to noise and motion
	Sensitive to noise and artifacts

that can lead to a difference in weighting factors by a factor of up to two.

When scoring one and the same data set on different workstations, the probability of getting different Agatston scores is quite high *(26,27)*. The quite complex description of the score makes it difficult to obtain a decisive conclusion, as it leaves in some points room for interpretation, while in others the programmers knowingly have tried to make the score more robust. However, these small differences obtained from the scoring software seem to be negligible, as the definition of the score itself is quite arbitrary and is not based on any physical fundamentals.

Besides the already mentioned strong dependence on small variations resulting from noise and motion, there are a number of other factors that have a serious effect on this scoring method. These include its dependence on absolute CT numbers, the number of slices per scan length, and its nonlinearity for increasing amounts of calcium, which is due to its reliance on nonlinear weighting factors. Furthermore, as the score does not correspond to any physical measure, it cannot be easily compared to "true" values for exactly defined calcifications.

A large amount of data has accumulated over the years with the use of the Agatston score, and the risk tables derived for coronary events *(28)* are the only, but of course very important, advantages of this score.

Even though the Agatston score shows a number of serious drawbacks and limitations, it has been used extensively in the past years and has established itself as a *de facto* standard for coronary calcium scoring. Some groups have suggested modifications for the Agatston score in order to improve its reproducibility *(29)* or sensitivity *(7)*, but all efforts were not rigorous enough and have not resulted in a better standard. Other groups made modifications to their EBCT scan protocols (e.g., different trigger positions than 80%, mean CT numbers instead of maximum CT numbers, or different thresholds were used), to achieve an increase in reproducibility or sensitivity *(29)*. Therefore, even for EBCT the data acquired during the last 13 yr are not necessarily validated and cannot be considered exactly comparable.

Compared to the known high interscan variability of calcium scores of up to 46% for small calcifications determined for EBCT and the Agatston score *(21)*, even conventional approaches without any dedicated improvements for motion-artifact reduction yielded similar results. For example, the intermodality variability in a study which compared conventional 0.75-s sequential scans without ECG triggering to EBCT was 42% *(6)*.

It is possible to adapt the Agatston score to a certain degree so that other scanners and other protocols yield similar absolute scoring results as EBCT (Fig. 4) if the scan protocols are carefully designed and corrections are applied when calculating the score. Nevertheless, not all effects that influence the Agatston score on different scanners or for different scan protocols can be taken into account.

VOLUME SCORES

Recent studies *(30)* based on estimating the volume of the calcification provide an alternative quantification method for coronary calcium. This scoring method, which can also be applied to EBCT, has become more and more popular as some studies indicate that it is more robust with respect to reproducibility *(25)*. The determination is very similar to the Agatston score. The volume score represents the volume V of the voxels of the calcification that lie above a certain threshold. A ROI is drawn around each calcified lesion, and for each lesion the number of voxels in the volume data set that lie above a certain threshold is multiplied by the volume of one voxel

$$V_{ij} = N_{\text{Voxel}} \cdot V_{\text{Voxel}} \tag{5}$$

The easiest segmentation approach again is to take all voxels above a certain threshold, e.g., again 130 HU.

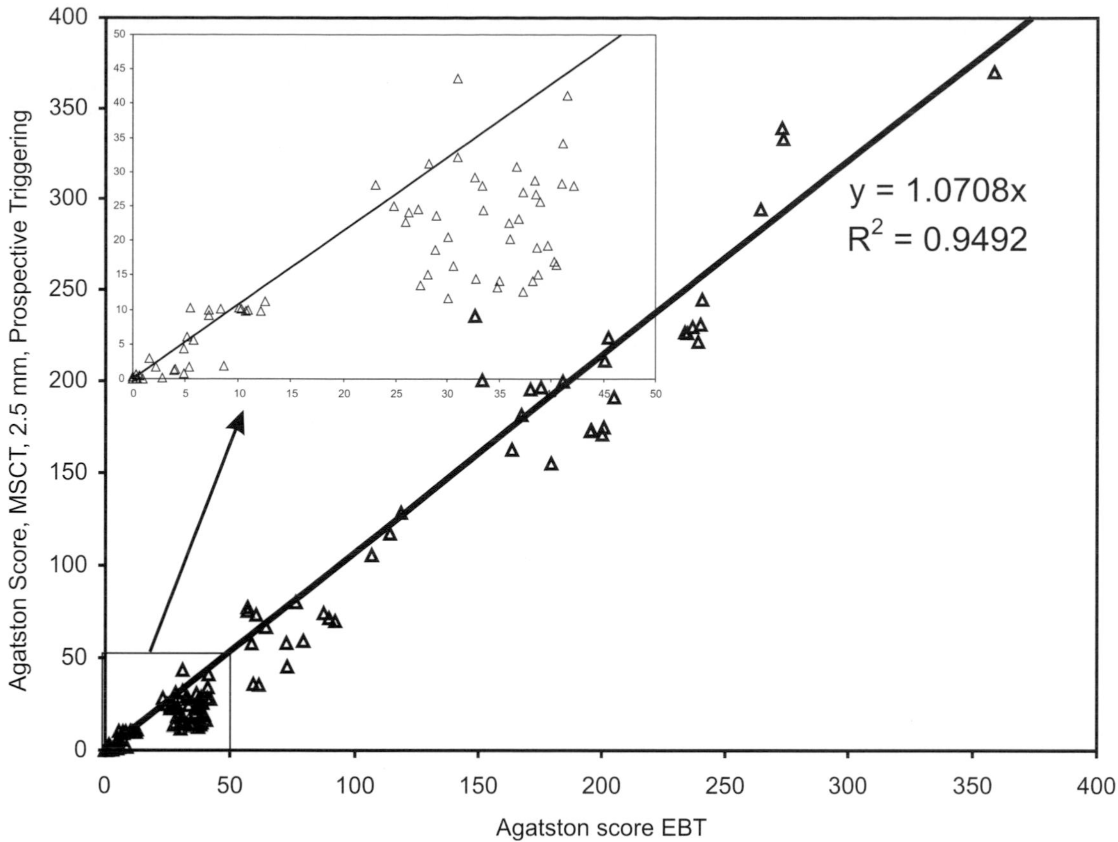

Fig. 4. Correlation of Agatston scores determined with two different scanners (EBCT and a conventional 4-slice scanner with prospective triggering). When the scan protocols on scanners other than EBCT are carefully designed and corrections are applied when calculating the Agatston score quite good agreement of scores on different machines can be achieved.

The total volume score is the sum of all individual lesions:

$$V_{tot} = \Sigma_{i,j} V_{ij}$$

Compared to the traditional scoring method—the Agatston score—this scoring method provides a higher reproducibility *(30)*. However, there are also a few disadvantages when using the volume score as a quantification method. For example, it should be noted that when using a relatively large slice thickness for small calcifications that have a high density, or when there is a fixed threshold, this score can lead to large deviations from the true volume of the calcification, caused by the partial-volume effects. Thus, the volume score may strongly over- or underestimate the real volume of the calcification. Also, as the volume score depends on the applied threshold, it is not a true physical representation of the volume of the calcification.

CALCIUM MASS

Another more rigorously defined scoring method aims at the determination of the absolute calcium mass, and thereby is the only scoring method that provides a truly quantitative measure for the amount of calcium, e.g., given in milligrams hydroxyapatite (HA) above a certain threshold. It possesses many advantages compared to the other two scoring methods. For instance, it can be easily determined, is comparable for different scanners and protocols, and shows an increased reproducibility compared to the Agatston score *(16,31)*. However, it also is dependent on the segmentation threshold.

The mean CT number $\overline{CT}$ of the calcification in each slice multiplied by the volume V of the calcification in that slice is directly proportional to the calcium mass m in that slice (Fig. 5).

$$m_i \propto \overline{CT_i} \cdot V_i \qquad (6)$$

The density of the calcification, and with it the calcium mass, is directly proportional to the mean CT number in the calcification (Fig. 5). It automatically corrects for linear partial-volume effects, as objects smaller than the slice thickness are displayed with accordingly decreased mean CT numbers. To obtain the complete mass of the calcification, the single masses for all slices are summed up. Although the value could serve as a measure for the calcium mass, it is desirable and much more descriptive to obtain absolute values for the calcium mass m.

To obtain absolute values for the calcium mass, a simple calibration measurement of a calcification with known HA density ρ_{HA} has to be carried out and a calibration factor c determined so that

$$m_{ij} = c \cdot \overline{CT_{ij}} \cdot V_{ij} \qquad (7)$$

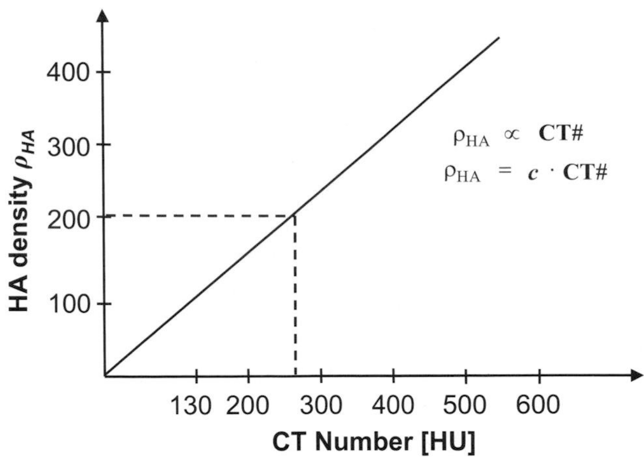

Fig. 5. The density of a calcification and with it the calcium mass is proportional to the mean CT number in the calcification. The absolute calcium mass can be determined with a simple calibration measurement carried out at a regular intervals for each scanner type and scan protocol.

Using the relation $m_{ij} = \rho_{HA} \cdot V$, the calibration factor c is calculated as

$$c = m/(\overline{CT} \cdot V) = (\rho_{HA} \cdot V)/(\overline{CT} \cdot V) = \rho_{HA}/\overline{CT}. \quad (8)$$

Equation 6 assumes that the mean CT number of water is 0 by definition. If an exact CT value for water is available from the same calibration measurement, and if it is not equal to 0, this can be taken into account by subtracting the CT value for water from the CT number of the calcification (baseline correction):

$$c = \rho_{HA} \left(\overline{CT} - \overline{CT}_{water} \right) \quad (9)$$

In practical cases, the CT number of water always has to be checked and taken into account. The calibration factor c therefore is given by the HA density ρ_{HA} of the known calcification divided by the mean CT number difference in the calibration measurement. Therefore, for each scanner and scan protocol, a specific calibration factor is obtained.

The mass score of individual lesions is summed up to obtain the total mass score:

$$m_{tot} = \Sigma_{i,j} m_{ij}.$$

TOOLS FOR QUALITY ASSURANCE IN CORONARY CALCIUM SCORING

Assessing important performance parameters such as reproducibility, accuracy, and comparability can be a difficult task, as there are many parameters that may vary. This is in particular so in patient studies where it might be ethically problematic to scan patients several times just to be able to obtain values for reproducibility or to compare calcium scores on different scanners. It is evident that it is necessary to design and develop appropriate phantoms that allow the investigation of such parameters. Furthermore, we will show that the anthropomorphic phantoms later introduced can be used as calibration standards for the assessment of absolute calcium mass values *(15,16,31)*.

The developed cardiac phantom has been manufactured in cooperation with the company QRM GmbH, in Möhrendorf, Germany. The exact dimensions of the phantom are shown in Fig. 6. In order to achieve maximum flexibility in the assessment of different image quality parameters, a modular concept has been chosen. In Fig. 7, an example of the phantom body with a calibration insert can be seen. The phantom consists of a phantom body that provides an anthropomorphic and reproducible environment, consisting of a cross-section of the human thorax with artificial lung tissue and a spine insert surrounded by tissue-equivalent material. At the position of the heart there is an empty 10-cm circular space that is able to hold different kinds of inserts. It allows for various quality assessment measurements in coronary calcium scoring, such as the investigation of spatial and temporal resolution, contrast and noise, patient dose and detection limits, reproducibility, and accuracy in coronary calcium scoring. Additionally, extension rings for the phantom were developed in order to mimic different patient sizes for the realistic assessment of image noise in larger patients (Fig. 8).

The phantom inserts representing different sizes and concentrations of calcium hydroxyapatite and two calibration inserts allow us to test both the calibration and accuracy of arbitrary scanners and scan protocols, and the reproducibility of the measurements.

Small, exactly defined calcifications, consisting of different HA densities immersed in water-equivalent plastic, can be inserted into the phantom body to simulate realistic calcifications. One example is a solid insert that contains nine small calcifications (1-, 3-, and 5-mm diameter) with three different HA densities (200, 400, and 800 mg HA/cm^3) (Fig. 9). Additionally, the insert contains two large cylinders, one consisting of water-equivalent material and one with an HA density of 200 mg HA/cm^3. These inserts can be used to determine the calibration factor c in equation 9 to calculate the calcium mass. Table 2 gives an overview of HA densities and the sizes of all cylindrical calcifications with their respective values for the areas of the circular cross-sections and the volumes of the cylinders and the HA masses inside the calcifications. One cannot expect to obtain exactly these values in measurements with the phantom, as the measured values strongly depend on scan parameters such as noise, slice thickness, and above all the segmentation threshold. They can be used in the calibration process, however, in order to provide more accurate scoring results.

An exemplary evaluation of all calcifications is given in Table 3. It shows among other findings an extremely high sensitivity, and that even for small calcifications with a calcium mass of less than 1 mg and a relatively large slice thickness of 2.5 mm, an acceptable quantification of the calcium can be performed. Nevertheless, thinner slices would improve the accuracy considerably.

In order to investigate the influence of cardiac motion, a setup was built using the anthropomorphic cardiac phantom with a water tank is placed inside the space reserved for inserts that also allows the movement of objects (e.g., calcifications) in an anthropomorphic manner. The setup is composed of a robot, seen at the back, which is able to mimic realistic heart

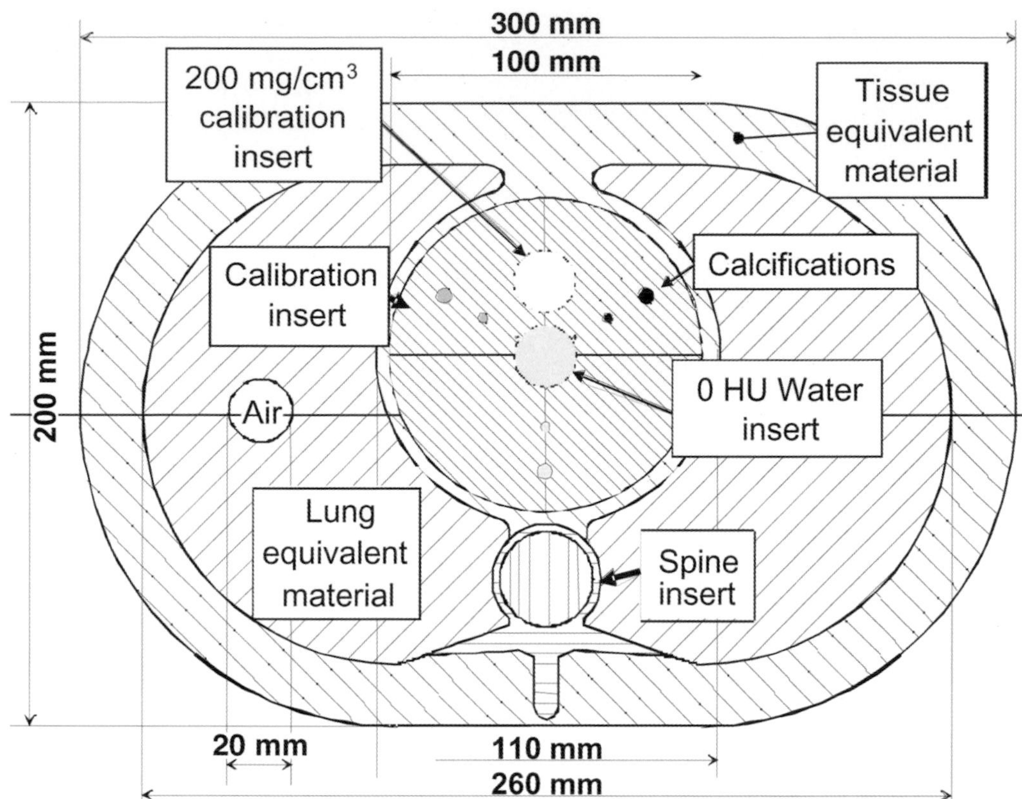

Fig. 6. Sketch of the anthropomorphic cardiac phantom for quality assurance and calibration purposes.

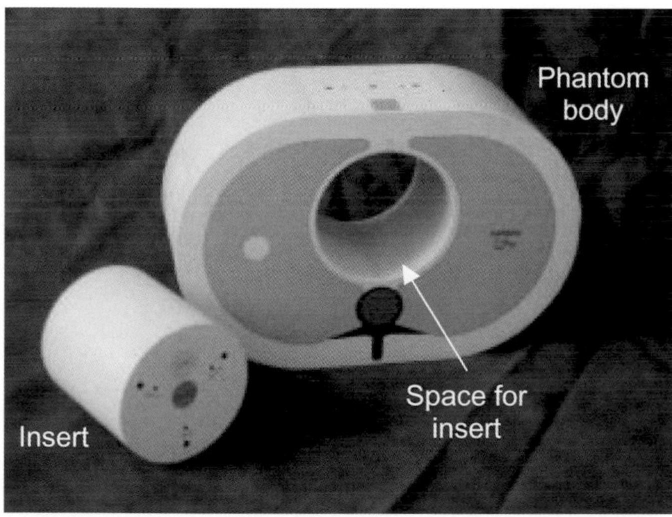

Fig. 7. A photo of the anthropomorphic phantom body with a calibration insert that can be placed inside the circular space in the center of the body phantom. The space can hold different kinds of static inserts for various quality assessment measurements.

movements in all three dimensions by simulating arbitrary 3D trajectories inside the water tank that is inserted into the anthropomorphic phantom body (Fig. 10A,B). The robot is controlled by means of a conventional PC or laptop, and its movements are coupled to an ECG monitor to simulate the required heartbeats later used for retrospective image reconstruction.

Realistic motion functions have been obtained from cine angiography. Figure 11 shows a 4D plot of such a motion function. A set of linear translation tables was assembled, which were mounted perpendicular to each other in order to reach all points in 3D space. A system of metal rods that reaches into the water tank was attached to one of the translation tables. The water-equivalent rods containing the respective test objects can be easily attached to this end of the metal rods. The setup also produces a corresponding ECG signal that can be directly fed into the ECG monitor used for triggering and gating reconstruction techniques. As an application example, a plastic rod with an immersed calcified specimen extracted from a cadaver was moved with a realistic 3D motion function at a heart rate of 60 beats per minute (bpm) and scanned on a spiral CT scanner with retrospective gating technique *(32)*. For the motion function that was used, the calcification is depicted nearly perfectly in a slow-motion heart phase at around 60% of the RR interval (Fig. 10C). In other phases the calcification is depicted with more or less severe motion artifacts, depending on the motion speed and amplitude. This or similar phantom setups are used in the validation of new approaches for cardiac imaging and in the comparison of the behavior of different scanners with respect to the depiction of the moving heart.

The described phantoms were used to show that comparable Agatston scores can be obtained on different scanners and with different scan protocols, but also that the calcium mass is an easier and more reproducible measure *(31)*. The calcium mass

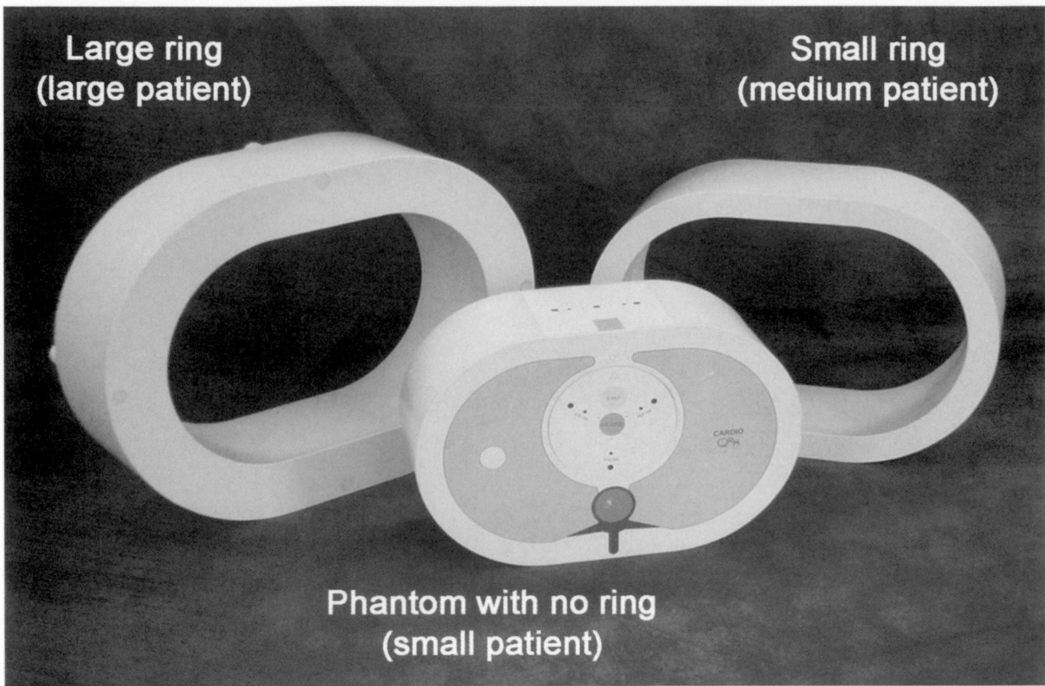

Fig. 8. Extension rings for the phantom body can mimic different patient sizes to investigate the influence of patient size on e.g., image noise and quantification results. The phantoms are manufactured in co-operation with QRM GmbH, Möhrendorf, Germany (www.qrm.de).

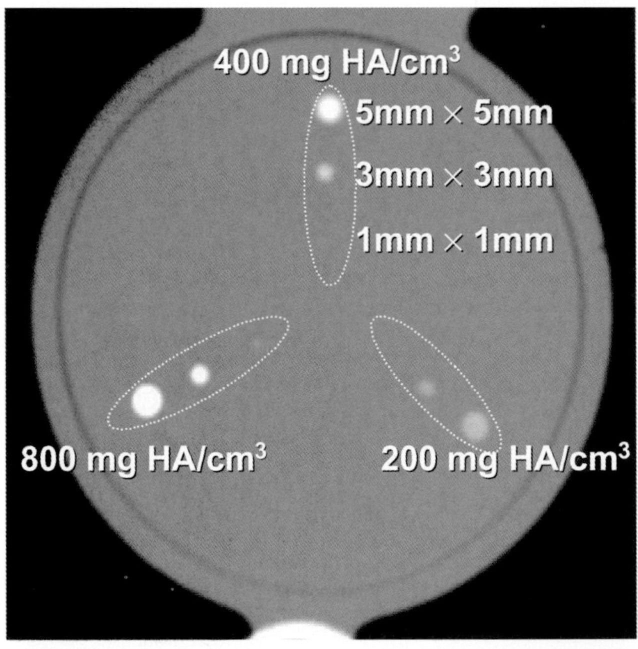

Fig. 9. Static insert for the phantom body that contains various calcifications of different sizes and HA densities. There are three different inserts for each of the three HA densities (200 mg HA/cm^3, 400 mg HA/cm^3, 800 mg HA/cm^3).

Table 2
Properties of the Cylindrical Calcifications Inside the Calibration Insert

HA density (mg/cm^3)	*Length (mm)*	*Diameter (mm)*	*Area (mm^2)^a*	*Volume (mm^3)*	*HA mass (mg)*
200	5.0	5.0	19.6	98.2	19.6
200	3.0	3.0	7.1	21.2	4.2
200	1.0	1.0	0.8	0.8	0.2
400	5.0	5.0	19.6	98.2	39.3
400	3.0	3.0	7.1	21.2	8.5
400	1.0	1.0	0.8	0.8	0.3
800	5.0	5.0	19.6	98.2	78.5
800	3.0	3.0	7.1	21.2	17.0
800	1.0	1.0	0.8	0.8	0.6

^{a}Area of the circular cross-section of the cylindric calcifications.

is correlated to the Agatston score, so that it is possible to roughly calculate the calcium mass from the Agatston score. The determination of the calcium mass and its accuracy with an EBCT scanner is depicted in Fig. 12. From the graph it can be easily shown that the calcium mass is quite well correlated to the Agatston score (R^2 = 0.9733) and that the mass can be accurately calculated from the Agatston score by multiplying it by a factor of, in this specific case, 0.1922. By achieving a good correlation between the two scores we are able to assure that old data collected over the past years would not be lost completely when switching to new quantification methods. Reproducibility for a moving calcification with different scores and scanning methods was investigated on three different scanners (EBCT Evolution C-150XP, Imatron; Volume Zoom, Siemens; SOMATOM Sensation 16, Siemens), in which the dependence of the Agatston score and HA mass on the heart

Table 3
Exemplary Determination of Agatston Score, Volume, and Calcium Mass for All Calcifications in the Calibration Insert

	Agatston score	*Volume (mm³)*			*Calcium mass (mg)*		
	measured	*measured*	*true value*	*deviation*	*measured*	*true value*	*deviation*
200 mgHA/cm3							
5 mm	86.33	118.45	98.17	21%	19.41	19.63	1%
3 mm	14.65	18.79	98.17	21%	19.41	19.63	1%
1 mm	—	—	0.79	—	—	0.16	—
400 mgHA/cm3							
5 mm	193.50	160.41	98.17	63%	42.11	39.27	7%
3 mm	43.18	42.25	21.21	99%	7.70	8.48	9%
1 mm	(0.53)[a]	1.34	0.79	70%	0.16	0.31	49%
800 mgHA/cm3							
5 mm	234.90	182.82	98.17	86%	92.79	78.54	18%
3 mm	83.47	52.17	21.21	146%	10.67	16.96	22%
1 mm	2.82	3.53	0.79	349%	0.53	0.63	15%

A sequence scan was carried out with 1.5-s rotation time and 2 × 10-mm slice collimation for the large calibration inserts and 4 × 2.5-mm slice collimation and 0.5-s rotation time for the small calcifications. For both measurements, the tube current was 150 mAs and the voltage 140 kVp. The field of view was chosen to be 100 mm with a 512 × 512 pixel matrix for both measurements.

[a]The area was below 1 mm^2. According to the original version of the Agatston score, the score is 0.

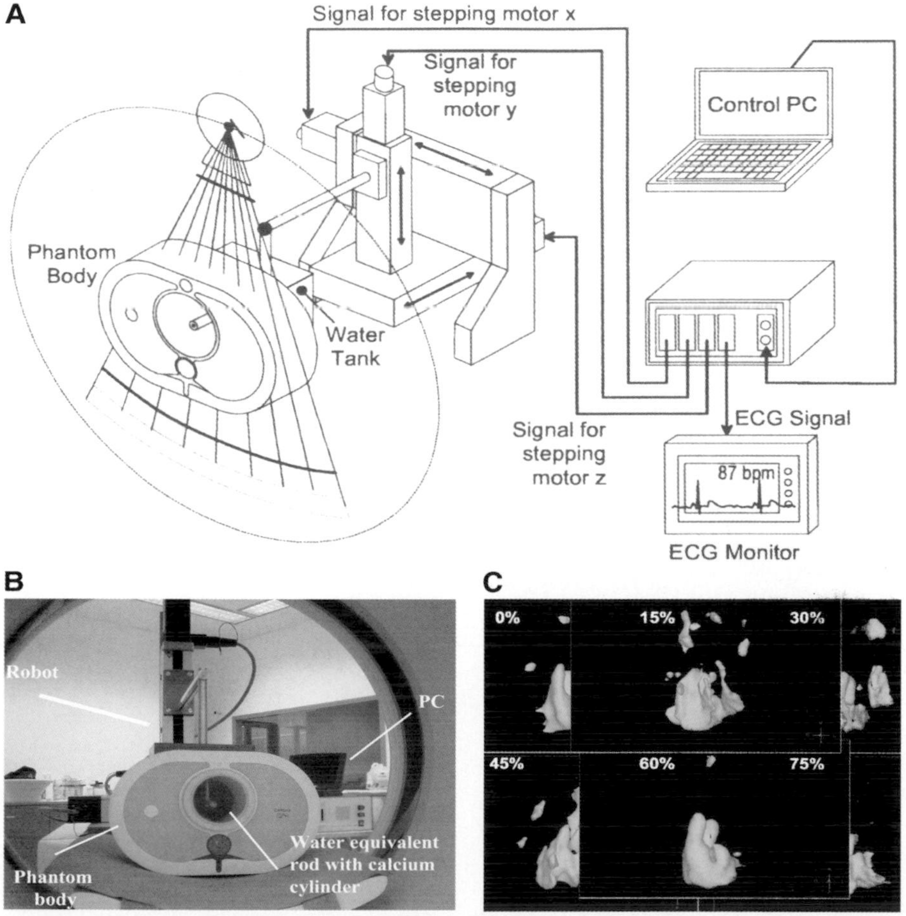

Fig. 10. Setup of a motion phantom. A robot setup can move arbitrary objects on realistic 3D trajectories to simulate cardiac motion. (**C**) shows an application example. A real specimen extracted from a cadaver scanned with a MSCT scanner and images were reconstructed at different positions in the RR interval. The shaded surface displays show motion artifacts in all phases except at 60% of RR for this motion function.

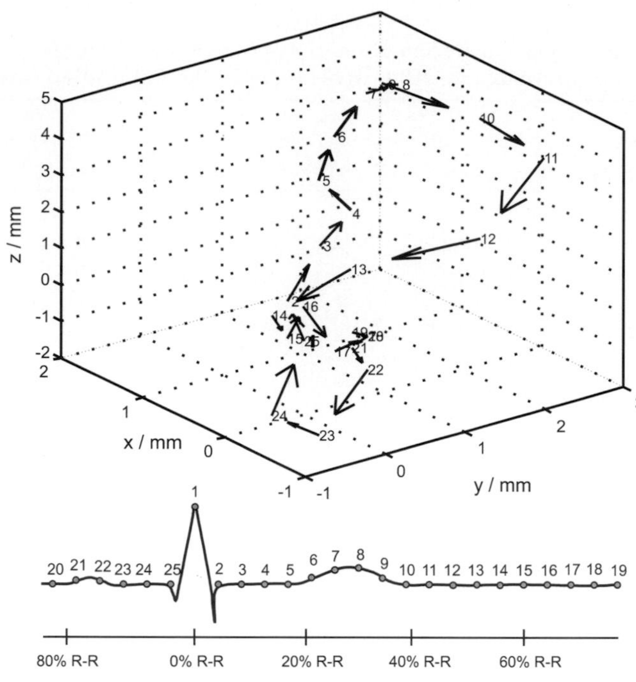

Fig. 11. A 4D plot of a realistic motion function.

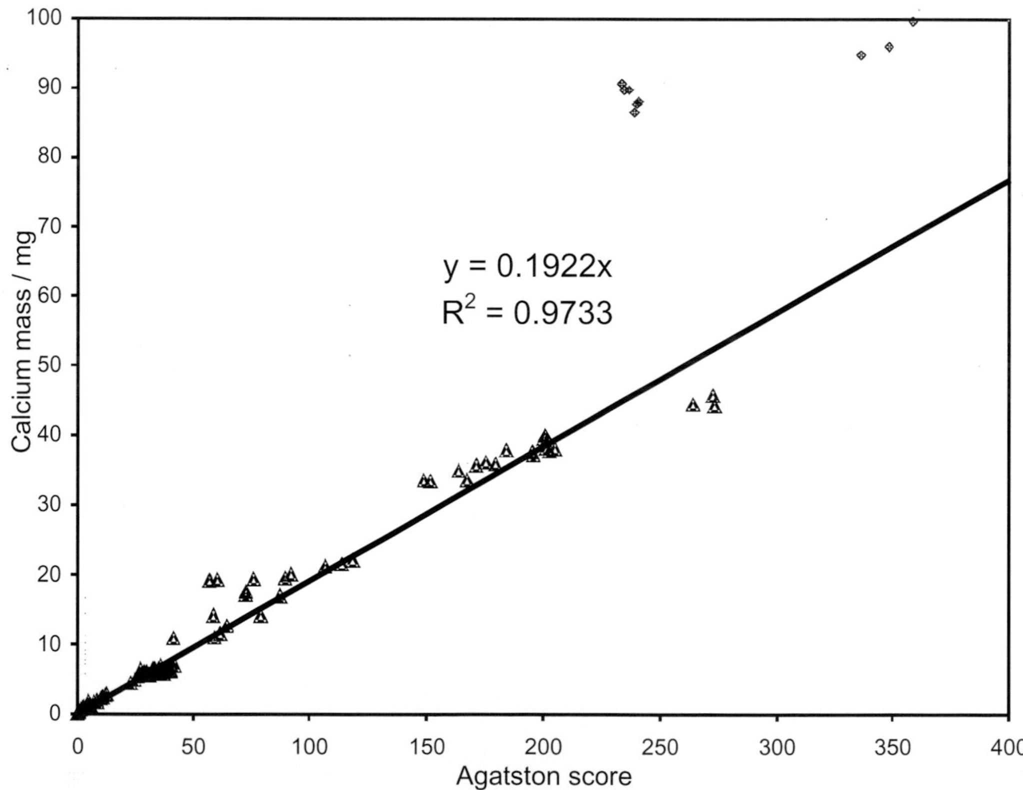

Fig. 12. Correlation of the calcium mass compared to the Agatston score for EBCT and artificial and real calcifications. The close correlation for calcifications that are not too dense allows a rough calculation of the mass from the Agatston score.

rate is depicted in Fig. 13 and Fig. 14. The results from the 16-slice CT scanner show an improvement over the 4-slice CT scanner when comparing the data with EBCT. The Sensation 16 shows a better behavior at higher heart rates than the Volume Zoom especially for retrospectively gated data. For the relationship of the calcium mass at various heart rates (Fig. 14) a similar behavior can be observed as for the Agatston score (Fig. 13). However, the error for the calcium mass is lower than

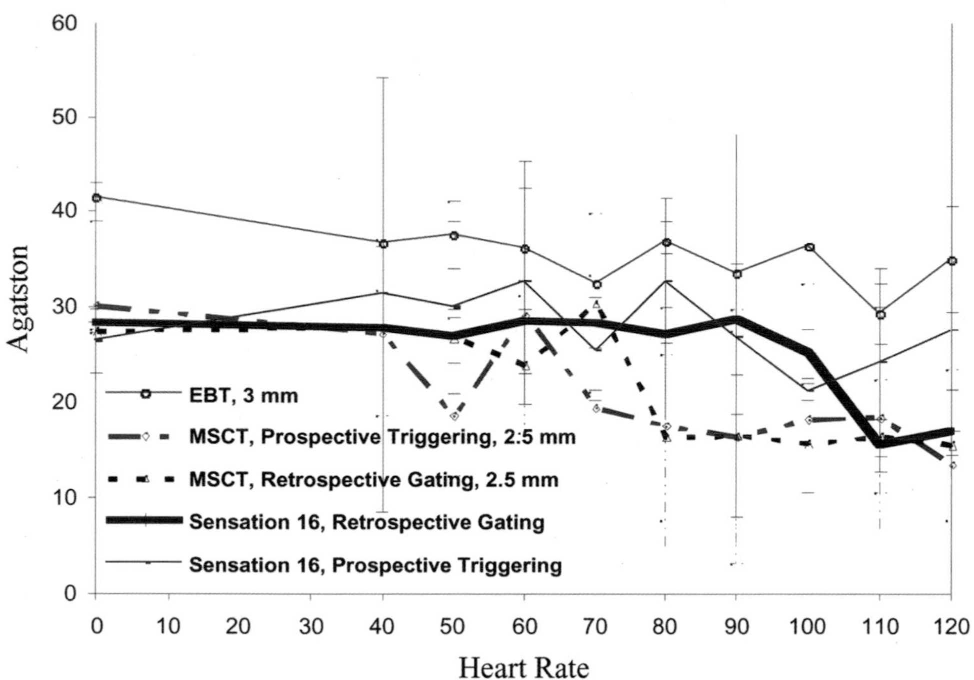

Fig. 13. Diagram showing the dependency of the Agatston score on the heart rate for different protrocols for the EBCT, the 4-slice MSCT, and a 16-slice MSCT scanner.

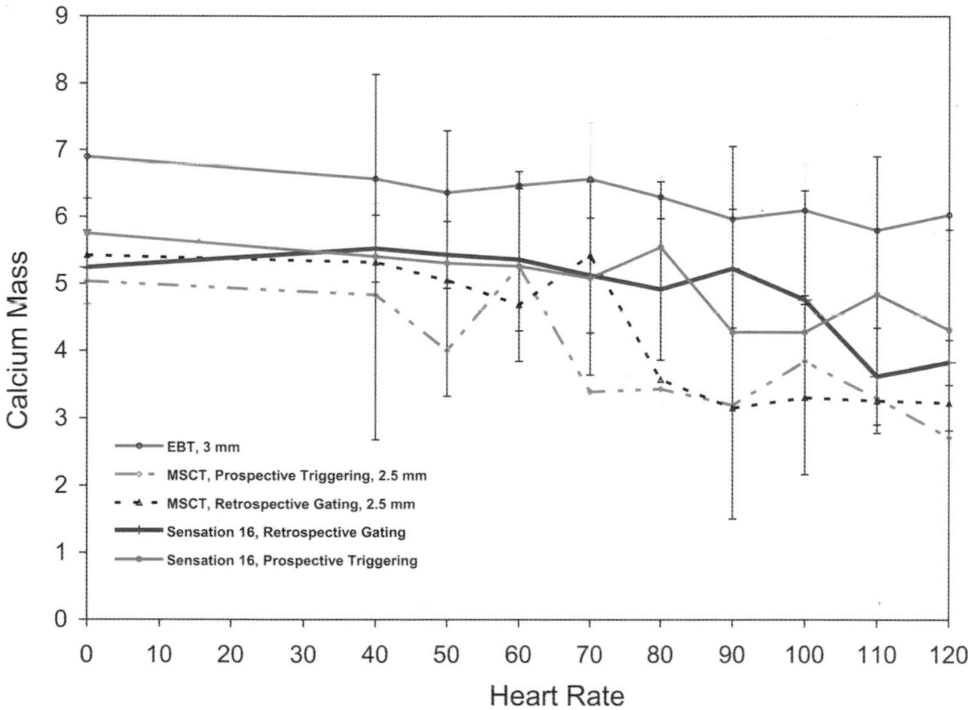

Fig. 14. Diagram showing the dependency of the calcium mass on the heart rate for different protocols on the EBCT, the 4-slice MSCT, and a 16-slice MSCT scanner.

for the Agatston score, making it much more suitable as an effective calcium quantification method.

More details and more investigations on reproducibility, detectability, and quality assurance in cardiac CT in general can be found in a recent PhD thesis *(31)*, peer reviewed articles *(16,33)*, and a recent textbook on computed tomography *(32)*.

FUTURE PERSPECTIVES

Several phantoms and concepts that have been developed for the evaluation of calcium scoring performance during the last four years are readily available at the Institute of Medical Physics at the University of Erlangen, Germany *(16,31,33,34)*. These phantoms have been widely accepted among CT manufacturers and within the scientific community during the last 4 yr and have been used in many studies that examined reproducibility and accuracy in the quantification of coronary calcium. The International Task Group on Standardization in Cardiac CT, consisting of representatives of all major CT manufacturers and experts from all over the world, was founded in 2002 and is trying to push forward these efforts.

The most important outcome of all investigations carried out with the phantoms up to now is that the calcium mass, as a true quantitative measure which corresponds to the amount of calcium, should be used for future clinical studies. It can be easily calculated for all CT scanners and scan protocols in a comparable way, it corresponds to the true amount of calcium, is more reproducible than the Agatston score, and it can roughly be calculated from the Agatston score for data acquired in the past. As many physicians are used to the old scoring method, the Agatston score can be given side by side during a transitional period.

However, it has to be stressed that the determination of calcium mass is not just another scoring method but appears to be the only reasonable physical quantification approach valid for arbitrary CT scanners. Adapting a scoring method like the Agatston score (with many disadvantages, developed for a special scanner) to new scanner types would introduce more errors and should be avoided.

Independently from the quantification method, it is mandatory for a scientific approach that the error of a method be known. In the case of the quantification of coronary calcium, this has been neglected in the past, and the goal should be that each manufacturer as well as each group that suggests a new approach (scanner, scan protocol, evaluation method) also validate it by giving the respective error for the method. As the error also depends on the characteristics of the calcifications (size, density, HA distribution) errors for typical calcifications and the detection limits of the method should be given.

For this purpose, the concepts and phantoms described in this chapter can be used in the future to check and improve accuracy and reproducibility of the quantification methods, to ensure uniform image quality for different approaches, and—an important aspect that has not been addressed in this chapter—to determine and limit patient dose *(35)*.

REFERENCES

1. Arad Y, Spadaro LA, Goodman K, Newstein D, Guerci AD. Prediction of coronary events with electron beam computed tomography. J Am Coll Cardiol 2000;36:1253–1260.
2. Raggi P, Callister TQ, Cooil B, et al. Identification of patients at increased risk of first unheralded acute myocardial infarction by electron-beam computed tomography. Circulation 2000;101: 850–855.
3. Wexler L, Brundage B, Crouse J, et al. Coronary artery calcification: pathophysiology, epidemiology, imaging methods, and clinical implications. A statement for health professionals from the American Heart Association. Writing Group. Circulation 1996;94:1175–1192.
4. Stanford W, Thompson BH, Weiss RM. Coronary artery calcification: clinical significance and current methods of detection. AJR Am J Roentgenol 1993;161:1139–1146.
5. Agatston AS, Janowitz WR, Hildner FJ, Zusmer NR, Viamonte Mj, Detrano R. Quantification of coronary artery calcium using ultrafast computed tomography. JACC 1990;15:827–832.
6. Becker CR, Knez A, Jakobs TF, et al. Detection and quantification of coronary artery calcification with electron-beam and conventional CT. Eur Radiol 1999;9:620–624.
7. Broderick LS, Shemesh J, Wilensky RL, et al. Measurement of coronary artery calcium with dual-slice helical CT compared with coronary angiography: evaluation of CT scoring methods, interobserver variations, and reproducibility. AJR Am J Roentgenol 1996;167:439–444.
8. Shemesh J. Spiral methods quantify coronary calcification. CT 1994:30–32.
9. Shemesh J, Apter S, Rozenman J, et al. Calcification of coronary arteries: detection and quantification with double-helix CT. Radiology 1995;197:779–783.
10. Shemesh J, Fisman EZ, Tenenbaum A, et al. Coronary artery calcification in women with Syndrome X: usefulness of double-helical CT for detection. Radiology 1997;205:697–700.
11. Shemesh J, Tenenbaum A, Fisman EZ, et al. Absence of coronary calcification on double-helical CT scans: predictor of angiographically normal coronary arteries in elderly women? Radiology 1996; 199:665–668.
12. Kachelriess M, Kalender WA. ECG-correlated image reconstruction from subsecond spiral CT scans of the heart. Medical Physics 1998;25:2417–2431.
13. Flohr T, Stierstorfer K, Bruder H, Simon J, Schaller S. New technical developments in multislice CT—Part 1: approaching isotropic resolution with sub-millimeter 16-slice scanning. Rofo Fortschr Geb Rontgenstr Neuen Bildgeb Verfahr 2002;174:839–845.
14. Flohr T, Bruder H, Stierstorfer K, Simon J, Schaller S, Ohnesorge B. New technical developments in multislice CT, part 2: sub-millimeter 16-slice scanning and increased gantry rotation speed for cardiac imaging. Rofo Fortschr Geb Rontgenstr Neuen Bildgeb Verfahr 2002;174:1022–1027.
15. Ulzheimer S, Kachelriess M, Kalender WA. New phantoms for quality assurance in cardiac CT. RSNA 1999;213(P):402.
16. Ulzheimer S, Kalender WA. Assessment of calcium scoring performance in cardiac computed tomography. Eur Radiol 2003;13: 484–497.
17. Miles KA. Measurement of tissue perfusion by dynamic computed tomography. Brit J Radiol 1991;64:409–412.
18. Bielak LF, Sheedy PF, 2nd, Peyser PA. Coronary artery calcification measured at electron-beam CT: agreement in dual scan runs and change over time. Radiology 2001;218:224–229.
19. Achenbach S, Ropers D, Mohlenkamp S, et al. Variability of repeated coronary artery calcium measurements by electron beam tomography. Am J Cardiol 2001;87:210–213, A8.
20. Becker CR, Knez A, Ohnesorge B, et al. Visualization and quantification of coronary calcifications with electron beam and spiral computed tomography. Eur Radiol 2000;10:629–635.
21. Devries S, Wolfkiel C, Shah V, Chomka E, Rich S. Reproducibility of the measurement of coronary calcium with ultrafast computed tomography. Am J Cardiol 1995;75:973–975.
22. Hernigou A, Challande P, Boudeville JC, Sènè V, Grataloup C, Plainfossè MC. Reproducibility of coronary calcification detection with electron-beam computed tomography. European Radiology 1996;6:210–216.
23. Shields JP, Mielke CH, Rockwood TH, Short RA, Viren FK. Reliability of electron beam computed tomography to detect coronary artery calcification. Am J Card Imaging 1995;9:62–66.
24. Wang S, Detrano RC, Secci A, et al. Detection of coronary calcification with electron-beam computed tomography: evaluation of interexamination reproducibility and comparison of three image-acquisition protocols. Am Heart J 1996;132:550–558.
25. Yoon HC, Greaser LE, Mather R, Sinha S, McNitt-Gray MF, Goldin JG. Coronary artery calcium: alternate methods for accurate and reproducible quantitation. Acad Radiol 1997;4:666–673.
26. Knollmann FD, Hum mel M, Spiegelsberger S, Bocksch W, Hetzer R, Felix R. Comparison of algorithms for coronary artery calcium scoring. Radiology 2000;217(P):588.

27. Adamzik M, Schmermund A, Reed JE, Adamzik S, Behrenbeck T, Sheedy PF, 2nd. Comparison of two different software systems for electron-beam CT-derived quantification of coronary calcification. Invest Radiol 1999;34:767–773.
28. O'Rourke RA, Brundage BH, Froelicher VF, et al. American College of Cardiology/American Heart Association Expert Consensus Document on electron-beam computed tomography for the diagnosis and prognosis of coronary artery disease. J Am Coll Cardiol 2000;36:326–340.
29. Shemesh J, Tenenbaum A, Kopecky KK, et al. Coronary calcium measurements by double helical computed tomography. Using the average instead of peak density algorithm improves reproducibility. Invest Radiol 1997;32:503–506.
30. Callister TQ, Cooil B, Raya SP, Lippolis NJ, Russo DJ, Raggi P. Coronary artery disease: improved reproducibility of calcium scoring with an electron-beam CT volumetric method. Radiology 1998; 208:807–814.
31. Ulzheimer S. Cardiac Imaging with X-ray computed tomography: new approaches to image acquisition and quality assurance. In: Kalender WA (ed), Reports from the Institute of Medical Physics, University of Erlangen-Nürnberg. Shaker Verlag, Aachen: 2001:123.
32. Kalender WA. Computed Tomography. Wiley and Sons, New York, NY: 2001.
33. Kachelrieß M, Ulzheimer S, Kalender WA. ECG-correlated imaging of the heart with subsecond multislice spiral CT. IEEE Trans Med Imaging 2000;19:888–901.
34. Ulzheimer S, Decker R, Kachelriess M, Kalender WA. ECG-correlated image reconstruction from subsecond multislice spiral CT scans of the heart: methodological investigations, phantom measurements and patient studies. 5th International SOMATOM CT Scientific User Conference, Zürich, 16./17.6.2000, 2000.
35. Schmidt B, Schmidt M, Kalender WA. A 3D voxel Monte Carlo program for scanner and patient specific dose calculations in CT. Eur Radiol 2000;10(Suppl 1):304.

CONTRAST-ENHANCED CT OF THE HEART: IV
MORPHOLOGY AND FUNCTION

14 CT of the Pericardium

Reinhard Groell, MD

INTRODUCTION

Because of its widespread availability and its cost-effectiveness, echocardiography represents the primary method of choice to image the pericardium. However, echocardiography is operator-dependent, and it often fails to detect the entire pericardium. Thus it is limited in the assessment of the severity of pericardial involvement in various diseases affecting the pericardium. Nataf et al. have demonstrated that echocardiography revealed thickened pericardium in only 62% of patients with constrictive pericarditis *(1)*. Additionally, ultrasound cannot penetrate calcifications that occur frequently in patients with constrictive pericarditis.

Magnetic resonance imaging (MRI) has a great potential in differentiating soft tissues of the pericardium and myocardium. In MRI of the heart, image quality strongly depends on the accuracy of cardiac gating. This can be problematic in the presence of arrhythmia, which frequently occurs in patients with pericardial diseases. Flow artifacts may compromise the evaluation of pericardial fluid during the cardiac cycle. Moreover, as a result of signal loss, the amount and distribution of pericardial calcifications cannot be determined accurately with MRI.

Fast computed tomography (CT) scanners that enable imaging of the entire pericardium with high temporal and spatial resolution in virtually every patient can overcome some of these limitations with echocardiography and MRI. More than ever, CT plays an important role in the diagnostic workup of pericardial diseases.

The pericardium is frequently involved in myocardial pathologies, and vice versa. Additionally, clinical symptoms of pericardial diseases may mimic those of myocardial pathologies. That is why CT imaging of the pericardium is generally combined with morphologic imaging of the entire heart, and a proper CT imaging protocol should follow these tasks. In our institution, we acquire subsecond, transverse CT sections of the heart during suspended respiration in the supine patient position, preferably using electrocardiogram (ECG) gating. Usually, a slice thickness of 1.5–3 mm is used, depending on the clinical question and the patient's capability to hold the breath.

From: *Contemporary Cardiology: CT of the Heart: Principles and Applications*
Edited by: U. Joseph Schoepf © Humana Press, Inc., Totowa, NJ

ANATOMY AND FUNCTION

The pericardium is a flask-like sac that surrounds the heart, and the neck of this sac is attached to the root of the great vessels at the base of the heart. The pericardium comprises an outer fibrous layer (the fibrous pericardium) and an inner serous sac (the serous pericardium) *(2)*. The serous pericardium consists of an inner visceral layer (the epicardium), which is intimately applied to the heart and the epicardial fat, and an outer parietal layer, which lines the fibrous pericardium. The visceral layer is reflected from the heart and the root of the great vessels onto the inner surface of the fibrous pericardium.

The pericardial cavity lies between the two layers of the serous pericardium. Under physiological conditions, it contains 20–25 mL of serous fluid; however, the amount of fluid may vary considerably among individuals, particularly in children and infants *(3)*. This fluid is an ultrafiltrate of plasma, which is produced by the monolayer of mesothelial cells of the serous pericardium. It is drained into the right lymphatic duct and the thoracic duct.

On its outside, the pericardium is connected anteriorly to the sternum, inferiorly to the diaphragm, and posteriorly to the esophagus, the thoracic aorta, and the spine *(2,4)*. The coronary vessels run in the subepicardial space between the epicardium and the myocardium, which is a connective tissue layer containing fat.

The pericardium is considered to prevent the ventricles from extreme distension and to control the mechanics of ventricular contractions *(5–7)*. However, it is known that even with congenital absence of the entire pericardium, subjects usually do not suffer from significant pathophysiological changes.

On computed tomography studies of the thorax, the normal pericardium appears as a thin band enveloping the heart (Fig. 1A,B). As the pericardium is surrounded by outer mediastinal and inner subepicardial fat, the visualization of the pericardium on CT strongly correlates with the amount of fat. In general, the more fat that is present, the better one can delineate the pericardium on CT; the presence of subepicardial fat is especially important for the depiction of the pericardium. Typically, subepicardial fat is well developed over the right ventricle, but it may be very thin or even invisible over the left ventricle. That is why it is often problematic to delineate the pericardium from the myocardium at the left lateral myocardial wall. The attachments to the sternum, diaphragm, or thoracic spine are rarely visualized, as they often do not represent dis-

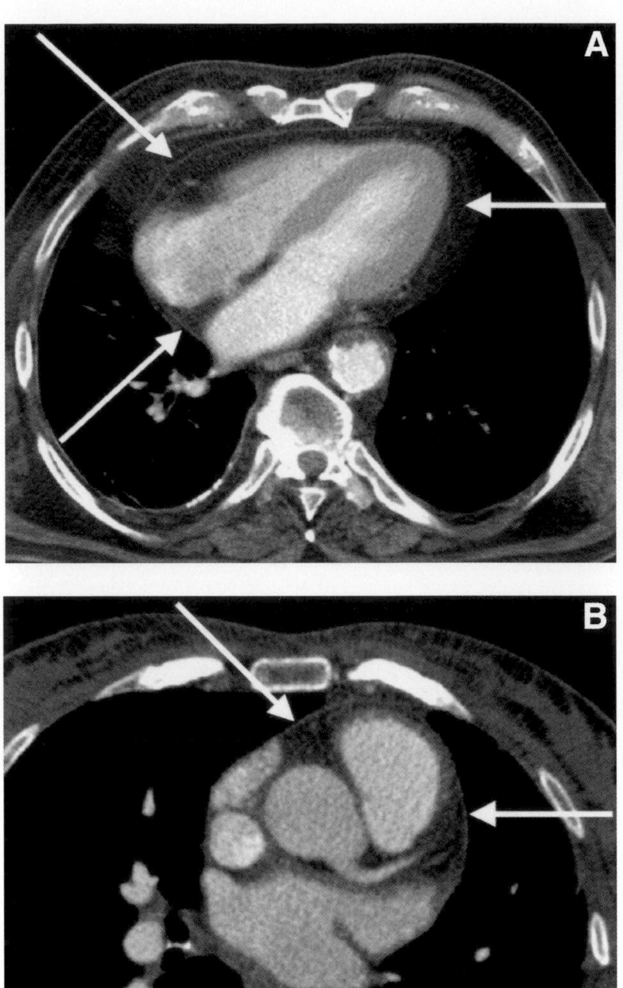

Fig. 1A,B. The pericardium (arrows) appears as a thin band enveloping the heart.

tinct anatomical ligaments but rather ill-defined fibrous strands within the mediastinal fat.

PERICARDIAL SINUSES AND RECESSES

At the serous reflections of the pericardium around the root of the great vessels at the base of the heart, the pericardial cavity forms the pericardial sinuses *(8,9)*. They are not separate compartments but represent extensions of the pericardial cavity. The *Nomina Anatomica* labels them the transverse sinus and the oblique sinus. Where the pericardium extends onto the great vessels, the pericardial cavity proper as well as the sinuses form recesses. Their differentiation is based on topographic landmarks, since there is no histological difference between the layers of the pericardial cavity, the sinuses, and the recesses.

Recesses of the Pericardial Cavity Proper

The right and left pulmonic vein recesses are extensions of the pericardial cavity proper located between the superior and inferior pulmonic veins on both sides. The postcaval recess lies behind and on the right lateral circumference of the superior vena cava.

Transverse Sinus

The transverse sinus is located above the left atrium and posterior to the ascending aorta and the pulmonary trunk. Between the ascending aorta and the superior vena cava, it is connected with the pericardial cavity proper. It extends upwards along the ascending aorta, where it forms the superior aortic recess. This superior aortic recess is frequently visible, and it was one of the first recesses described in CT studies of the mediastinum; it can be divided into an anterior, posterior, and right lateral portion *(10)*. The anterior and right lateral portions are directly related to the thymus, the posterior portion to tracheobronchial lymph nodes. On unenhanced CT images and on magnetic resonance imaging studies, the superior aortic recess may also simulate aortic dissection or intramural hematoma (Fig. 2). The left pulmonic recess is located below

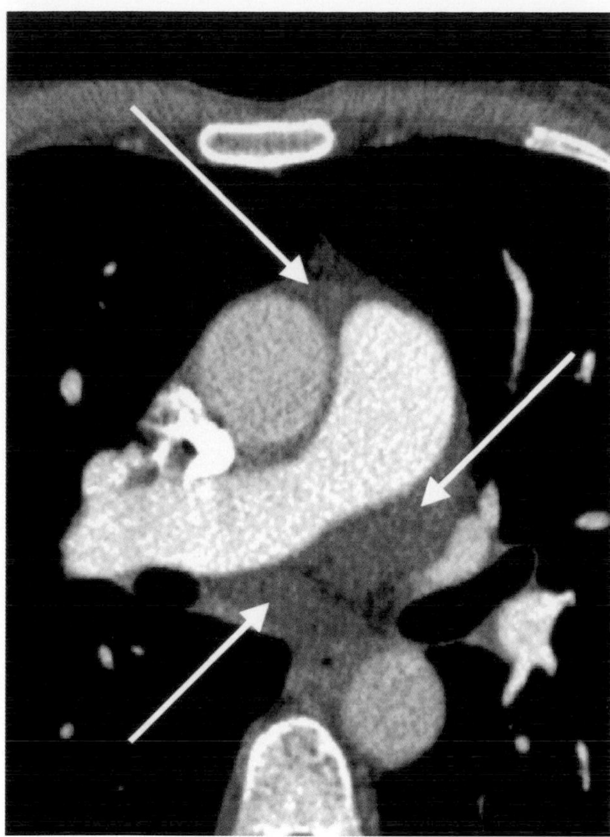

Fig. 2. Pericardial sinuses and recesses (arrows) are located at the pericardial reflections around the root of the great vessels.

the left pulmonary artery and posterolateral to the proximal portion of the right pulmonary artery. The right pulmonic recess lies below the right pulmonary artery and above the left atrium. Its posterior circumference is directly related to inferior tracheobronchial lymph nodes. The inferior aortic recess is situated between the ascending aorta and the inferior portion of the vena cava superior or the right atrium, respectively. It may extend down to the level of the aortic valve.

Oblique Sinus

The oblique sinus lies behind the left atrium. It is separated from the transverse sinus by a double reflection of the pericardium between the right and left superior pulmonic veins. On CT, the transverse sinus (including the right and left pulmonic recess) is always clearly separated from the oblique sinus (including the posterior pericardial recess) by a fat plane. The upper, right lateral extension of the oblique sinus is named the posterior pericardial recess. It is located behind the distal right pulmonary artery and medial to the bronchus intermedius. The esophagus runs posterior to the oblique sinus, and inferior tracheobronchial lymph nodes are in close proximity to these structures.

In general, pericardial sinuses and recesses are frequently observed on CT studies of the heart. They may be problematic in the differentiation from lymph nodes, esophageal or thymic processes, or vascular abnormalities. The knowledge of their typical location and appearance helps the radiologist avoid a misdiagnosis of lymphadenopathy and of other mediastinal pathologies. Rarely, pericardial cysts or tumors that can mimic cardiac tumors may develop in these sinuses and recesses *(3)*. As the pericardial sinuses and recesses represent extensions of the pericardial cavity proper, it is very likely that pericardial fluid might move from one area to another during the cardiac cycle or during respiration *(11)*.

DEVELOPMENTAL ANOMALIES

ABSENCE OF THE PERICARDIUM

Congenital absence of the pericardium may be partial or complete, with a prevalence of 0.01% in postmortem studies *(12,13)*. The majority of cases consists of a partial defect of the pericardium located over the left ventricle or left-lateral to the left atrium and left auricle. Partial defects at the right side of the pericardium or at the diaphragmatic parts are much less common, and complete absence of the pericardium is extremely rare. In 30% of the patients, congenital defects of the pericardium may be associated with malformations of the heart such as tetralogy of Fallot, atrial septal defects, or patent ductus arteriosus, or with congenital pulmonary malformations such as bronchogenic cyst and lung sequestration. In most patients, total absence of the left-sided pericardium does not result in clinical symptoms; the same is true for very small defects. However, medium-sized defects carry the risk of cardiac herniation and even strangulation, particularly of the left atrial appendage. In our institution we have examined a patient after left-sided pneumectomy and pericardiectomy, whose heart herniated into the left thoracic space, resulting in compression of the great vessels, which resulted in subsequent cardiac failure (Fig. 3). The symptoms resolved after subsequent re-operation with closure of the left-sided pericardial defect. It is also reported that pericardial defects may predispose the heart to pulmonary or mediastinal infections.

Frequently, the left ventricle is not surrounded by excessive fatty tissue, which makes the delineation of the left-sided pericardium difficult even in normal subjects. Thus, defects of the left-sided pericardium are often not directly encountered on CT. More frequently, these defects are recognized indirectly by a shift of the heart to the left or—when the defect is smaller—by left-lateral prominence or herniation of the left atrium or left atrial appendage.

PERICARDIAL CYSTS AND DIVERTICULA

Pericardial cysts and diverticula are rare clinical entities *(12,14,15)*. They represent well-demarcated fluid collections that blend with the pericardium. Most often they occur in the right cardio-phrenic angle (Fig. 4); alternative locations in the left cardio-phrenic angle or at the base of the heart are extremely uncommon. Usually they remain constant in size, but slow progression has also been described. Rarely, calcifications may be present in the wall of a pericardial cyst. While pericardial cysts represent encapsulated collections of fluid, diverticula are herniations of the pericardial cavity through a defect of the parietal pericardium (Fig. 5). Although pericardial cysts and diverticula may reach a size of several centimeters, they rarely cause clinical problems. Their radiological importance lies in the differentiation against clinically relevant pathologies such

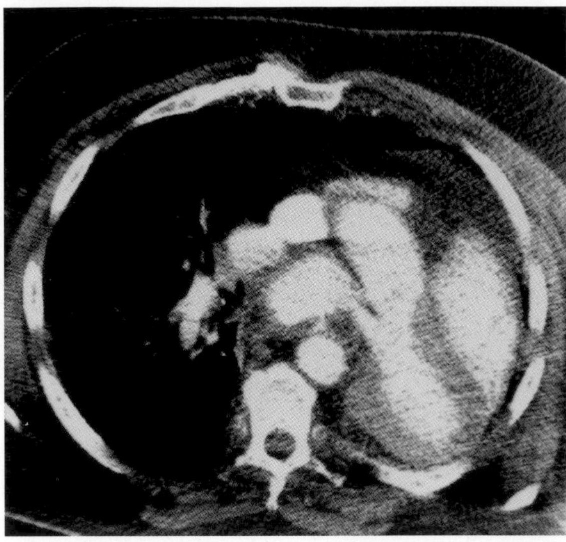

Fig. 3. Dislocation of the heart to the left after left-sided pericardiectomy and pneumectomy, resulting in acute postoperative cardiac failure. The symptoms resolved after surgical repositioning of the heart with fixation of the pericardial defect.

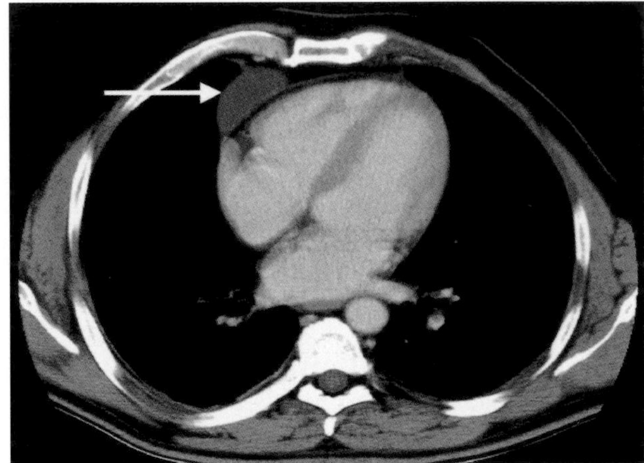

Fig. 4. Pericardial cyst (arrow) represents well-demarcated fluid collection that is typically located in the right cardio-phrenic angle.

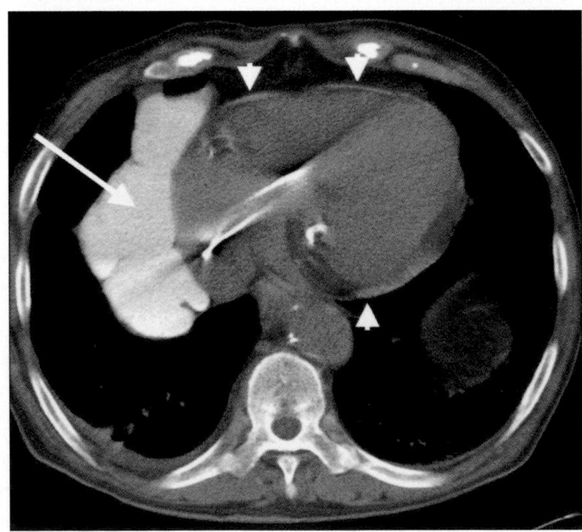

Fig. 5. Pericardial diverticulum (long arrow) with open communication between the diverticulum and the pericardial cavity. Note contrast material in the pericardial cavity proper (short arrows) after transthoracic puncture of the diverticulum and installation of diluted contrast material.

as diaphragmatic hernias, abscesses, or bronchogenic cysts. Uncommonly, pericardial cysts and diverticula may be acquired, such as after severe chest trauma or surgery.

On CT, pericardial cysts and diverticula present as water-equivalent, round or oval fluid collections surrounded by a thin wall without significant wall enhancement at the above-mentioned typical locations.

PERICARDIAL EFFUSION

The etiology of pericardial effusion comprises a variety of clinical entities such as inflammation (e.g., viral, bacterial, or fungal infections); collagenous and autoimmune disorders (e.g., lupus erythematosus); metabolic diseases (e.g., uremia); tumors; radiation, drug, or toxic reactions; and trauma *(16–18)*. Within the first days following transmural myocardial infarction, acute hemopericardium and tamponade may occur as a result of cardiac rupture, which is associated with a high mortality rate. Subacute cardiac tamponade may occur after even nontransmural myocardial infarction. Postinfarct pericarditis and Dressler's syndrome may appear from one week to several months after myocardial infarction, but it rarely leads to cardiac tamponade. Chylopericardium is extremely uncommon and mainly occurs after surgical or traumatic tears of the thoracic duct or in association with neoplastic duct stenoses.

While rapid accumulation of 150–250 mL of fluid may lead to cardiac tamponade, much higher volumes can be tolerated without significant hemodynamic disturbances when they collect over a longer period of time.

Usually, pericardial effusion is of low density in the range from 0 to 20 Hounsfield Units (HU). When it contains higher amounts of protein, such as in bacterial infections, or when it is hemorrhagic, its density may rise to 50 HU and more. Fig. 6 shows two patients with high-density pericardial effusions resulting from hemopericardium. In inflammation, the pericardial layers may show contrast enhancement *(16)*.

PERICARDIAL THICKENING AND CONSTRICTION

PERICARDIAL THICKENING

On CT studies, the thickness of the normal pericardium is 1–2 mm when measured at the levels of the great vessels or the cardiac chambers *(9,19,20)*. Inferiorly, near the diaphragmatic portion of the pericardium, it may appear slightly thicker, owing to partial-volume effects and the insertion of fibers for its diaphragmatic attachment.

That is why measurements of pericardial thickness should be performed at more cranial, midventricular levels. Pericardial thickening is frequently observed after operation, radiation therapy, or inflammation, and it may occur with or without accompanying effusion and calcifications. On autopsy, regional thickening and calcifications of the pericardium are frequent findings, and in the majority of cases they are not associated with prior symptoms of constriction. Doppman et al. have demonstrated that most thickened pericardia they observed on CT studies of the chest were hemodynamically insignificant *(21)*. It is important to consider that pericardial thickening alone without clinical symptoms of cardiac constriction does not establish the diagnosis of constrictive pericarditis *(22)*.

PERICARDIAL CONSTRICTION

Pericardial constriction is defined as fibrotic or calcific thickening and scarring of the pericardium, which then loses its compliance and impairs diastolic filling of the cardiac chambers *(22–24)*. It also leads to dissociation of intracardiac and intrathoracic pressures during respiration.

Pericardial constriction is a rare but potentially curable clinical entity. Pericardiectomy is the only known treatment. Pericardial constriction is most often idiopathic, but it also may occur after surgery, radiation therapy, or inflammation—particularly after tuberculosis, especially in developing countries. In most patients, pericardial constriction presents with insidious symptoms of venous congestion and is therefore difficult to diagnose and differentiate from other cardiac diseases. In particular, pericardial constriction may mimic restrictive cardiomyopathy, which is why their differentiation has to rely on imaging studies that allow exact assessment of peri- and myocardial structures.

According to the topographical distribution of pericardial thickening and calcifications, global forms of constriction can be differentiated from partial forms, in which the pericardium is affected over the right or left side of the heart or in the atrioventricular grooves (annular constriction) (Fig. 7) *(25)*. In the majority of patients, calcifications are present in the thickened pericardium, and often these calcifications extended into the pericardial reflection zones at the root of the great vessels. It is particularly important to the surgeon to know the extent and the topographic distribution of pericardial fibrosed and calcified plaques, not only to establish the diagnosis but also to determine the optimal approach and sites (sternotomy vs thoracotomy) for pericardiectomy. Frequently, the calcifications may invade the right- or left-ventricular myocardium (Fig. 8). CT is able to assess such possible myocardial invasion of pericardial calcifications, which is a high risk factor during pericardiectomy and which is not easily visible to the surgeon during surgery. Exact visualization of the subepicardial fat layer on CT helps the surgeon determine the sites of potential resectability with relatively low risks. Occasionally pericardial constriction is accompanied by myocardial fibrosis or atrophy. Knowledge of such areas of myocardial atrophy and fibrosis is also crucial for the cardiac surgeon, owing to a high risk of intraoperative ventricular aneurysms when the pericardium is resected over segments of myocardial fibrosis and atrophy *(25)*. Adequate assessment of pericardial calcifications is important in the diagnostic work-up of patients with constrictive pericarditis, since calcifications are considered to be an independent risk factor concerning pericardiectomy *(26)*. Knowledge of the topographic distribution of calcifications helps surgeons plan and calculate the risks of pericardiectomy. Secondary CT signs of pericardial constriction include dilatation of the superior/inferior vena cava and of the right/left atrium as well as deformity of ventricular or septal contours.

TUMORS OF THE PERICARDIUM

Primary tumors of the pericardium are very rare. Among the primary benign tumors of the pericardium are lymphangioma, hemangioma, lipoma, and teratoma *(27)*. The most frequent

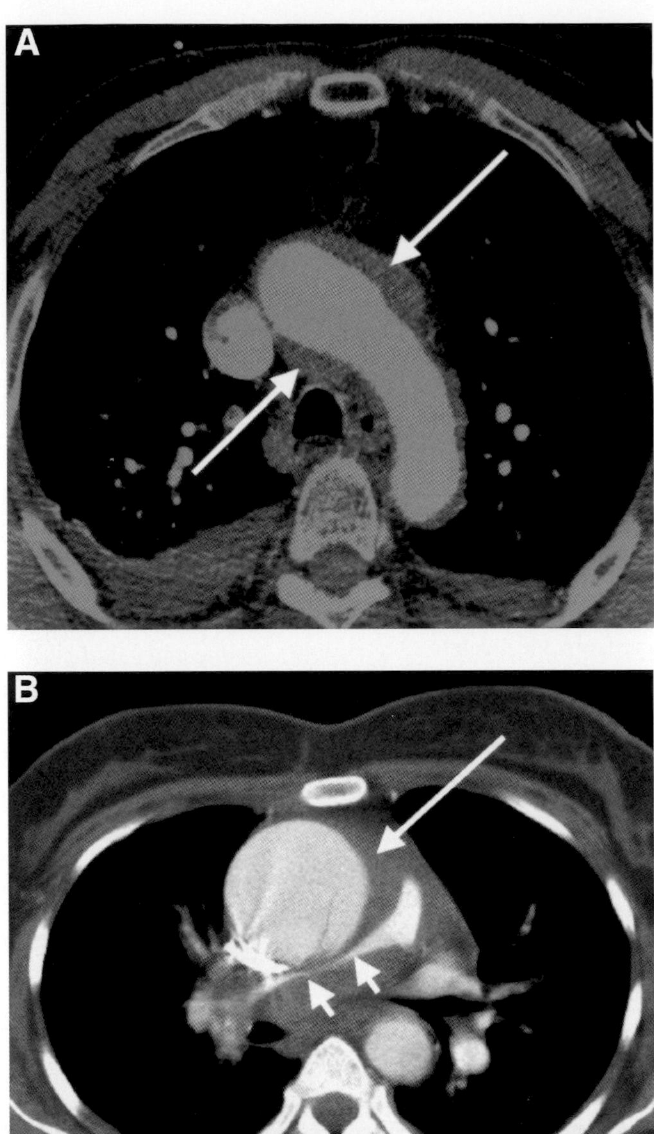

Fig. 6. (A) Hemopericardium (arrows) with hemorrhagic distension of the superior aortic recess of the pericardium. **(B)** Hemopericardium (long arrow) resulting from a ruptured ascending aortic aneurysm. Note compression of the right pulmonary artery (small arrows).

primary malignant pericardial tumor is pericardial malignant mesothelioma; other malignant primary tumors include hemangiosarcoma, fibrosarcoma, malignant teratoma, and liposarcoma. Apart from fat-containing tumors like lipoma and liposarcoma, CT usually cannot characterize these tumors; their definitive characterization has to rely on biopsy.

By far the majority of pericardial tumors are secondary neoplasms *(28)*. The pericardium is frequently involved in hematogeneous or lymphatic dissemination from various extrapericardial malignant tumors, such as malignant lymphoma or melanoma (Fig. 9). In autopsy examinations, pericardial metastases occur frequently in patients with malignancies, and generally more often than usually recognized. The pericardium may also be directly infiltrated from adjacent tumors, such as carcinoma of the lung, breast, or esophagus. Apart from solid components, malignant tumors of the pericardium are often associated with hemorrhagic pericardial effusion and possible tamponade. Usually, the amount of effusion does not directly correlate with tumor volumes. Finally, malignancies of the pericardium may invade the myocardium and vice versa. Similar to constrictive pericarditis, infiltration of the myocardium is indicated by nonvisualization of the subepicardial fat space.

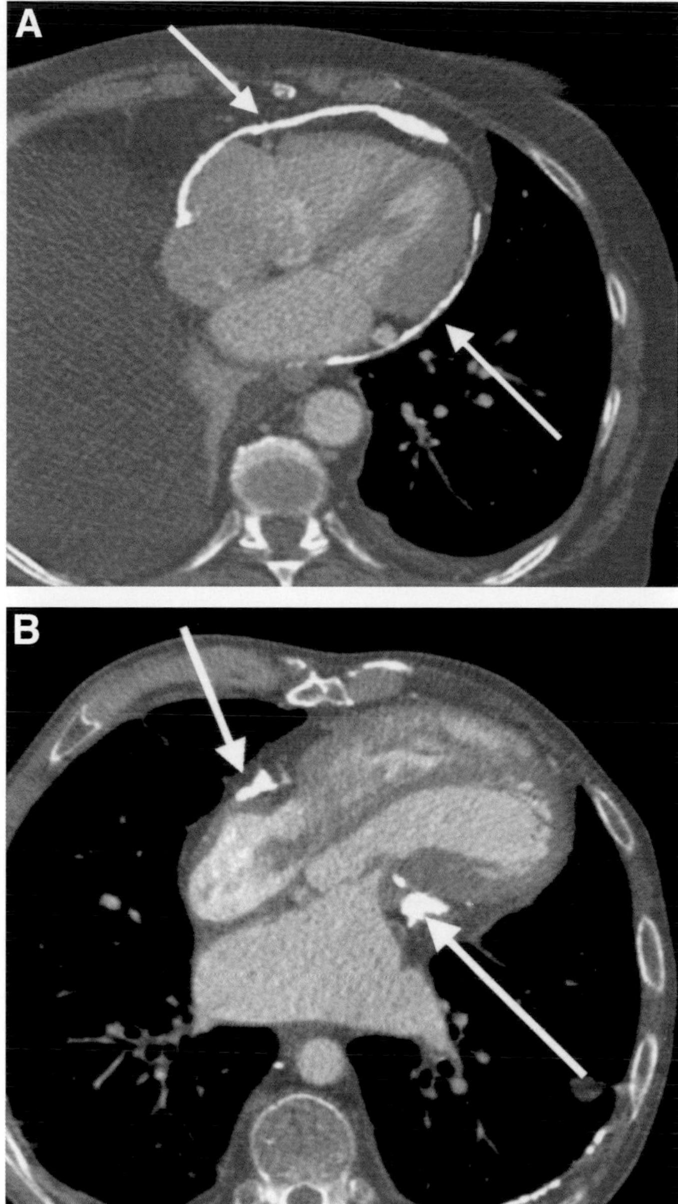

Fig. 7. Global (**A**) and annular (**B**) forms of pericardial constriction (arrows). Dilatation of the atria (**A,B**) and deformity of ventricular and septal contours (**B**) represent secondary CT signs of constriction. Persistent visualization of a subepicardial fat space (**A**) indicates potential surgical respectability of calcified plaques.

CONCLUSION

With the advent of CT technologies during the last decade providing high temporal and spatial resolution, CT gained more and more influence in imaging the pericardium. The latest spiral and electron beam CT scanners enable the imaging of the normal pericardium and the most relevant diseases of the pericardium with excellent image quality and almost free of motion artifacts. Although echocardiography still represents the first-line imaging modality in assessing pericardial morphology and pathology, some of the inherent limitations of echocardiography can be overcome by CT, such as operator dependence, restricted field of view not covering the entire pericardium, or nonpenetration of calcified plaques.

CT is especially important in the examination of patients with constrictive pericarditis, since exact knowledge of the extent and location of fibrosed and calcified plaques is crucial to the cardiac surgeon to determine the optimal sites and the possible risks of pericardiectomy.

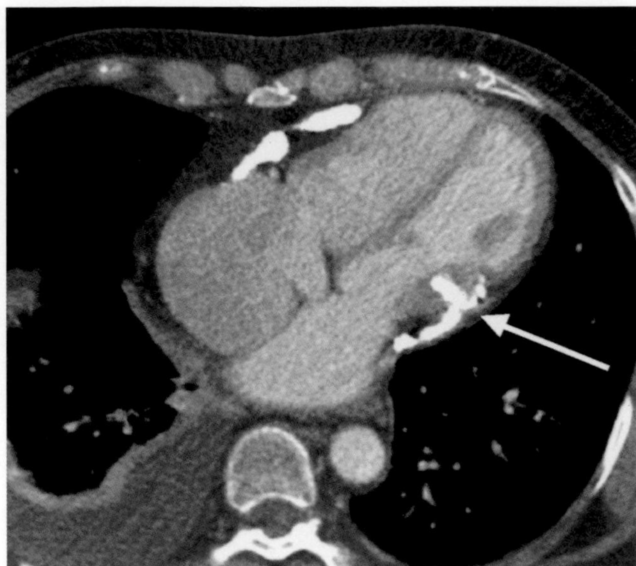

Fig. 8. Myocardial infiltration of calcified plaques (arrow) is frequently encountered in constrictive pericarditis. Surgical attempts to remove such infiltrating plaques are associated with high risks of developing intraoperative ventricular aneurysms.

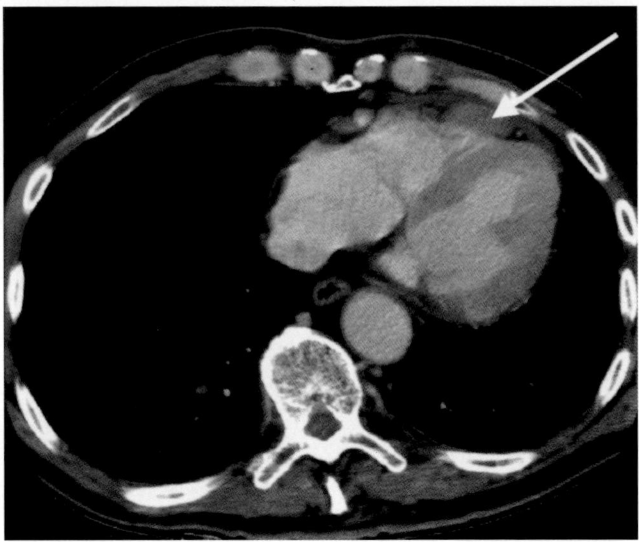

Fig. 9. Pericardial metastasis (arrow) from malignant lymphoma.

REFERENCES

1. Nataf P, Cacoub P, Dorent R, et al. Results of subtotal pericardiectomy for constrictive pericarditis. Eur J Cardiothorac Surg 1993;7: 252–255.
2. Shabetai R. Anatomy. In: The Pericardium. Grune and Stratton, New York, NY: 1981;1–32.
3. Moncada R, Baker M, Salinas M, et al. Diagnostic role of computed tomography in pericardial heart disease: congenital defects, thickening, neoplasms, and effusions. Am Heart J 1982;103: 263–282.
4. Hoit BD. Imaging the pericardium. Cardiol Clin 1990;8:587–600.
5. Shabetai R. Function of the pericardium. In: The Pericardium. Grune and Stratton, New York, NY: 1981;33–107.
6. Freeman GL. The effects of the pericardium on function of normal and enlarged hearts. Cardiol Clin 1990;8:579–586.
7. Borrego JM, Ordonez A, Gutierrez E, et al. Integrity of the pericardium. Its beneficial effects on the protection of the right ventricle in the presence of acute pulmonary hypertension. Ann Thorac Cardiovasc Surg 1998;4:332–335.
8. Vesely TM, Cahill DR. Cross-sectional anatomy of the pericardial sinuses, recesses and adjacent structures. Surg Radiol Anat 1986; 8:221–227.
9. Groell R, Schaffler GJ, Rienmueller R. The pericardial sinuses and recesses: findings on ECG-triggered electron-beam CT studies. Radiology 1999;212:69–73.
10. Kubota H, Sato C, Ohgushi M, Haku T, Sasaki K, Yamaguchi K. Fluid collection in the pericardial sinuses and recesses: thin-section helical computed tomography observations and hypothesis. Invest Radiol 1996;31:603–610.
11. Suolen RL, Lapayowker MS, Cortes FM. Distribution of pericardial fluid: dynamic and static influences. AJR Am J Roentgenol 1968; 103:583–588.
12. Shabetai R. Congenital malformations of the pericardium. In: The Pericardium. Grune and Stratton, New York, NY: 1981;366–373.

13. Jacob JL, Souza Jr. AS, Parro A, Jr. Absence of the left pericardium diagnosed by computed tomography. Int J Cardiol 1995;47: 293–296.
14. Olson MC, Posniak HV, McDonald V, Wisniewski R, Moncada R. Computed tomography and magnetic resonance imaging of the pericardium. Radiographics 1989;9:633–649.
15. Kutlay H, Yavuzer I, Han S, Cangir, AK. Atypically located pericardial cysts. Ann Thorac Surg 2001;72:2137–2139.
16. Hackney D, Slutsky RA, Mattrey R, et al. Experimental pericardial inflammation evaluated by computed tomography. Radiology 1984;151:145–148.
17. Breen JF. Imaging of the pericardium. J Thorac Imaging 2001;16: 47–54.
18. Suchet IB, Horwitz TA. CT in tuberculous constrictive pericarditis. J Comput Assist Tomogr 1992;16:391–400.
19. Delille JP, Hernigou A, Sene V, et al. Maximal thickness of the normal human pericardium assessed by electron-beam computed tomography. Eur Radiol 1999;9:1183–1189.
20. Ling LH, Oh JK, Tei C, et al. Pericardial thickness measured with transesophageal echocardiography: feasibility and potential clinical usefulness. J Am Coll Cardiol 1997;29:1317–1323.
21. Doppman JL, Rienmuller R, Lissner J. Computed tomography in constrictive pericarditis. J Comput Assist Tomogr 1981;5:1–11.
22. Fowler NO. Constrictive pericarditis: its history and current status. Clin Cardiol 1995;18:341–350.
23. Myers RB, Spodick DH. Constrictive pericarditis: clinical and pathophysiologic characteristics. Am Heart J 1999;138:219–232.
24. Ling LH, Oh JK, Schaff HV, et al. Constrictive pericarditis in the modern era: evolving clinical spectrum and impact on outcome after pericardiectomy. Circulation 1999;100:1380–1386.
25. Rienmüller R, Gürgan M, Erdmann E, Kemkes BM, Kreutzer E, Weinhald C. CT and MR evaluation of pericardial constriction: a new diagnostic and therapeutic concept. J Thoracic Imaging 1993;8: 108–121.
26. Ling LH, Oh JK, Breen JF, et al. Calcific constrictive pericarditis: is it still with us? Ann Intern Med 2000;132:444–450.
27. McAllister HA, Jr. Tumors of the heart and pericardium. In: Silver MD (ed.) Cardiovascular Pathology. Churchill Livingstone, New York, NY: 1983:909–943.
28. Chiles C, Woodard PK, Gutierrez FR, Link KM. Metastatic involvement of the heart and pericardium: CT and MR imaging. Radiographics 2001;21:439–449.

15 Multidetector-Row CT for Assessment of Cardiac Valves

Jürgen K. Willmann, MD and Dominik Weishaupt, MD

INTRODUCTION

Imaging of the heart with computed tomography (CT) is challenging because the heart is continuously moving during data acquisition. As a result of the limited temporal resolution, the use of single-detector helical CT for noninvasive cardiac imaging was limited and resulted often in images with a high content of artifacts. The introduction of multidetector-row CT (MDCT) scanners by the end of 1998 laid the foundation for increased clinical use of CT for cardiac imaging. Partial view acquisition and retrospectively electrocardiogram (ECG)-gated helical reconstruction offered by 4-channel MDCT scanners, allow for a temporal resolution of up to 125 ms, combined with both a high spatial resolution and a high signal-to-noise ratio *(1)*. Last-generation 16-channel MDCT scanners permit scanning of the whole heart with an even higher temporal resolution of up to 105 ms within a convenient short breath-hold of about 18 s *(2)*. Apart from visualization of coronary artery lumen and stenosis as well as detection and quantification of coronary calcification *(3,4)*, these technical developments in CT technology also improved visualization of morphological details of the heart including the cardiac valves *(5,6)*.

In this chapter, we describe the potential clinical and research applications of MDCT, with special focus on the assessment of the aortic and mitral valves.

CONVENTIONAL IMAGING TECHNIQUES

CONVENTIONAL ANGIOGRAPHY

Conventional angiography allows assessment of functional data, including measuring the transvalvular pressure gradient as well as calculating the valve area using the Gorlin formula *(7)*. However, in patients with valvular regurgitation, conventional angiography has been demonstrated to be inaccurate. In addition, conventional angiography does not allow precise quantification of valvular calcification.

TRANSTHORACIC AND TRANSESOPHAGEAL ECHOCARDIOGRAPHY

Transthoracic echocardiography is a widely available, noninvasive, and safe imaging modality which allows an expeditious assessment of the anatomic and functional status of the cardiac valves. In patients with stenotic aortic and mitral disease, precise quantification of mean and maximum transvalvular pressure gradients as well as determination of valve area can be performed. Alternatively, transesophageal echocardiography can be performed, in particular in patients with poor transthoracic acoustic windows, such as patients with large and thick chest walls, small hearts, chest deformities, or in elderly patients. Transthoracic as well as transesophageal echocardiography allow assessment of the entire spectrum of valvular disease, in particular visualization of infective endocarditis and its sequelae, including perivalvular abscesses. However, both transthoracic and transesophageal echocardiography permit only a rough quantification of valvular calcification, as only indirect signs of calcification, including increased echogenicity and thickening of the valves, may be used for quantification *(8)*.

MDCT

RATIONALE

Aortic valve stenosis is the most common cardiac valve lesion in the developed countries, with a prevalence of 2% to 7% in the population above 65 yr of age *(9)*. Degeneration and calcification of the aortic valve cusps and the aortic annulus are the most common cause of aortic valve stenosis *(10)*. Several studies have identified the presence and extent of aortic valve calcification as a strong predictor both for the progression as well as for the outcome of aortic valve stenosis *(11,12)*. The positive therapeutic effect of a lipid-lowering pharmacological therapy with HMG-CoA reductase inhibitors on the natural history of calcific aortic valvular disease has been demonstrated recently *(13)*. Therefore, an imaging modality for quantification of aortic valve calcium in patients with aortic valve stenosis is desirable. From a surgical point of view, preoperative knowledge about anatomic details of the aortic valve is of particular interest, since the procedure of aortic valve surgery itself and the choice of the type of valve prosthesis to be implanted depend on various parameters, including the aortic valve morphology (tricuspid vs bicuspid), its diameter, as well as the presence and extent of aortic valve and annulus calcification *(14–16)*. Moreover, the presence of aortic valve calcification extending to the interventricular septum as a surgical finding at aortic valve replacement predicts the need for permanent pacing postoperatively *(17)*. Similarly, two studies

From: *Contemporary Cardiology: CT of the Heart: Principles and Applications*
Edited by: U. Joseph Schoepf © Humana Press, Inc., Totowa, NJ

have demonstrated that mitral annulus calcification may be used as a marker for the severity of atherosclerosis and may be helpful to identify patients with a higher likelihood of diffuse vascular atherosclerotic processes *(18,19)*.

Since CT is a sensitive and objective method for the detection of calcifications, imaging of the aortic and mitral valve with MDCT combines both assessment of aortic and mitral valve morphology and quantification of aortic valve and mitral valve annulus calcifications *(5,6)*.

TECHNICAL CONSIDERATIONS

MDCT for assessment of the cardiac valves may be performed either with or without administration of intravenous contrast agents. Usually, for assessment of valvular morphology, a contrast-enhanced CT scan is performed. For mere determination of valvular calcification, a nonenhanced CT scan is sufficient.

The scan is planned on a low-dose anteroposterior scout view (120 kV, 50 mAs) from the ascending aorta to the apex of the heart. Four-channel MDCT acquisition is performed with 4 × 1-mm collimation (1.25-mm slice width for reconstruction), 500-ms rotation time, table feed of 2.5–4.5 mm per rotation, 300 mA at 120 kV, and a 0.6- to 0.8-mm image reconstruction increment. The acquisition parameters for a 16-channel MDCT acquisition include a 12 × 0.75-mm collimation (0.75-mm slice width for reconstruction), a table feed of 6.7 mm/s, a gantry rotation time of 420 ms, and a reconstruction increment of 0.4 mm. For retrospective reconstruction of the MDCT data set, a digital ECG file from the patient is simultaneously recorded during MDCT scanning. Image reconstruction is performed with a medium-sharp body convolution kernel in the mid- to end-diastolic phase of the cardiac cycle using between 50% and 70% relative delay to the R waves of the ECG signal. With 4-channel MDCT scanning, this results in a voxel size of 0.35 × 0.35 × 1.25 mm^3 (field of view [FOV], 18 cm; matrix size, 512 × 512 pixels). For 16-channel MDCT, the resulting voxel size is 0.35 × 0.35 × 0.75 mm^3. For data analysis, the reconstructed MDCT data are best transferred to an independent workstation, which allows multiplanar reconstructions in sagittal, coronal, and oblique planes. For assessment of the valvular morphology and quantification of valvular calcium, routine reconstruction of volume renderings or multiplanar reformations is not necessary.

If the MDCT scanning is performed with intravenous administration of an iodinated contrast agent, we first determine the optimal scan delay using the test bolus method. For this purpose, a test bolus of 20 mL of iodinated contrast agent followed by a 50-mL chaser of saline is injected by a power injector. Delay times are determined by visually evaluating the contrast material at the level of the aortic valve by using ten consecutive transverse images obtained every 2 s without table feed. The MDCT scan is then performed after administering 120 mL of nonionic contrast material through a 20-gage needle placed in an antecubital vein at 3–5 mL/s followed by a 50-mL saline chaser bolus. Alternatively, the delay time can be obtained by using a bolus-tracking technique (e.g., CARE-Bolus, Volume Zoom Navigator, Siemens). For this purpose, a single nonenhanced low-dose scan (10 mAs) at the level of the ascending aorta is performed. Based on this transverse image, a region of interest (ROI) with an area of 10–15 mm^2 is placed in the lumen of the ascending aorta. This ROI serves as a reference for the following dynamic measurements of contrast enhancement after administration of 120 mL of nonionic iodinated contrast medium. Repetitive low-dose monitoring scans (120 kV; 10 mAs; 0.5 s scanning time; 1 s interscan delay) are then performed 10 s after the beginning of the contrast material injection. After reaching the preset contrast enhancement level of 100–120 HU, the MDCT scan is initiated automatically.

VALVULAR MORPHOLOGY

MDCT allows reliable differentiation between bicuspid and tricuspid aortic valves. In a prospective study of 25 patients with aortic valve stenosis, Willmann et al. *(5)* have shown that contrast-enhanced MDCT is highly accurate for prediction of valve morphology when compared to surgery and echocardiography. Using contrast-enhanced MDCT there was a 100% agreement between MDCT and surgical or echocardiographic findings with regard to the morphology of the aortic valve (Fig. 1) *(5)*. On nonenhanced MDCT data sets, the aortic valve could be correctly classified in 87% of the cases *(5)*. MDCT also allows for a precise measurement of the diameter of the aortic valve annulus (Fig. 2). In the same study by Willmann et al. *(5)*, the diameter of the aortic valve annulus as measured on contrast-enhanced 4-channel MDCT images correlated highly with the intraoperative measurement with only an overestimation by 0.7 mm on contrast-enhanced MDCT data sets *(5)*.

The morphology of the mitral valve and its apparatus, including the mitral valve annulus, mitral valve leaflets, tendinous cords, and papillary muscles can also be visualized on MDCT (Fig. 3). Recently, our group reported on the preliminary experience with mitral valve imaging in 20 patients *(6)*. Good-to-excellent image quality of the mitral valve annulus and its leaflets were obtained in 15 of 20 consecutive patients (75%). In 19 of 20 patients (95%) papillary muscles could also be visualized to good or excellent advantage. However, visibility of tendinous cords was inferior. In 14 of 20 patients (70%) tendinous cords were not or only moderately visible *(6)*.

VALVULAR CALCIFICATION

MDCT is in particular helpful for the assessment of aortic valve calcification. According to the echocardiographic grading of aortic valve calcifications *(11)*, we use a four-point grading scale for assessment of the degree of the calcification of the aortic valve. This grading scale is as follows: grade 1, no calcification; grade 2, mild calcification (small, isolated spots of calcification); grade 3, moderate calcification (multiple larger spots of calcification); and grade 4, heavy calcification (extensive calcification of all aortic valve leaflets) (Figs. 4 and 5). By using this grading scale there was an 84% agreement between contrast-enhanced MDCT findings and the true calcification status of the aortic valves as assessed during surgery *(5)*.

As with the aortic valve, the calcifications of the mitral valve may be located either on the mitral valve annulus or on the mitral valve leaflets. MDCT yielded a 95–100% agreement compared to echocardiography and intraoperative findings with regard to assessment of calcifications of the mitral valve annulus and mitral valve leaflets *(6)*.

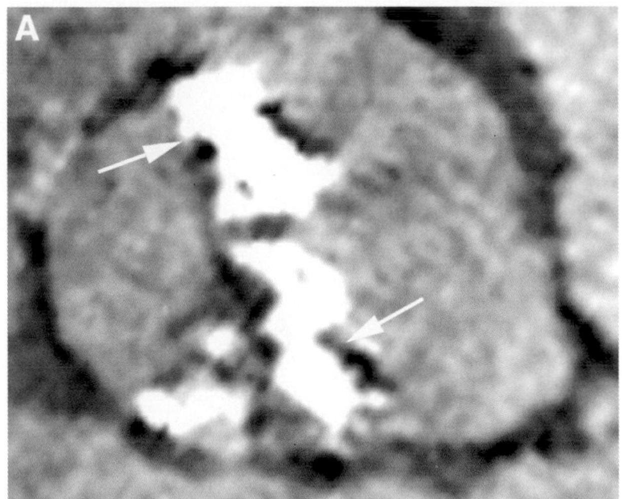

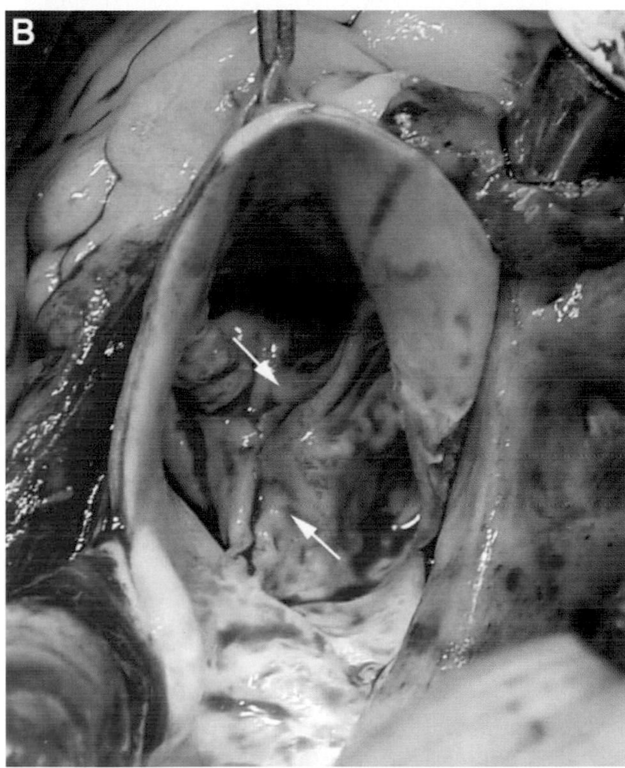

Fig. 1. **(A)** 57-yr-old male with severe aortic valve stenosis who underwent contrast-enhanced retrospectively electrocardiogram-gated multidetector-row CT (MDCT) before surgery. Double oblique reconstruction shows heavily calcified bicuspid aortic valve with large calcific deposit (arrows). **(B)** Image obtained during surgery shows excellent agreement between both MDCT and intraoperative status. Note presence of bicuspid aortic valve with large deposits of calcium at the free edges of the aortic valve (arrows).

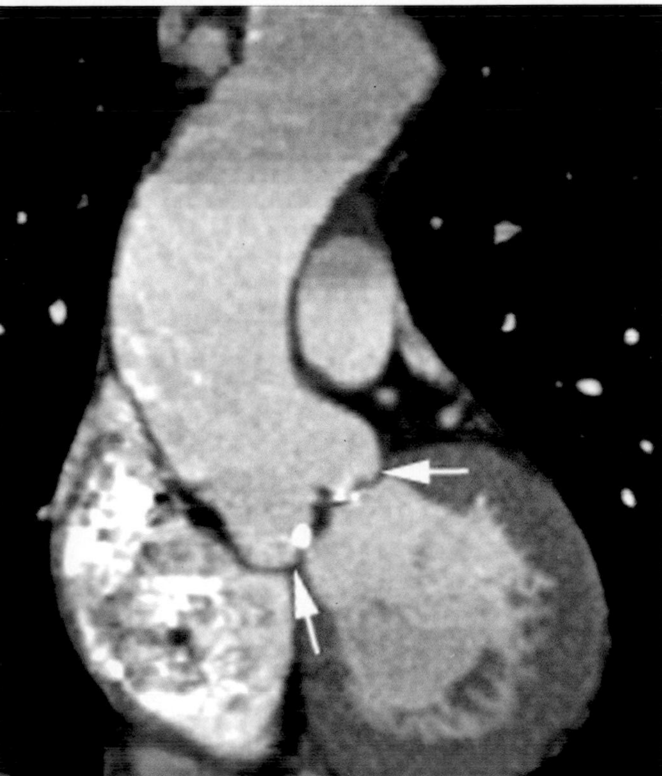

Fig. 2. Precise assessment of aortic valve diameter is possible with contrast-enhanced, retrospectively electrocardiogram-gated multidetector-row CT (MDCT). Preoperative assessment was performed on a sagittal oblique reconstruction of the heart in this 63-yr-old female with aortic valve stenosis. There was only a minimal difference between the diameter as assessed by MDCT and the diameter as measured during surgery.

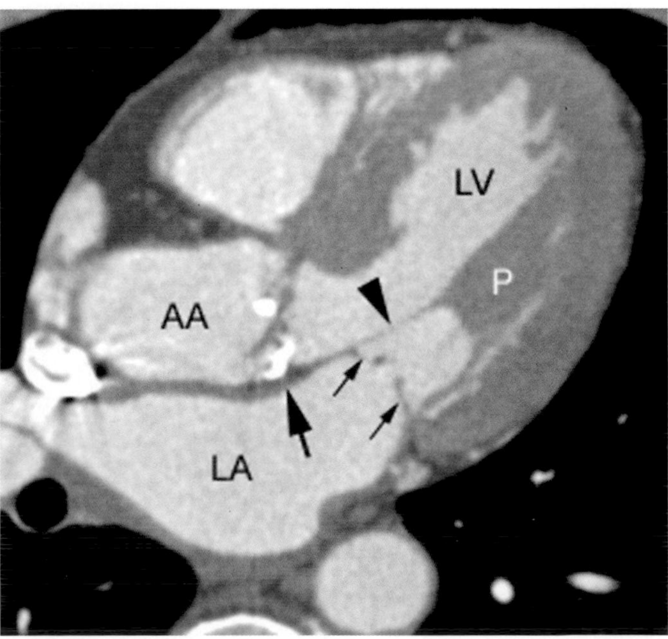

Fig. 3. 73-yr-old female with mitral regurgitation. Long-axis view reconstruction contrast-enhanced, retrospectively electrocardiogram-gated multidetector-row CT data set demonstrates anterior mitral valve annulus (large arrow), mitral valve leaflets (small arrows), tendinous cord (arrowhead), and the anterior papillary muscle (P). LV, left ventricle; LA, left atrium; AA, ascending aorta.

All these findings imply the potential of MDCT for a longitudinal monitoring of patients with aortic and mitral valve calcifications by measuring the change of valvular calcification over time. Apart from a visual semi-quantitative assessment of valvular calcification, future studies will demonstrate whether MDCT imaging may also allow an absolute quantification of valvular calcium. In vitro studies with absolute determination

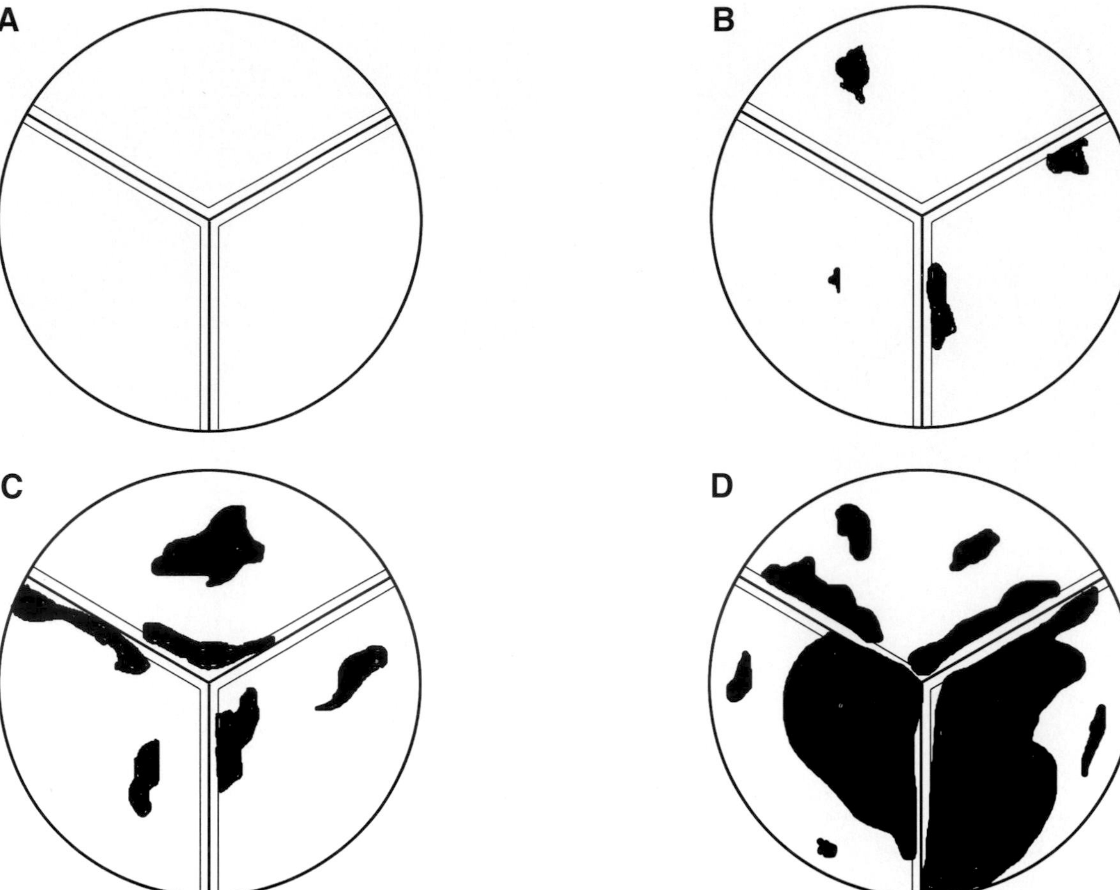

Fig. 4. Diagrams of different grades of aortic valve calcification (modified from ref. *5*). (**A**) Grade 1, no calcification; (**B**), grade 2, mild calcification (small isolated spots of calcification); (**C**), grade 3, moderate calcification (multiple larger spots of calcification); and (**D**), grade 4, heavy calcification (extensive calcification of all aortic valve leaflets).

of aortic valve calcium by ashing or enzymatic digesting of noncalcified areas of the aortic valve and subsequent measurement of the mass of the remaining aortic valve calcium are warranted to correlate the real amount of calcium and the calcium obtained on MDCT. Furthermore, the reliability of different calcium scores used for quantification of coronary artery calcium need to be evaluated when quantifying aortic valve calcium, including the Agatson score *(20)*, the volume score *(21)*, the mass equivalent score, as well as the calibrated mineral mass score *(22)*.

LIMITATIONS OF MDCT IMAGING

So far, MDCT imaging has demonstrated its capability only for evaluation of the morphology of mitral and aortic valves, including the semi-quantitative assessment of calcifications. As a result of the limited temporal resolution of 4-channel MDCT scanners, functional assessment of cardiac valves as well as quantification of valvular area, in particular of the aortic valve, has not been possible yet. With the introduction of 16-channel scanners, as well as further reduction of the rotation time of the CT tube, additional improvement of spatial and temporal resolution may also allow accurate assessment of valvular area.

A second limitation includes the radiation dose, which is inherent to CT scanning. Since the data are acquired with an overlapping helical pitch and continuous radiation exposure, there is a considerable applied radiation dose. Mean effective dose values of up to 13 mSv have been calculated for imaging the entire heart using a 4-channel MDCT scanner *(23)*. Compared to the mean effective dose values calculated for conventional coronary angiography (usually between 2.1 and 2.5 mSv), the mean effective dose caused by MDCT angiography is higher by a factor of about 5 *(23)*. However, by reducing the tube output during heart phases that are not likely to be targeted by the ECG-gated reconstruction (i.e., reconstruction intervals excepting 50–70% of the cardiac cycle), a dose reduction of up to 48% is possible *(24)*. Furthermore, improvements of dose utilizations of recent generation 16-channel MDCT scanners may also help in reducing radiation dose *(25)*.

CONCLUSION AND FUTURE DIRECTIONS

MDCT is an emerging tool for noninvasive imaging of the heart. Apart from evaluation of the coronary arteries, a comprehensive work-up of the heart also includes assessment of morphological details of the heart chambers, including cardiac valves. Preliminary studies have shown that the aortic and

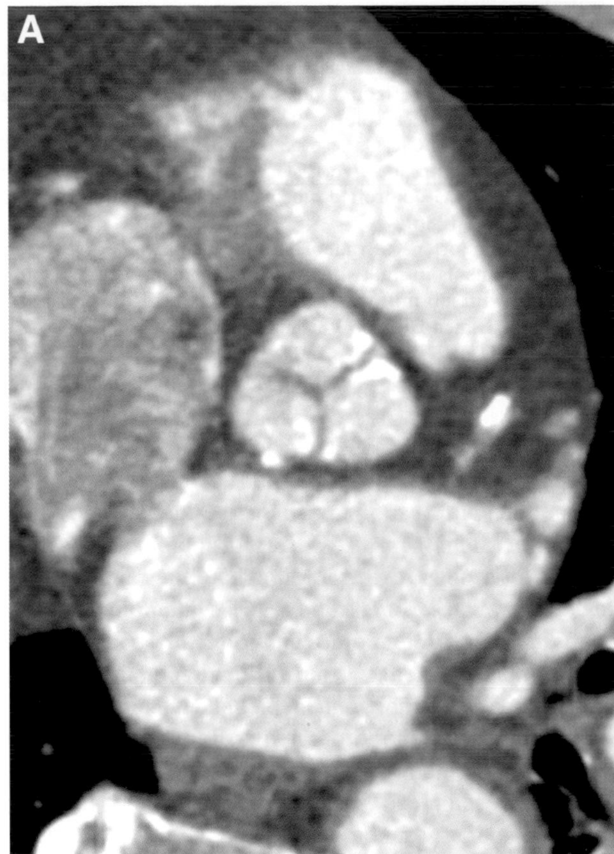

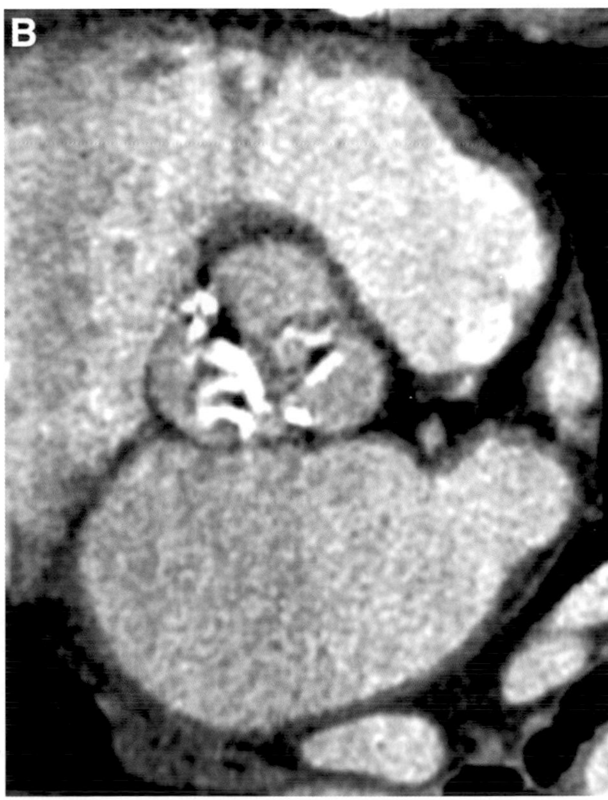

Fig. 5. Two examples of two different grades of aortic valve calcifications. Double-oblique reconstruction of multidetector-row CT angiographic data set demonstrates small isolated spots of calcification (grade 2, [**A**]) as well as multiple larger spots of calcification (grade 3, [**B**]).

mitral valves can be visualized with high quality. At this point, MDCT of the aortic valve seems to be of special interest for the assessment of aortic valvular calcification. Future studies are warranted to exploit the potential of MDCT for evaluation of the pulmonary and tricuspidal valves as well as to establish tools for quantitative analysis of valvular function and quantification of the calcium deposits.

REFERENCES

1. Ohnesorge B, Flohr T, Becker C, et al. Cardiac imaging by means of electrocardiographically gated multisection spiral CT: initial experience. Radiology 2000;217:564–571.
2. Flohr T, Bruder H, Stierstorfer K, Simon J, Schaller S, Ohnesorge B. New technical developments in multislice CT, part 2: sub-millimeter 16-slice scanning and increased gantry rotation speed for cardiac imaging. Rofo Fortschr Geb Rontgenstr Neuen Bildgeb Verfahr 2002;174:1022–1027.
3. Achenbach S, Giesler T, Ropers D, et al. Detection of coronary artery stenoses by contrast-enhanced, retrospectively electrocardiographically-gated, multislice spiral computed tomography. Circulation 2001;103:2535–2538.
4. Becker CR, Kleffel T, Crispin A, et al. Coronary artery calcium measurement: agreement of multirow detector and electron beam CT. AJR Am J Roentgenol 2001;176:1295–1298.
5. Willmann JK, Weishaupt D, Lachat M, et al. Electrocardiographically gated multi-detector row CT for assessment of valvular morphology and calcification in aortic stenosis. Radiology 2002;225: 120–128.
6. Willmann JK, Kobza R, Roos JE, et al. ECG-gated multi-detector row CT for assessment of mitral valve disease: initial experience. Eur Radiol 2002;12:2662–2669.
7. Gorlin R, Gorlin SG. Hydraulic formula for calculation of the area of the stenotic mitral valve, other valves and central circulatory shunts. Am Heart J 1951;41:1–29.
8. Otto CM, Lind BK, Kitzman DW, Gersh BJ, Siscovick DS. Association of aortic-valve sclerosis with cardiovascular mortality and morbidity in the elderly. N Engl J Med 1999;341:142–147.
9. Stewart BF, Siscovick D, Lind BK, et al. Clinical factors associated with calcific aortic valve disease. Cardiovascular Health Study. J Am Coll Cardiol 1997;29:630–634.
10. Otto CM, Burwash IG, Legget ME, et al. Prospective study of asymptomatic valvular aortic stenosis. Clinical, echocardiographic, and exercise predictors of outcome. Circulation 1997;95: 2262–2270.
11. Rosenhek R, Binder T, Porenta G, et al. Predictors of outcome in severe, asymptomatic aortic stenosis. N Engl J Med 2000;343: 611–617.
12. Otto CM. Timing of aortic valve surgery. Heart 2000;84:211–218.
13. Shavelle DM, Takasu J, Budoff MJ, Mao S, Zhao XQ, O'Brien KD. HMG CoA reductase inhibitor (statin) and aortic valve calcium. Lancet 2002;359:1125–1126.
14. Adams DH, Chen RH, Kadner A, Aranki SF, Allred EN, Cohn LH. Impact of small prosthetic valve size on operative mortality in elderly patients after aortic valve replacement for aortic stenosis: does gender matter? J Thorac Cardiovasc Surg 1999;118:815–822.
15. Delius RE, Samyn MM, Behrendt DM. Should a bicuspid aortic valve be replaced in the presence of subvalvar or supravalvar aortic stenosis? Ann Thorac Surg 1998;66:1337–1342.
16. Luciani GB, Casali G, Mazzucco A. Risk factors for coronary complications after stentless aortic root replacement. Semin Thorac Cardiovasc Surg 1999;11:126–132.
17. Boughaleb D, Mansourati J, Genet L, Barra J, Mondine P, Blanc JJ. [Permanent cardiac stimulation after aortic valve replacement: incidence, predictive factors and long-term prognosis]. Arch Mal Coeur Vaiss 1994;87:925–930.
18. Adler Y, Fink N, Spector D, Wiser I, Sagie A. Mitral annulus calcification—a window to diffuse atherosclerosis of the vascular system. Atherosclerosis 2001;155:1–8.

In children between ages 6 and 12, we usually test the breath-hold two or three times before the acquisition, in order to ensure thoracic immobility during the scanning process.

NEONATES AND YOUNG INFANTS

In neonates or young infants, breath-hold is not possible, and we do not use ECG-gated acquisition, for four main reasons:

1. Respiratory artifacts are responsible for substantial degradation of images. These respiratory artifacts cause more important artifacts than heart motion does. ECG-gated acquisition is much slower than nongated acquisitions, causing more respiratory artifacts.
2. In babies, normal heart rate is over 100 beats per minute (bpm), which is too fast to prevent any heart motion artifacts. First reports on cardiac CT showed that artifacts are frequent in adults when cardiac rhythm is over 64 (4-slice technology) or 70 bpm (16-slice technology) *(3)*. In babies with cyanotic CHD, cardiac rhythm is much higher, generally between 140 and 180 bpm.
3. Generally, the clinical question concerns extracardiac anatomy. Images of extracardiac structures are less sensitive to heart motion than heart images are.
4. ECG-gated cardiac retrospective acquisitions require much higher radiation doses than nongated thoracic CT, because only a part of the dose (i.e., dose delivered during diastole) is used for creating images. If a standard cardiac adult protocol were applied for a 3-kg baby, dose delivered would be about 50 times more than the dose we currently use in these conditions. In babies, organ sensitivity to radiation is much higher than in adults. In addition, better imaging quality is not guaranteed, because of the two first points mentioned above, and a risk of developing cancer in the future could not be totally ruled out *(4)*.

In our experience, the principle "go as fast as possible" was adequate to get good image quality in neonates with CHD. Short acquisition time is the best way to minimize respiratory artifacts. With a 4-slice CT (Volume Zoom, Siemens), we currently scan the thoraxes of babies in 3 or 4 s, using 2.5-mm collimation and a table speed of 20 mm/s (pitch 8). The images are of superior quality to those using 1-mm slice thickness, which also require longer acquisition time and cause more respiratory artifacts. Very short acquisition times (5 s or less) make apnea possible in intubated babies. In these cases, images were found free from respiratory artifacts. With the 16-slice CT, we may choose now either to scan the thorax of a baby in about 4 s using 0.75-mm slices or in 2 s using 1.5-mm collimation.

CHILDREN OVER SEVEN YEARS OF AGE, AND ADULTS

In this group of older children and young adults, two options are possible: (1) breath-hold angio-CT acquisition; or (2) ECG-gated acquisition. In this group, the protocol must be chosen depending on the clinical questions. If, for example, coronary visualization is required to look for a possible anatomical variant, ECG-gated protocols are recommended. In the other cases, ECG gating is often not mandatory. In any case, one should always keep in mind that the radiation dose delivered is much higher when using ECG-gated acquisition.

DOSE CONSIDERATIONS

Radiation exposure is a major public health issue. CT contributes greatly to the population dose arising from medical exposure, accounting for 35% of the dose delivered during diagnostic examinations, although representing 4% of those studies *(5)*. Multislice CT offers even more diagnosis capabilities but tends to increase the radiation dose as a result of routine use of thinner slice thicknesses, extension of the volume of acquisition, or multiple phase acquisitions. Following the As Low As Reasonably Achievable (ALARA) principle, dose reduction is necessary but examination quality must be preserved without losing diagnostic information. The thorax is a low-attenuation region, though substantial dose reduction during chest CT is feasible because of the high inherent contrast. In August 2001, the ALARA conference of the Society for Pediatric Radiology raised the question of dose reduction by reduction of kilovoltage *(6)*.

In our center, we decided to apply the ALARA principle as far as possible in neonates and babies with CHD, and then apply some systematic rules:

- No preview scan (responsible for unnecessary additional radiation dose). Scan length is calculated with laser.
- Systematic use of 80-kV settings.
- Adaptation of the mAs to child's weight.
- Only one phase acquisition when possible.
- Systematic protection of nonscanned organs.

80-kV protocols have not been developed yet, although in our experience, it is possible to scan the thorax in adults of less than 75 kg without substantial loss of image quality. Reducing the kilovoltage from 120kVp to 80 kVp decreases the radiation dose by 65% at constant current setting, as radiation dose varies with the square of kV. This setting is sufficient for good quality images, as long as the mAs are adjusted according to the child's weight.

We always use 80 kV as the standard kilovoltage setting in children. Current exposure is adapted to the body weight in neonates and infants, using the following rule:

3 kg: 30 mAs
4 kg: 35 mAs
5 kg: 40 mAs
6 kg: 45 mAs

Using this protocol, radiation exposure is estimated under 1 mSv for a neonate. 1 mSv in equivalent to less than 6 mo natural radiation. Even lower dose may be used in premature babies or when high quality images are not mandatory for diagnosis. 80 kV and 17 mAs is the minimum exposure setting allowed with the 16-slice CT from Siemens (Sensation 16). A previous study compared radiation dose with electron beam CT (EBCT) and conventional angiography, which were favourable from far to EBCT *(7)* (25 to 50 times less skin exposure than with conventional angiography as estimated by the authors). Anatomical data acquired from CT may be judiciously used to limit the number of views acquired with angiography, and sometimes replace conventional angiography. CT may be then advantageous to reduce global radiation exposure in CHD patients.

The other advantage of 80 kV settings is the possibility for reduction of amount of contrast medium injection, because low kilovoltage is more sensitive to contrast (iodine has a high atomic number) than standard 120 or 140 kV settings.

INJECTION PROTOCOL

Dose injection must be adapted to the baby's weight. We currently use 2 cc per kg in our institution, which was sufficient in all cases encountered. Sometimes CT is performed just after conventional angiography, in order to benefit from central venous access. The limit of the total contrast amount of the two procedures may be up to of 8 cc/kg without complication in our experience.

Basic protocol of injection for pulmonary arteries or systemic vascular enhancement:

Using 80 kV, rate of injection can be as low as 0.6 cc per second in neonates with catheter placed in the vein of the hand. Higher rate may be used in case of central catheter (femoral or jugular). Power injector is currently used to ensure a continous and regular flow rate. Our current rules used for rate of injection are as follows:

3 kg: 30 mAs
4 kg: 35 mAs
5 kg: 40 mAs
6 kg: 45 mAs

The start delay in neonates and infants is 15 s for peripheral injection, 10 s for central venous injection. To be sure of having vascular contrast during the acquisition, we sometimes slightly increase the amount of contrast medium in order to follow this rule:

Time of injection = start delay + time of acquisition

Using this rule, acquisition is never "too late" for good vascular enhancement, because acquisition ends with the end of injection, so contrast medium is still in the peripheral veins when acquisition ends.

Precautions for Venous Access

Peripheral venous access is performed in the pediatric unit. Right arm injection is preferable (but not mandatory) to avoid striking artifacts on the innominate left brachio-cephalic vein. In some cases, venous connections are congenitally different or surgically modified. This information, when available, is important before the scan procedure, as it may change the scan injection protocol. Venous visualization may be realized at first pass, with a high concentration of contrast medium, or sometimes later, at the time of venous return. The optimal injection protocol depends on each particular venous anatomy.

Catheter permeability is checked before injection. It is essential to avoid any air injection during the scan procedure. All bubbles should be removed when connecting catheter to power injector. Because many patients with CHD have right to left shunt, air injection through venous access could cause air systemic embolism, with possible fatal consequences.

Sedation

General anesthesia is never necessary in our experience. In neonates we do not use any sedative drugs. In infants, we recommend oral or intrarectal sedation (or both) before CT procedure, to prevent baby agitation during the acquisition, which may be responsible for poorer image quality and occasionally require re-examination. Sedation is not always mandatory if the baby is quiet. Experienced technologists are necessary in the CT room for good management of the babies: precise knowledge of baby management and a quiet attitude is of primary importance.

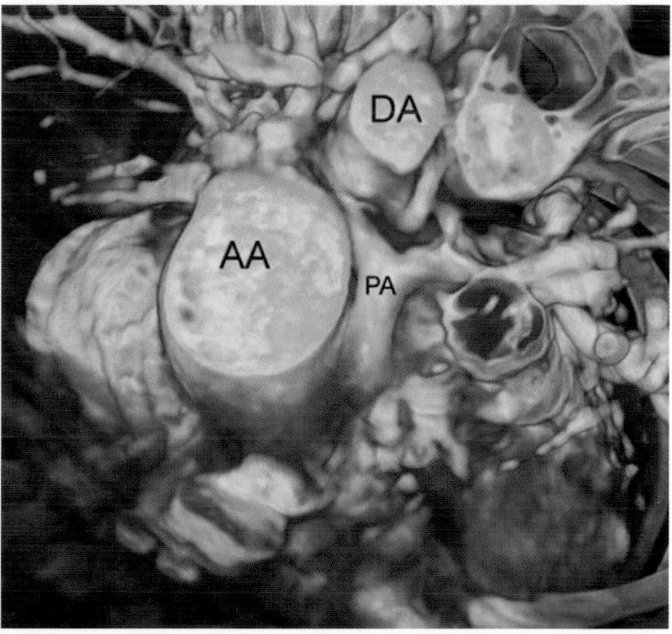

Fig. 1. Pulmonary atresia with ventricular septal defect: Multislice CT showed small but confluent pulmonary arteries ("seagull sign") in a 8-yr-old patient. These pulmonary arteries were not seen with conventional angiography. This finding has been of fundamental importance for surgical decision (staged repair). Complete repair was finally obtained with normalization of blood oxygen saturation.

Our sedation protocol in infants includes intrarectal: midazomal at 0.3 mg/kg, given 15 min before examination. Additional sedative drugs may be useful (hydroxyzine at 1 mg/kg, per os, 1 h before examination). With experienced technologists, mean total examination time in the CT room is 20 min. Qualified medical monitoring may sometimes be necessary during the examination, depending on the clinical conditions of the babies. In all cases, oxygen saturation should be closely monitored.

ANATOMICAL ASSESSMENT

Although CHDs may be a difficult topic for radiologists who are not familiar with the exploration of these pathologies, the main clinical question for which the CT is performed is often simple, making interpretation of the image accessible to any radiologist. Examples of questions include: What is the status of the pulmonary artery (present, absent, or stenotic)? What is the size of the aorta? Where are the collateral arteries originating? Do these collaterals cross behind or beyond the central airways? Where are the pulmonary venous connections situated? We identified several main follow-up questions to be raised, which include: pulmonary artery status and morphology, coronary artery origins, aorta and collaterals, suspicion of airway compression of vascular origin, suspicion of anomalous venous return, and postoperative evaluation. Questions may sometimes be multiple, so protocols should be adapted accordingly.

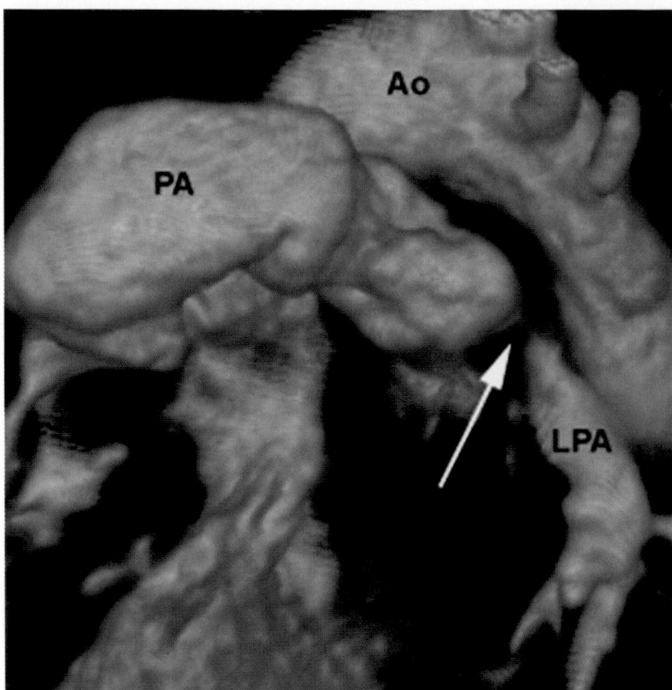

Fig. 2. Tetralogy of Fallot: 3D visualization of severe left pulmonary artery (LPA) stenosis in an infant (10 mo, 8 kg). PA, pulmonary artery; Ao, aorta.

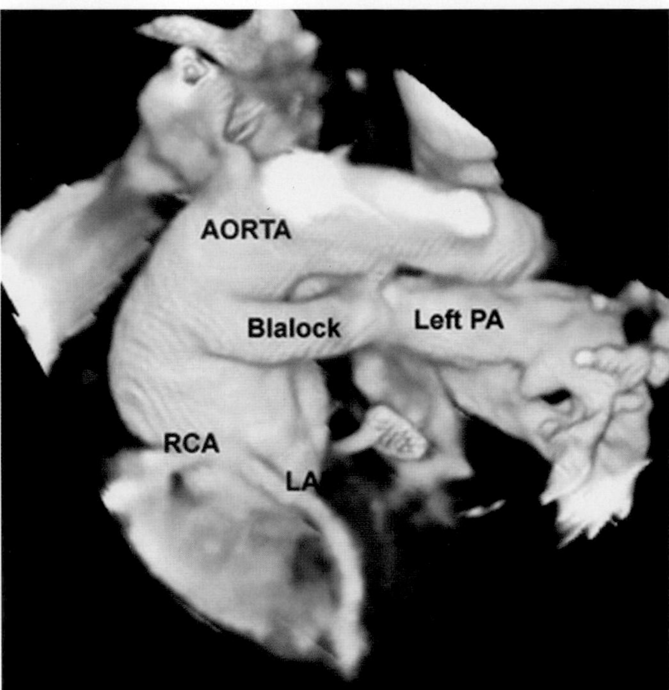

Fig. 4. Left anterior descending (LAD) coronary artery arising from the right coronary artery (RCA) in an infant (5 mo, 4.5 kg) with pulmonary atresia with ventricular septal defect.

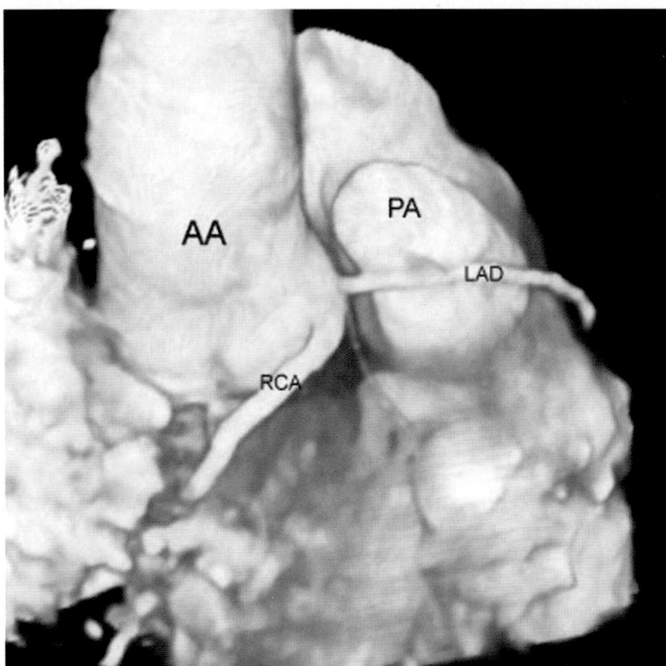

Fig. 3. Right and left pulmonary artery (PA) stenosis after complete repair of pulmonary atresia with ventricular septal defect: control following endovascular kissing stents (arrowheads) implantation in a 14-yr-old patient.

PULMONARY ARTERIES

Pulmonary artery evaluation is a priority in pulmonary atresia with ventricular septal defect (PAVSD) (Fig. 1), tetralogy of Fallot (Figs. 2 and 3), truncus arteriosus, or suspicion of pulmonary sling. For pulmonary artery visualization, we usually do not use ECG-gated acquisition. With a 4-slice CT, we use 2.5-mm collimation (3-mm slice width) with an increment of 1.5 mm in order to get fast acquisitions (of less than 5 s in babies), for reduction of motion and respiratory artifacts on pulmonary arteries. With a 16-slice CT, we usually use 0.75-mm collimation and get 1-mm slice width with an increment of 0.5 mm. Compared to 4-slice acquisition, images of higher resolution are acquired in a similar acquisition time. High resolution is advantageous for pulmonary artery stenosis evaluation. For neonates or infants before 7 yr of age, start delay is either 15 s (peripheral venous access) or 10 s (central venous access). In patients over 6 yr of age, we sometimes use the bolus tracking technique for optimization of start delay. For reconstructions, 3D images are currently performed using maximum intensity projection, multiplanar reformations, and volume-rendering technique.

CORONARY ARTERIES

Anomalous coronary arteries are frequently associated with CHD. The most frequent anomalous finding is a left coronary artery originating from right coronary sinus (Fig. 4), but many variants are possible, even coronary artery originating from pulmonary arteries. The "normal" position of coronary origins may be different from usual in PAVSD or in tetralogy of Fallot, because of rotation of the aorta: the origin of the left main is typically at 6 o'clock, and the origin of the right coronary artery at 1 o'clock. Detection of an anomalous origin of coronaries is especially important before surgery when a ventriculotomy is planned, as accidental lesion of the coronary artery crossing the right ventricle during intervention can be fatal.

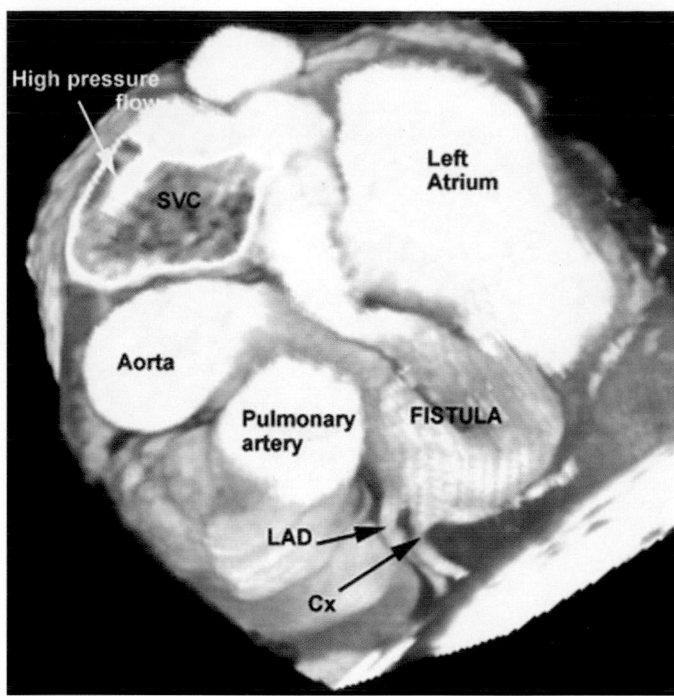

Fig. 5. Multislice CT shows a large fistula connecting the left main coronary artery and the superior vena cava (SVC) in an adult patient. Cx, left circumflex artery;. LAD, left anterior descending coronary artery.

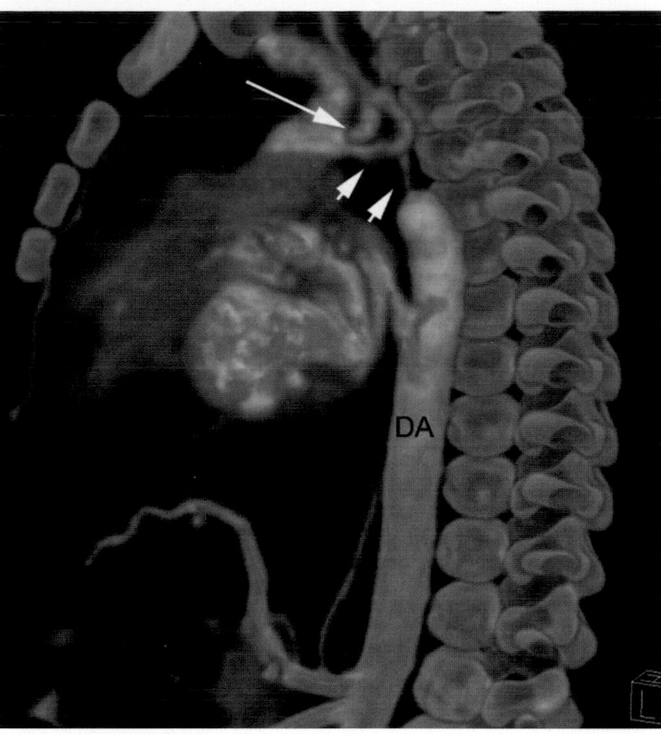

Fig. 7. Severe aortic coarctation in a newborn (4 d, 3 kg). Multislice CT showed absence of opacification of aortic arch after the origin of supra-aortic trunks (arrowheads). A severe stenosis of left carotid artery was also depicted (arrow). DA, descending aorta.

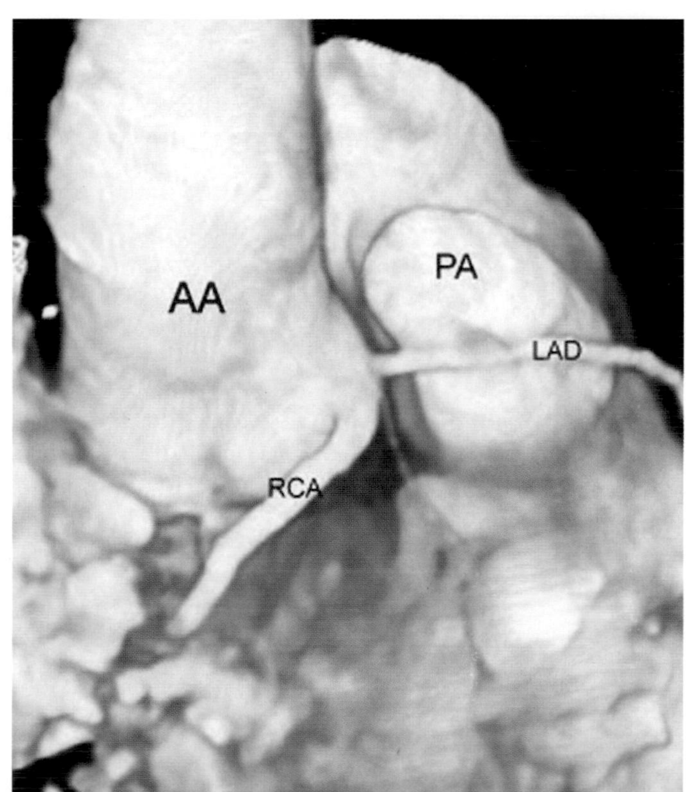

Fig. 6. Anomalous origin of coronary arteries in a patient with Tetralogy of Fallot: left anterior descending (LAD) coronary artery is originating from right coronary sinus. RCA, right coronary artery. AA, ascending aorta; PA, pulmonary artery.

In neonates we usually do not use ECG-gated acquisition because the heart rate is too high and also to prevent excessive radiation dose. Using the same protocol of injection as for pulmonary arteries, coronary origins can be clearly seen in about 70% of the cases, but visualization remains difficult in babies of less than 4 kg. The value of multislice CT for detection of anomalous coronaries has not yet been assessed.

In older CHD patients, if the patient can hold his or her breath for a sufficient time, ECG-gated acquisition may be the technique of choice. Visualization is then possible free of motion artifact, making possible the precise evaluation of the coronary artery tree. To avoid heart motion artifacts, heart rate must be regular and below 70 per minute; excellent results are generally obtained at 55–60 bpm. We usually use ECG-pulsing technique, in order to reduce radiation dose by about 35% (author's data), all other factors being constant. If axial and maximum-intensity projection images are sufficient for diagnosis, volume-rendering technique may provide comprehensive imaging of the coronary artery anomaly (Figs. 5 and 6).

AORTA AND COLLATERALS

Aortic anatomy evaluation is essential in case of aortic coarctation (Fig. 7) or for suspicion of aortic arch anomalies; complete or incomplete double aortic arch (Fig. 8), right aortic arch, or cervical arch are very clearly seen with 3D CT images. In case of PAVSD, major aorto-pulmonary collateral arteries (MAPCA) often originate from the descending aorta (Fig. 9); evaluation of size and spatial relationship of these arteries is of primary importance for planning surgical intervention.

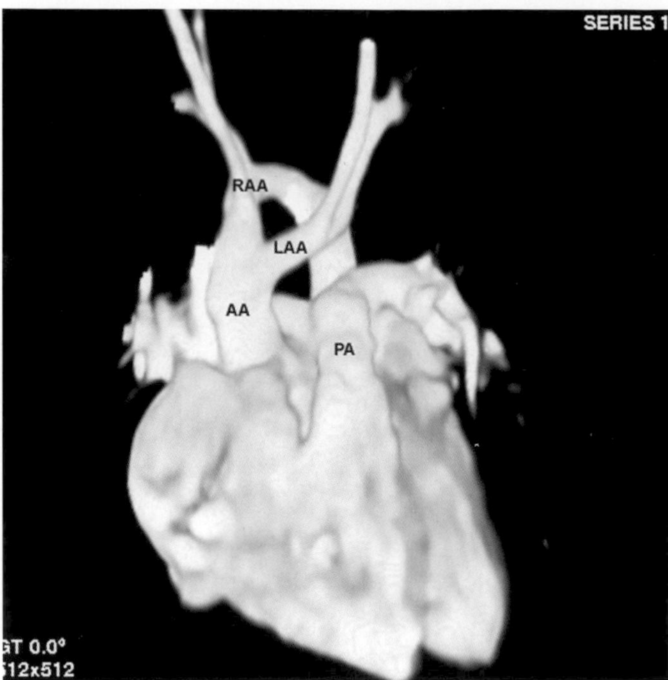

Fig. 8. Severe respiratory distress in a newborn: multislice CT showed clearly a complete double aortic arch responsible for tracheal compression (2-mo-old patient, 4 kg). RAA, right aortic arch; LAA, left aortic arch; AA, ascending aorta; PA, pulmonary artery.

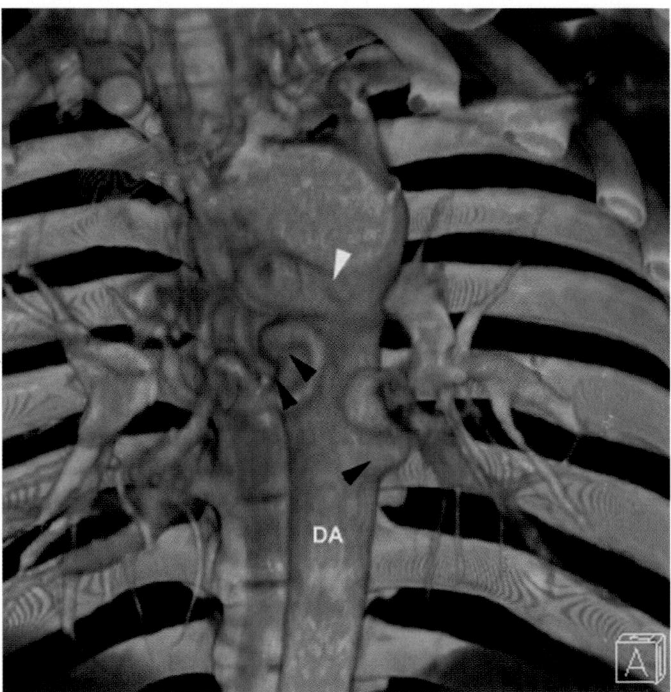

Fig. 9. Multislice CT shows four major aorto-pulmonary collateral arteries (arrowheads) originating from descending aorta (DA), in a patient with pulmonary atresia with ventricular septal defect. Three-dimensional evaluation of the course of each collateral was of primary importance for surgical planning.

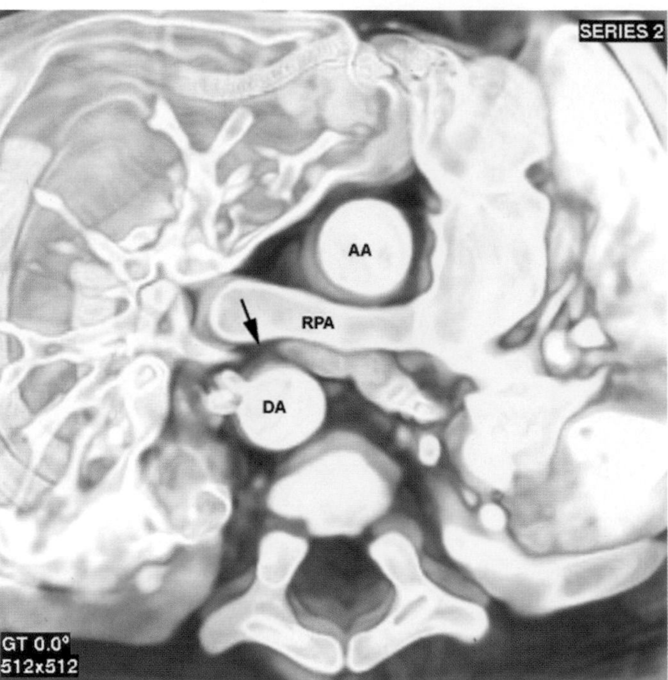

Fig. 10. Severe respiratory distress in a newborn (20 d, 3.8 kg) with pulmonary valves agenesis with ventricular septal defect. Multislice CT showed a compression of the right bronchus between the dilated right pulmonary artery (RPA) and the right sided aorta. DA, descending aorta; AA, ascending aorta.

For aorta visualization, we usually not use ECG-gated acquisition for babies, infants, or adult patients. Thin collimation (1 mm with a 4-slice CT, 0.75 mm with a 16-slice CT), is used to get high-resolution images. High-resolution images are useful for aorta stenosis evaluation, especially in case of aortic coarctation, for a better evaluation of vessel narrowing. For neonates or children before 7 yr of age, start delay is either 15 s (peripheral venous access) or 10 s (central venous access). In patients over 6 yr of age, we usually use the bolus tracking technique for optimization of start delay. The ROI is placed at the center of the ascending aorta. For reconstructions, 3D images are currently performed using maximum-intensity projection, mutliplanar reformations, and volume-rendering technique.

UPPER AIRWAYS EVALUATION

Compression of central airways from vascular origin may result from various situations; the most frequently observed are aortic arch anomalies, pulmonary artery sling, dilated pulmonary arteries, posteriorly displaced aorta (switch intervention), and so on. In 20 consecutive cases of vascular compression, we observed six cases of aortic arch anomalies (four double aortic arch, one incomplete vascular ring, one circling aorta), five cases of dilatation of pulmonary arteries (one case of pulmonary valve agenesia [Fig. 10], and four cases of pulmonary hypertension associated with ventricular septal defect), three cases of posteriorly displaced aorta after intervention for transposition of great vessels, three cases of left main bronchus compression by descending aorta, one pulmonary artery sling, and two compressions by a brachio-cephalic artery.

Nonenhanced CT is sufficient to look for a stenosis of central airways, but contrast enhancement is mandatory to search for a vascular origin. In babies, we currently use the same protocol as for pulmonary artery or aorta visualization. In addition

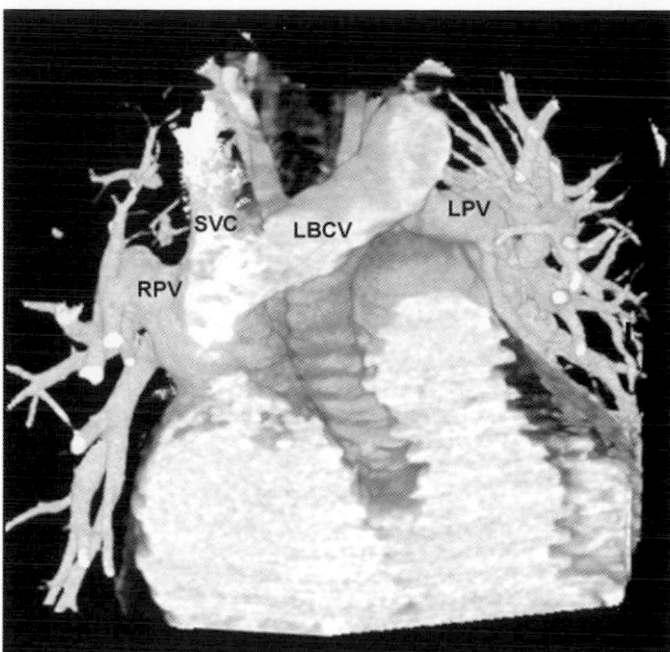

Fig. 11. Multislice CT using 3D rendering technique showed total abnormal pulmonary venous return in the superior vena cava (SVC) and left brachio-cephalic vein (LBVC). LPV, left pulmonary vein; RPV, right pulmonary vein.

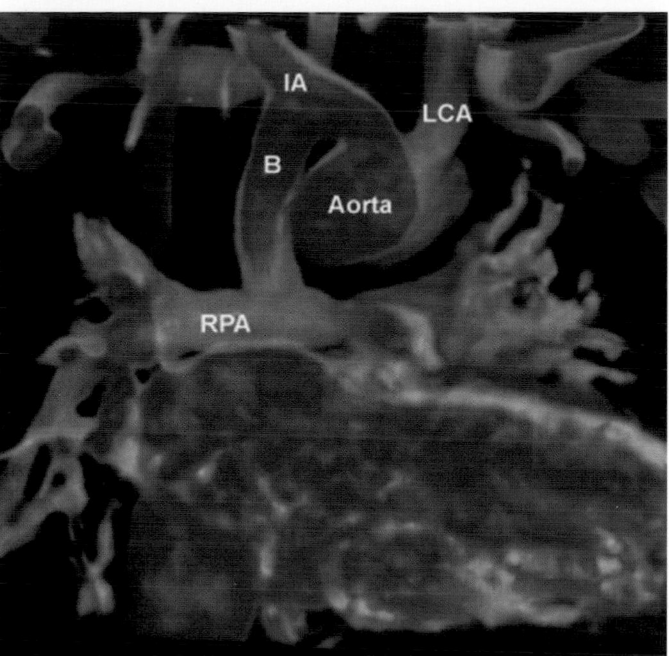

Fig. 13. Postoperative control of a Blalock (B) anastomosis between the innominate artery (IA) and the right pulmonary artery (RPA) in a newborn with tetralogy of Fallot (15 d, 3.5 kg). LCA, left carotid artery.

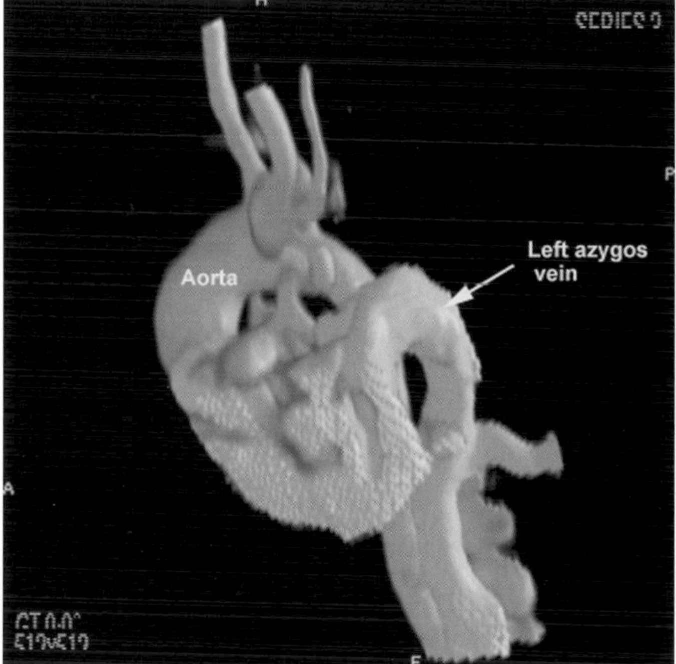

Fig. 12. Demonstration of anomalous systemic venous return in a newborn patient with tetralogy of Fallot: multislice CT showed absence of right superior vena cava and anomalous left azygos vein ending in the coronary sinus (15-d-old patient, 1.9 kg).

to maximum intensity projection (MIP) reconstructions, volume-rendering technique (VRT) is very effective to show central airway narrowing (Fig. 10). Using VRT, it is easy to colorize low-density airway structures and high-density vascular structures to get high-contrast images, making diagnosis of vascular compression easy. However, airway compression can be more distal: in this case, diagnosis of vascular compression may be difficult. Evidence of air trapping on parenchymal windowing may be of interest for distal compressions.

ANOMALOUS VENOUS RETURN

CT and MRI are very efficient imaging techniques to detect pulmonary or systemic anomalous venous return. Both techniques allow 3D visualization of these anomalies. Three-dimensional images can be used as a primary method for diagnosis (Figs. 11 and 12). ECG-gated acquisitions are usually not necessary because venous structures are not very sensitive to cardiac motion. Injection site and timing for acquisition must be chosen carefully, because time for best opacification depends on the venous drainage, and any anomalous venous drainage may interfere with the optimal timing. An additional delayed acquisition may be necessary to opacify the whole venous system. To avoid striking artifacts from concentrated contrast medium in the veins, it is preferable to reduce the rate of injection.

POSTINTERVENTIONAL EVALUATION

Postoperative evaluation includes various clinical situations, such as evaluation of bypass patency (Fig. 13), suspicion of mediastinitis, suspicion of airway compression (Fig. 14), and pulmonary embolus (Fig. 15). The CT protocol should be adapted to the question. Generally speaking, radiation exposure can often be reduced, because there is generally no need for detailed anatomic information. For example, for a mediastinitis search, only one delayed (3–5 min) acquisition may be enough to evidence a mediastinal collection. Conversely, control of conduit patency can be carried out with an acquisition at the arterial phase alone. CT evaluation of new vascular anatomy may be useful after complex surgical repair (Fig. 16).

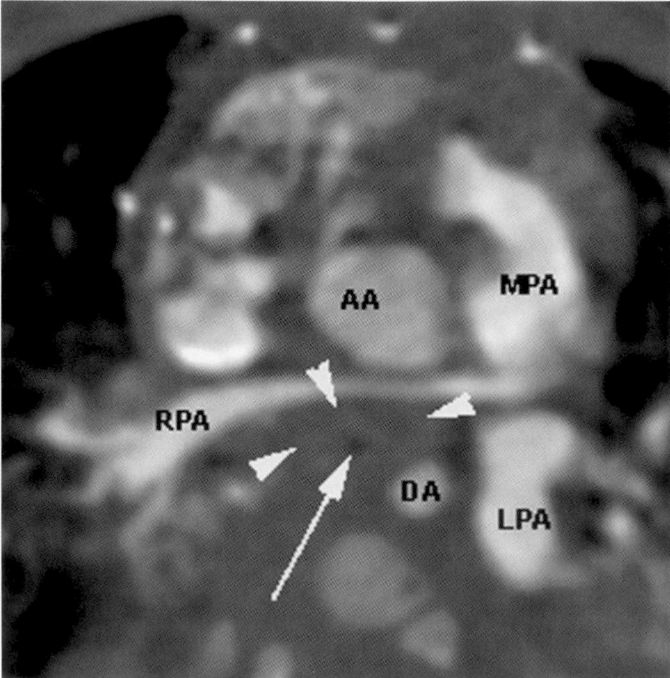

Fig. 14. External tracheal compression by dense material (found to be biological glue) following complete repair of aortic coarctation and ventricular septal defect. Note that the right pulmonary artery (RPA) is also narrowed due to the presence of the glue. DA, descending aorta; AA, ascending aorta; LPA, left pulmerary artery; MPA, main pulmonary artery.

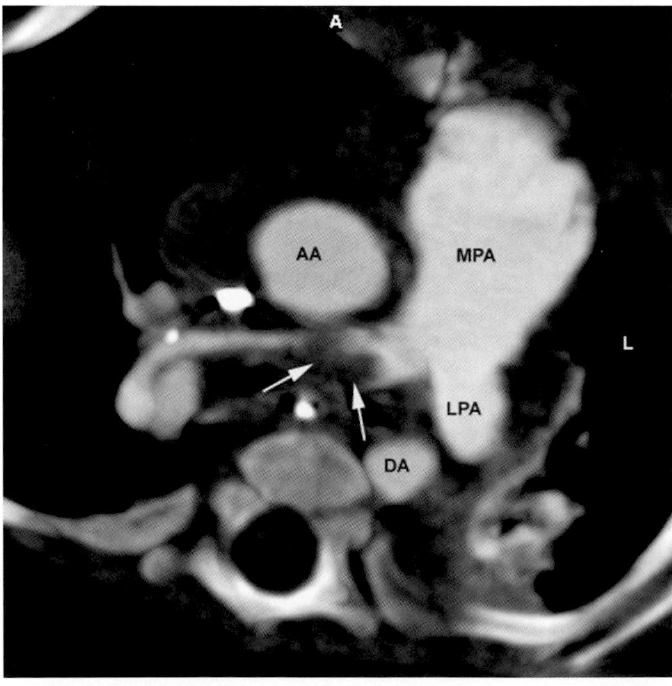

Fig. 15. Persistent hypoxia following surgery in a 13-mo-old baby: multislice CT using axial MIP view showed an obstructive thrombus at the origin of the right pulmonary artery (arrows). DA, descending aorta; AA, ascending aorta; LPA, left pulmonary artery; MPA, main pulmonary artery.

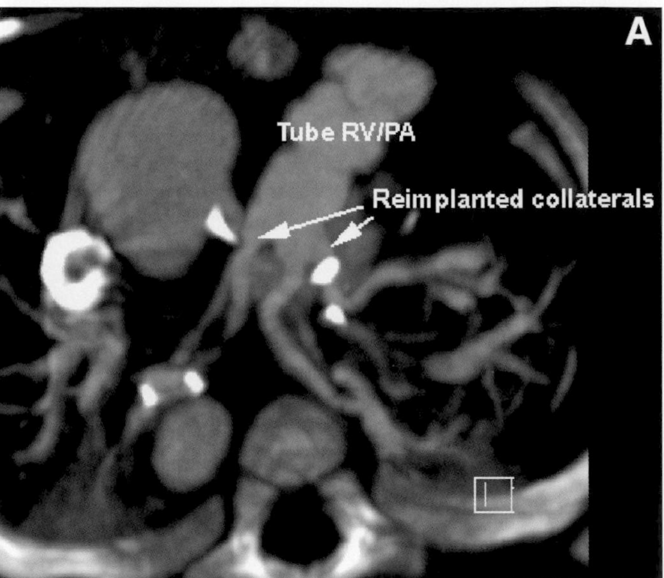

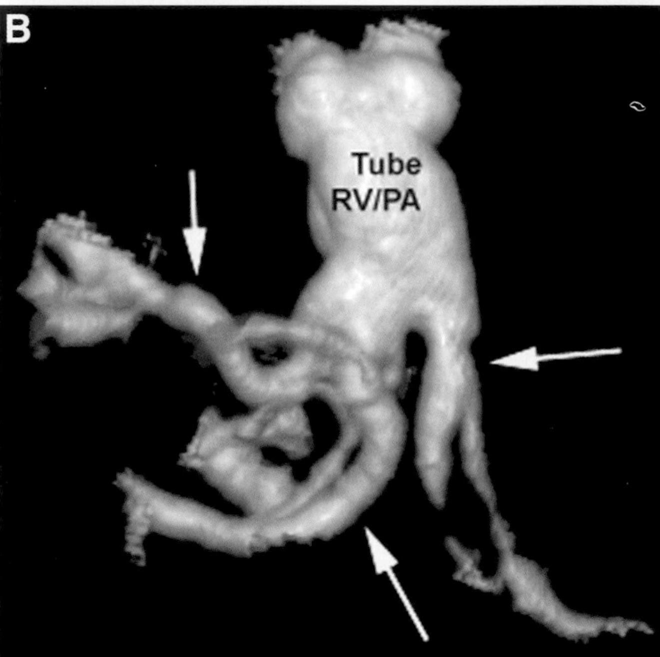

Fig. 16. Complete unifocalization in an infant (3 mo, 4 kg) with pulmonary atresia with ventricular septal defect and no confluent pulmonary arteries: the major aortopulmonary collaterals were unifocalized and connected to the right ventricle with a tube. (A) Maximum intensity projection view in axial plane. (B) Volume-rendering technique view allowing evaluation of the surgical repair from any angle.

EVALUATION OF MAIN CHD WITH MULTISLICE CT

PULMONARY ATRESIA WITH VENTRICULAR SEPTAL DEFECT

Status of Pulmonary Arteries

- Presence or absence pulmonary arteries
- Confluent pulmonary arteries ("seagull sign," Fig. 1).
- Size of the pulmonary arteries
- Presence of pulmonary artery stenosis
- Patent ductus arteriosus

Status of MAPCA
- Number and location (Fig. 9)
- Stenosis (usually proximal)
- Position in front of or behind the central airways (essential for surgical planning)

Coronary Arteries
- Left anterior descending artery originating from right coronary artery (Fig. 4)
- Double LAD (anterior and posterior)

Others
- Venous connections
- Bronchial anomalies

Follow-up
- Increase of PA
- Patency of conduits
- New pulmonary anatomy (unifocalization) (Fig. 16)

TETRALOGY OF FALLOT

Status of pulmonary arteries
- Size of pulmonary arteries
- Presence of pulmonary artery stenosis
- Pulmonary artery stenosis (evaluation of stenosis and planning before stent placement [Fig. 2])

Coronary arteries
- Left anterior descending artery originating from right coronary artery (contraindication for ventriculotomy)
- Double LAD (anterior and posterior)

Follow-up
- Size of PA
- Patency of conduits or stent (Fig. 3 and 13)

Others
- Venous connections
- Bronchial anomalies

Transposition of Great Arteries
- Long-term follow-up
- Position of aorta and pulmonary artery
- Pulmonary artery stenosis
- Re-implanted coronary arteries

Atrial Septal Defect
- Generally the defect is not well visible
- CT may be useful to detect associated anomalous venous return

Double Aortic Arch
- Size of both arches (Fig. 8)
- Right or left sided anterior arch
- Right or left sided descending aorta

Aortic Coarctation
- Type of coarctation: preductal, juxtaductal, or postductal (Fig. 7)
- Degree of narrowing
- Presence of thrombus
- Visualisation of collateral arteries
- Associated anomalies

Anomalous Pulmonary Venous Return
- 3D visualization of anomalous venous return (Figs. 11, 12)
- Distance from left atrium for evaluation of surgical repair possibilities

CONCLUSIONS

Precise 3D visualization of anomalous extracardiac anatomy can be routinely carried out using multislice CT in CHD patients. Multislice CT angiography represents an important additional low-invasive diagnostic tool for evaluation of CHD, and may be used occasionally as an alternative to angiography. Dose consideration is the only relative limitation of this technique, especially in neonates and infants, but excellent image quality may be achieved using very low exposure parameters.

REFERENCES

1. The clinical role of magnetic resonance in cardiovascular disease. Task Force of the European Society of Cardiology, in collaboration with the Association of European Paediatric Cardiologists. Eur Heart J 1998;19:19–39.
2. Kawano T, Ishii M, Takagi J, et al. Three-dimensional helical computed tomographic angiography in neonates and infants with complex congenital heart disease. Am Heart J 2000;139:654–660.
3. Schroeder S, Kopp AF, Kuettner A, et al. Influence of heart rate on vessel visibility in noninvasive coronary angiography using new multislice computed tomography: experience in 94 patients. Clin Imaging 2002;26:106–111.
4. Brenner D, Elliston C, Hall E, Berdon W. Estimated risks of radiation-induced fatal cancer from pediatric CT. AJR Am J Roentgenol 2001;176:289–296.
5. Nagel HD et al. In: Radiation exposure in computed tomography: Fundamentals, influencing parameters, dose assessment, optimization, scanner data, terminology. 2nd ed. Offizin Paul Hartung Druck, Hamburg, Germany: 2002;1–3.
6. Slovis TL. ALARA conference proceedings. The ALARA concept in paediatric CT: intelligent dose reduction (Editorial). Pediatr Radiol 2002; 32:217–231.
7. Westra SJ, Hurteau J, Galindo A, McNitt-Gray MF, Boechat MI, Laks H. Cardiac electron-beam CT in children undergoing surgical repair for pulmonary atresia. Radiology 1999;213:502–512.

17 Imaging of Cardiac and Paracardiac Masses and Pseudotumors

Bernd J. Wintersperger, MD

INTRODUCTION

Although the use of computed tomography (CT) in cardiac imaging mainly focuses on coronary artery disease and its sequelae, there are many more indications in which CT can provide excellent and valuable information. This has already been reported based on studies with electron beam CT (EBCT). The rapidly emerging and vastly growing interest and knowledge in cardiac CT today is mainly caused by the development and widespread use of multidetector-row CT (MDCT) systems. Initially introduced in 1992 (Elscint CT-Twin), MDCT led to a more widespread use of CT in cardiac imaging, starting with 4-row MDCT. Within recent years, further technical developments have led to the use of 8-, 16-, and 64-row MDCT systems. Cardiac imaging has been one of the major and most exciting focuses of MDCT since then. Although the focus of interest in cardiac MDCT is again coronary artery disease and its prevention, most of the information provided by EBCT can also be revealed by MDCT *(1–4)*.

Compared to other referrals, imaging of cardiac or paracardiac masses is a rather rare request for a CT study. The examination of and screening for cardiac tumors is among the rare causes for performing cross-sectional cardiac imaging studies. The modality of choice in screening for cardiac masses is still 2D echocardiography *(5–7)*. Because of its real-time approach, echocardiography can detect cardiac and even small cardiac valve-attached masses and their impact on valve and global cardiac function within the same examination *(8)*. However, there are certain restrictions to echocardiography affecting its clinical use. Although echocardiography can be easily performed in any patient with bedside capabilities, image quality is mainly dependent on the patient's habitus and the examiner's skills. Besides restrictions caused by limited acoustic windows due to obesity, right-ventricle assessment may be hampered by pulmonary emphysema. In addition, tissue characterization is often not possible even though tumors may present with typical echocardiographic signs. EBCT and MDCT are cross-sectional techniques for acquiring images with high spatial and temporal resolution to freeze cardiac motion and to follow the cardiac cycle *(9,10)*. Although tumor studies are not the primary focus of cardiac CT imaging, CT is a valuable tool in the work-up of patients with suspected cardiac tumors.

As noninvasive cross-sectional imaging modalities, EBCT and MDCT offer a large field of view without major limitations based on the patient's constitution. In addition, with the use of retrospectively electrocardiogram (ECG)-gated data acquisition techniques, MDCT provides a 3D data set that enables secondary reconstruction of any desired image plane. These features overcome the limitation of providing only transaxial images in CT or the approximation of individual cardiac axes in EBCT. With the recent advent of 16-row MDCT, even submillimeter collimated images are possible within a short breath-hold of 17–20 s. However, temporal resolution of EBCT is superior to that of MDCT and also allows visualizing very tiny valve-attached tumors, although this still remains a challenge *(11)*.

IMAGING TECHNIQUES

CT imaging of cardiac masses is basically not different from other cardiac applications like coronary artery imaging or cardiac morphology in congenital heart disease (CHD). Detailed information and background about cardiac CT imaging algorithms using EBCT and MDCT can be found in Part II, "Technical Background."

However, depending on the individual scanner and data acquisition settings, a few basics have to be considered for imaging of cardiac masses.

DATA ACQUISITION

Especially in MDCT cardiac imaging, different algorithms and data acquisition techniques can be used. However, to allow a 3D assessment of the heart with adaptation to individual cardiac axis cardiac chambers, retrospective ECG-gated algorithms are strongly recommended, although they basically lead to a higher radiation exposure. Recently developed techniques allow again for a subsequent reduction of redundant radiation without losing the benefits of retrospective gating. In the assessment of coronary artery calcifications, Jakobs et al. showed a significant reduction of 45–50% without change in image quality *(12)*. As there are major differences in basic techniques, only general recommendations can be given. Technical backgrounds and imaging algorithms of EBCT and MDCT are

From: *Contemporary Cardiology: CT of the Heart: Principles and Applications*
Edited by: U. Joseph Schoepf © Humana Press, Inc., Totowa, NJ

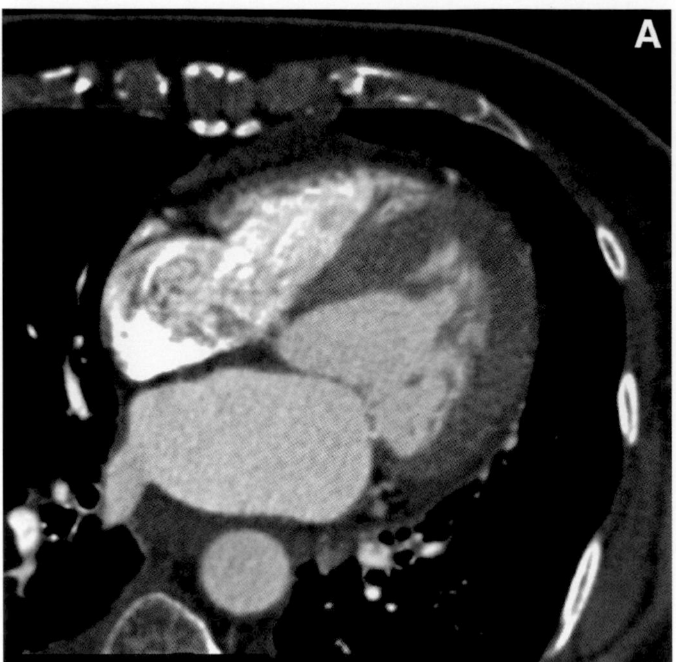

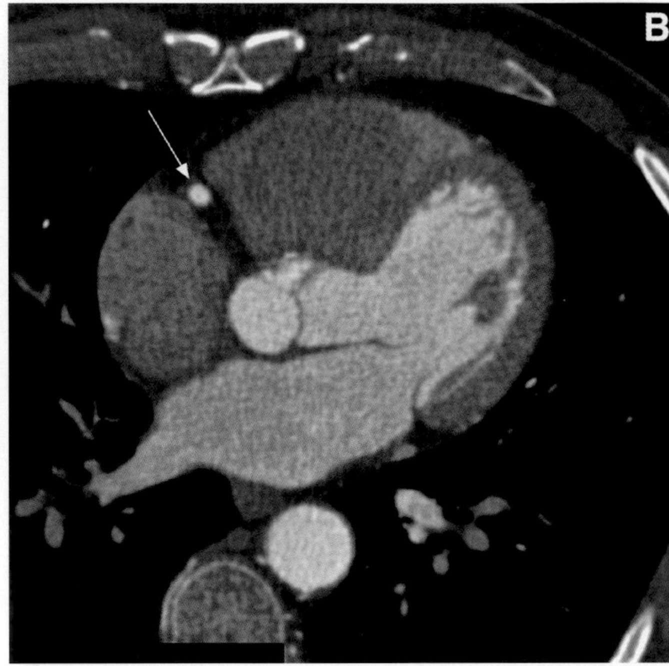

Fig. 1. Axial multidetector-row CT (MDCT) image of a 4-row MDCT scanner system showing artifacts within the right atrium and ventricle due to contrast influx (**A**). By optimization of contrast application using 16-row MDCT these artifacts can be avoided, leading to a better depiction of the right coronary artery (arrow). However, for mass depiction, an enhancement of all cardiac chambers would be necessary.

substantially different. This implies differences in the exact scanning protocol used. However, there are basic demands and requirements for assessment of cardiac masses in CT that determine the details of the imaging protocol.

MDCT allows for very thin collimated slices in the range of 1 mm or even less. This is favorable for the assessment of coronary arteries but is usually unnecessary for the assessment of cardiac masses. This can also satisfactorily be done with a slice thickness in the range of 2–3 mm. This allows for a cutoff in data acquisition time that makes it even possible to be performed easily within a short breath-hold on 4-row MDCT. With overlapping slice reconstruction, multiplanar reformations (MPR) can be used to determine the exact location and extent of tumors.

Although infrequently used at present, dynamic ECG-triggered or -gated scanning can provide dynamic tumor enhancement and may provide further information concerning tumor type. However, to date there has been no study published focusing on such an imaging strategy in CT.

CONTRAST APPLICATION

Although some features of cardiac tumors (e.g., fatty tissue, calcifications) may even be visible on plain scans without application of contrast agents, allocation of these features and mass diagnosis necessitates the use of iodinated contrast media. There is extensive literature on the optimization of contrast injection regimens, primarily focusing on the assessment of coronary arteries. With the use of 16-row MDCT, contrast agent volume could be reduced, therefore avoiding streak artifacts from high contrast influx within the right atrium and ventricle affecting the assessability of the proximal right coronary artery *(10)* (Fig. 1A,B). However, using these injection protocols, opacfication of the right atrium and ventricle is not guaranteed and mass diagnoses may fail.

Therefore, modification of injection protocols is necessary in order to ensure opacification of all cardiac chambers. Especially where right atrial tumors are suspected, additional delayed scanning during the second or third pass of contrast media will improve the homogeneity of atrial opacification and help to avoid misinterpretation of influx of nonopacified blood from the inferior vena cava.

EPIDEMIOLOGY OF CARDIAC MASSES

Basically, when talking about cardiac masses, primary and secondary tumors have to be differentiated. Primary tumors typically originate within the heart, whereas secondary tumors most commonly result from metastasis of malignancies primarily located outside the heart or from direct tumor spread and invasion of masses located adjacent to the heart (e.g., bronchgenic carcinoma). Primary tumors of the heart are by far less common that secondary tumors. Autopsy studies report a prevalence of primary masses in the range of 0.0017%–0.33% *(13)*. However, although there is a wide range of variation between different studies mainly based on the year of publication and inclusion criteria, primary cardiac masses can definitely be considered as rare tumors when compared to other types. Secondary cardiac tumors on the other hand are about 20–40 times more frequent than primary ones *(13)*. Modern noninvasive imaging modalities such as echocardiography in particular, but also CT and magnetic resonance imaging (MRI), now allow mass diagnosis prior to death and allow for therapy planning. In addition to real neoplasms, no matter whether benign or malignant, primary, or secondary, CT imaging is also increasingly performed when cardiac thrombi are suspected. In

Table 1
Frequency of Benign Cardiac Tumors (adapted from ref. *13*)

Benign tumors	*Approximate frequency (%)*
Myxoma	29
Papillary fibroelastoma	8
Rhabdomyoma	5
Fibroma	5
Hemangioma	4
Lipoma	4
Others	8
Total	63

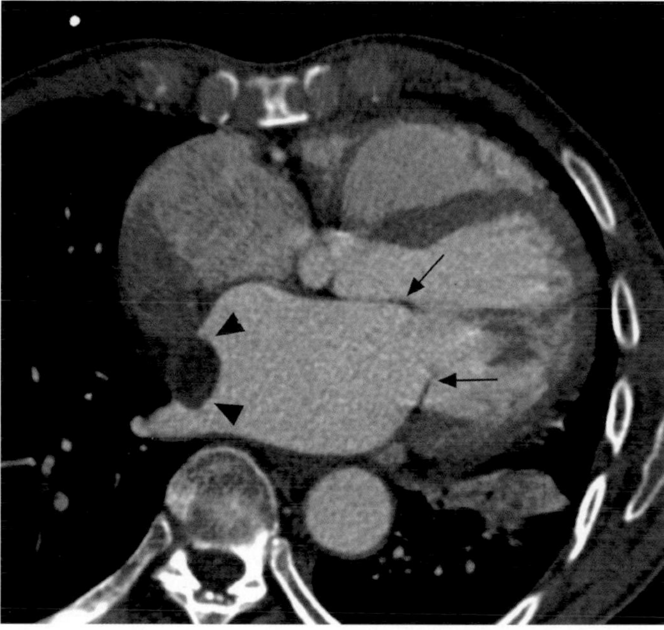

Fig. 2. Patient with a hypodense round mass within the left atrium attached to the interatrial septum (arrow heads). Mass was proven as a myxoma at surgery. Reconstruction was performed during mid-diastole with open mitral valve leaflets (arrows).

addition to imaging features and appearance, cardiac masses can often be differentiated based on location and morphology.

BENIGN CARDIAC TUMORS

Approximately 60–70% of primary cardiac tumors are benign *(13)*. Cardiac myxoma accounts for about half of all benign tumors, followed by papillary fibroelastoma, fibroma, and lipoma (Table 1) *(13)*. However, there is also a difference in frequency of benign tumors based on a patient's age. Whereas myxoma represents the most common tumor type in adults, in childhood, rhabodomyoma accounts for the majority of cases.

Myxomas can be found in all cardiac chambers; however, in approx 75% of the cases, the mass is located within the left atrium (Fig. 2). Another 20% of myxomas are located within the right atrium, whereas only 5% arise within either the left or the right ventricle. In rare instances, myxomas can be found at multiple locations within the heart. Although most cases of cardiac myxoma are sporadic, possibly part of the Carney complex, an autosomal dominant syndrome of cardiac myxomas has been associated with a variety of hyperpigmented skin lesions *(14)*. Also, the development of other, extracardiac tumors and endocrine abnormalities may occur *(15)*.

Although the diagnosis can be easily made using different imaging modalities, patients with cardiac myxoma can be symptomatic for a long time before myxomas are considered as a potential differential diagnosis *(16)*. Patients may present with a triad of symptoms including constitutional symptoms, signs of valvular obstruction (based on myxoma prolapse), and embolic events. The target vasculature of embolic events is strongly dependent on the location of the tumor. Embolic phenomena of left-sided myxomas, considered the most severe complication, may lead to ischemia of either the extremities or the viscera. In case of supra-aortic emboli, symptoms of acute stroke, transient ischemic attacks, or seizures may occur. In right atrial myxomas, symptoms are less frequent.

Atrial myxoma often shows a pedunculated appearance, with its origin in the area of the oval fossa, although the stalk may not be identified with CT (Fig. 3A,B). With increasing size, those mobile masses can even prolapse into the mitral annulus, leading to changes in cardiac hemodynamics. Right-sided myxomas are less frequently attached to the oval fossa. Myomas can even present as a mass within the area of the oval fossa extending to both atria.

Intracavitary tumor masses usually appear as filling defects within the opacified blood pool (Figs. 2 and 3). This necessitates homogeneous contrast distribution and cavitary opacification. However, especially within the right atrium, inflow artifacts need to be differentiated. Mass appearance in CT is strongly dependent on gross pathologic features. Based on their gelatinous nature, myxomas usually have heterogeneous low attenuation at CT (Figs. 2 and 3). Regressive changes may lead to recurrent hemorrhage and calcification, which is frequently seen in CT *(17)* (Fig. 3A). In addition, adherent thrombi can occur. The mobility of myxomas can be demonstrated by either the cine mode in EBCT or multiple data reconstructions at different time points of the cardiac cycle in MDCT with retrospective ECG gating.

Although papillary fibroelastomas represent the second most common benign primary cardiac neoplasm, they are rarely demonstrated with CT modalities. They usually appear at endocardial surfaces and are most commonly located (90%) on valve surfaces. The vast majority of these tumors are less than 1 cm in diameter *(18)*. Their appearance on the rapidly moving valves and their small size makes it rather difficult to identify those lesions using CT, although they are easily detected at echocardiogaphy. Whereas MDCT techniques currently cannot easily follow valve movement because of the rather bad temporal resolution (approx 100–250 ms), EBCT may allow the depiction of those tumors *(11)* (Fig. 4). Recently published MDCT data report the depiction of even small valvular pathology *(19,20)*. However, at present, especially in diagnosis of fibroelastomas, echocardiography is usually far superior to CT. Although symptoms are less frequent than in cases of myxoma, papillary fibroelastomas may also lead to embolic events. This is mostly based on adherent thrombo-embolic material. Although the suspicion of a fibroelastoma cannot be consid-

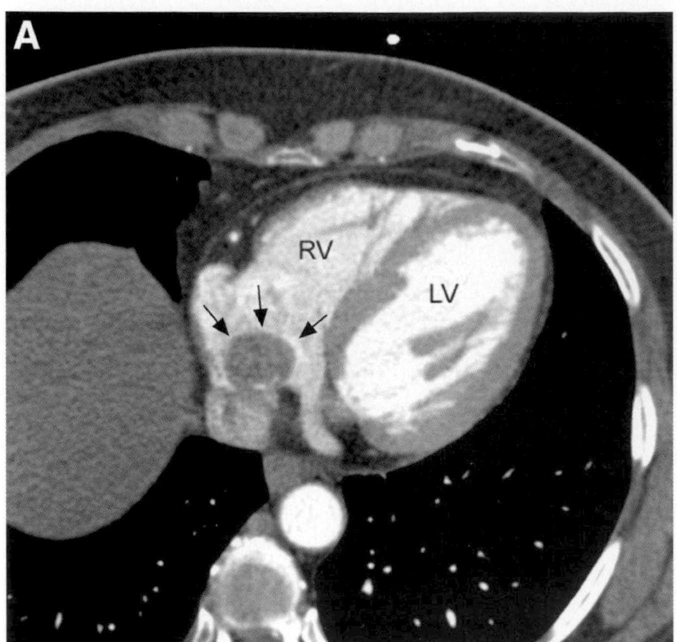

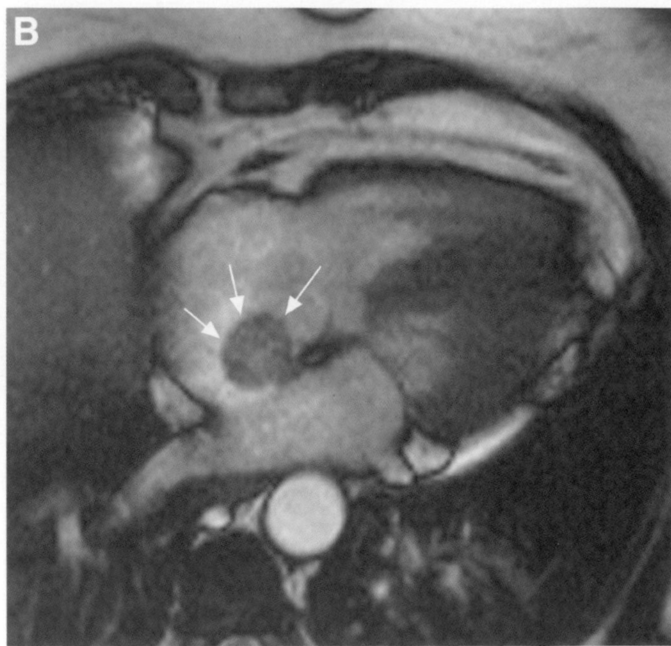

Fig. 3. (A) Round-shaped myxoma of the right atrium with small calcifications (arrows). RV, right ventricle; LV, left ventricle. **(B)** Corresponding magnetic resonance imaging in long-axis orientation show the stalk of the myxoma (arrows) attached to the oval fossa.

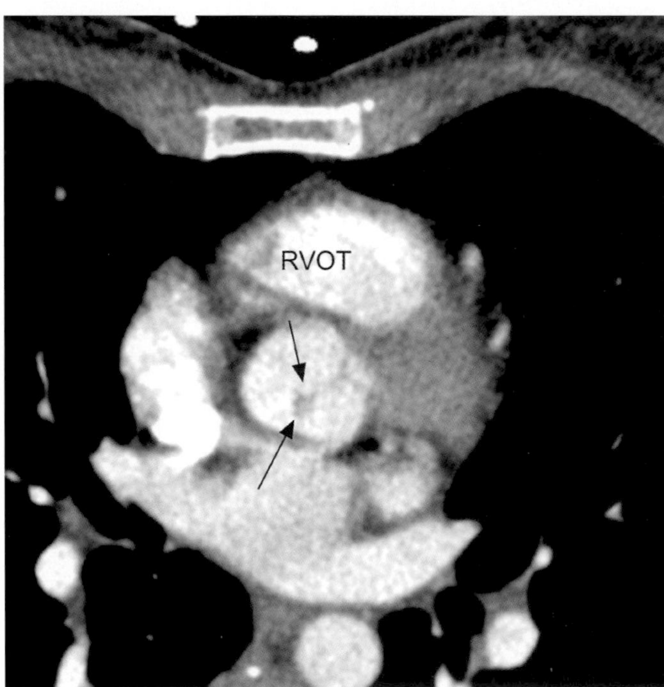

Fig. 4. Axial image of an electron beam CT data set at the level of the aortic valve. A small papillary fibroelastoma can be depicted at the tip of the aortic valve cusps (arrows). RVOT, right-ventricular outflow tract.

ered as a reason for cardiac CT scanning, CT may be helpful to exclude thrombi within the cardiac cavities.

Based on the typical appearance of fatty tissue, lipomatous tumors are usually easily diagnosed using CT. Based on pathology findings, two different types have to be differentiated—lipomas and lipomatous hypertrophy of the interatrial septum.

Contrary to other tumors, lipomas are usually found on the epicardial surface, and may present at any site of the atria or ventricles. However, lipomas may also extent intracavitary. In combination with other tissues, e.g., in angiolipoma, typical image features of fatty tissue may disappear and therefore hamper diagnosis (Figs. 5A–C and 6A,B).

Lipomatous hypertrophy of the interatrial septum consists of an accumulation of mature fat as well as of adipose cells resembling brown fat cells. Deposits at the level of the oval fossa with a diameter larger than 2 cm are considered lipomatous hypertrophy (Fig. 7). These changes may be accompanied by arrhythmias. Similar to lipomas, lipomatous hypertrophy usually shows typical homogeneous low attenuation at CT, which can be found even in nonenhanced scans *(21,22)*.

Other benign tumors such as rhabdomyoma and fibroma usually appear within the ventricular wall or the interventricular septum. They usually show a density comparable to normal myocardium, which precludes easy diagnosis and delineation. Rhabdomyoma is the most frequent tumor in infancy and childhood, and is often associated with tuberous sclerosis *(23)*. Up to 50% of patients with rhabdomyoma suffer from tuberous sclerosis syndrome, and 60% of children with tuberous sclero-

Fig. 5. (A) *(right and page 176)* Axial slices of an extensive mass arising from the right atrial roof, narrowing the right pulmonary artery and the superior vena cava. The mass shows heterogeneous enhancement with central necrosis and calcifications. The mass was proven to be a benign angiomyolipoma based on several tissue probes using CT-guided needle biopsy and open thoracotomy. **(B)** The sagittal reconstruction also shows central necrosis and calcification (arrow). VC, vena cava. Fatty tissue is found only at the very bottom of the mass (arrow heads).

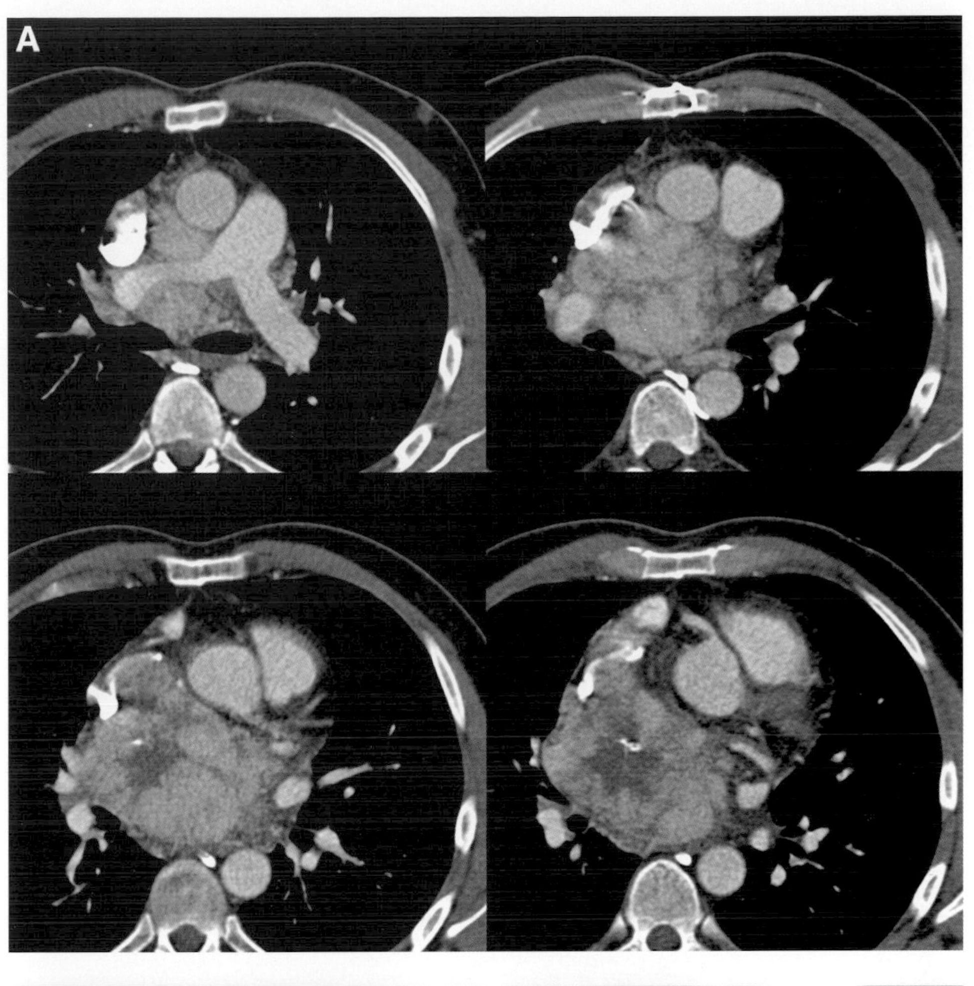
A

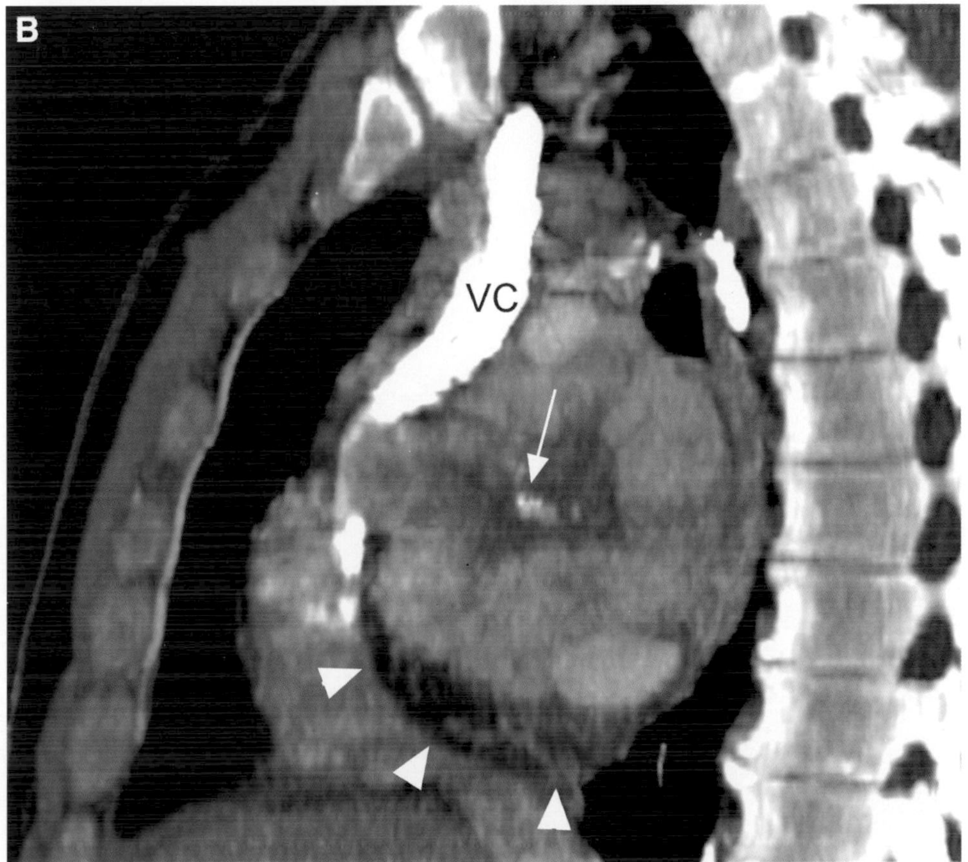
B
VC

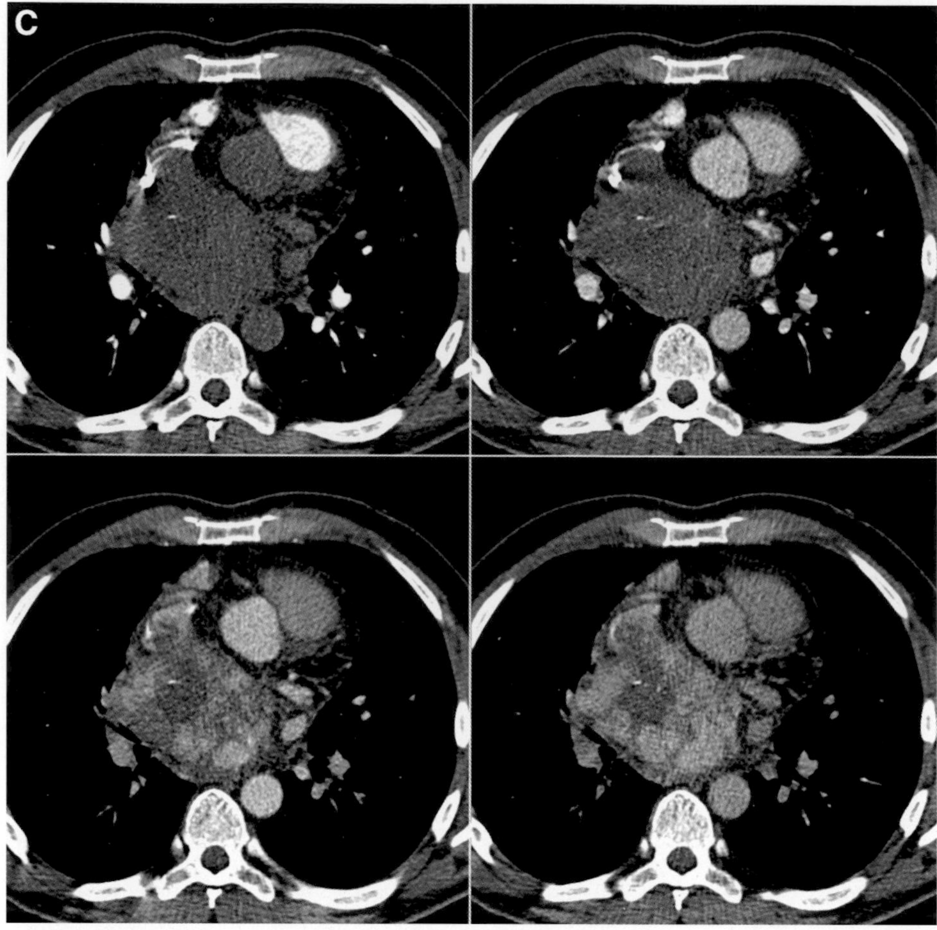

Fig. 5. *(Continued from page 174)* **(C)** Sequential electrocardiogram-triggered axial multidetector-row CT images at a constant level of the tumor shows a marked enhancement of most parts of the mass. This is based on the high degree of vascularization in this angiomyolipoma.

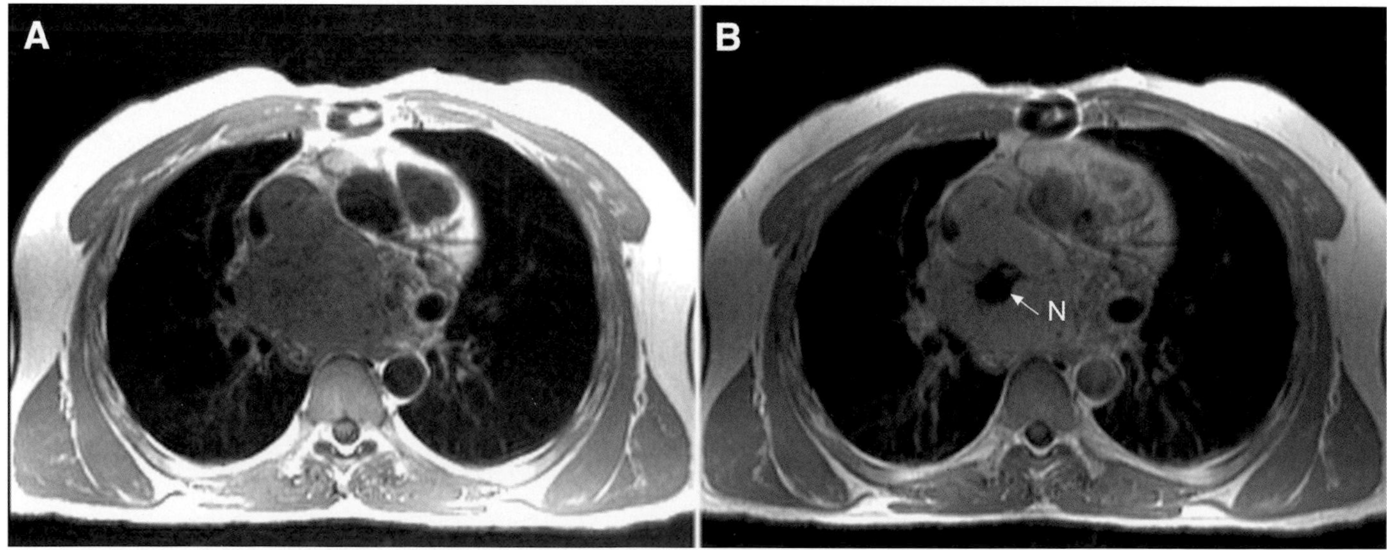

Fig. 6. Corresponding T1 weighted axial magnetic resonance imaging sections before **(A)** and after **(B)** contrast administration show massive enhancement of most tumor parts except a central necrosis (N).

sis have detectable cardiac masses *(24)*. Fibroma also primarily affects children and is often detected in infants or in utero by ultrasound *(25)*.

Beside these solid tumors, pericardial cysts represent a benign lesion that needs to be differentiated from other tumors.

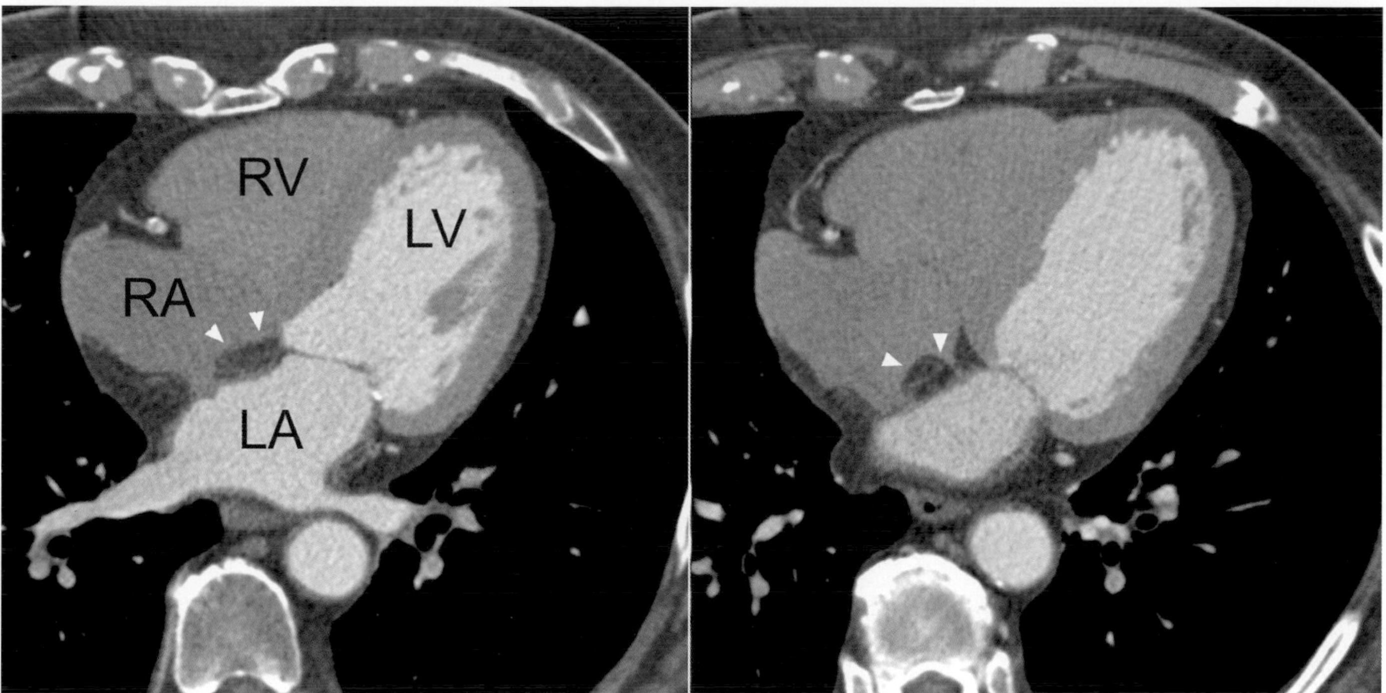

Fig. 7. Axial multidetector-row CT images of a patient with lipomateous hypertrophy of the atrial septum. Note the thickened septum and the low-density mass between both atria, consistent with fatty tissue (arrow heads). RA, right atrium; LA, left atrium; RV, right ventricle; LV, left ventricle.

MALIGNANT CARDIAC TUMORS

PRIMARY CARDIAC TUMORS

Primary cardiac malignancies are rather rare. Only 25% of all primary cardiac tumors are malignant *(13)*. In addition, they are much more uncommon than metastatic lesions to the heart. The distribution and frequency of different types varies within published data *(13)*. Primary cardiac malignancies represent a clinical dilemma. They are often asymptomatic until they become large, and even then they produce nonspecific symptoms *(26)*. Before the advent of cross-sectional imaging, primary cardiac malignancies were rarely diagnosed before death. Nowadays they are being diagnosed within living patients, allowing for conservative or even surgical treatment, including heart transplantation *(27)*. However, based on the usual delayed diagnosis of then extended disease including metastasis, these tumors show a rather bad outcome. CT can be used to accurately image the heart and the surrounding mediastinum, and therefore to evaluate the extent of disease.

Angiosarcoma represents the most common (approx 35–40%) cardiac sarcoma. Patients usually present with right-sided heart failure or tamponade based on its tendency to occur within the right atrium and to invade the pericardium (Fig. 8). Approximately 75% of angiosarcomas are located within the right atrium *(28)*. Based on their composition, they usually show a major contrast uptake, which may be combined with areas of necrosis. In contrast to angiosarcoma, rhabdomyosarcomas do not show a predominant location within the heart. On nonenhanced scans, they may show a density identical to normal myocardium, whereas they can usually be well differentiated from myocardium in enhanced scans. They may even invade cardiac valves, and tend to recur after resection (Fig. 9A,B). There are numerous other types of malignant primary cardiac tumors, including malignant fibrous histiocytomas, osteosarcomas, hemangiopericytomas, and lymphomas (Fig. 10). The approximate frequency of different types of malignant tumors is shown in Table 2.

Both CT and MRI are used in follow-up of malignant tumors after chemotherapy, resection, or even cardiac transplantation. When focusing on the primary lesion itself, cardiac gating is recommended, whereas in examinations for assessment of metastatic lesions from primary cardiac tumors, nongated techniques are adequate. Compared to MRI, CT allows for a comprehensive appreciation of the primary lesion and possible tumor spread with a single injection of contrast agent. Beside time-saving considerations, work-flow and patient management have to be taken into account

SECONDARY CARDIAC TUMORS

Secondary malignancies are 20–40 times more frequent than primary ones. As already mentioned, not only metastatic disease but also direct tumor involvement and invasion of the heart from primary lesions adjacent to the heart account for these cases. In addition to direct invasion, tumor spread to the heart can also arise via predefined venous structures, from hepatocellular carcinomas or renal cell carcinomas, for example. Based on their proximity to the heart, the most common tumors affecting the heart by direct invasion are bronchogenic carcinomas and breast tumors. An overview of the frequency of cardiac or pericardial involvement of different tumor types is given in Table 3. Imaging features of secondary cardiac malignancies are often but not mandatory, similar to those of the primary lesion.

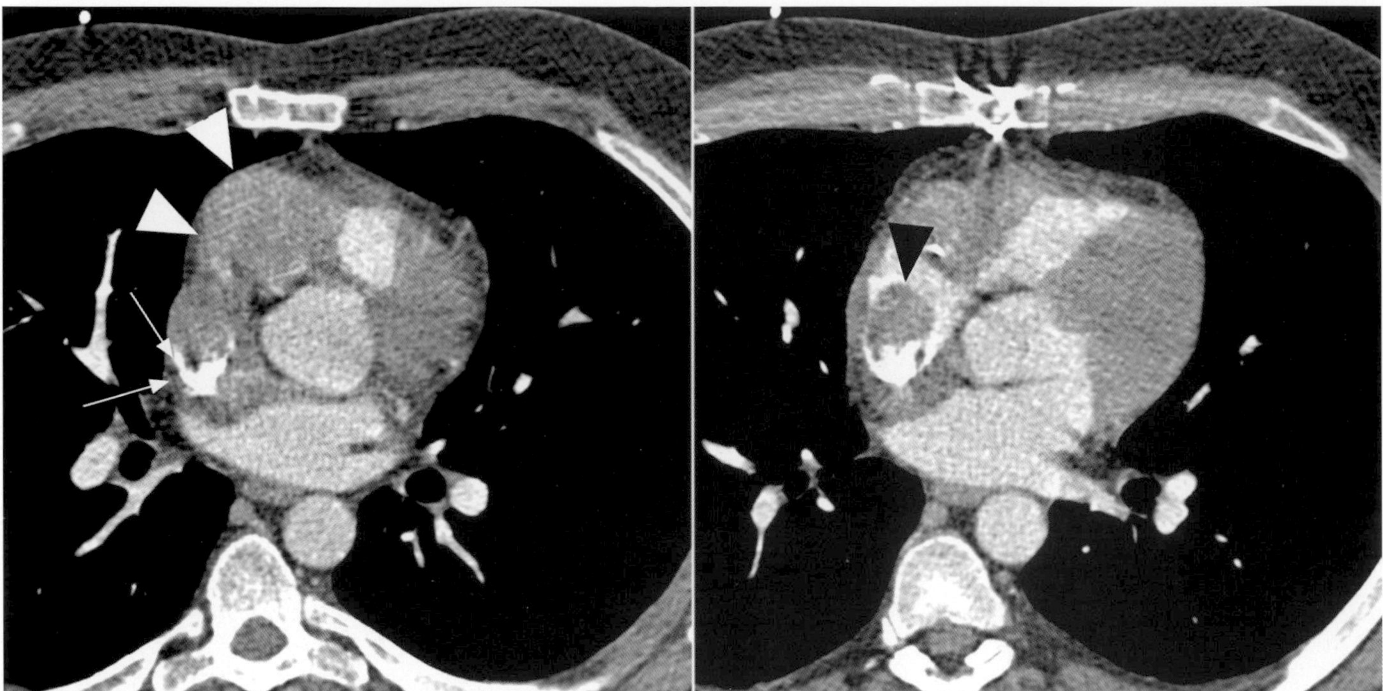

Fig. 8. Multidetector-row CT images of a patient with recurrent angiosarcoma involving the right atrium and parts of the right ventricle (arrow heads). The mass almost occludes the superior vena cava (arrows).

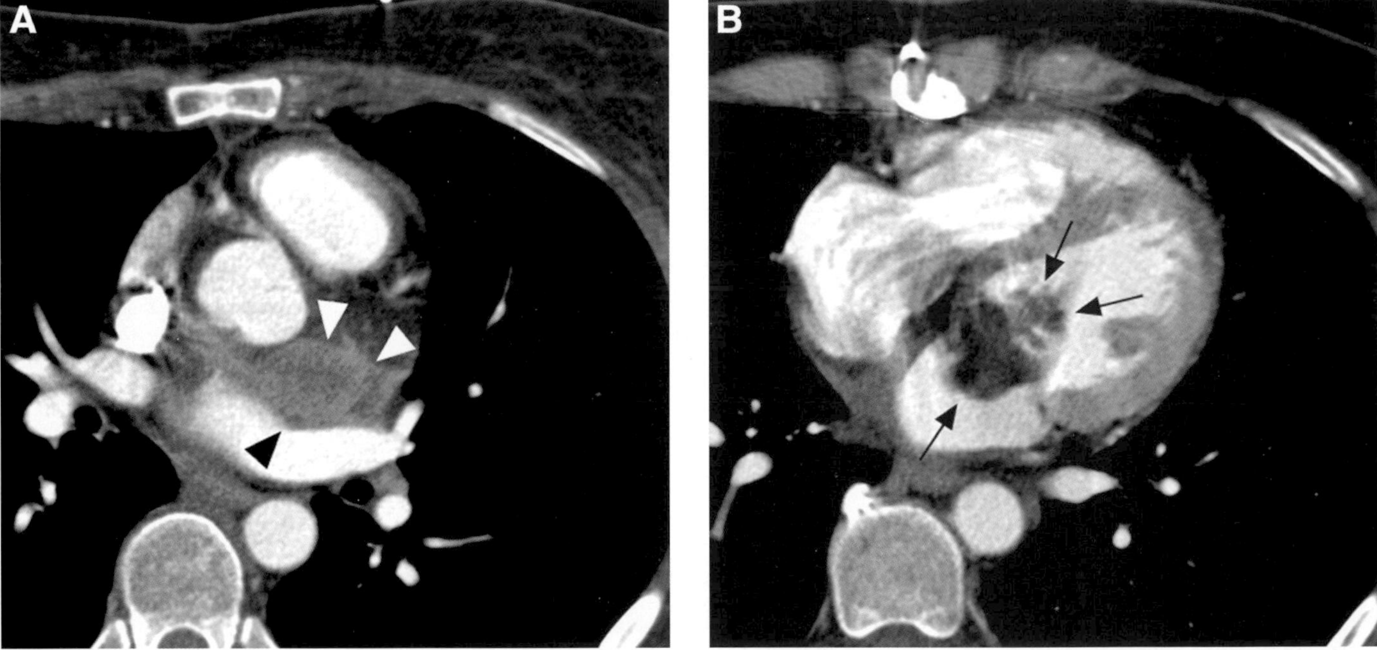

Fig. 9. (**A**) Recurrence of a rhabdomyosarcoma within the left atrium (arrow heads). (**B**) In addition to the tumor within the left atrium, the mass infiltrates the mitral valve and extends to the left ventricle (arrows).

IMAGING OF CARDIAC THROMBI

Thrombotic deposits within the heart are often referred to as pseudotumors or pseudomasses. Intracardiac thrombi may be caused by a variety of different pathologies and may occur in any cardiac chamber. They are responsible for approx 15% of all ischemic strokes and put patients at a major risk of stroke. Therefore, early identification with subsequent therapy is of paramount importance.

Occurring in virtually any part of the vascular system, the development of thrombotic clots may be based either on changes of surface properties, flow dynamics, or changes in blood coagulation. Patients with artificial devices (e.g., pros-

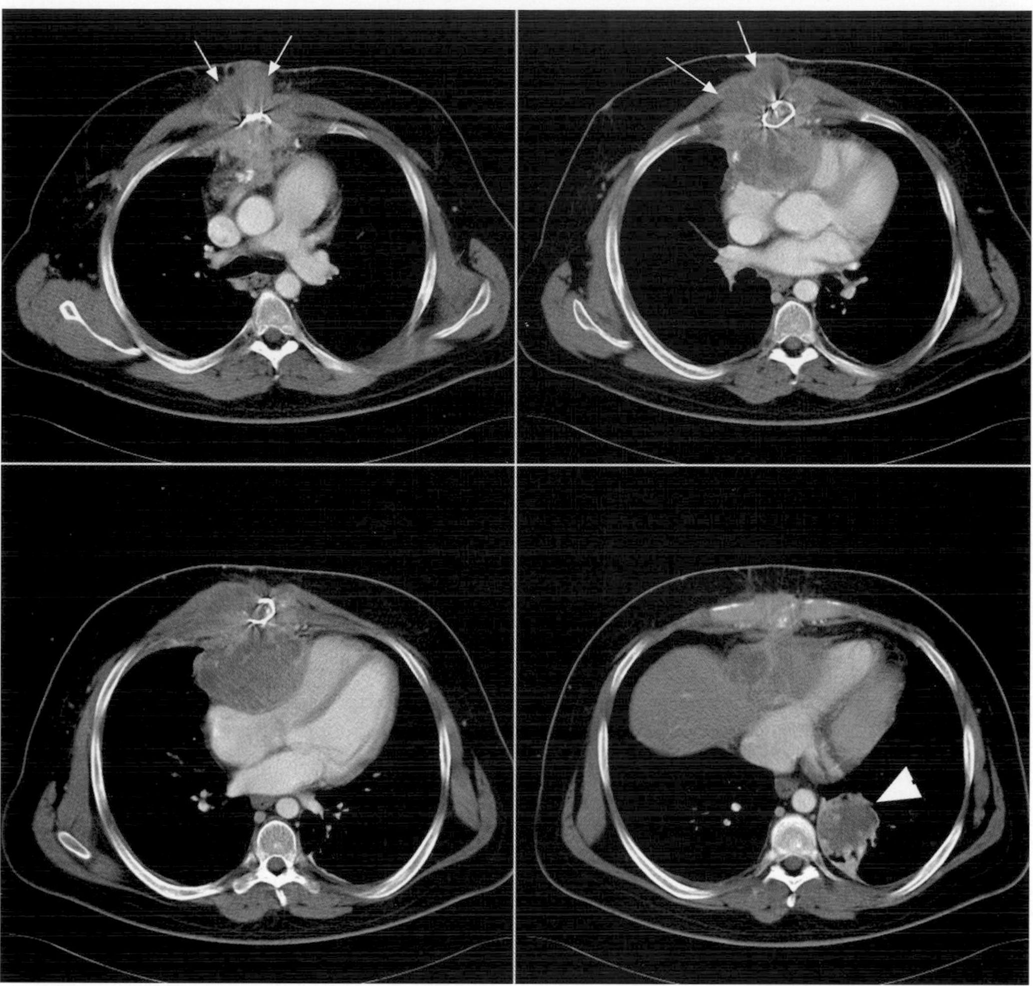

Fig. 10. A set of axial multidetector-row CT images of a malignant hemangiopericytoma involving the right coronary artery and the chest wall (arrows). The tumor encases the right atrium and ventricle. Within the left lower lobe of the lungs, metastatic disease in shown.

Table 2
Distribution and Frequency of Primary Cardiac Malignancies (adapted from ref. *13*)

Malignant tumors	*Approximate frequency (%)*
Angiosarcoma	9
Malignant fibrous histiocytoma	4
Osteosarcoma	3
Leimyosarcoma	3
Rhabdomyosarcoma	2
Lymphoma	2
Others	14
Total	37

Table 3
Frequency of Cardiac/Pericardial Involvement in Cases of Extracardiac Malignancies (adapted from ref. *13*)

Malignant tumors	*Frequency (%)*
Melanoma	49
Germinoma	42
Leukemia	34
Bronchogenic carcinoma	28
Sarcomas	22
Lymphomas	21
Breast Cancer	20
Esophageal carcinoma	17
Renal cell carcinoma	15
Thyroid carcinoma	12

thetic valves, pacemakers), atrial fibrillation, or wall motion abnormalities (including ventricular aneurysms) are at special risk. As already stated, thrombotic layers may also occur at the surface of myxomas or papillary fibroelastomas.

Thrombi may be solitary or multiple, and present as filling defects within opacified cardiac chambers. Their appearance depends on location. In regions of wall motion, abnormalities, or ventricular aneurysms after myocardial infarction, they usually lie adjacent to the areas of infracted myocardium. They can usually be differentiated from normal myocardium based on their rather low attenuation. However, in close contact to scar tissue in chronic infarction, the exact extent may be overesti-

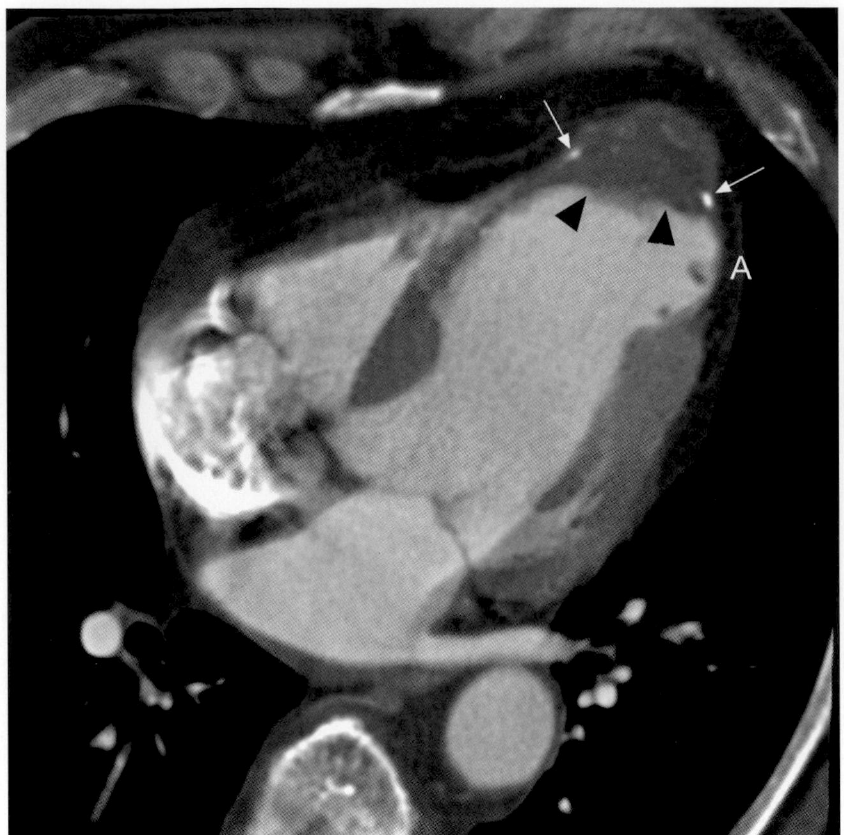

Fig. 11. Four-chamber view of a multidetector-row CT data set. Ventricular aneurysm (A) within the apex after myocardial infarction and a thrombus can be delineated (arrow heads). The thrombus show tiny calcifications (arrows).

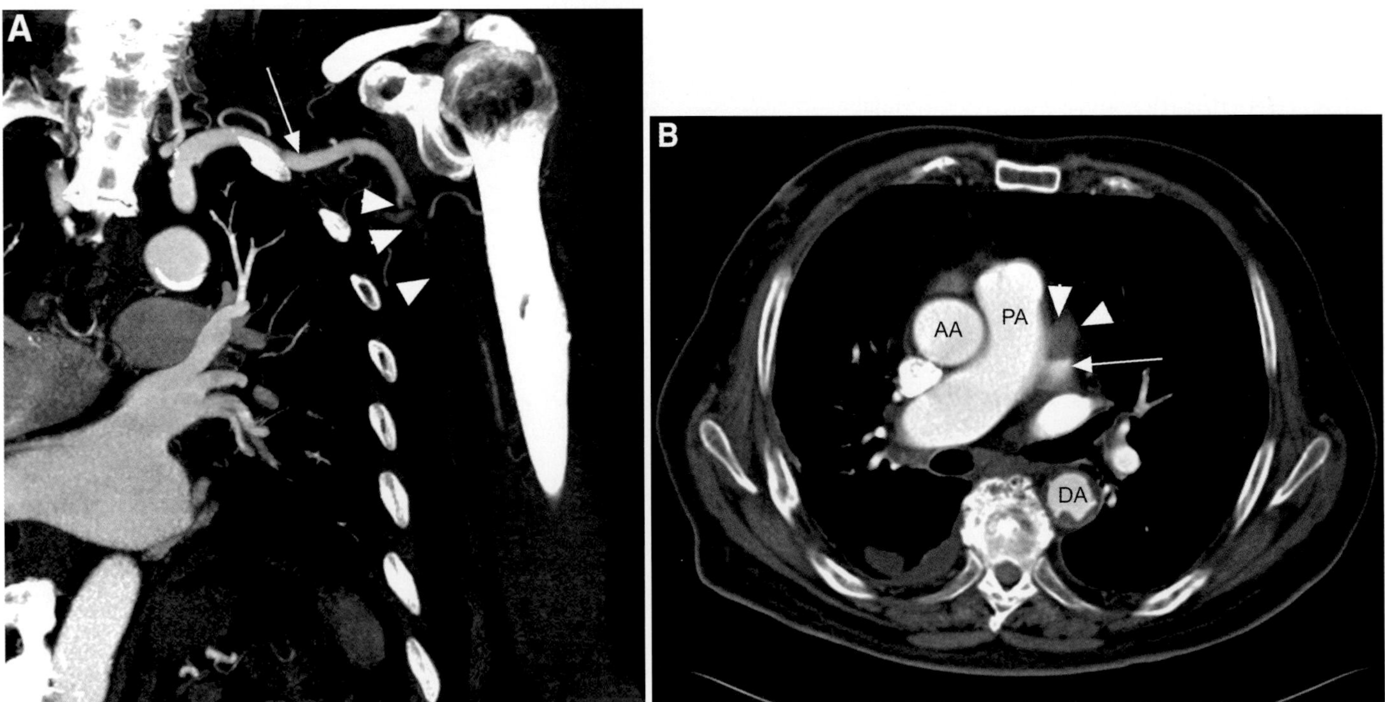

Fig. 12. (**A**) Multiplanar reformation (MPR) of the left upper extremity with an acute embolic occlusion of the axillary artery (arrow heads). The subclavian artery shows normal diameter and patency (arrow). (**B**) Reconstruction of the same data set focused in the chest shows residual thrombus (arrow heads) within the left atrial appendage (arrow). AA, ascending aorta; DA, descending aorta; PA, pulmonary artery.

mated. Long-standing thrombi tend to get organized and may calcify (Fig. 11). Clots within the atria are commonly related to contraction abnormalities (e.g., atrial fibrillation). They may often be found within the atrial appendages (Fig. 12A,B).

Echocardiography represents the basic modality for thrombus screening. However, based on the large field of view, cardiac CT allows for reliable depiction or occlusion of thrombi. Although not primarily used for cardiac imaging, routine CT of the chest may reveal unknown cardiac thrombi.

CONCLUSION

Cardiac CT shows promise in the assessment of cardiac masses. Especially with the widespread use of MDCT, this modality is rapidly growing in cardiac imaging. Its use in imaging of cardiac masses and thrombi represents only a niche indication. However, the requirements are less demanding than those of coronary CT angiography and can also be performed with less sophisticated MDCT scanner generations. However, as a prerequisite for cardiac CT imaging, ECG-based data acquisition strategies and algorithms are necessary. With the use of MDCT, a new modality of cardiac imaging competes with MRI. The acquisition of 3D data sets even allows for multiplanar imaging of cardiac tumors. There are specific features of tumors (e.g., calcifications) that may be visualized and depicted only in CT. On the other hand, CT may be inferior to MRI in exact evaluation of the tumor type in most cases, based on its lower soft-tissue contrast properties.

REFERENCES

1. Knez A, Becker CR, Leber A, et al. Usefulness of multislice spiral computed tomography angiography for determination of coronary artery stenoses. Am J Cardiol 2001;88:1191–1194.
2. Nieman K, Oudkerk M, Rensing BJ, et al. Coronary angiography with multi-slice computed tomography. Lancet 2001;357:599–603.
3. Nieman K, Cademartiri F, Lemos PA, Raaijmakers R, Pattynama PM, de Feyter PJ. Reliable noninvasive coronary angiography with fast submillimeter multislice spiral computed tomography. Circulation 2002;106:2051–2054.
4. Ropers D, Baum U, Pohle K, et al. Detection of coronary artery stenoses with thin-slice multi-detector row spiral computed tomography and multiplanar reconstruction. Circulation 2003;107: 664–666.
5. Felner JM, Knopf WD. Echocardiographic recognition of intracardiac and extracardiac masses. Echocardiography 1985;2:3.
6. Salcedo EE, Cohen GI, White RD, Davison MB. Cardiac tumors: diagnosis and management. Curr Probl Cardiol 1992;17:73–137.
7. Link KM, Lesko NM. MR evaluation of cardiac/juxtacardiac masses. Top Magn Reson Imaging 1995;7:232–245.
8. Olson LJ, Tajik AJ. Valvular heart disease. In: Skorton DJ, Schelbert HR, Wolf GL, Brundage BH. (eds.) Cardiac Imaging. 2nd ed. Saunders Company, Philadelphia: 1996;365–394.
9. MacMillan RM. Magnetic resonance imaging vs. ultrafast computed tomography for cardiac diagnosis. Int J Card Imaging 1992;8: 217–227.
10. Wintersperger BJ, Nikolaou K, Jakobs TF, Reiser MF, Becker CR. Cardiac multidetector-row computed tomography: initial experience using 16 detector-row systems. Crit Rev Comput Tomogr 2003;44: 27–45.
11. Wintersperger BJ, Becker CR, Gulbins H, et al. Tumors of the cardiac valves: imaging findings in magnetic resonance imaging, electron beam computed tomography, and echocardiography. Eur Radiol 2000;10:443–449.
12. Jakobs TF, Becker CR, Ohnesorge B, et al. Multislice helical CT of the heart with retrospective ECG gating: reduction of radiation exposure by ECG-controlled tube current modulation. Eur Radiol 2002;12:1081–1086.
13. Burke A, Virmani R. Tumors of the heart and great vessels. Armed Forces Institute of Pathology; Washington D.C.: 1995.
14. Carney JA, Gordon H, Carpenter PC, Shenoy PV, Go VL. The complex of myxomas, spotty pigmentation and endocrine overactivity. Medicine 1985;64:270–283.
15. Casey M, Mah C, Merliss AD, et al. Identification of a novel genetic locus for familial cardiac myxomas and Carney complex. Circulation 1998;98:2560–2566.
16. Burke AP, Virmani R. Cardiac myxomas: a clinicopathologic study. Am J Clin Pathol 1993;100:671–680.
17. Tsuchiya F, Kohno A, Saitoh R, Shigeta A. CT findings of atrial myxoma. Radiology 1984;151:139–143.
18. Abu Nassar SG, Parker JC, Jr. Incidental papillary endocardial tumor. Its potential significance. Arch Pathol 1971;92:370–376.
19. Willmann JK, Kobza R, Roos JE, et al. ECG-gated multi-detector row CT for assessment of mitral valve disease: initial experience. Eur Radiol 2002;12:2662–2669.
20. Willmann JK, Weishaupt D, Lachat M, et al. Electrocardiographically gated multi-detector row CT for assessment of valvular morphology and calcification in aortic stenosis. Radiology 2002;225:120–128.
21. Kamiya H, Ohno M, Iwata H, et al. Cardiac lipoma in the interventricular septum: evaluation by computed tomography and magnetic resonance imaging. Am Heart J 1990;119:1215–1217.
22. Hayashi H, Wakabayashi H, Kumazaki T. Ultrafast computed tomography diagnosis of an epicardial lipoma in the pericardial sac: the split pericardium appearance. J Thorac Imaging 1996;11: 161–162.
23. Smythe JF, Dyck JD, Smallhorn JF, Freedom RM. Natural history of cardiac rhabdomyoma in infancy and childhood. Am J Cardiol 1990;66:1247–1249.
24. Smith HC, Watson GH, Patel RG, Super M. Cardiac rhabdomyomata in tuberous sclerosis: their course and diagnostic value. Arch Dis Child 1989;64:196–200.
25. Beghetti M, Gow RM, Haney I, Mawson J, Williams WG, Freedom RM. Pediatric primary benign cardiac tumors: a 15-year review. Am Heart J 1997;134:1107–1114.
26. Araoz PA, Eklund HE, Welch TJ, Breen JF. CT and MR imaging of primary cardiac malignancies. Radiographics 1999;19:1421–1434.
27. Uberfuhr P, Meiser B, Fuchs A, et al. Heart transplantation: an approach to treating primary cardiac sarcoma? J Heart Lung Transplant 2002;21:1135–1139.
28. Janigan DT, Husain A, Robinson NA. Cardiac angiosarcomas: a review and a case report. Cancer 1986;57:852–859.

18 Multidetector-Row CT Assessment of Left-Ventricular Function

Kai Uwe Juergens, MD and Roman Fischbach, MD

INTRODUCTION

For the diagnosis, disease stratification, treatment planning, and prognosis of different cardiac diseases clinically presenting with myocardial dysfunction and regional or global ischemia, respectively, the accurate and reproducible determination of left-ventricular myocardial function is fundamental. Heart failure afflicts about 4.5 to 5 million people in the United States, with more than 500,000 new cases developing each year. Clinical assessment with regard to left-ventricular function is generally difficult; although an entirely normal electrocardiogram (ECG) provides a close correlation to normal systolic function, electrographical findings are nonspecific. The ideal imaging modality to determine left-ventricular function in a clinical setting would be noninvasive, accurate, reproducible, easily available, as well as cost and time effective *(1–3)*.

The analysis of left-ventricular myocardial function includes the determination of *regional* and *global* function characteristics. Regional function parameters are *myocardial wall thickness* and *wall thickening*, calculated as end-diastolic and end-systolic wall thickness, systolic wall thickening, and percent systolic wall thickening. Clinical information on global left-ventricular function are determined from measurements of diastolic and systolic left-ventricular volumes and consecutively calculated *ejection fraction*, *stroke volume*, and *cardiac output*. With regard to reproducibility and accuracy of global functional parameters, an imaging modality is only as good as its measurements of left-ventricular volumes.

ESTABLISHED TECHNIQUES FOR ASSESSING LEFT-VENTRICULAR FUNCTION

Various noninvasive imaging modalities (such as echocardiography, radionuclide ventriculography, gated perfusion single photon emission computed tomography [SPECT], electron-beam computed tomography [EBCT], and cardiac magnetic resonance imaging [MRI]) and invasive techniques (such as cine ventriculography [CVG]) are in use for the determination of regional and global left-ventricular function.

From: *Contemporary Cardiology: CT of the Heart: Principles and Applications*
Edited by: U. Joseph Schoepf © Humana Press, Inc., Totowa, NJ

Transthoracic echocardiography is a widely available imaging modality, relatively cheap and mobile; however, image acquisition is acoustic-window and operator dependent. Owing to geometric assumptions of the left-ventricular shape, accuracy in regards to quantitative assessment of left-ventricular function is hampered in remodeled hearts with complex irregular shape changes. Good visualization of the entire endocardial border cannot always be provided using conventional 2D echocardiography, resulting in a high amount of subjectivity and dependency on the operator's clinical experience. Thus, reliable measurement of myocardial thickness and thickening is frequently elusive. Three-dimensional echocardiography has improved its clinical impact; however, dependency of acoustic windows and clinical practicability have to be evaluated in further studies. Analysis of left-ventricular volume-time curves by real-time 3D echocardiography provides quantitative data on global left-ventricular function, such as filling rates *(4)*.

CVG while performing coronary catheter angiography is currently a clinically accepted standard for the assessment of cardiac volumes and function. However, this method is invasive and is limited as a result of geometric assumptions made from projection images.

Radionuclide ventriculography is commonly used to measure cardiac function in terms of left-ventricular ejection fraction; however, it is rarely performed clinically, because it is hampered by limited temporal and spatial resolution, and preparation and scanning times are relatively prolonged *(5)*. Gated perfusion SPECT is not used to measure ventricular function alone, although it enables 3D assessment of cardiac function and is especially useful when perfusion needs to be assessed with a high reproducibility. Its diagnostic accuracy might be limited both in small and large ventricles due to limited spatial resolution. Owing to very low counts, it is difficult to define ventricular borders in left-ventricular areas with circumscript thinning as a result of transmural infarction. In both nuclear techniques, the need for repeated radionuclide doses in sequential studies is problematic due to radiation exposure. Using ^{99m}Tc-tetrofosmin, the dose equivalent for myocardium and a blood pool marker is about 8×10^{-1} mSv per 100 MBq. In a clinical setting, about 750 to 900 MBq ^{99m}Tc-tetrofosmin are commonly used to perform a first-pass radionuclide ventriculography.

Table 1
Left-Ventricular (LV) Parameters (mean ± 1 SD) With 95% Confidence Interval (1.96 SD) in Parentheses[a]

	ALL *(N = 75)*	*Males* *(N = 47)*	*Females* *(N = 28)*
LV end-diastolic volumes [mL]	121 ± 34 (55–187)	136 ± 30 (77–195)	96 ± 23 (52–141)
LV end-diastolic volumes BSA [mL/m^2]	66 ± 12 (44–89)	69 ± 11 (47–92)	61 ± 10 (41–81)
LV end-systolic volumes [mL]	40 ± 14 (13–67)	45 ± 14 (19–72)	32 ± 9 (13–51)
LV ejection fraction [%]	67 ± 5 (57–78)	67 ± 5 (56–78)	67 ± 5 (56–78)
LV stroke volume [mL]	82 ± 23 (36–127)	92 ± 21 (51–83)	65 ± 16 (33–97)

[a] Derived from reference method cardiovascular magnetic resonance imaging. BSA, body surface area; SD, standard deviation. *N* = 75. Modified from ref. *11*.

EBCT scanners providing a temporal resolution down to 50–100 ms have been successfully used for noninvasive coronary calcium measurements, coronary arteriography, and determination of left-ventricular (LV) mass and function data. However, these systems are costly, and the limited number of scanners available restricts access to this modality *(6,7)*. Prospectively ECG-triggered sequential single-slice scanning is performed with a selected delay from the preceding R peak of the ECG. This prospective triggering technique renders the images vulnerable to sudden changes in heart rate or cardiac rhythm. The fixed setup of an EBCT scanner impairs assessing LV functional parameters in the anatomically true short-axis orientation, as it is applied in echocardiography and cardiac MRI.

In comparison to other noninvasive imaging techniques, cardiac MRI is now widely accepted as the reference standard of noninvasive assessment of cardiac function, being accurate and reproducible in normal and also in abnormal ventricles using conventional breath-hold turbo-gradient echo sequences (TGrE) as well as newly developed steady-state free precession (SSFP) cine sequences *(8–10)*. Cardiac MRI provides an excellent temporal and spatial resolution, with image acquisition in any desired plane (e.g., in vertical and horizontal long-axis and short-axis views). Image acquisition can be performed rapidly to allow visual and qualitative assessment of global and regional left-ventricular function. A synopsis of global left-ventricular functional parameters in healthy volunteers *(11)* as determined by cardiac MRI is given in Table 1.

ASSESSMENT OF LEFT-VENTRICULAR FUNCTION USING CT

Application of conventional CT to cardiac imaging has long been limited by insufficient temporal resolution as a result of slow gantry rotation, and long total acquisition time resulting from slow volume coverage with single-slice imaging. Analysis of cardiac function has been possible only in experimental setups and was restricted to a transaxial slice orientation *(12,13)*. Cardiac imaging using conventional single-slice CT scanners had become available with the introduction of subsecond rotation in 1994. Initial promising results were achieved using prospective ECG-triggering technique combined with a possible temporal resolution of 500 ms. As in EBCT, prospective ECG-triggering techniques enable determination of volumetric data of the heart from sequential scans, which are started following a predefined delay to the onset or the R waves of the patient's ECG. A major drawback of prospectively ECG-triggered image acquisition, however, is its vulnerability to cardiac arrhythmia or changes in heart rate.

Continuous imaging of the heart volume with spiral technique and ECG-synchronized image reconstruction was severely hampered because of limited volume coverage in the patient-longitudinal (z) axis when only one detector line was available. In contrast, multidetector spiral CT technique enables scanning of larger anatomical volumes at a given scan time or smaller volumes at a narrower collimation, resulting in a higher axial resolution. Thus, high-quality data sets for 3D postprocessing are provided. The entire volume of the heart can be scanned within a single breath-hold. Motion of the heart can be virtually frozen using retrospective ECG-gating technique, when the ECG signal of the patient is recorded simultaneously during spiral CT data acquisition. The method of retrospective ECG gating enables greater robustness with regard to arrhythmia, because prospective estimation of the heart rate is not needed for the trigger's placement *(14)*. In the clinical setting, left-ventricular function information can be derived from multidetector-row CT (MDCT) coronary angiography data sets. From axial thin-section CT spiral data sets acquired during the entire cardiac cycle, images at diastolic and systolic window can be subsequently reconstructed using retrospective ECG-gating technique (*see* "Data Acquisition and Image Reconstruction" below).

DETERMINATION OF LEFT-VENTRICULAR VOLUMETRIC DATA

For clinical and research purposes, left-ventricular volumetric data are determined using different anatomical and geometric models. The standard approaches for reliable and reproducible volumetrics are the *area-length method* based on the long-axis view as well as the *Simpson's method* applied to contiguous short-axis reformations (Fig. 1). For reproducible assessment of volumetric data, the imaging of the left ventricle along to the *cardiac imaging axes* is advantageous, because the body axes—i.e., transverse, sagittal, and coronal planes (Figs. 2–4)—are not perpendicular to the left-ventricular cavity or the myocardial wall, resulting in an overestimation of true left-ventricular dimensions owing to partial-volume effects and obliqueness of those axes. High z-axis resolution nearly approaching isotropic voxels, provided by MDCT technique, enables multiplanar reformations (MPRs) from primary axial image reconstructions—in particular, the left-ventricular

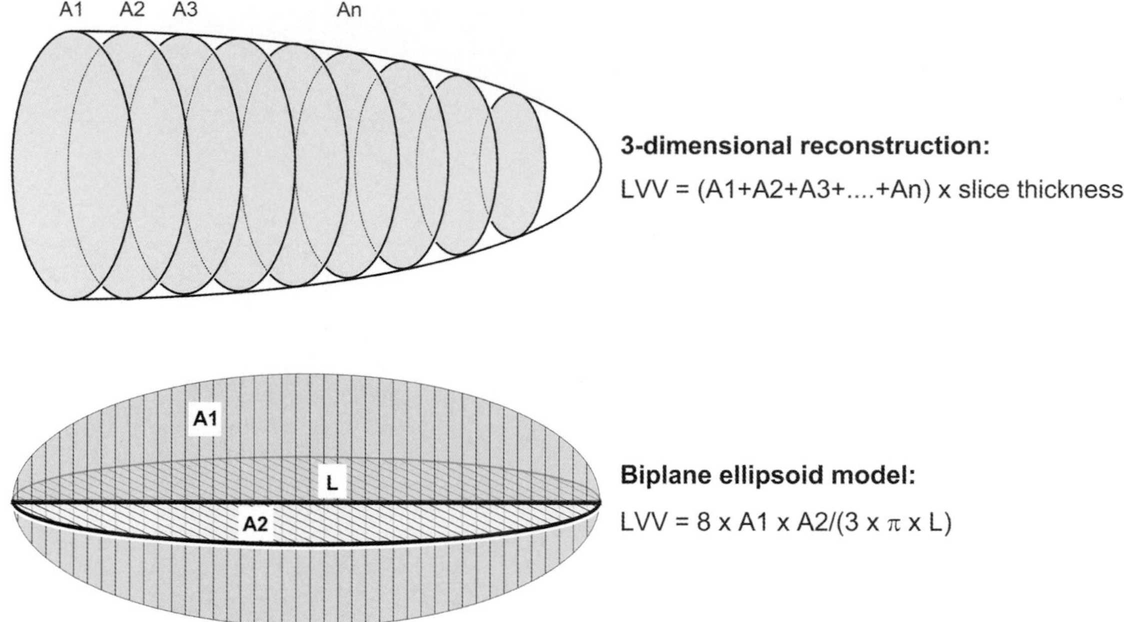

Fig. 1. Diagram showing two different geometric models for determination of left-ventricular volumetric data: the standard approaches for reliable and reproducible volumetric are the Simpson's method applied to contiguous short-axis reformations using 3D reconstruction (**A**) as well as the area-length method based on the long-axis view of the heart using the biplane ellipsoid model (**B**). A = cross-sectional area within endocardial borders determined from one section (modified from *9*).

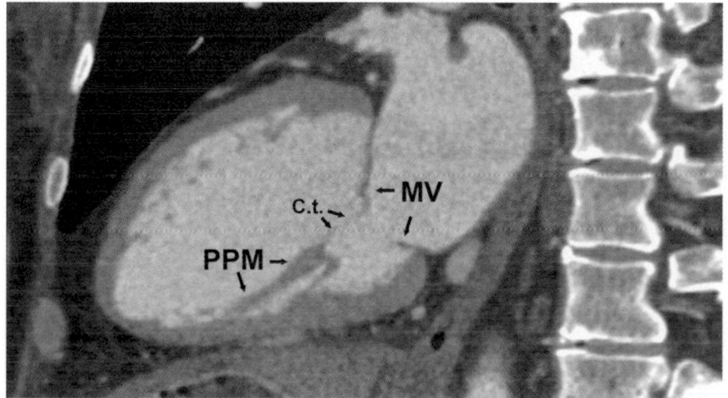

Fig. 2. Multidetector CT postprocessing and generation of multiplanar reformations in an anatomically optimized vertical long-axis view. C.t., chordae terdinae; MV, mitral valve; PPM, posterior papillary muscle.

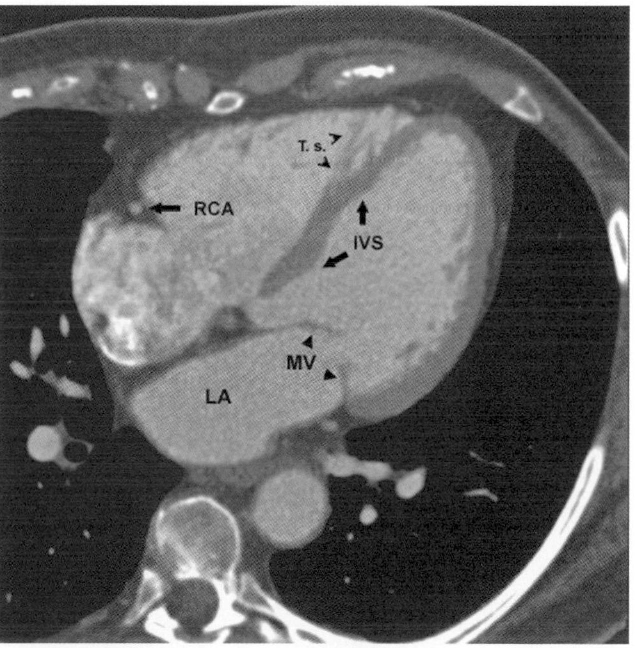

Fig. 3. Multidetector CT postprocessing and generation of multiplanar reformations in an anatomically optimized horizontal long-axis view. IVS, intraventricular septum; LA, left atrium; MV, mitral valve; RCA, right coronary artery; T.s., Trabecular septomarginalia.

long axis and the *short-axis* plane: starting with axial reconstructions, a *vertical long-axis* plane is obtained connecting the left-ventricular apex and the middle of the atrioventricular junction. A further plane connecting the left-ventricular apex and the middle of the mitral valve ring is chosen, resulting in a *horizontal long-axis* plane. Perpendicular to the horizontal long axis, the stack of double-oblique *short-axis* images are orientated by an inclination parallel to the mitral-valve ring. Secondary MPRs in horizontal and vertical long-axis and true short-axis orientation, respectively, can be performed from diastolic and systolic reconstructions, enabling determination of left-ventricular end-diastolic and end-systolic volumes (Figs. 5 and 6). Consecutively, the calculation of left-ventricular ejection fraction and stroke volume is feasible as follows:

Area-length method. From a long-axis view, the area A within traced endocardial contours and the length L from the left-ventricular apex to the level of mitral valve ring are used to calculate the LV volume (V_{LA}) according to equation 1:

$$V_{LA} = (8/3) \times A^2/\pi L \qquad (1)$$

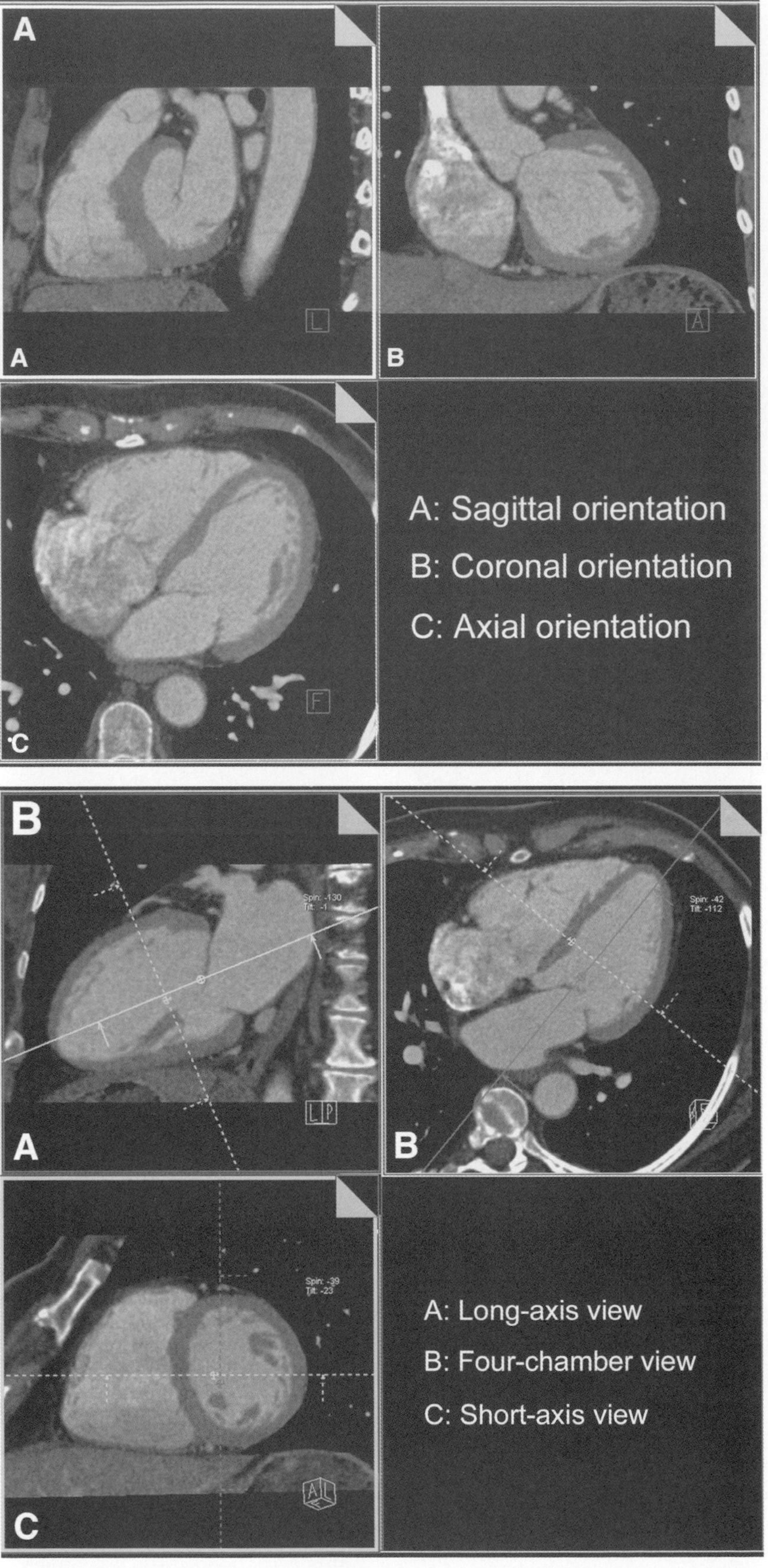

Fig. 4. (**A**) The standard sagittal, coronal, and axial orientation of multiplanar reformations (MPR) as provided by standard postprocessing software. Based on those standard angulations, MPR in the long-axis view and four-chamber view can be generated, resulting in a true short-axis orientation (**B**). With regard to functional analysis, a stack of double contiguous short-axis-orientated sections (thickness 8 mm without any intersection gap) is acquired.

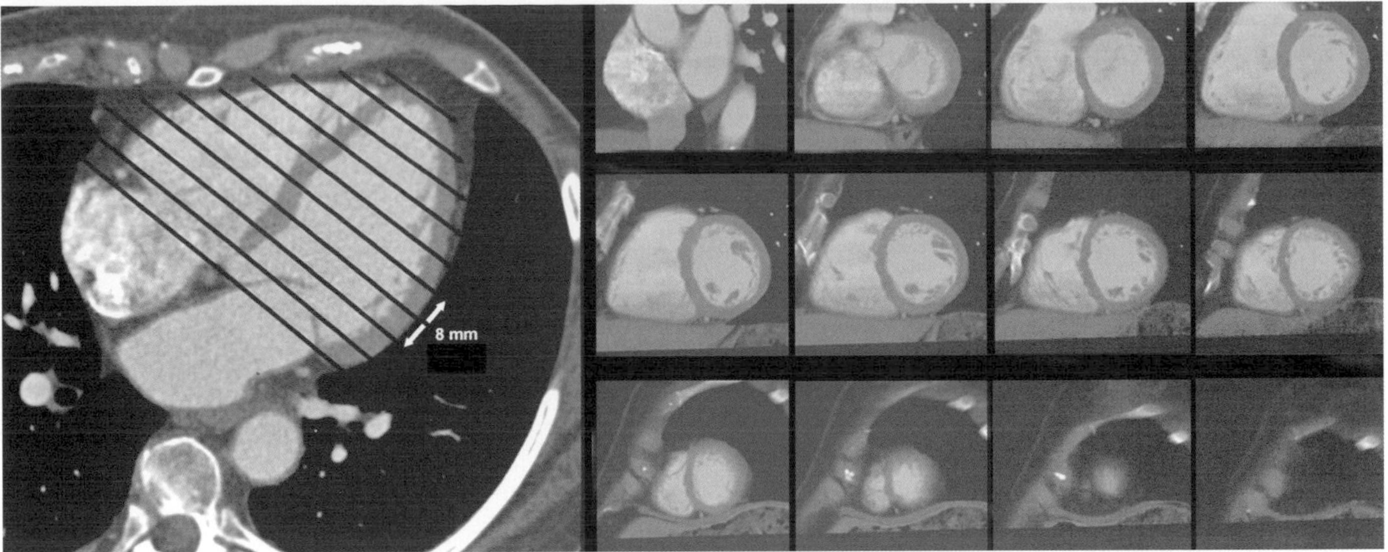

Fig. 5. Ten to eighteen sections are used to encompass the entire left ventricle from base to apex.

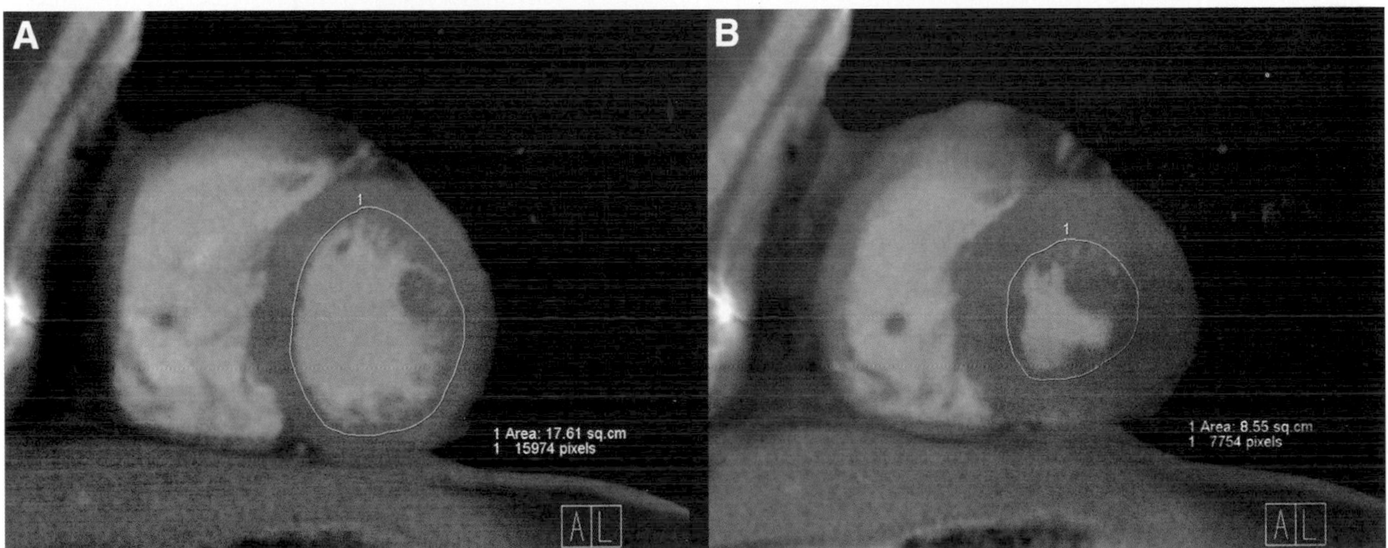

Fig. 6. Endocardial contours were manually traced using standard planimetric software implemented in the workstation. Midventricular short-axis multidetector-row CT (MDCT) images in end diastole (**A**) and end systole (**B**) showing the manually traced endocardial borders and the respective cross-sectional areas (A: 17.61 cm^2, B: 8.55 cm^2) in a patient with arrhythmogenic right-ventricular cardiomyopathy. Coronary artery disease was ruled out using MDCT coronary angiography; global left-ventricular (LV) function was normal (LV-ejection fraction 72.9%). Calculation of diastolic and systolic left-ventricular volumes using Simpson's method based on the short-axis reformations.

Simpson's method. Endocardial contours of all short-axis images showing left-ventricular cavity are traced with papillary muscles being included into the left-ventricular cavity to calculate the cross-sectional area A of each section. Left-ventricular volumes (V_{SA}) are calculated by adding all measured cross-sectional areas A_N multiplied by the intersection thickness S:

$$V_{SA} = \Sigma A_N \times S \quad (2)$$

Left-ventricular ejection fraction (LV-EF) is calculated for both, long-axis and short-axis reformations, from end-diastolic (LV-EDV) and end-systolic (LV-ESV) volumes according to equation 3

$$\text{LV-EF} = [(LV_{EDV} - LV_{ESV})/\text{LV}_{\text{EDV}}] \times 100\% \quad (3)$$

PRACTICAL GUIDE TO FUNCTIONAL MDCT—SCAN PROTOCOL, IMAGE ACQUISITION, AND DATA ANALYSIS

DATA ACQUISITION AND IMAGE RECONSTRUCTION

In initial studies, left-ventricular function data have been determined from MDCT coronary angiography studies using standard technique. The preparation and carrying-out of the MDCT studies are performed according to the manufacturer's recommendations. For optimal contrast bolus timing, the use of a bolus tracking technique is not necessary; however, a good contrast between endocardium and left-ventricular cavity is mandatory, enabling optimized delineation of endocardial contours. Following CT data acquisition, retrospectively ECG-gated image reconstruction in axial orientation is performed using standard reconstruction parameters in overlapping slices (increment < slice thickness) in set increments.

In order to calculate volumetric data, the maximal systolic constriction and diastolic relaxation phase of the left ventricle are identified by performing an axial image test series at midventricular level in 5% steps through the entire RR interval. It is recommended that axial images show the anterior left-ventricular papillary muscles as well as the anterior and posterior leaflet of the mitral valve (Fig. 7). End-diastolic and end-systolic phase are identified electrocardiographically and controlled visually as the images showing the largest and smallest left-ventricular cavity area, respectively. The reconstruction windows determined in this way finally are used for diastolic and systolic image calculation. According to a current study, a mean reconstruction window for diastolic image series was 83.1 ± 4.1% (range 75 to 90) of the RR interval, whereas systolic image reconstructions from MDCT data sets were performed at 23.1 ± 3.8% (range 20 to 35) of the RR interval *(15)*.

From axial image reconstructions, short-axis orientated MPRs are created for diastolic and systolic image series. To encompass the entire left ventricle from the base of the heart to its apex, usually ten to eighteen sections of short-axis-orientated MPRs are needed. In principle, any section thickness is possible. A section thickness of 8 mm using no intersection gap seems to be sufficient, according to experiences from cardiac MRI (Fig. 5 and 6).

DATA ANALYSIS OF LEFT-VENTRICULAR VOLUMETRY AND FUNCTION

Left-ventricular volumetric analysis can be performed from MPRs orientated to left-ventricular long axis and short axis, respectively, using standard 3D postprocessing software as provided by several manufacturers. Recently, dedicated analysis software enabling semiautomated contour detection might has been developed as an alternative for clinical and research purposes.

DATA ANALYSIS USING STANDARD 3D SOFTWARE

Diastolic and systolic left-ventricular volumes can be calculated using standard planimetric software provided by the different manufacturers according to the area-length method based on the long-axis view as well as to Simpson's method applied to contiguous short-axis reformations (see "Assessment of Left Ventricular Function Using CT" above). The tracing of left-ventricular endocardial contours as well as the determination of left-ventricular area and length in the long-axis view are done using standard software tools with manual interaction. As in cardiac MRI, papillary muscles and endocardial trabeculae should be included in the left-ventricular cavity and excluded from the left-ventricular volume.

DATA ANALYSIS USING DEDICATED ANALYSIS SOFTWARE

Alternatively, left-ventricular volumes can be determined by analysis software adapted from cardiac MRI, which has been validated in research and clinical studies for the past decade. Following data acquisition and postprocessing, MPRs are performed in short-axis orientation. For diastolic and systolic MPRs, basal and apical sections are visually identified and manually marked. To ensure reproducible data analysis, the first short-axis orientated section should be placed at the heart's base, covering the most basal portion of the left ventricle just forward of the atrioventricular ring. Endocardial borders are traced semiautomatically in both image series, starting with a software-generated ellipsoid or circular figure placed in the middle of the left-ventricular cavity. Contours are visually reviewed for correctness and, if necessary, are manually adjusted to endocardial contours.

ACCURACY AND REPRODUCIBILITY OF MDCT ASSESSMENT OF LEFT-VENTRICULAR FUNCTION

So far, only initial results have been reported from studies with small numbers of patients evaluating left-ventricular volume and function assessment from MDCT in comparison to such established techniques as CVG *(16–19)*, echocardiography *(20)*, and cardiac MRI *(15,21–23)*.

As has been demonstrated for cardiac MRI, an early study comparing MDCT and biplane CVG determination of left-ventricular ejection fraction found a better correlation if Simpson's method on short-axis reformations was used in comparison to the area-length method. Regions with previous myocardial infarction could clearly be delineated, showing a thinned LV wall and reduced or missing systolic myocardial wall thickening *(16)*. Those results were confirmed by others *(17–19)*, showing that 3D data assessed from retrospectively ECG-gated MDCT studies enable calculation of left-ventricular volumes to estimate systolic function. All authors consistently found an overestimation of left-ventricular end-systolic volumes, resulting in underestimation of left-ventricular ejection fraction in MDCT. In comparison to transthoracic echocardiography, no significant differences in left-ventricular volumes and ejection fraction were detected from MDCT in patients with both ischemic and nonischemic cardiomyopathies *(20)*. Measurements of end-diastolic and end-systolic volumes as determined by MDCT revealed a close correlation to respective cardiac MRI measurements (Figs. 8–11, Table 2). Acceptable limits of agreement between the two modalities were found, demonstrating a mean difference below 1% and 1.5 mL regarding determination of left-ventricular ejection fraction and stroke volume (Fig. 12), respectively *(16,22,23)*.

The use of MDCT for the analysis of global left-ventricular function has been limited by the lack of standardized analysis software in clinical practice. Semi-automated or automated methods of border detection have been developed in such cardiac imaging techniques as echocardiography or monoplane and biplane CVG *(24)*. An initial study demonstrated that evaluation of MDCT data sets lasted 10–15 min using analysis software to perform semi-automated contour detection. Although

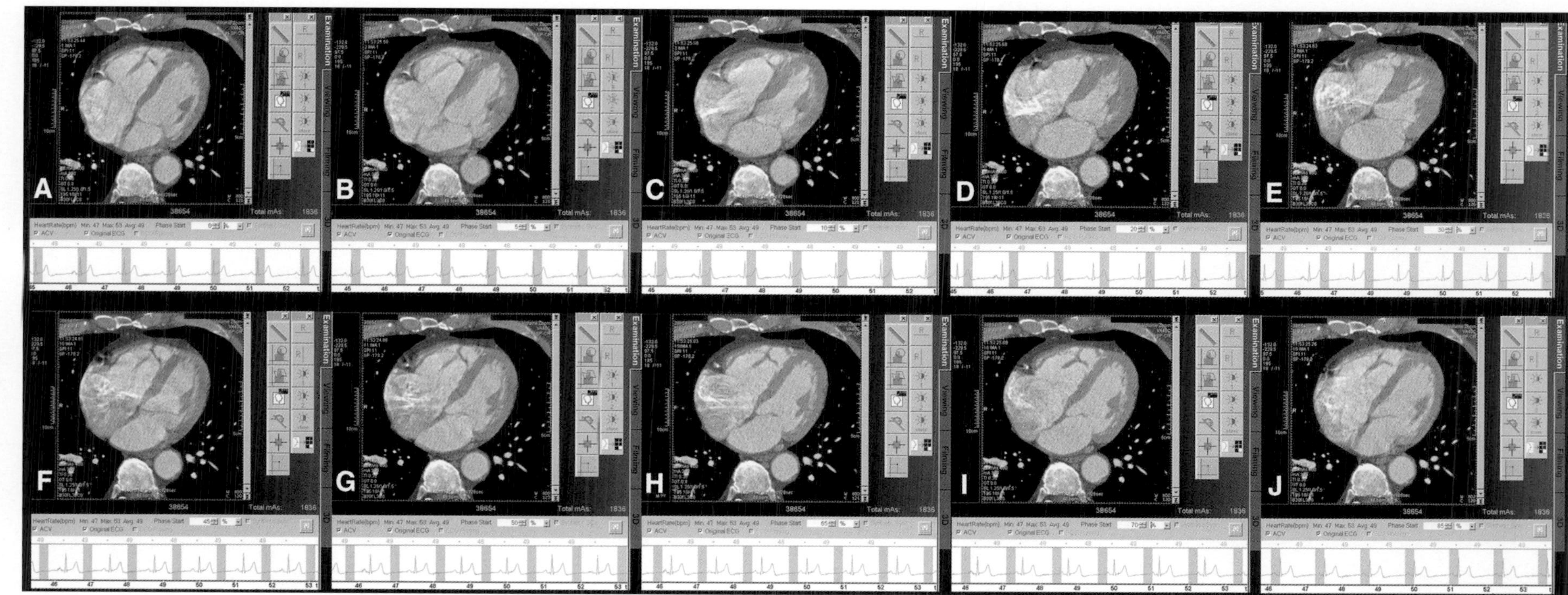

Fig. 7. Screenshots acquired from the scanner's main workstation (Navigator®) illustrating an axial-image-orientated test series in 5% steps (**A–J**) through the entire RR interval at midventricular level. Axial sections show the anterior left ventricular papillary muscles as well as the anterior and posterior leaflet of the mitral valve. End-diastolic and end-systolic phase were identified electrocardiographically and controlled visually as the images showing the largest and smallest left-ventricular cavity area, respectively. The corresponding reconstruction window was used for image calculation.

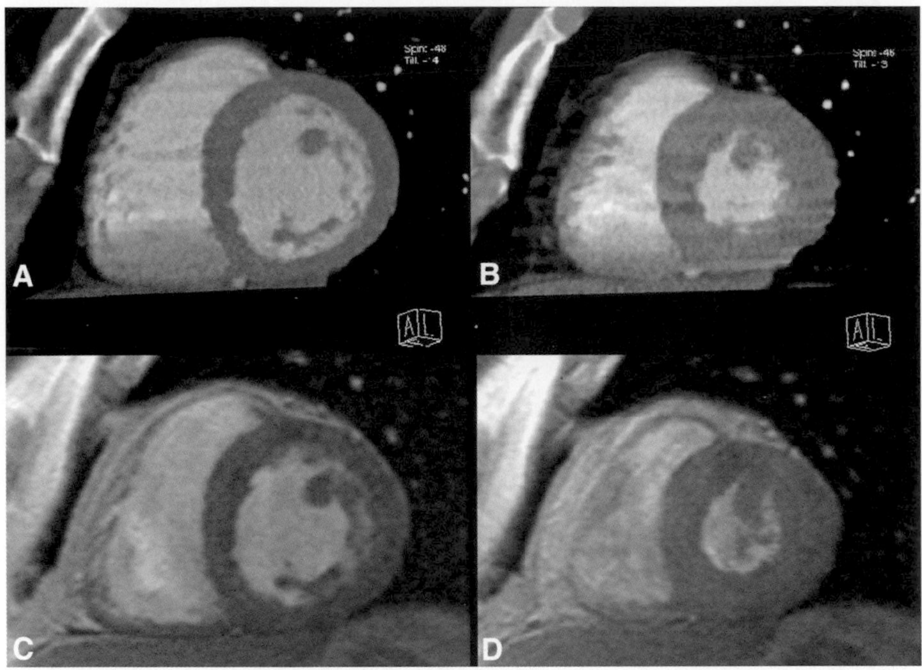

Fig. 8. Short-axis reformations comparing four-slice multidetector-row CT (MDCT) technology (**A** and **B**) to cardiac magnetic resonance imaging (MRI) (**C** and **D**) using conventional turbo gradient-echo sequences. (**A**) MDCT diastole; (**B**) MDCT systole (minor stair step artifacts resulting from a mean heart rate of 69 beats per minute); (**C**) MRI diastole; (**D**) MRI systole. Left-ventricular ejection fraction was 51.8% as determined from MDCT study in comparison to 57.9% as calculated from cine MRI.

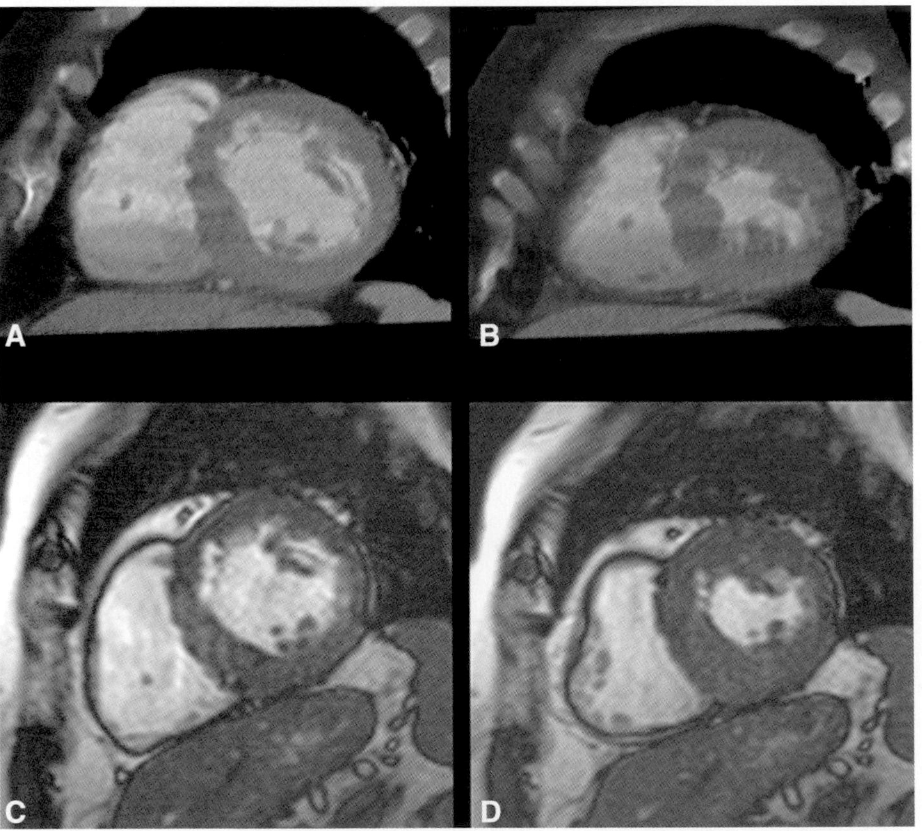

Fig. 9. Short-axis reformations comparing four-slice multidetector-row CT (MDCT) technology and cardiac magnetic resonance imaging (MRI) using steady-state free precession (SSFP) cine sequences. Diastolic (**A,C**) and systolic (**B,D**) short-axis reformations from MDCT (**A,B**) and SSFP cine magnetic resonance imaging (MRI: **C,D**) studies from a 58-yr-old female patient with one-vessel coronary artery disease. Normal dimensions of both ventricles and myocardial wall thickness, normal global left-ventricular function (left-ventricular ejection fraction = 67.5% MDCT vs 67.6% MRI).

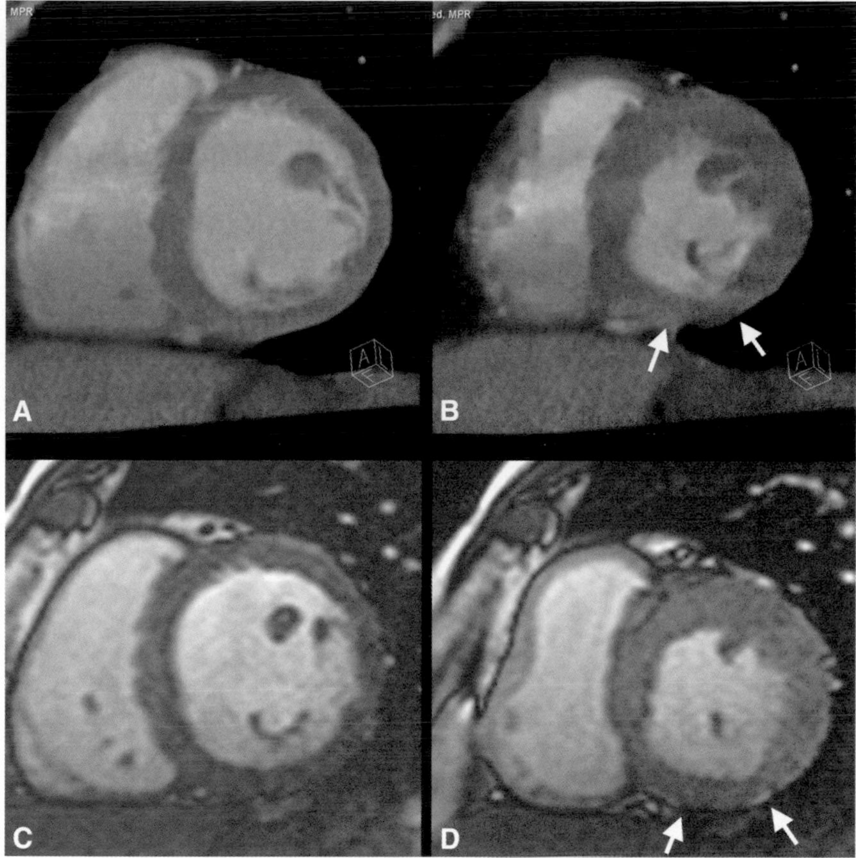

Fig. 10. Diastolic (**A,C**) and systolic (**B,D**) short-axis reformations from multidetector-row CT (MDCT) (**A,B**) and steady-state free precession cardiac magnetic resonance imaging MRI (**C,D**) studies obtained in a 72-yr-old male patient with three-vessel coronary artery disease who had experienced previous inferior myocardial infarction. Hypokinetic infero-septal and akinetic inferior wall of left ventricle can be clearly identified (white arrow; left-ventricular ejection fraction = 64.1% MDCT vs 62.9% MRI).

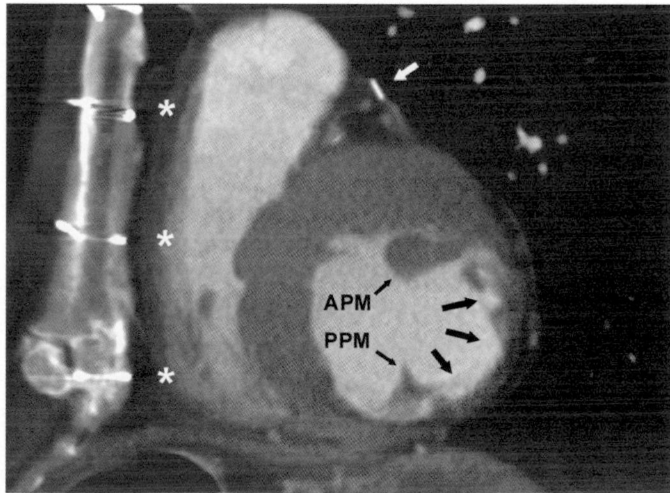

Fig. 11. Systolic short-axis reformation from sixteen-slice multidetector CT at midventricular level from a 72-yr-old man with a history of three-vessel coronary artery disease having undergone bypass surgery (white arrow indicates a tiny vascular clip from a bypass to the left descending coronary artery). As a result of recurrent myocardial infarction the multiplanar reformation in the short-axis demonstrates an absent regional contraction of left-ventricular myocardium in the lateral and inferior wall of left-ventricular myocardium including the posterior papillary muscles (dark arrows). APM, anterior papillary muscle; PPM, posterior papillary muscle.

endocardial left-ventricular contours had to be manually corrected in some cases, there was not a relevant difference in comparison to cardiac MRI data sets, with a mean analysis time of approx 10 min. Thus, in selected patients evaluated for coronary artery disease, semiautomated analysis software enabled reliable left-ventricular volumetric measurements and function analysis from MDCT data sets (Table 3) in comparison to SSFP cardiac MRI *(15)*.

With regard to left-ventricular end-diastolic and end-systolic volumes as well as ejection fraction as determined by MDCT studies, an inter-observer variability between 6 and 8% was reported *(16,22)*.

It has been generally accepted that a temporal resolution of 50 ms—achievable by established techniques as CVG, nuclear techniques, EBCT, and cardiac MRI—is mandatory for a reproducible evaluation of global left-ventricular function. Currently available MDCT techniques achieve a temporal resolution down to 105 ms, depending on the patient's heart rate. However, initial studies published by different investigators suggest that left-ventricular volumetric and functional evaluation by MDCT gives reliable results in comparison to reference modalities. A current study compared data of patients with a mean heart rate below and above 65/min, respectively, revealing no significant differences with regards to reliability of volumetric measurements *(15)* by MDCT (Table 4).

Table 2
Comparison of Left-Ventricular Volumetric and Functional Parameters As Determined From MDCT of the Heart in Comparison to CVG and MRI Using TGrE and SSFP Cine Sequences

Reference	*N*	*Modality compared to MDCT*	*LV-EDV*	*LV-ESV*	*LV-EF*	*LV-EF: MDCT vs other modality*
Juergens et al. *(22)*	28	TGrE-MRI	0.92	0.90	0.90	–7.9 ± 5.6 %
Wintersperger et al. *(17)*	25	CVG	0.59	0.88	0.82	–17 ± 9 %
Hundt et al. *(19)*	30	CVG	0.72	0.88	0.76	–13.7 ± 11 %
Erhard et al. *(27)*	7	SSFP-MRI	0.93	0.95	0.83	–3.8 ± 9.4 %
Mahnken et al. *(23)*	16	SSFP-MRI	0.99	0.99	0.98	–0.9 ± 3.6 %
Juergens et al. *(15)*	30	SSFP-MRI	0.93	0.94	0.89	–0.25 ± 4.9 %

CVG, cine ventriculography; MDCT, multidetector-row computed tomography; MRI, magnetic resonance imaging; SSFP, steady-state free precession; TGrE, Turbo gradient-echo.

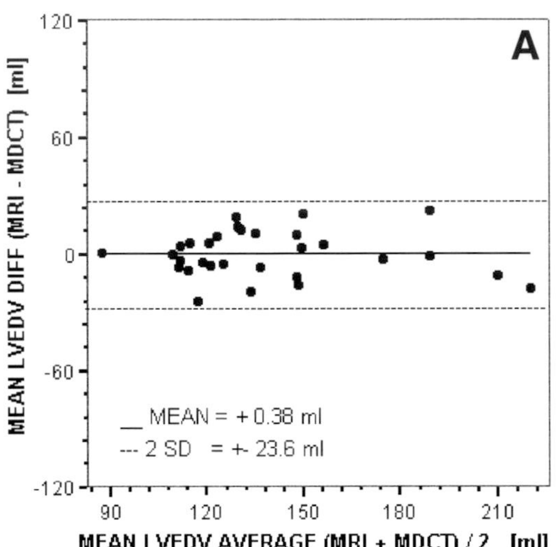

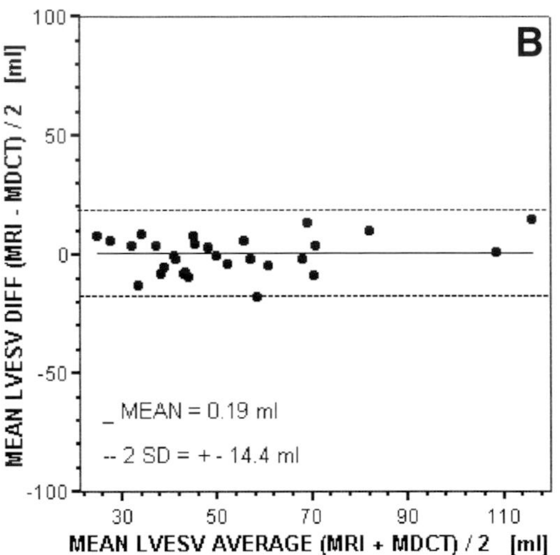

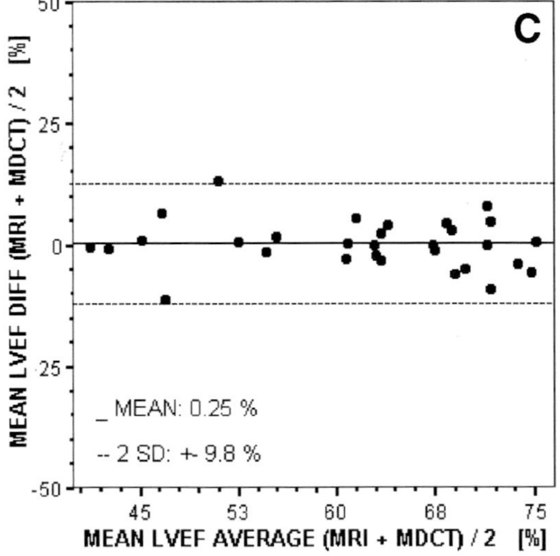

Fig. 12. Bland-Altman plots of left-ventricular end-diastolic volume (LVEDV) (**A**), left-ventricular end-systolic volume (LVESV) (**B**), and left-ventricular ejection fraction (LVEF) (**C**), showing the relation between differences and means between multidetector-row CT (MDCT) and cine steady-state free precession magnetic resonance imaging (MRI) for each parameter. The difference (*y* axis) between each pair ([mean MDCT] – [mean MRI]) is plotted against the average value (*x* axis) of the same pair ([(mean MDCT) + (mean MRI)]/2). (**A–C**: solid lines = mean value of differences; short dotted lines = mean value of differences ± 2 standard deviation.)

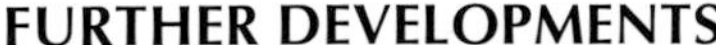

FURTHER DEVELOPMENTS

Progress concerning a more accurate determination of end-systolic frames, and possibly analysis of regional myocardial function, can be expected from MDCT systems with reduced gantry rotation time (below 500 ms) and a concomitant increase in temporal resolution (down to 105 ms). As a result of physical limitations, however, a further significant increase in temporal resolution may be realized only by separating physiological and physical acquisition time. Multisegment-reconstruction algorithms have become available for MDCT that process data from several gantry rotations and can reduce the temporal resolution down to 70–90 ms *(25,26)*. Initial results, however, suggest that the resulting decrease in spatial resolution limits left-ventricular function analysis by multisegment-algorithms in comparison to cardiac MRI.

MDCT VS CARDIAC MRI

In comparison to MDCT, the advantages of cardiac MRI are the lack of radiation exposure, avoidance of iodinated contrast media, and better temporal resolution. Furthermore, short-axis

Table 3
Volumetric and Functional Left-Ventricular Parameter As Determined by Means of MDCT and SSFP Cine MRI, N = 30

	MDCT		*SSFP Cine MRI*		*MDCT vs MRI*	
	Mean±SD	*Range*	*Mean±SD*	*Range*	*r =*	*p <*
LV-EDV [mL]	138±31	87–228	142±32	88–211	0.93	0.001
LV-ESV [mL]	53±21	20–108	54±22	27–123	0.94	0.001
LV-EF [%]	61±10	40–77	62±10	41–75	0.89	0.001
LV-SV [mL]	84±20	48–140	86±21	51–142	0.88	0.001

CI, confidence interval; LV-EDV, left-ventricular end-diastolic volume; LV-ESV, left-ventricular end-systolic volume; LV-EF, left-ventricular ejection-fraction; LV-SV, left-ventricular stroke volume; MDCT, multidetector-row computed tomography; MRI, magnetic resonance imaging; SD, standard deviation; SSFP, steady-state free precession. From ref. *15*.

Table 4
Volumetric and Functional Left-Ventricular Parameter As Determined by MDCT and SSFP Cine MRI[a]

	HR < 65/min N = 20 Mean ± SD			*HR ≥ 65/min N = 10 Mean ± SD*		
HR—Mean	58.1 ± 5.5			71.2 ± 6.2		< 0.001
HR—Range	47–64			65–88		< 0.001
	MDR-CT	*Cine MRI*	*p*	*MDR-CT*	*Cine MRI*	*p*
LV-EDV (mL)	142.7 ± 32.8	143.7 ± 34.3	n.s.	129.3 ± 22.3	134.6 ± 25.8	n.s.
LV-ESV (mL)	57.3 ± 20.9	56.5 ± 23.8	n.s.	45.9 ± 17.3	48.1 ± 17.7	n.s.
LV-EF (%)	58.9 ± 10.6	61.2 ± 10.4	n.s.	65.3 ± 9.8	64.7 ± 8.9	n.s.

HR, heart rate; LV-EDV, left-ventricular end-diastolic volume; LV-ESV, left-ventricular end-systolic volume; LV-EF, left-ventricular ejection-fraction; MDCT, multidetector-row computed tomography; MRI, magnetic resonance imaging; SD, standard deviation; SSFP, steady-state free precession; n.s., not statistically significant.

[a]Comparison of MDCT data sets reconstructed by biphasic adaptive cardiac volume algorithm with regard to mean HR of below 65/min vs ≥ 65/min. From ref. *15*.

images are readily available, and time-consuming secondary reformations as required in MDCT are not needed. Therefore, the software-assisted automatic or even the interactive creation of short-axis orientated reformations during data acquisition, as provided by state-of-the art cardiac MR scanners, would lead to an improved applicability of global left-ventricular volumetric and functional measurements in a clinical setting.

Considering contrast media application, radiation exposure, and limited temporal resolution, the use of MDCT solely for analysis of cardiac function parameters seems not unreasonable at present time. Regarding radiation exposure, a substantial reduction may be achieved by the application of an ECG-triggered tube current modulation. However, the combination of noninvasive coronary artery imaging and determination of global left-ventricular function within one single breath-hold MDCT study, however, might be an interesting approach to a fast and conclusive cardiac workup in different cardiac diseases, e.g., patients with suspected coronary artery disease. This application of MDCT might be of clinical relevance for patients who are not suitable for cardiac MRI because of specific contraindications.

SUMMARY

The assessment of global functional and volumetric left-ventricular parameters has become feasible using MDCT studies of the heart. Although this application is still in an experimental stage, initial studies from different study groups have revealed promising results in comparison to established techniques as CVG, echocardiography, and cardiac MRI. Recent developments in postprocessing and analysis software have improved clinical applicability.

REFERENCES

1. White HD, Norris RM, Brown MA, Brandt PWT, Whitlock RML, Wild CJ. Left ventricular end-systolic volume as the major determination of survival after recovery from myocardial infarction. Circulation 1987;76:44–51.
2. Schocken DD, Arrieta MI, Leaverton PE, Ross EA. Prevalence and mortality rate of congestive heart failure in the United States. J Am Coll Cardiol 1992;20:301–305.
3. Gerber TC, Behrenbeck T, Allison T, Mullan BP, Rumberger JA, Gibbons RJ. Comparison of measurement of left ventricular ejection fraction by Tc-99 m sestamibi first-pass angiography with electron beam computed tomography in patients with anterior wall acute myocardial infarction. Am J Cardiol 1999;83:1022–1026.

4. Zeidan Z, Erbel R, Barkhausen J, Hunold P, Bartel, Buck T. Analysis of global systolic and diastolic left ventricular performance using volume-time curves by real-time three-dimensional echocardiography. J Am Soc Echocardiogr 2003;16:29–37.
5. Lethimonnier F, Furber A, Balzer P, et al. Global left ventricular cardiac function. Comparison between magnetic resonance imaging, radionuclide angiography, and contrast angiography. Invest Radiol 1999;34:199–203.
6. Lipton MJ, Higgins CB, Boyd DP. Computed tomography of the heart: evaluation of anatomy and function. J Am Coll Cardiol 1985;5: 55S–69S.
7. Woo P, Mao S, Wang S, Detrano RC. Left ventricular size determined by electron beam computed tomography predicts significant coronary artery disease and events. Am J Cardiol 1997;79:1236–1238.
8. Bloomgarden DC, Fayad ZA, Ferrari VA, Chin B, St. John Sutton M, Axel L. Global cardiac function using fast breath-hold MRI: validation of new acquisition and analysis techniques. Magn Reson Med 1997;37:683–692.
9. Thiele H, Paetsch I, Schnackenburg B, et al. Improved accuracy of quantitative assessment of left ventricular volume and ejection fraction by geometric models with steady-state-free precession. J Cardiovasc Magn Reson 2002;4:327–339.
10. Miller S, Simonetti OP, Carr J, Kramer U, Finn JP. MR imaging of the heart with cine true fast imaging with steady-state precession: influence of spatial and temporal resolutions on left ventricular functional parameters. Radiology 2002;223:263–269.
11. Lorenz CH, Walker ES, Morgan VL, Klein SS, Graham TP Jr. Normal human right and left ventricular mass, systolic function, and gender differences by cine magnetic resonance imaging. J Cardiovasc Magn Reson 1999;1:7–21.
12. Harell GS, Guthaner DF, Breiman RS, et al. Stop-action cardiac computed tomography. Radiology 1977;123:515–517.
13. Lackner K, Thurn P. Computed tomography of the heart: ECG-gated and continuous scans. Radiology 1981;140:413–420.
14. Flohr T, Ohnesorge B. Heart rate adaptive optimization of spatial and temporal resolution for electrocardiogram-gated multislice spiral CT of the heart. J Comput Assist Tomogr 2001;25:907–923.
15. Juergens KU, Grude M, Maintz D, et al. Multi-detector row CT of left ventricular function with dedicated analysis software versus MR imaging: initial experience. Radiology 2004;230(2):403–410.
16. Juergens KU, Grude M, Fallenberg EM, et al. Using ECG-gated multidetector CT to evaluate global left ventricular myocardial function in patients with coronary artery disease. Am J Roentgenol 2002; 179:1545–1550.
17. Wintersperger BJ, Hundt W, Knez A, et al. Left ventricular systolic function assessed by ECG gated multirow-detector spiral computed tomography (MDCT): comparison to ventriculography. Eur Radiol 2002;12:S192.
18. Herzog C, Mehtap A, Abolmaali N, Balzer JO, Schaller S, Vogl TJ. Value and reproducibility of multidetector-row CT in the assessment of cardiac function. Eur Radiol 2002;12:S192.
19. Hundt W, Siebert K, Becker C, Knez A, Rubin GD, Reiser MF. Assessment of global left ventricular function: comparison of multidetector computed tomography with left ventriculography. Radiology 2002;252:388(P).
20. Sakuma T, Nishioka M, Fukuda K. Noninvasive determination of left ventricular volumes and ejection fraction assessed by multidetector-row CT. Radiology 2001;221:452(P).
21. Halliburton S, Petersilka M, Schvartzman P, Obuchowski N, White R. Validation of left ventricular volume and ejection fraction measurement with multi-slice computed tomography: comparison to cine magnetic resonance imaging. Radiology 2001;221:452(P).
22. Juergens KU, Fischbach R, Grude M, et al. Evaluation of left ventricular myocardial function by retrospectively ECG-gated multislice spiral CT in comparison to cine magnetic resonance imaging. Eur Radiol 2002;12:S191.
23. Mahnken AH, Spüntrup E, Wildberger JE, et al. Quantification of cardiac function with multislice spiral CT using retrospective ECG-gating: comparison with MRI. Fortschr Röntgenstr 2003;175: 83–88.
24. Waiter GD, McKiddie FI, Redpath TW, Semple SIK, Trent RJ. Determination of normal regional left ventricular function from cine-MR images using a semi-automated edge detection method. Magn Reson Imag 1999;17:99–107.
25. Boese JM, Bahner ML, Albers J, van Kaick G. Optimization of temporal resolution in CT using retrospective ECG-gating. Radiologe 2000;40:123–129.
26. Halliburton SS, Boese JM, Flohr TG, Lieber ML, Kuzmiak SA, White RD. Improved volumetric analysis of left ventricle using cardiac multi-slice computed tomography (MSCT) with high temporal resolution image reconstruction. Radiology 2002;252: 389(P).
27. Ehrhard K, Oberholzer K, Gast K, Mildenberger P, Kreitner KF, Thelen M. [Multi-slice CT (MSCT) in cardiac funciton imaging: threshold-value-supported 3D volume reconstructions to determine the left ventricular ejection fraction in comparison to MRI] [Article in German]. Rofo Fortschr Geb Rontgenstr Neuen Bildgeb Verfahr. 2002;174(12):1566–1569.

19 Imaging Intramyocardial Microcirculatory Function Using Fast Computed Tomography

Stefan Möhlenkamp, MD, Axel Schmermund, MD, Birgit Kantor, MD, Raimund Erbel, MD, and Erik L. Ritman

WHY IMAGE CORONARY MICROVASCULAR FUNCTION?

Coronary arterial disease is currently diagnosed and treated primarily on the basis of its impact on the large-diameter epicardial arteries. A structural change, usually a localized narrowing (stenosis) of a coronary artery lumen, is generally detected and quantitated by selective coronary angiography. However, by the time the epicardial artery stenosis results in reduced epicardial flow and the patient becomes symptomatic, it is generally too late to arrest (much less reverse) the disease process in that artery. Therefore, a noninvasive test that identifies presymptomatic, subclinical disease should result in initiation of therapy at a time when the disease process is still reversible. Causal risk factors—i.e., dyslipidemia, arterial hypertension, diabetes mellitus, and smoking—are responsible for the majority of coronary artery disease cases, and risk-factor modification in high-risk asymptomatic individuals has been shown to improve outcome *(1)*. Early risk stratification, aggressive preventive counseling, and therapy in high-risk subjects is therefore recommended *(2,3)*. However, limited economic resourses warrant careful patient selection and appropriate therapeutic aggressiveness. Hence, any imaging tool for this purpose is required (1) to allow identification and quantification of early disease, and (2) to be sensitive enough to ascertain therapeutic efficacy over time to justify continuation or modification of the initiated therapy.

Coronary atherosclerosis affects the intramyocardial arterial microcirculation early in the disease process, well before the epicardial vessels are hemodynamically compromised *(4–6)*. If symptoms are present, they frequently cannot sufficiently be explained by the degree of epicardial lumen narrowing. Even a "normal" coronary angiogram may be associated with typical angina pectoris and inducible ischemia in noninvasive stress tests *(7,8)*, which is usually attributed to microvascular functional impairment and termed *Syndrome X (9) or* microvascular angina *(10)*. Risk factors can frequently be identified, that can induce endothelial dysfunction and hence be responsible for a reduced vasomotor capacity of intramyocardial coronary microvessels *(11–15)*. Accordingly, risk factor-induced epicardial atherosclerosis is frequently, but not always, preceded by impaired vasomotion of coronary microvessels *(16–18)*. Different risk factors, coronary atherosclerosis, and also other diseases such as aortic valve stenosis or cardiomyopathies may all ultimately result in reduced coronary flow reserve, but their functional impact on the coronary microvasculature, which predominantly regulates regional myocardial blood flow *(4,19–22)*, is markedly different.

We have explored fast X-ray computed tomography (CT) as a minimally invasive method to quantitate intramyocardial microcirculatory function in different "clinically relevant" settings, and we propose to use the blood volume-to-flow relationship to identify characteristic changes in the functional behavior of the coronary microcirculation.

FAST CT-BASED INDICES OF INTRAMYOCARDIAL MICROVASCULAR FUNCTION

The intramyocardial microcirculation consists of arteries that are up to 0.5 mm in lumen diameter and progressively branch to the 5-μm-diameter capillaries. Unfortunately, these small microvessels cannot be individually visualized by clinically applicable imaging methods. Consequently, some indirect estimates of microvascular vasomotion must be made. We do this using the intramyocardial intravascular blood volume-to-flow relationship. Minimally invasive estimates of microvascular blood volume and perfusion in absolute numbers can be obtained from the analysis of whole-body CT images using intravascular contrast-medium dilution curves. The principles of indicator dilution techniques using X-ray CT and contrast agent as the indicator have been described in detail elsewhere *(23–25)*. Its basis is the Stewart–Hamilton Equation *(26–31)*:

$$\text{Blood volume (BV)} = \text{Flow (F)} \cdot \text{Mean transit time (MTT)}$$

With the development of fast-CT technology such as the dynamic spatial reconstructor (DSR) *(32)* and electron beam CT (EBCT) scanners (GE-Imatron, South San Francisco, CA) *(33)*, quantitative estimates of intramyocardial fractional blood volume and perfusion in vivo have been obtained in the beating heart *(24,25,34–43)* and other organs like the kidney *(44–46)*, the brain *(23,47)*, the liver *(48)*, and the lung *(49–50)*.

To estimate intramyocardial (fractional) blood volume and flow in the beating heart in vivo, we used the following equa-

From: *Contemporary Cardiology: CT of the Heart: Principles and Applications*
Edited by: U. Joseph Schoepf © Humana Press, Inc., Totowa, NJ

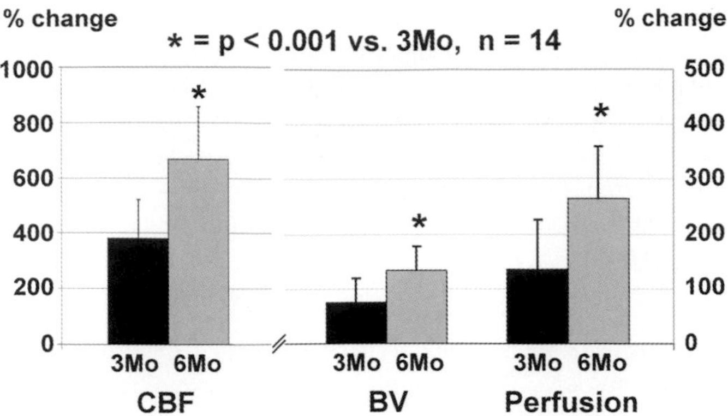

Fig. 2. Quantitation of long-term changes in microvascular functional response to adenosine infusion at baseline (3-mo-old pigs) and at follow-up (6-mo-old pigs). Within the baseline and follow-up studies separately, Doppler-ultrasound-based intracoronary blood flow (CBF), EBCT-based blood volume (BV), and perfusion significantly increased in response to adenosine (p < 0.001, respectively). The increases in BV and perfusion at follow-up in response to adenosine were significantly greater compared to baseline, consistent with CBF measurements (p < 0.001, respectively) (*see* text for details; modified from ref. *41*).

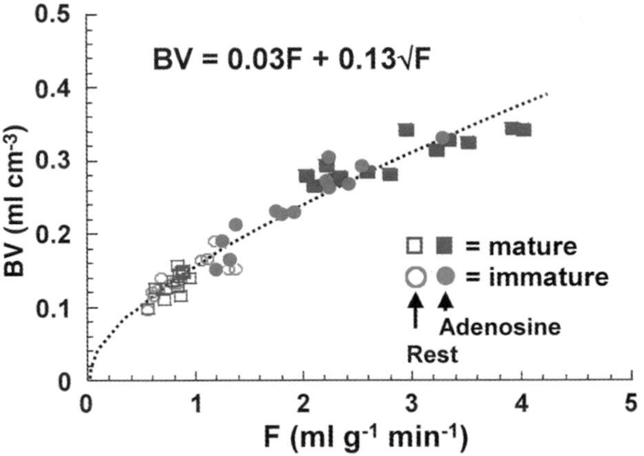

Fig. 3. Fast CT-based blood volume (BV) to flow (F) relationship in normal hearts imaged twice before and after 3 mo (same data as in Fig. 2). Values are given at baseline (resting conditions = open red circles, adenosine = closed red circles) and at follow-up (resting conditions = open blue squares, adenosine = closed blue squares). Despite a different microvascular functional response to adenosine at baseline and follow-up, all values follow the same curvilinear line (*see* text for details; modified from ref. *41*).

MICROVASCULAR ENDOTHELIAL DYSFUNCTION IN HYPERCHOLESTEROLEMIA

Imaging Diseased Coronary Microvascular Function in Chronic Hypercholesterolemia

Chronic hypercholesterolemia (HC) leads to endothelial damage and dysfunction, as well as impaired coronary microvascular function. Using a porcine model of chronic hypercholesterolemia, EBCT technology was used to evaluate the degree to which it is able to detect, discriminate, and quantify microvascular permeability and blood volume in the different functional components of the coronary microcirculation in normal compared to hypercholesterolemic pigs *(40,59,60)*.

Intramyocardial microvascular functional reserve in response to selective intracoronary infusion of adenosine was impaired in hypercholesterolemic vs normal control pigs, consistent with our intracoronary Doppler ultrasound measurements (Fig. 4) and experimental and clinical observations by others *(59,67)*. In contrast to our findings in young presumably immature normal control pigs (above), the BV-to-F relationship demonstrated a significantly attenuated increase in blood volume per increase in perfusion in hypercholesterolemic versus normal mature control pigs (Fig. 5), which can be explained by HC-induced endothelial dysfunction and its consequences for microvascular vasomotion: in hypercholesterolemia it is primarily the oxidized low-density lipoprotein- and free oxygen radicals-induced inhibition of nitric oxide (NO)-dependent vasorelaxation *(68,69)*, in combination with reduced NO bioavailability *(70,71)*, that plays a key role for the observed endothelial microvascular dysfunction both in animal experiments and in humans *(72,73)*. Stepp et al. demonstrated that flow-induced vasodilation in arteries with diameters >160 μm is also regulated to some degree by endothelial NO release *(74)*. This explains the observed effects of adenosine, a substance that results in vasodilation of resistance and conducting microvessels *(21,75)* and capillary recruitment *(76)*, predominantly via endothelium-independent mechanisms.

At rest, blood volume in the recruitable component was decreased, but it was increased in the nonrecruitable component in hypercholesterolemic pigs *(40)*. Lerman et al. previously reported a similar change in microvascular blood volume distribution after administration of N^G-monomethyl-L-arginine (L-NMMA), a competitive inhibitor of NO synthase *(39)*. Since experimental hypercholesterolemia is associated with a decrease in endogenous NO bioavailability *(70,71)*, it probably induces physiological effects similar to those with L-NMMA. In response to 5-min continuous infusion of nitroglyceride (NTG), we observed an increase in both the recruitable and nonrecruitable microvascular component in control pigs, although NTG primarily acts on microvessels >200 μm in diameter. These findings can be explained by a modulating effect of upstream resistance vessel function on capillary recruitment *(40)*. In hypercholesterolemic pigs however, blood volume remained unchanged in both the recruitable and the nonrecruitable component, likely a result of impaired resistance vessel vasomotion.

The characteristic behavior of different functional microvascular components in hypercholesterolemic animals as imaged by fast CT is consistent with experimental observation by others using different methodology, which supports the ability of fast CT to obtain meaningful information on intracoronary microvessels in chronic diseases that alter microvascular function.

Imaging Therapeutic Reversal of Coronary Microvascular Dysfunction in Chronic HC

Using the same porcine model of hypercholesterolemia and similar methodology, the effect of HC with and without high-dose antioxidants (vitamins E and C) and statins on fast-CT-

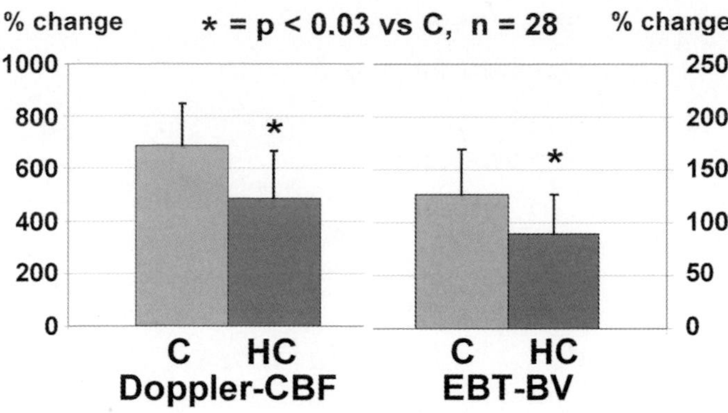

Fig. 4. Quantitation of changes in microvascular functional response to adenosine infusion in normal control pigs (C) and chronic hypercholesterolemic (HC) pigs (HC). Doppler-ultrasound-based intracoronary blood flow (CBF) and electron beam CT-based blood volume (BV) significantly increased in response to adenosine ($p < 0.001$, respectively). However, the increase in microvascular response to adenosine was significantly blunted in HC-pigs compared to normal controls (*see* text for details; modified from ref. *40*).

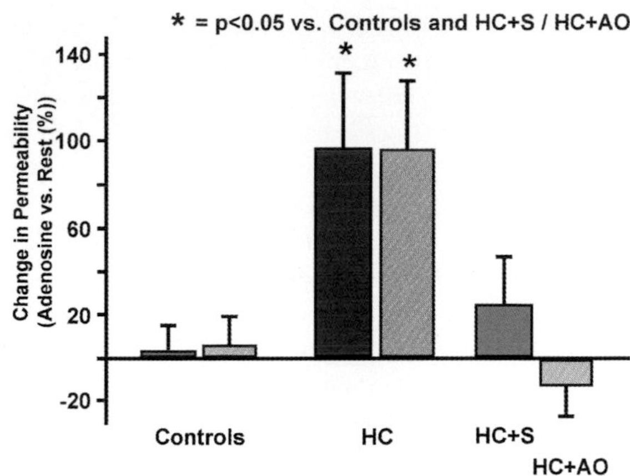

Fig. 6. Relative change (percent compared with resting conditions) of microvascular permeability in response to intravenous adenosine in three groups: normal controls, hypercholesterolemic (HC) pigs, and HC pigs treated with statins (S) or antioxidants (AO, vitamins E and C). Microvascular permeability is significantly increased in HC pigs, but long-term therapy preserves permeability (*see* text for details; modified from refs. *59* [shaded bars] and *60* [full colors]).

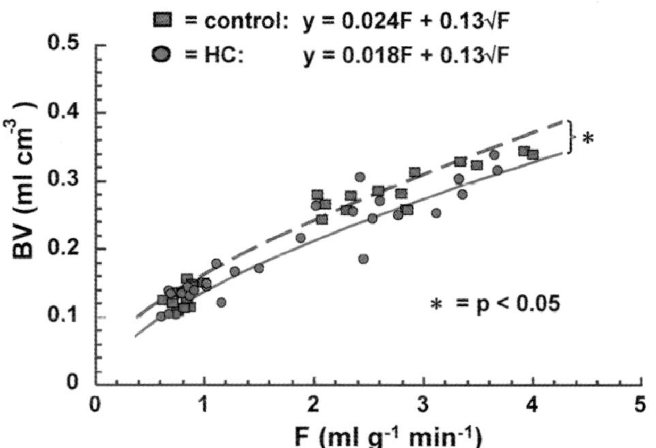

Fig. 5. Blood volume-to-flow relationship in normal controls and hypercholesterolemic (HC) pigs. A 3-mo high-cholesterol diet led to endothelial dysfunction with significant impairment in mobilization of microvascular blood volume for any given perfusion value (*see* text for details; modified from ref. *40*)

based myocardial perfusion and microvascular permeability has been assessed at rest and during intravenous infusion of adenosine *(59,60)*. These studies found a significant increase in myocardial perfusion and unaltered microvascular permeability in response to adenosine in normal control pigs, whereas in hypercholesterolemic animals, myocardial perfusion remained unaltered after adenosine infusion and microvascular permeability significantly increased (Fig. 6). However, animals treated with antioxidants and statins showed a response to adenosine comparable to normal control pigs *(59,60)*, which is consistent with clinical observations *(77–79)*. Since statins do not alter plasma cholesterol levels to the same degree as they do in humans *(80)*, preservation of microvascular (endothelial) function is likely independent of their lipid-lowering properties *(81)*. In accordance with previous studies *(82,83)* and with the established role of lipid oxidation in endothelial dysfunction, it was suggested that the beneficial effects are mediated via antioxidative, vasoprotective properties of statins.

The above findings are in accordance with our own observations in hypercholesterolemic pigs and also support the ability of fast-CT technology to quantitatively assess coronary microvascular dysfunction in chronic diseases such as HC. Most importantly, these studies demonstrate that reversal of HC-induced endothelial dysfunction using statins and vitamins can be quantitated using minimally invasive fast-CT image analysis.

CORONARY MICROVASCULAR DYSFUNCTION IN SUBCLINICAL CORONARY ARTERY STENOSIS

Coronary angiography remains the "gold standard" to assess advanced stages of epicardial coronary artery disease. While there is no doubt about the hemodynamic relevance of high-grade lesions *(84)*, functional assessment of apparently mild or intermediate lumen diameter reductions (50–75%) remains difficult *(85,86)*. Lumen narrowing less than 50% is frequently associated with a normal epicardial flow reserve and therefore considered clinically nonsignificant. However, such "nonsignificant" lesions may already be associated with functional microvascular alterations *(17)*. In a canine study, Wu et al. demonstrated that intramyocardial blood volume increases with increasing pressure gradients across a nonsignificant stenosis ($\Delta P \leq 40$ mmHg ≅ Stenosis ≤ 55%), while perfusion initially remains unaltered *(58,87)*. When the pressure gradient across a more severe epicardial stenosis rises to values much above 50 mmHg, compensatory mechanisms will exhaust and regional blood flow drops in proportion to a decrease in blood volume *(58)*. Similar results have been found using echocardiography in a canine open-chest model *(88)*. These observations are consistent with intramyocardial release of adenosine in response to mild local ischemia, leading to compensatory vasodilation of resistance vessels and preservation of regional perfusion *(89)*. The increase in microvascular blood volume in nonsignificant epicardial lumen reduction in order to preserve microvascular perfusion is also reflected in the BV-to-F relationship (Fig. 7) *(87)*, which may be a more sensitive index for microvascular impairment than the coronary flow reserve in early CAD *(87)*.

CORONARY MICROVASCULAR DYSFUNCTION IN CORONARY MICROEMBOLIZATION

Data from large clinical trials suggest that embolization of plaque material or microthrombi from dysfunctional epicardial arterial endothelium into the distal coronary microcirculation has long been an underappreciated, possibly common, event *(90-92)*, particularly during acute coronary syndromes *(93,94)* and intravascular coronary interventions *(95,96)*. Interestingly, resting epicardial arterial blood flow may even be elevated despite being associated with myocardial ischemia, necrosis, and contractile dysfunction—a phenomenon termed *perfusion-contraction mismatch (92,97)*. The functionally "frustrate" increase in coronary flow was attributed to vasodilation of adjacent nonembolized vessels in response to adenosine release from the surface of embolized myocardium *(98–100)*. It may be accompanied by a reduction in maximum achievable epicardial coronary blood flow despite normal or restored coronary artery lumen diameter *(101)*, suggesting involvement of the coronary microvasculature for these observations.

In another porcine study, we assessed the degree to which different sized coronary microvessels contribute to the pathophysiological changes observed after microembolization *(43)*. Specifically, we studied the consequences of embolization of 10 μm and 100 μm intramyocardial arteries and arterioles on microvascular blood volume, perfusion, and transit time in vivo. We found appreciable differences in microvascular blood volume and perfusion dynamics depending on the size of embolized microvessels and the initial perfusion state (Fig. 8). At rest, injection of small amounts of 10 μm microspheres initially result in a very brief decrease in coronary blood flow, which is soon followed by increases in blood volume and perfusion. This hyperemic response usually lasts for several minutes *(92)*. As previously observed in a canine model, the hyperemic response progressively diminishes with increasing doses of small microspheres (Fig. 8) *(98,102)*. In canines and in pigs, the local hyperemic response can be attributed to adenosine release, because it was prevented by the adenosine receptor antagonist theophylline *(98,99)* and the α 1-adrenoceptor antagonist prazosin *(103)*. Unlike the response to 10 μm microspheres, resting blood volume and perfusion was not preserved with injection of 100 μm microspheres. When the microvasculature was maximally dilated before injection of microspheres, blood volume and perfusion also decreased immediately and progressively with repetitive injections of microspheres, irrespective of microsphere size, both in porcine and canine myocardium *(43,98)*.

Our EBCT-based findings support the concept of mobilization of a functional arteriolar and capillary blood volume and perfusion reserve in response to microspheres injection. The increase in blood volume and perfusion after injection of low amounts of 10 μm-microspheres at resting conditions may be

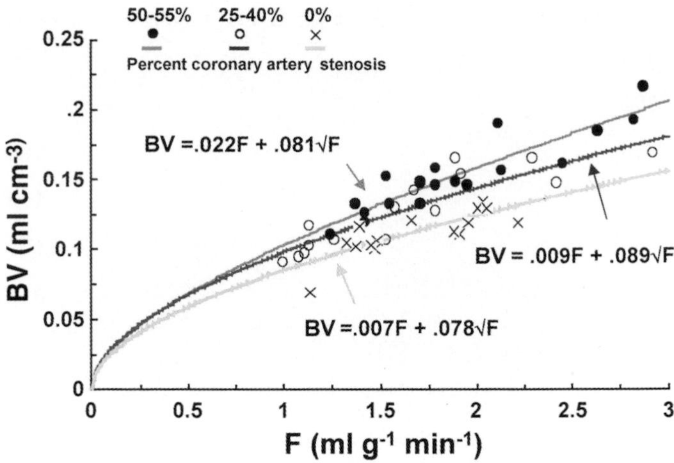

Fig. 7. Effect of experimental canine coronary artery stenosis on myocardial blood volume and perfusion. Increasing nonsignificant stenosis, which is not associated with decreased epicardial flow reserve, leads to a progressive increase in blood volume relative to perfusion values. This is characteristically different from changes observed in microvascular disease (*see* text for details; modified from ref. *87*).

explained by the increase in blood volume and perfusion within neighboring terminal arterioles and capillaries that is greater than the loss of blood volume and perfusion resulting from the embolized vessels. Such an excess mobilization of microvascular functional reserve may be required to compensate for the greater intercapillary distance between the recruited effective capillary exchange surface area and the tissue previously perfused by the embolized microvessel. When microspheres are injected during adenosine infusion, the already mobilized microvascular functional reserve cannot counteract the loss of microvessels so that blood volume and perfusion decrease even after injection of small amounts of small microspheres. When large diameter microspheres embolize, then a large contiguous volume of myocardium is deprived of flow. As the functional capillary reserve can now be mobilized only at the surface of the embolized perfusion territory, this limited increase in capillary blood volume and perfusion cannot overcome the loss of capillaries at the center of the embolized perfusion territory *(43,100)*.

When microvascular blood volume progressively decreased from maximum vasodilation to resting state by infusing decreasing adenosine concentrations, transit time significantly increased in nonembolized myocardium. In contrast, when intramyocardial blood volume decreased in response to microvascular embolization, transit time remained unchanged (Fig. 9). Because transit time is inversely related to perfusion, this leads to perfusion values higher than expected for the given volume of perfused microvessels and hence to "pseudo-preservation" of microvascular perfusion. This may contribute to a perfusion-contraction mismatch *(97)* by reducing the time available for nutrient exchange at the capillary level. Our findings are consistent with the previously reported microspheres-induced decrease in arterio-venous O_2 difference and lactate extraction *(98)*, and may, in part, explain microembolization-

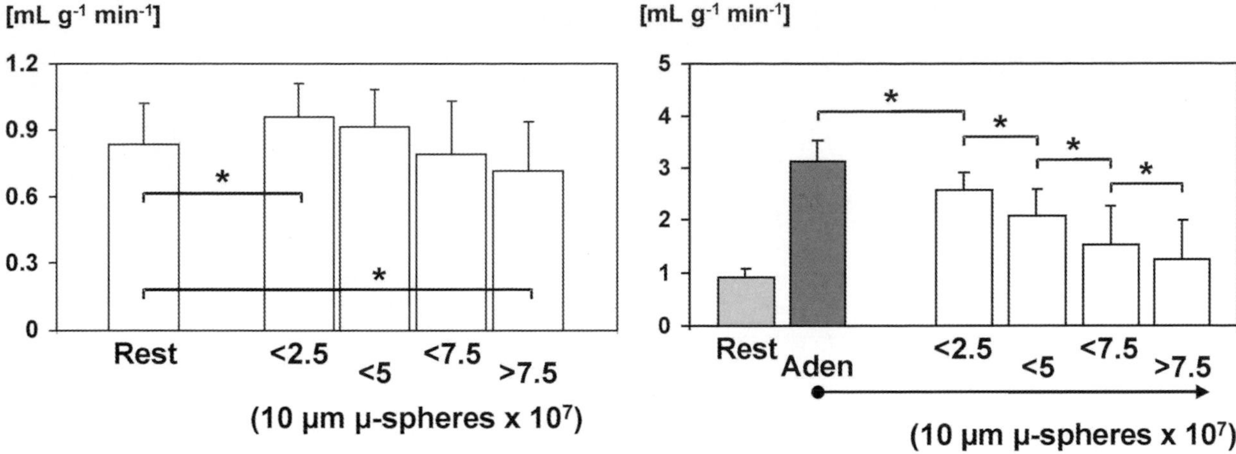

Fig. 8. Myocardial perfusion in response to selective injections of 10-µm microspheres into the left anterior descending coronary artery. Injection of small amounts of small microspheres at rest leads to an initial increase in myocardial perfusion, which then decreases with further injections (left panel). When microspheres are injected at maximum vasodilation, the microvasculature cannot compensate for the loss of embolized microvessels, and perfusion decreases even after small amounts of microspheres are injected (right panel). Injection of larger microspheres leads to immediate decrease in perfusion and blood volume also at resting conditions (not shown) (*see* text for details; modified from ref. *43*).

related regional contractile dysfunction despite (pseudo-) normal regional flow. The degree to which myocardial perfusion is preserved is described by the BV-to-F relationship (Fig. 10A,B) *(104)*.

Our study demonstrated the ability of fast CT to image acute changes in microvascular function, which in this experiment was induced by selective injection of microspheres. The technique provided new and unique insight into microvascular functional behavior in vivo. The alterations in response to different sized microspheres of blood volume, perfusion, and transit time, and the way in which these parameters are interrelated, were highly specific for coronary microembolization.

QUANTITATION AND ASSESSMENT OF MYOCARDIAL MICROVASCULAR FUNCTIONAL HETEROGENEITY

Under normal conditions, intramyocardial blood volume and perfusion have been shown to be heterogeneously distributed in adjacent regions of interest (= spatial heterogeneity) and over time (= temporal heterogeneity) *(105–107)*. It was recently suggested that increased heterogeneity may be present in early atherosclerosis *(108)*. Assuming a bifurcation at every coronary artery branch *(109)*, myocardial heterogeneity can be well represented by a fractal process *(19,110)* and can be measured by relating the relative dispersion (= standard deviation divided by the mean = the coefficient of variation) to the size of the region of interest (ROI) *(111,112)*. It has been shown that the logarithm of the coefficient of variation between contiguous ROIs within the myocardium varies linearly with the logarithm of the size of those ROIs: log [SD/mean] = (1-D) log [area ROI], with 1-D being the slope and "D" being the fractal dimension *(111,113)*. The value of D is expected to increase with increasing heterogeneity both in normal and diseased myocardium.

Under resting conditions, and using 4 to 16 contiguous myocardial ROIs, the range of perfusion values has been shown to be between 2.0 and 5 mL/g/min, and the blood volume has a corresponding range in values *(114)*. Importantly, the BV-to-F relationship generated from the BV and F values obtained from those multiple ROIs follows the same $BV = aF + b\sqrt{F}$ relationship compared to the one that can be generated with a single large ROI sampled in scans repeated under resting and vasodilated states (Fig. 11).

Consequently, the BV-to-F relationship that characterizes the myocardial microcirculatory function can be generated from a single scan sequence, which reduces both radiation and contrast material exposure.

CONCLUSION

Using fast X-ray CT and indicator dilution principles, indices of intramyocardial fractional blood volume, myocardial perfusion, and microvascular transit time can be quantitated with minimal invasiveness in vivo in absolute numbers. These data provide important information on coronary microvascular function in healthy and diseased myocardium, and contribute to a better understanding of the role of the coronary microvasculature in different physiological and pathophysiological settings.

Our data provide evidence that the BV-to-F relationship is sensitive enough to detect characteristic differences in the behavior of healthy compared to diseased coronary microvascular function, and specific enough to identify distinct differences in microvascular function between different diseases. In healthy myocardium, blood volume relative to flow always follows a single curvilinear line. A reduced response to adenosine results in reduced increases in blood volume and perfusion, but shows no deviation of values from the relationship seen in a presumably healthy microvasculature. In contrast, epicardial and microvascular alterations lead to characteristic deviations

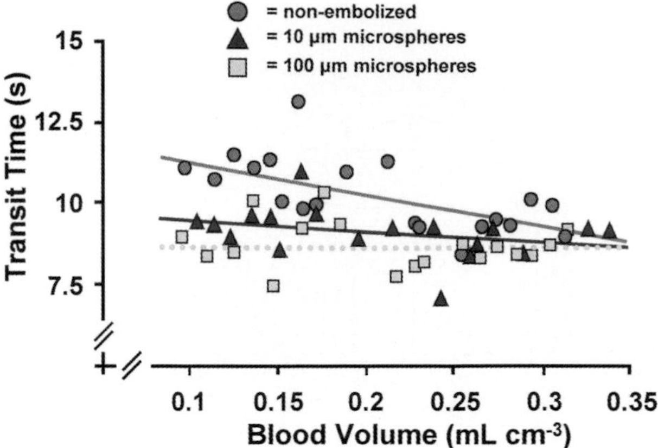

Fig. 9. Blood volume (BV)-to-transit time relationship in normal, nonembolized myocardium and in myocardium embolized with 10-µm and 100-µm microspheres. In normal, nonembolized myocardium, transit time increases when maximal functionally available blood volume decreases. However, when functionally available volume of myocardium is progressively reduced by embolization with increasing amounts of 10-µm and 100-µm microspheres, transit times remain unaltered, leading to "pseudo-preservation" of myocardial perfusion (from ref. *43*).

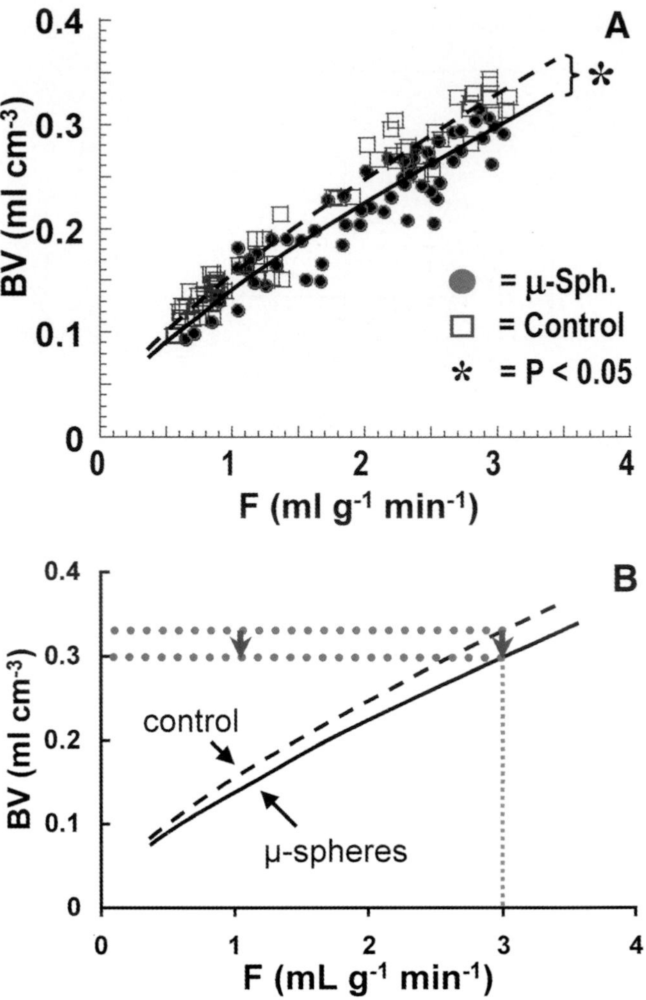

Fig. 10. Blood volume-to-flow (BV-to-F) relationship normal controls compared to repetitive selective injection of microspheres into the left anterior descending coronary artery (LAD). Microembolization—i.e., plugging of intramyocardial microvessels—leads to a reduced number of patent microvessels and hence to a decrease in fractional blood volume. Despite the decrease in fractional blood volume, perfusion values are preserved within limits, which are described by the BV-to-F relationship (*see also* Fig. 9 and text for details; from ref. *104*).

from this "normal" relationship. In mild epicardial coronary stenosis, coronary microvessels are recruited to increase the transstenotic pressure gradient and hence to preserve flow, which leads to an increase in blood volume for any given amount of microvascular blood flow.

Our approach to the evaluation of microvascular function is not limited to fast X-ray CT. Other imaging techniques, especially cardiac ultrasound and magnetic resonance imaging , are under extensive investigation and continuous refinement in their ability to obtain absolute values of microvascular blood volume and perfusion *(115–118)*. Once blood volume and perfusion are both accurately and concurrently quantifiable, then the subsequent use of the BV-to-F relationship easily follows, irrespective of the imaging modality.

Evaluating myocardial microvascular function should be useful in other clinically relevant settings. In nondiseased myocardium, the approach may be used to quantify the long-term effect of physiological stimuli such as aging and exercise on normal coronary microvascular functional reserve *(64,119)*. It is likely that other diseases that affect intramyocardial microvessels (e.g., diabetes mellitus, arterial hypertension, or cardiomyopathies) *(20)* also show characteristic patterns in the BV-to-F relationship. Fast CT may further be used to monitor the efficacy of therapeutic strategies that target the coronary microcirculation such as medication *(120,121)*, or potentially transmyocardial laser revascularization *(122)* and gene therapy to induce myocardial angiogenesis in ischemic myocardium *(123)*. Preliminary reports on the assessment of coronary microvascular function in patients *(38,124)* suggest a potential of fast-CT technology to evaluate early microvascular disease also in clinical practice, and may become a useful adjunct to noninvasive assessment of epicardial coronary calcium quantitation *(125)* and noninvasive coronary angiography *(126)*.

REFERENCES

1. Grundy SM. Primary prevention of coronary heart disease. Integrating risk assessment with intervention. Circulation 1999;100: 988–998.
2. Smith SC, Greenland P, Grundy SM. Prevention Conference V—Beyond secondary prevention: Identifying the high-risk patient for primary prevention—executive summary. Circulation 2000;101: 111–116.
3. Greenland P, Smith SC, Grundy SM. Improving coronary heart disease risk assessment in asymptomatic people. Role of traditional risk factors and non-invasive cardiovascular tests. Circulation 2001; 104:1863–1867.
4. Marcus, ML, Chilian WM, Kanatsuka H, et al. Understanding the coronary circulation through studies at the microvascular level. Circulation 1990;82:1–7.
5. Naseri A, Crea KF, Crainflone D. Myocardial ischemia caused by distal coronary vasoconstriction. Am J Cardiol 1992;7:1602–1605.

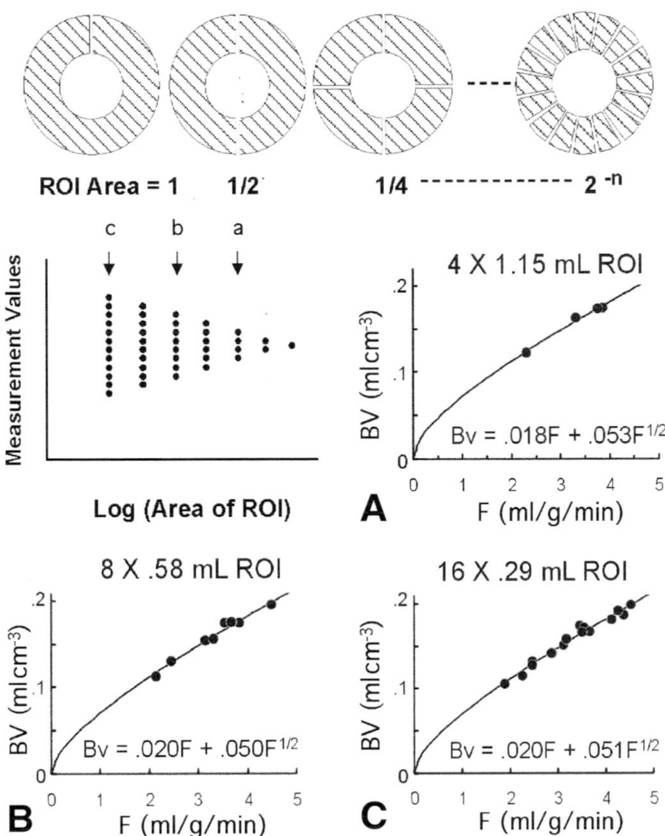

Fig. 11. "Multiple-ROI" analysis of blood volume and perfusion heterogeneity: to measure blood volume (BV) and flow (F) heterogeneity, one large myocardial region of interest (ROI) is consecutively halved (top). BV and F are determined within each ROI. Because of the fractal nature of BV and F, variation of measurements (or relative dispersion) increases around the mean value within progressively smaller ROIs (middle left). These values have been shown to follow the BV-to-F relationship, which can therefore be determined individually based on just one image sequence (middle right and bottom, **A–C**) (*see* text and refs. *112* and *114* for details).

6. Hasdai D, Sangiorgi G, Spagnoli LG, et al. Coronary artery apoptosis in experimental hypercholesterolemia. Atherosclerosis 1999; 142:317–325.
7. Kemp HG, Kronmal RA, Vliestra RE, Frey RL. Seven year survival of patients with normal or near normal coronary arteriograms: a CASS registry study. J Am Coll Cardiol 1986;7:479–483.
8. Hasdai D, Gibbons RJ, Holmes DR Jr., Higgano ST, Lerman A. Coronary endothelial dysfunction in humans is associated with myocardial perfusion defects. Circulation 1997;96:3390–3395.
9. Kemp HG. Left ventricular function in patients with angina and normal coronary angiograms. Am J Cardiol 1973;32:375–376.
10. Cannon R, Epstein S. "Microvascular angina" as a cause of chest pain with angiographically normal coronary arteries. Am J Cardiol 1988;43:1338–1343.
11. Schachinger V, Britten MB, Elsner M, et al. A positive family history of premature coronary artery disease is associated with impaired endothelium-dependent coronary blood flow regulation. Circulation 1999;100:1502–1508.
12. Nahser PJ, Brown RE, Oskarsson H, et al. Maximal coronary flow reserve and metabolic coronary vasodilation in patients with diabetes mellitus. Circulation 1995;91:635–640.
13. Kaufmann PA, Gnecci-Ruscone T, DiTerlizzi M, et al. Coronary heart disease in smokers—vitamin C restores coronary microcirculatory function. Circulation 2000;102:1233–1238.
14. Nitenberg A, Valensi P, Sachs R, et al. Impairment of coronary vascular reserve and ACh-induced coronary vasodilation in diabetic patients, angiographically normal arteries and normal left ventricular systolic function. Diabetes 1993;42:1017–1025.
15. Bartel T, Yang Y, Müller S, Wenzel RR, Baumgart D, Philipp T, Erbel R. Non-invasive assessment of microvascular function in arterial hypertension by transthroacic Doppler harmonic echocardiography. J Am Coll Cardiol 2002;39(12):2012–2018.
16. Baumgart D, Haude M, Liu F, et al. Current concepts of coronary flow reserve for clinical decision making during cardiac catheterization. Am Heart J 1998;136:136–149.
17. Ge J, Qian J, Bhate R, et al. Prevalence of microvascular dysfunction in patients with severe coronary artery disease. Eur Heart J 1999;20(Suppl):476–482.
18. Kuo L, Davies MJ, Cannon MS, Chilian WM. Pathophysiological consequences of atherosclerosis extend to the microcirculation. Circ Res 1992;70:465–476.
19. Chilian WM, Eastham CL, Layne SM, Marcus ML. Small vessel phenomena in the coronary microcirculation: phasic intramyocardial perfusion and coronary microvascular dynamics. Prog Cardiovasc Dis 1988;31:17–38.
20. Chilian WM. Coronary microcirculation in health and disease. Summary of an NHLBI workshop. Circulation 1997;95:522–528.
21. Kuo L, Davies MJ, Chilian WM. Longitudinal gradients for endothelium-dependent and -independent vascular responses in the coronary microcirculation. Circulation 1995;92:518–525.
22. Kanatsuka H, Lamping KG, Eastham CL, Marcus ML. Heterogenous changes in epimyocardial microvascular size during graded coronary stenosis. Circ Res 1990;60:389–396.
23. Axel L. Cerebral blood flow determination by rapid-sequence computed tomography. A theoretical analysis. Radiology 1980;137: 679–686.
24. Wang T, Wu S, Chung N, Ritman EL. Myocardial blood flow estimates by synchronous, multislice high-speed CT. IEEE Transact Med Imag 1989;8(1):70–77.
25. Rumberger JA, Bell MR. Measurement of myocardial perfusion using electron beam (ultrafast) computed tomography. In: Marcus ML (ed), Cardiac Imaging. A Companion to Braunwald's Heart Disease. WB Saunders, Philadelphia: 1996;835–852.
26. Stewart GN. Researches on the circulation time and on the influences that affect it. IV. The output of the heart. J Physiol 1897;22: 159–183.
27. Hamilton WF, Moore JW, Kinsman JM, Spurling RG. Studies on circulation IV. Further analysis of the injection method and of changes in hemodynamics under physiological and pathophysiological conditions. Am J Physiol 1932;99:534–551.
28. Meier P, Zierler KL. On the theory of the indicator-dilution method for measurement of blood flow and volume. J Appl Physiol 1954; 6(12):731–744.
29. Zierler KL. A simplified explanation of the theory of indicator dilution for measurement of fluid flow and volume and other distributive phenomena. Bull Johns Hopkins Hosp 1958;103:199–217.
30. Zierler KL. Theoretical basis of indicator-dilution methods for measuring flow and volume. Circ Res 1962;10:393–407.
31. Zierler KL. Equations for measuring blood flow by external monitoring of radioisotopes. Circ Res 1965:16(4):309–321.
32. Ritman EL, Kinsey JH, Robb RA, Harris LD, Gilbert BK. Physics and technical considerations in the design of the DSR: a high temporal resolution volume scanner. AJR 1980;135:369–374.
33. Boyd DP, Lipton MJ. Cardiac computed tomography. Proc IEEE 1983;71(3):298–307.
34. Wolfkiel CJ, Ferguson JL, Chomka EV, et al. Measurement of myocardial blood flow by ultrafast CT. Circulation 1987;76(6): 1262–1273.
35. Liu YH, Bahn RC, Ritman EL. Dynamic intramyocardial blood volume: evaluation with a radiological opaque marker method. Am J Physiol 1992;263:H963–H967.
36. Liu YH, Bahn RC, Ritman EL. Microvascular blood volume to flow relationship in porcine heart wall: Whole body CT evaluation in vivo. Am J Physiol 1995;269(38):H1820–1826.

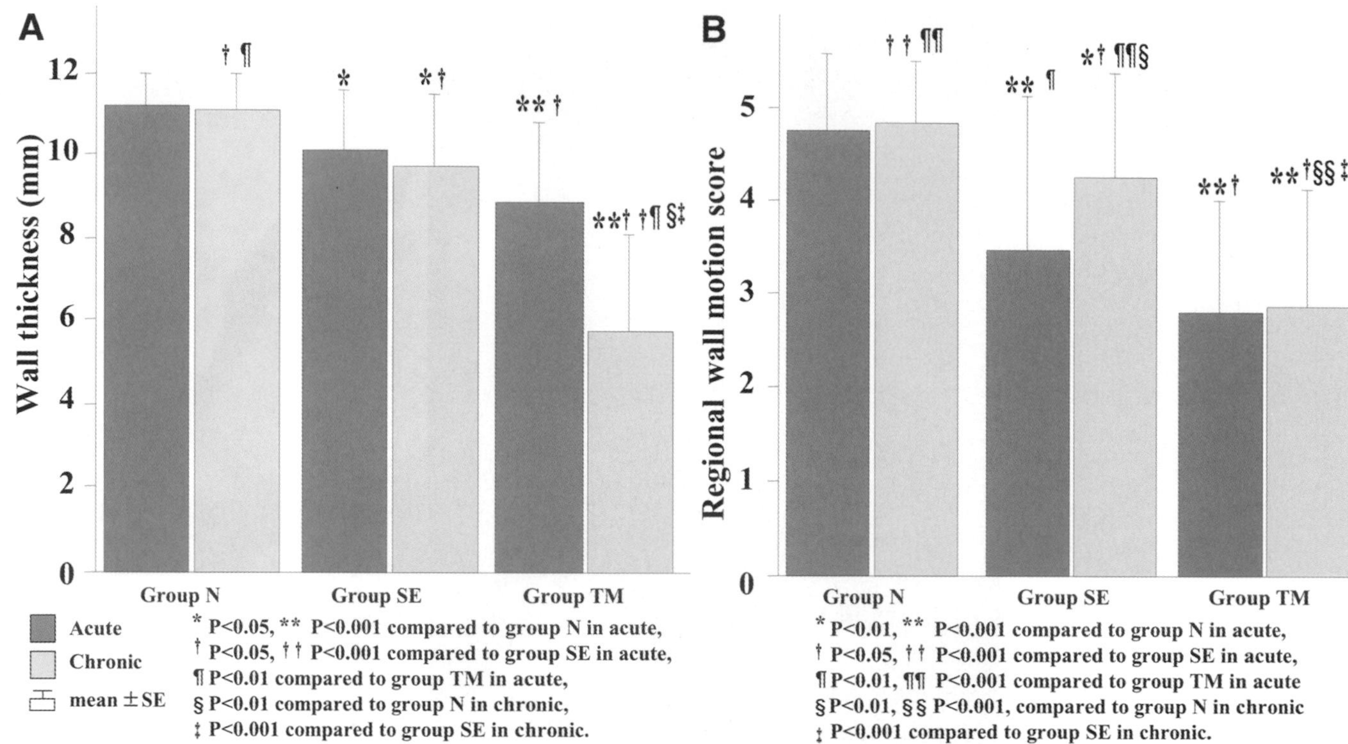

Fig. 4. **(A)** Wall motion (regional wall motion score, RWM) in the chronic phase (1 mo) in Group-N, Group-SE, and Group-TM). RWM in group-SE improved, while in Group-TM it became worse. **(B)** Wall thickness in the chronic phase (1 mo) in Group-N, Group-SE, and Group-TM). As the depth of early defect increased, wall thickness decreased in the chronic phase.

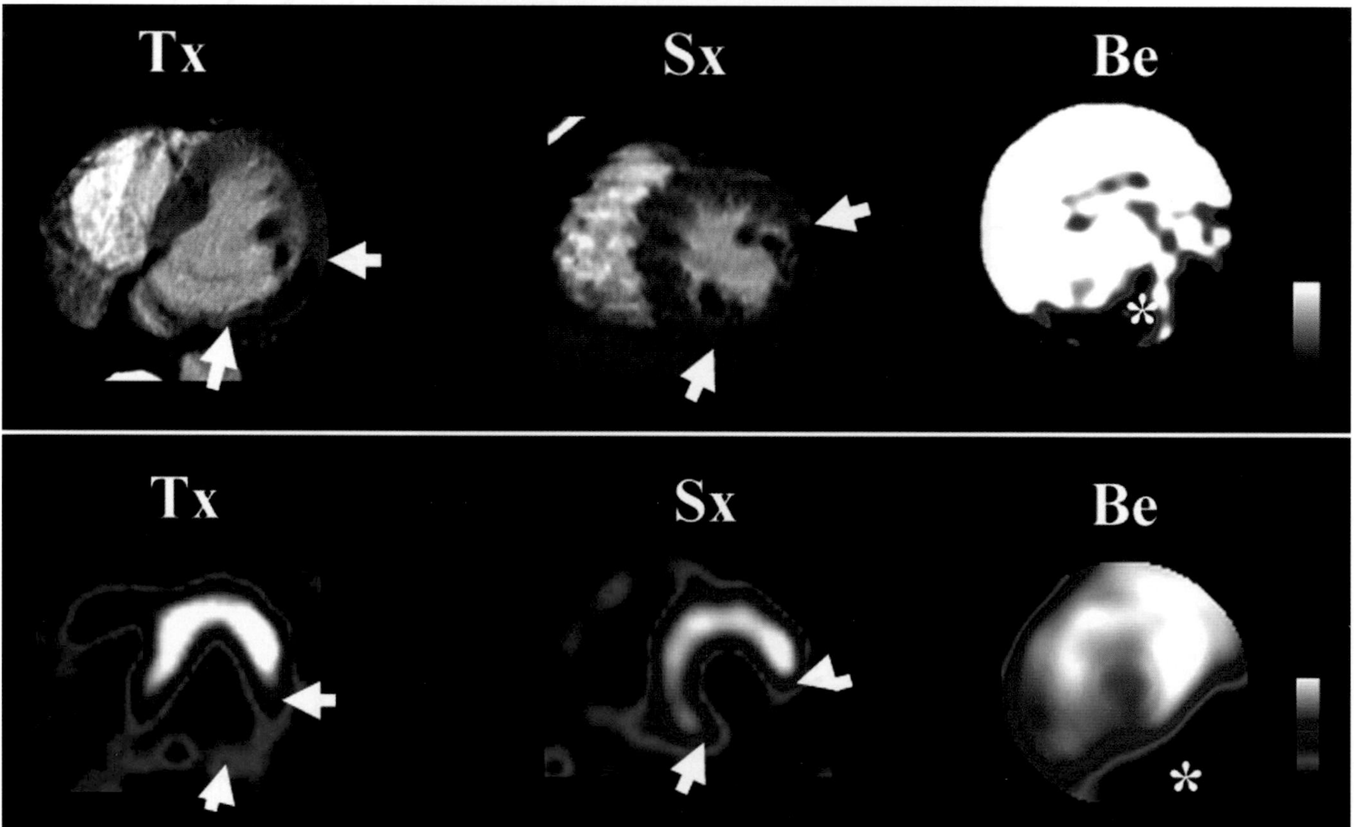

Fig. 5. A case of infero-lateral transmural acute myocardial infarction after successful primary percutaneous coronary intervention. Location and extent of the perfusion defects were well concordant. The hypoenhanced (dark) region between arrows indicates the perfusion defect by contrast-enhanced CT. Note that the perfusion defect by CT is similar in extent and location to the perfusion defect on Tl-201 myocardial perfusion single photon emission CT. Tx = transaxial image; Sx = short axis; and Be = Bull's eye map.

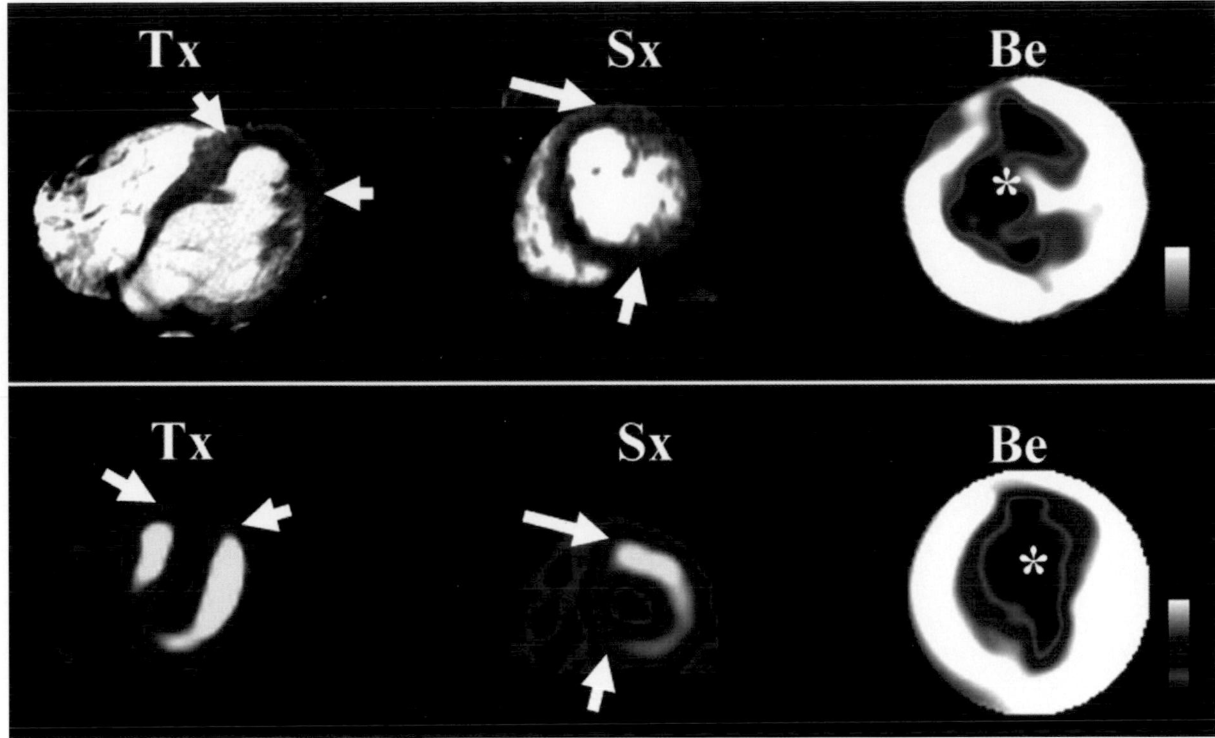

Fig. 6. A case of antero-septal transmural acute myocardial infarction after successful primary percutaneous coronary intervention. Location and extent of the perfusion defects were well concordant. The hypoenhanced (dark) region between arrows indicates the perfusion defect by contrast-enhanced CT. Note that the perfusion defect by CT is similar in extent and location to the perfusion defect on Tl-201 myocardial perfusion single photon emission CT. Tx, transaxial image; Sx, short axis; and Be, Bull's eye map.

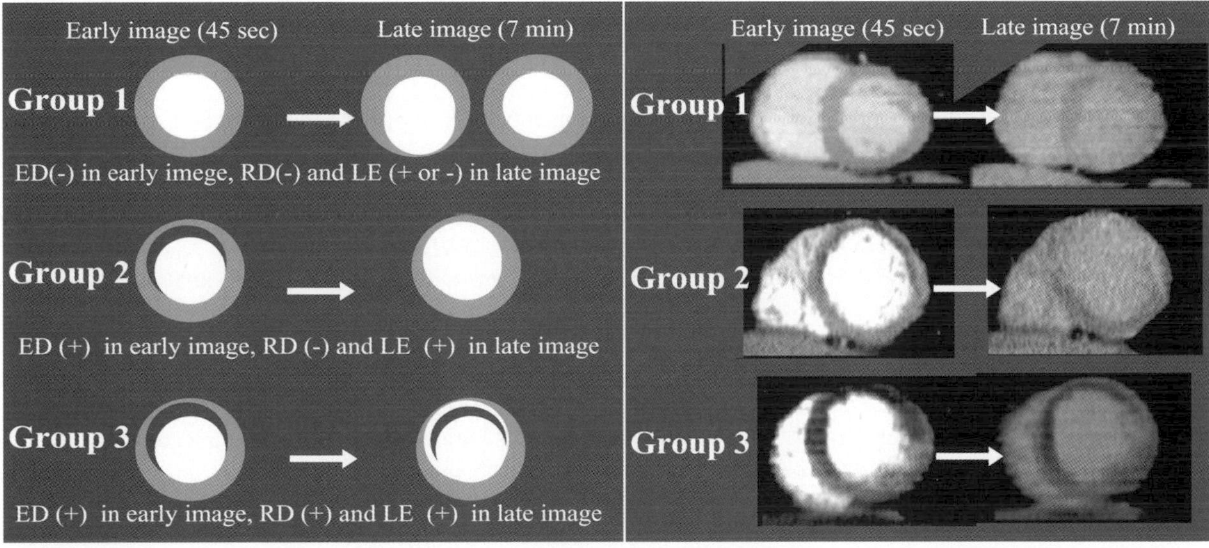

Fig. 7. Three enhancement patterns. Illustration (**A**) and typical cases (**B**). Group 1: the absence of early defect (ED) in the early phase, and the presence of late enhancement (LE) without residual defect (RD) in the late phase. Group 2: the presence of ED in the early phase, and the presence of LE without RD in the late phase. Group 3: the presence of ED in the early phase, and the presence of both LE and RD.

yield a more detailed prediction of functional recovery in the chronic phase.

The protocol for the contrast-enhanced CT was as follows. A nonion iodine contrast medium (300 mg iodine/mL) was intravenously administrated at a rate of 1.5 mL/s for the first (early) scan, with the early image being taken 45 s after the start of the administration. Then the same contrast medium was infused at a rate of 0.1 mL/s for the second scan to acquire the late image, which was taken 7 min after the start of the administration. A total of 150 mL of the contrast medium was used.

CLASSIFICATION OF ENHANCEMENT PATTERNS

Enhancement patterns can be classified into three groups (Fig. 7): Group 1, the absence of ED in the early phase, and the presence of LE without RD in the late phase; Group 2, the

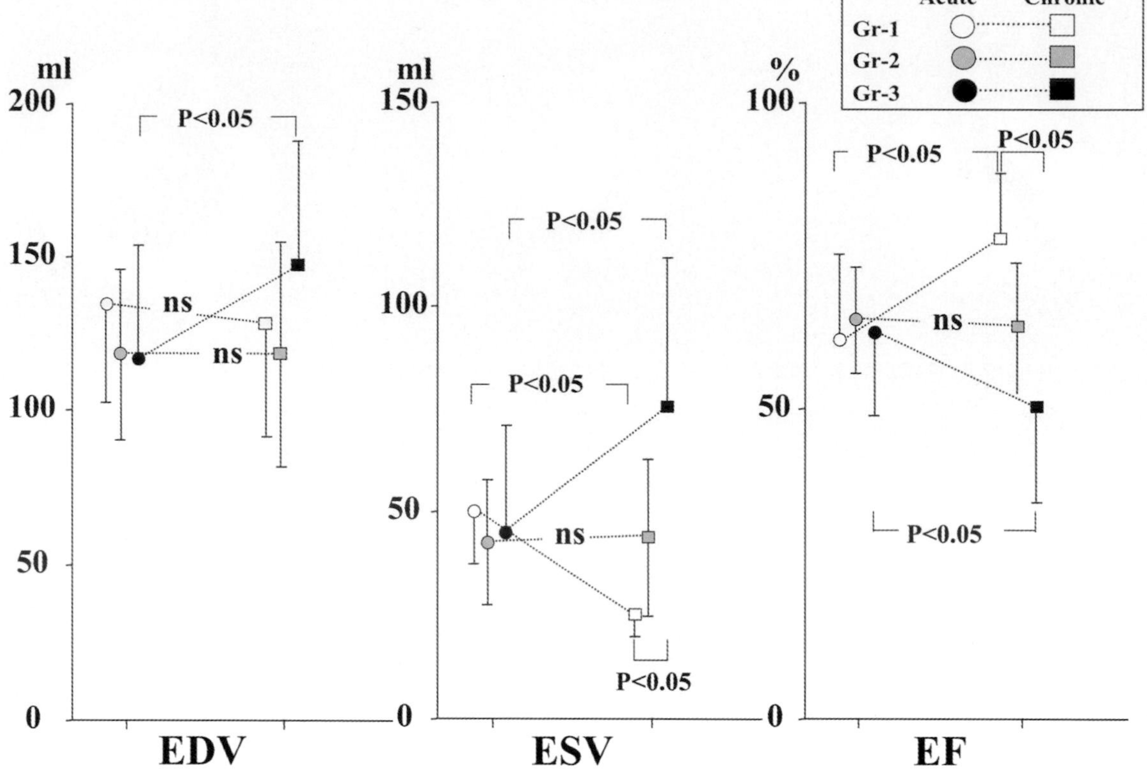

Fig. 8. Left-ventricular volume (end-diastolic volume [EDV], end-systolic volume [ESV] and functional parameters (left-ventricular ejection fraction) in Group 1 to 3 are summarized. In Group 1, the ejection fraction (EF) significantly improved from 61 ± 14% to 78 ± 10% ($p < 0.05$). In Group 2, the EF was not significantly different. In Group 3, the EDV significantly increased from 117 ± 38 mL to 147 ± 41 mL and the EF significantly decreased from 63 ± 13% to 51 ± 15%.

presence of ED in the early phase, and the presence of LE without RD in the late phase; and Group 3, the presence of ED in the early phase, and the presence of both LE and RD in the late phase. Figure 7B shows typical cases of the enhancement patterns.

ENHANCEMENT PATTERNS ON TWO-PHASE CONTRAST-ENHANCED CT VS LEFT-VENTRICULAR FUNCTION AND VOLUME IN THE CHRONIC PHASE *(17)*

Thirty AMI patients, after successful PCI (4.3 ± 1.2 h after onset), underwent a two-phase contrast-enhanced CT (37 ± 4 h after direct angioplasty). Conventional LVG was performed immediately after the PCI as the acute study. They had both coronary angiography (CAG) and LVG as the chronic study (28 ± 3 d).

COMPARISON OF LEFT-VENTRICULAR VOLUME AND FUNCTION IN EACH GROUP BY CONVENTIONAL LVG

The left-ventricular volume and functional parameters (end-diastolic volume [EDV], end-systolic volume [ESV], and ejection fraction [EF]) in each group are summarized in Fig. 8. In Group 1, the left-ventricular ejection fraction (LV-EF) improved. In Group 2, the LVEF was not significantly different. In Group 3, the EDV increased and the LV-EF decreased.

The lack of evidence of the ED, as seen in Group 1, indicates a functional improvement in the chronic phase. Residual defect, as seen in Group 3, indicates the worst functional outcome, i.e., deterioration in the chronic phase. Diminishment of the ED, as seen in Group 2, exhibited an intermediate functional recovery between Group 1 and Group 3. Thus, two-phase contrast-enhanced CT predicts left-ventricular functional recovery in patients with AMI after successful reperfusion therapy.

ENHANCEMENT PATTERNS ON TWO-PHASE CONTRAST-ENHANCED CT VS ^{201}TL/^{99M}TC-PYROPHOSPHATE DUAL-ISOTOPE SPECT

Patients with RD > LE zones showed a perfusion defect of ^{201}Tl and strong uptake of ^{99m}Tc-pyrophosphate (*see* Note 3). Patients with RD < LE zones showed an overlap of ^{201}Tl and ^{99m}Tc- pyrophosphate.

A few patients with subendocardial-early defects, having only wide LE without RD, showed normal perfusion without ^{99m}Tc-pyrophsphate accumulations. Thus, a large RD compared with LE indicates the least viability. In other words, RD in the late image suggests an abundance of necrotic tissue injured by AMI. Fig. 9 shows a comparison of two-phase contrast-enhanced CT with ^{201}Tl/^{99m}Tc-pyrophosphate dual isotope SPECT.

THE MEANING OF EACH ENHANCEMENT PATTERN

SIGNIFICANCE OF AN ED

The contrast medium is thought to reach the microvascular bed in the early phase after an intravenous administration. An EBCT study *(13)* reported that myocardial enhancement in the early phase reflected the volume of the vascular bed.

Recently, reduced signal intensity on first-pass MRI contrast images has been shown to indicate reduced blood flow *(18)*. Therefore, the ED observed on CT would also reflect a

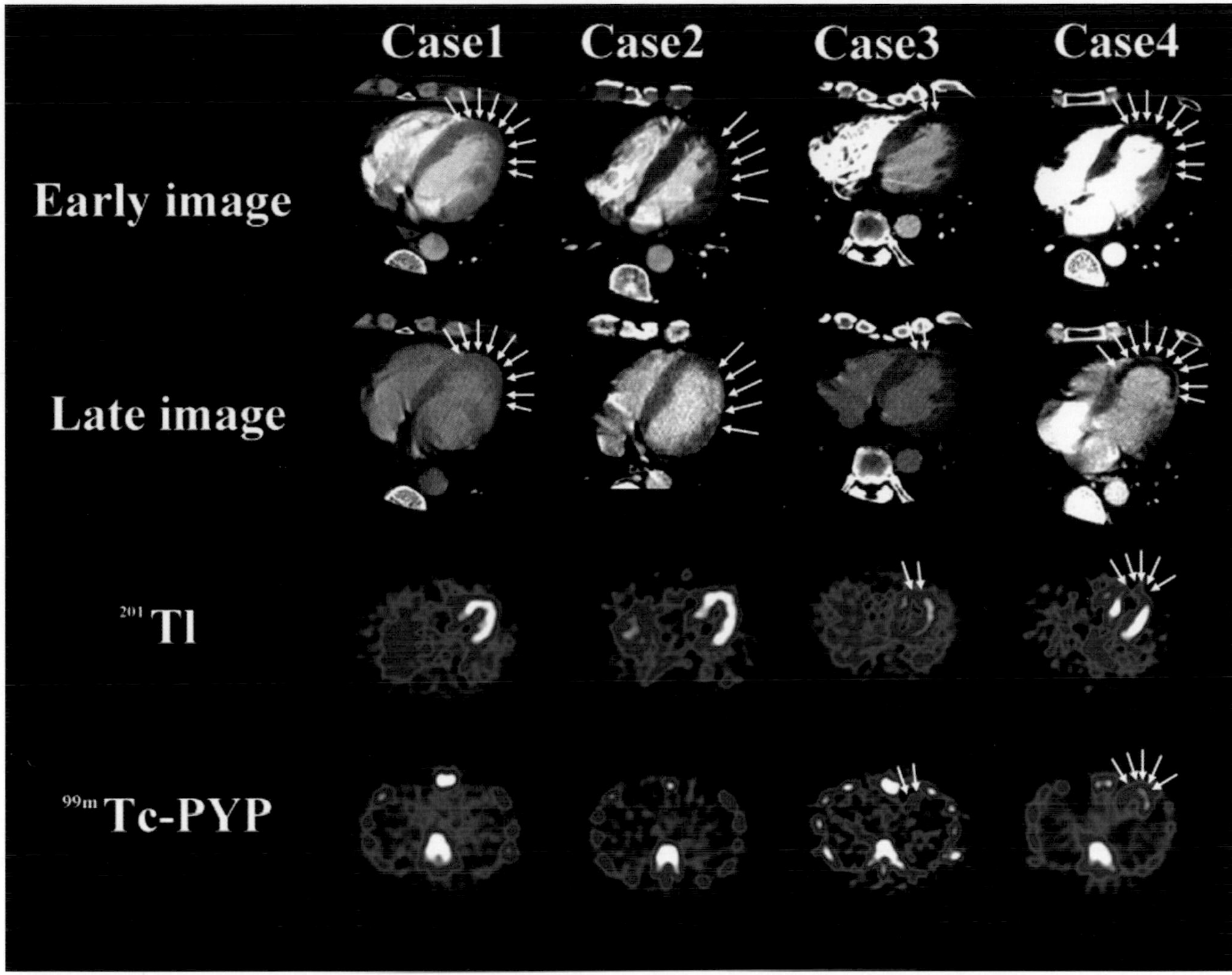

Fig. 9. Comparison of two-phase contrast-enhanced CT with ^{201}Tl/^{99m}Tc-pyrophosphate dual isotope single photon emission CT. Case 1 was a patient with acute myocardial infarction (AMI) after left ascending coronary artery reperfusion (white arrows), such as Group 1 (an almost normal enhancement pattern of CT), who had a normal uptake of ^{201}Tl and an absence of ^{99m}Tc-pyrophosphate (^{99m}Tc-PYP) accumulations. Case 3 was a patient with AMI after left ascending coronary artery reperfusion, and Case 4 was a patient with AMI after left ascending coronary artery reperfusion, such as Group 3 (early defect [ED] (+), late enhancement [LE] (+), residual defect [RD] (+)). The ED is similar to the uptake of ^{201}Tl. However, subendo-ED of Case 2, who was a patient with AMI after circumflex coronary artery reperfusion, such as Group 2 (ED [+], LE [+], RD [-]), had a mismatch of uptake of ^{201}Tl and ED. Especially the infracted area of LE in Case 2 had an absence of ^{99m}Tc-PYP, on the other hand, the infarct area of LE with small RD of Case 3 had a small accumulation of ^{99m}Tc-PYP. That is, LE was not the necrotic area of AMI. RDs in Case 3 and Case 4 appear to be the necrotic areas, because these RD areas correlated well with the accumulation of ^{99m}Tc-PYP. These findings are important in evaluating the myocardial viability of using CT.

decrease in the volume of the vascular bed, i.e., a decrease of the myocardial blood flow.

Using an experimental infarct-reperfusion model in dogs, Braunwald et al. *(19)* classified the condition of myocardial tissue into four layers from the endocardial side. The first layer corresponded to a viable and very thin myocardium, receiving oxygen directly from the left ventricle; the second layer to myocardial necrosis with extensive capillary (microcirculation) disorder; the third layer to myocardial necrosis, in which blood supply was preserved to some extent; and the fourth layer to stunned myocardium that had escaped from necrosis.

The ED in our study may correspond to myocardial necrosis with extensive capillary (microcirculation) disorder, or to myocardial necrosis in which blood supply was preserved to some extent—that is, tissue showed mild to severe microvascular damage and myocardial necrosis, owing to the wall thickness in Group 2 and Group 3, showing that the ED was significantly reduced.

SIGNIFICANCE OF RD AND LE

After the contrast medium reaches the microvascular bed, it gradually flows into the interstitium (extracellular space), remains for some time, and then washed out slowly. Therefore, myocardial enhancement in the late phase mainly reflects the characteristics of the interstitium—that is, the volume of the interstitial space *(12,13)*.

When the RD was detected, as in Group 3, functional recovery was not observed. However, when ED turned into LE, as in Group 2, deterioration of left-ventricular function was minimal, or less than that observed in Group 3. We speculate that the area of the RD might correspond to myocardial necrosis with extensive capillary disorder—i.e., microvascular no-reflow—and that LE might correspond to the layer where blood supply was preserved to some degree, indicating the possibility of residual myocardial viability, although microvascular flow was disturbed by edema within 48 h after PCI.

Considering the findings of SPECT studies and our results, we conclude that the RD indicated a necrotic area as a result of severe microvascular obstruction "microvascular no-reflow" by red blood cells and necrotic debris *(20)*, as seen in the "wave front" phenomenon of ischemic necrosis *(21,22)*. Since the presence of ^{99m}Tc-pyrophosphate in Group 3 was well correlated with RD, the myocardial enhancement pattern in Group 3 indicates less antegrade microvascular flow beyond the point of microvascular obstruction than seen in Group-2. As a result of the incomplete perfusion in the microvascular level, the necrotic area of Group 3 increased among three groups.

Basically, the pharmacokinetic properties of X-ray contrast agents are similar to those of the well-known gadolinium complexes *(23–25)* for MRI. Judd et al. reported that the hyperintense regions observed on delayed MRI images were generally smaller than the risk region and larger than regions of necrosis as defined by triphenyltetrazolium chloride staining *(26)*. This would indicate that at least part of the delayed hyperintense region was viable myocardium. Yokota et al. investigated Gd-enhanced MRI images 5 to 10 min after an intravenous gadopentate dimeglumine (Gd-DTPA) injection in patients with nonreperfused myocardial infarction *(27)*. They qualitatively analyzed Gd-enhanced MRI findings in relation to peak creatine phosphokinase levels, wall motion, and coronary angiography, and concluded that subendocardial or transmural hyper-enhancement could reflect the existence of viable myocardium, while subendocardial hypoenhancement was associated with necrotic myocardium.

In general, there is a consensus that delayed hyper-enhancement on MRI reflects nonviable myocardium *(28)*. But in our study, the LE presented both in Group 1 and in Group 2, indicating that the LE included viable myocardium, at least in contrast-enhanced CT studies within 48 h after reperfusion therapy, as seen in our results in this chapter.

The myocardium and the microvasculature changes dynamically during the healing stage in the acute phase after successful reperfusion; therefore, timing of the CT study after reperfusion therapy is important in order to assess the myocardial enhancement pattern with contrast-enhanced CT.

RELATIONSHIP BETWEEN ED, RD, AND THE NO-REFLOW PHENOMENON

The causes of the no-reflow phenomenon include experimental obstruction of the lumen of vascular vessels by neutrophils or platelets, compression towing to edema of myocardial cells out of the vascular vessels, and a change in the viscosity of blood *(29)*.

In our study, the ED and RD existed even after successful reperfusion at the epicardial coronary artery level and improvement of coronary blood flow, indicating that the circulation disorder at the level of coronary microcirculation level, that is, the no-reflow at the regional microcirculation level, still persisted after successful reperfusion. Additionally, in patients showing RD in our study, this no-reflow phenomenon exists, regardless of its various degrees and causes, in the coronary microcirculation system after successful reperfusion in coronary arteriography. We believe that the no-reflow at the level of regional microcirculation is involved in decreases in cardiac function and wall motion in the chronic phase.

We conclude that contrast-enhanced CT is useful in evaluating myocardial enhancement, which may serve as a predictor of changes in wall motion and thickness, left-ventricular function, and myocardial viability after PCI in patients with AMI.

PITFALLS OF ENHANCEMENT PATTERNS

In the assessment of perfusion, there are some pitfalls.

In patients with old myocardial infarction, or re-AMI, we may also detect lipid degeneration in the left-ventricular myocardium (Fig. 10A). This is always clearly detectable in plain images without the administration of a contrast medium. This should not be interpreted as ED or RD on two-phase contrast-enhanced CT. In patients with old myocardial infarction, or re-AMI, we may detect a thrombus in the left ventriculum (Fig. 10B), which is always clearly detectable in both early and late images. This should not be misinterpreted as ED or RD. In patients with old myocardial infarction or re-AMI, we may even detect calcium in the left-ventricular myocardium (Fig. 10C). This is clearly detectable in plain CT, and should not be misinterpreted as LE on two-phase contrast-enhanced CT.

STUDY LIMITATIONS AND FUTURE OF MDCT

ADVANTAGES OF CARDIAC CT FOR PATIENTS WITH AMI

The advantages of cardiac CT are generally as follows: (1) no blind area; (2) shorter acquisition time (less than 30 s); (3) metal devices such as an infusion pump, pacemaker, and intra-aortic balloon pump (IABP) are acceptable, whereas they are commonly contraindicated for MRI, and therefore the CT is able to utilize them for the acute phase of AMI; (4) coronary arteries can be evaluated with the same data.

DISADVANTAGES OF CT FOR PATIENTS WITH AMI

The disadvantages of CT over other noninvasive modalities are the use of an iodine contrast medium (however, there were neither major nor minor complications in this study) and X-ray exposure of the two-phase contrast CT. Although the two-phase study requires double dose compared to the single-phase study, overlapping reconstruction does not increase the radiation dose—i.e., it is exactly the same as nonoverlapping reconstruction. The exposed range for cardiac CT (12 cm) is smaller than that of whole-lung or abdominal CT scans. Therefore, the radiation dose is not a limitation.

CLINICAL IMPLICATIONS OF CARDIAC CT

Although cardiac CT is a retrospective analysis, and not a real-time analysisas is echocardiography, it provides a lot of information from data obtained during a 30-s breath-hold acquisition *(30–35)*. The assessment of the myocardial enhance-ment patterns was one of clinical implications of cardiac CT.

NOTES

1. TIMI grade: grade 0 perfusion is no antegrade flow beyond the point of occlusion; grade 1 is minimal incomplete per-

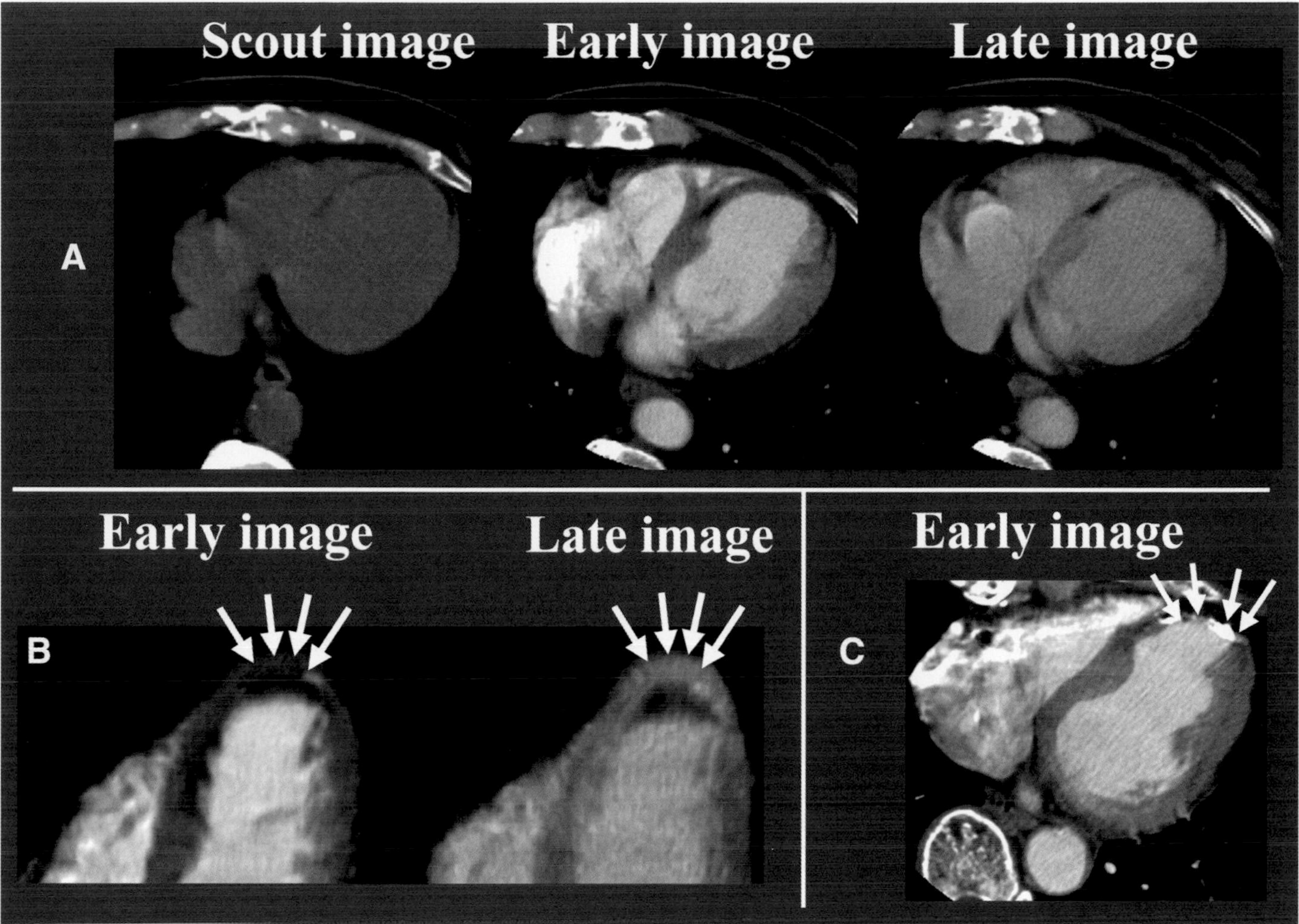

Fig. 10. Pitfalls of enhancement patterns. Fatty degeneration in old myocardial infarction (**A**). Left-ventricular thrombus (**B**). Left-ventricular calcium deposit (**C**).

fusion of the contrast medium around the clot; grade 2 (partial perfusion) is complete but delayed perfusion of the distal coronary bed with contrast material; and grade 3 (complete perfusion) is antegrade flow to the entire distal bed at a normal rate.

2. TIMI myocardial perfusion grade (TMPG): in TMPG 0, there is minimal or no myocardial blush; in TMPG 1, dye stains the myocardium and this stain persists until the next injection; in TMPG 2, dye enters the myocardium but washes out slowly so that the dye is strongly persistent at the end of the injection; and in TMPG 3, there is normal entrance and exit of dye in the myocardium so that dye is mildly persistent at the end of the injection.
3. ^{99m}Tc-pyrophosphate localizes to denatured proteins within the mitochondria in areas of myocardial necrosis, highlighting AMI region during the 7 to 10 d after the onset.

ACKNOWLEDGMENTS

We are grateful to Taketoshi Ito, MD, Hiroshi Matsuoka, MD, Hiroshi Higashino, MD, Hideo Kawakami., MD, Jun Aono, MD, Kana Sakamoto, MD, and Junko Kato, MD, in the Department of Cardiology and Radiology, Imabari Hospital; Kazuhisa Nishimura, MD, Hideki Okayama, MD, Takumi Sumimoto, MD, in the Kitaishikai Hospital; and Shigru Nakata, RT, Katsuji Inoue, MD, Tsuyoshi Matsunaka, MD, and Jitsuo Higaki, MD, the Chairman of the 2nd Department of Internal Medicine in Ehime University School of Medicine, for their excellent assistance in publication. We are very grateful to Masaya Doi, RT, Masato Imai, RT, Yasuyuki Takahashi, RT, Hideyuki Chiba, RT, Takashi Okamoto, RT, Isao Ouchi, RT, and Hiroshi Miguchi, RT, for their excellent technical assistance.

REFERENCES

1. Gibson CM, Cannon CP, Murphy SA, et al. Relationship of TIMI myocardial perfusion grade to mortality after administration of thrombolytic drugs. Circulation 2000;101:125–130.
2. Abe M, Kazatani Y, Fukuda H, Tatsuno H, Habara H, Shinbata H. Left ventricular volumes, ejection fraction, and regional wall motion calculated with gated technetium-99m tetrofosmin SPECT in reperfused acute myocardial infarction at super-acute phase: comparison with left ventriculography. J Nucl Cardiol 2000;7:569–574.
3. Watanabe K, Sekiya M, Ikeda S, Miyagawa M, Kinoshita M, Kumano S. Comparison of adenosine triphosphate and dipyridamole in diagnosis by thallium-201 myocardial scintigraphy. J Nucl Med 1997;38:577–581.
4. Al-Saadi N, Nagel E, Gross M, et al. Noninvasive detection of myocardial ischemia from perfusion reserve based on cardiovascular magnetic resonance. Circulation 2000;101:1379–1383.

5. Rogers WJ Jr, Kramer CM, Geskin G, et al. Early contrast-enhanced MRI predicts late functional recovery after reperfused myocardial infarction. Circulation 1999;99:744–750.
6. Pislaru SV, Ni Y, Pislaru C, et al. Noninvasive measurements of infarct size after thrombolysis with a necrosis-avid MRI contrast agent. Circulation 1999;99:690–696.
7. Bogaert J, Maes A, Van de Werf F, et al. Functional recovery of subepicardial myocardial tissue in transmural myocardial infarction after successful reperfusion: an important contribution to the improvement of regional and global left ventricular function. Circulation 1999;99:36–43.
8. Ito H, Tomooka T, Sakai N, et al. Lack of myocardial perfusion immediately after successful thrombolysis. A predictor of poor recovery of left ventricular function in anterior myocardial infarction. Circulation 1992;85:1699–1705.
9. Scherrer-Crosbie M, Liel-Cohen N, Otsuji Y, et al. Myocardial perfusion and wall motion in infarction border zone: assessment by myocardial contrast echocardiography. J Am Soc Echocardiogr 2000;13:353–357.
10. Lepper W, Hoffmann R, Kamp O, et al. Assessment of myocardial reperfusion by intravenous myocardial contrast echocardiography and coronary flow reserve after primary percutaneous transluminal coronary angioplasty [correction of angiography] in patients with acute myocardial infarction. Circulation 2000;101:2368–2374.
11. Hamada S, Naito H, Takamiya M. Evaluation of myocardium in ischemic heart disease by ultrafast computed tomography. Jpn Circ J 1992;56:627–631.
12. Naito H, Saito H, Takamiya M, et al. Quantitative assessment of myocardial enhancement with iodinated contrast medium in patients with ischemic heart disease by using ultrafast x-ray computed tomography. Invest Radiol 1992;27:436–442.
13. Naito H, Saito H, Ohta M, Takamiya M. Significance of ultrafast computed tomography in cardiac imaging: usefulness in assessment of myocardial characteristics and cardiac function. Jpn Circ J 1990; 54:322–327.
14. Koyama Y, Matsuoka H, Higashino H, et al. Wall motion and wall thickness analysis of after receiving successful reperfusion therapy in acute myocardial infarction: an assessment of early perfusion defect by enhanced helical CT. Jpn J Interv Cardiol 2001;16: 233–242.
15. Koyama Y, Matsuoka H, Higasino H, et al. Assessment of Myocardial Infarct Volume by Contrast Enhancement CT. The Radiological Society of North America 87th Scientific Assembly and Annual Meeting November 25–30, 2001 Supplement to Radiology 2001; 221(P):196.
16. Koyama Y, Matsuoka H, Higasino H, et al. Assessment of Myocardial Infarct Size by Contrast Enhanced CT. American Heart Association Scientific Sessions 2001, November 11–14, 2001 Supplement to Circulation 2001;104(17):II-477.
17. Koyama Y, Matsuoka H, Higasino H, et al. Early Myocardial Perfusion Defect and Late Enhancement on Enhancement CT Predict Clinical Outcome in Patients with Acute Myocardial Infarction after Reperfusion Therapy. The Radiological Society of North America 87th Scientific Assembly and Annual Meeting November 25–30, 2001. Supplement to Radiology 2001;221(P):196.
18. Rochitte CE, Lima JA, Bluemke DA, et al. Magnitude and time course of microvascular obstruction and tissue injury after acute myocardial infarction. Circulation 1998;98:1006–1014.
19. Braunwald E, Kloner RA. Myocardial reperfusion: a double-edged sword? J Clin Invest 1985;76:1713–1719.
20. Engler RL, Schmid-Schonbein GW, Pavelec RS. Leukocyte capillary plugging in myocardial ischemia and reperfusion in the dog. Am J Pathol 1983;111:98–111.
21. Reimer KA, Lowe JE, Rasmussen MM, Jennings RB. The wavefront phenomenon of ischemic cell death. 1. Myocardial infarct size vs duration of coronary occlusion in dogs. Circulation 1977;56:786–794.
22. Reimer KA, Jennings RB. The "wavefront phenomenon" of myocardial ischemic cell death. II. Transmural progression of necrosis within the framework of ischemic bed size (myocardium at risk) and collateral flow. Lab Invest 1979;40:633–644.
23. Mutzel W, Speck U, Weinmann HJ. Pharmacokinetics of iopromide in rat and dog. Fortschr Geb Rontgenstrahlen Nuklearmed Erganzungsbd 1983;118:85–90.
24. Allard M, Doucet D, Kien P, Bonnemain B, Caille JM. Experimental study of DOTA-gadolinium. Pharmacokinetics and pharmacologic properties. Invest Radiol 1988;23 Suppl 1:S271–274.
25. Tauber U, Mutzel W, Schulze PE. Whole body autoradiographic distribution studies on nonionic x-ray contrast agents in pregnant rats. Fortschr Geb Rontgenstrahlen Nuklearmed Erganzungsbd 1989;128:215–219
26. Judd RM, Lugo-Olivieri CH, Arai M, et al. Physiological basis of myocardial contrast enhancement in fast magnetic resonance images of 2-day-old reperfused canine infarcts. Circulation 1995;92: 1902–1910.
27. Yokota C, Nonogi H, Miyazaki S, et al. Gadolinium-enhanced magnetic resonance imaging in acute myocardial infarction. Am J Cardiol 1995;75:577–581.
28. Wu K, Zerhouni E, Judd R, et al. Prognostic significance of microvascular obstruction by magnetic resonance imaging in patients with acute myocardial infarction. Circulation 1998;97:765–772.
29. Engler RL, Schmid-Schönbein GW, Pavelec RS. Leukocyte capillary plugging in myocardial ischemia and reperfusion in the dog. Am J Pathol 1983;111:98–111.
30. Becker CR, Ohnesorge BM, Schoepf UJ, Reiser MF. Current development of cardiac imaging with multidetector-row CT. Eur J Radiol 2000;36:97–103.
31. Mochizuki T, Murase K, Higashino H, et al. Two- and three-dimensional CT ventriculography: a new application of helical CT. AJR 2000;174:203–208.
32. Mochizuki T, Murase K, Koyama Y, Higashino H, Ikezoe J. LAD stenosis detected by subsecond spiral CT. Circulation 1999;99:1523.
33. Mochizuki T, Koyama Y, Tanaka H, Ikezoe J, Shen Y, Azemoto S. Left ventricular thrombus detected by two- and three-dimensional computed tomographic ventriculography: a new application of helical CT. Circulation 1998;98:933–934.
34. Koyama Y, Matsuoka H, Higasino H, et al. Four-dimensional cardiac image by helical computed tomography. Circulation 1999;100:e61–e62.
35. Koyama Y, Matsuoka H, Higashino H, et al. Left ventricular hypertrophy demonstrated by four-dimensional myocardiography by helical computed tomography. Circulation 2001;103:e15–e17.

CONTRAST-ENHANCED CT OF THE HEART: V

CORONARY ARTERIES

21 Anatomy of the Coronary Arteries and Veins in CT Imaging

Robert J. M. van Geuns, MD and Filippo Cademartiri, MD

INTRODUCTION

The cardiologist and radiologist interpreting coronary computed tomography angiography (CTA) should be familiar with coronary artery anatomy. It has a standard logical structure with some common variations and only a few rare abnormalities. In a conventional selective coronary angiography, blood in the chambers and coronary veins does not interfere with the visualization of the coronary arteries. In addition, myocardium and other soft tissues are hardly seen because of their low absorption of X-rays. Invasive selective coronary angiograms use projections performed in various orientations so that the cardiologist can perceive the 3D anatomy of the coronary arteries. This is quite different for imaging techniques such as CTA. In CTA the contrast agent is intravenously injected, which results in enhancement of the myocardium and blood in the cavities, and projection techniques such as maximum intensity projection (MIP) are therefore of limited use. Overlap of structures that obscure coronary imaging can be avoided by multiplanar reformation (MPR) using thin slices in any desired orientation. However, in that case much of the 3D information is not used. With modern postprocessing tools, such as MIP or the volume-rendering technique (VRT), 3D impressions on a 2D surface can be created. These images look much like the gross anatomy of the heart, but they do not resemble the images known from invasive selective coronary angiography. In this chapter we will therefore review the normal coronary artery and venous anatomy as it may be seen on MPR and VRT images of CTA. We will also review the anomalies that may be encountered during investigations for coronary artery disease.

CORONARY ARTERY ANATOMY

LEFT CORONARY ARTERY

The left main coronary artery (LCA) arises from the left posterior aortic sinus. In tomographic imaging, the preferred orientation displays the left of the patient in the right side of the images, as when the patient is viewed from the feet. In such images the LCA starts at the right side of the aorta just posterior to the right-ventricular outflow tract (Fig. 1). Its length is variable, but usually 1–2 cm *(1)*. In a small proportion of cases, the LCA is very short and bifurcates almost immediately. In 0.41% of the cases, the LCA is not developed and there are two orifices in the left coronary sinus *(2)*. In two-thirds of the subjects, the main LCA divides beneath the left atrial appendix, into the left anterior descending (LAD) and the circumflex arteries. When using VRTs for off-line evaluation, the atrial appendix is usually excluded from the data set (Fig. 2) *(3)*. The LAD artery passes to the left of the pulmonary trunk and turns forwards to run downwards in the anterior interventricular groove towards the apex. When MPR is used for evaluation of CTA data sets, a series of parallel slices or curved MPR along the intraventricular groove have to be created for optimal visualization of the vessel (Fig. 3). The LAD artery provides two main groups of branches. First, the septal branches, which supply the anterior two-thirds of the septum, and second, the diagonal branches, which lie on the lateral aspect of the left ventricle. The septal branches arise form the LAD at approximately 90-degree angles. They vary in size, number, and distribution. The first large septal branch may divide into a fork where both branches run parallel into the septum. In other cases, a septal branch may run parallel to the LAD through the myocardium of the septum. By convention, the first septal branch separates the proximal LAD from the middle part of the LAD. The diagonals also vary in number and course (Fig. 4). Usually at least one diagonal is present, and if none is visualized, a total occlusion may be expected. A normal variation of the large diagonal is a parallel course to the LAD. In the majority of the patients, the LAD itself courses around the apex to reach the inferior wall and septum. In the other cases, the distal right coronary artery (RCA) is larger and supplies the blood flow for the apex. This is one of the potential collateral routes if either the RCA or LAD is occluded. The left circumflex artery (LCx) turns backwards shortly beyond its origin to run downwards in the left arterioventricular groove. It too gives rise to a variable number of branches, which lie on the lateral aspect of the left ventricle (the marginal branches, Fig. 4). In one-third of the subjects, the left main coronary artery trifurcates into the aforementioned branches and an intermediate artery, which follows a course between the circumflex and LAD arteries over the anterolateral wall of the left ventricle (Fig. 5) *(3)*. Additional branches of the LCx are small atrial branches that supply the lateral and posterior regions of the left atrium.

From: *Contemporary Cardiology: CT of the Heart: Principles and Applications*
Edited by: U. Joseph Schoepf © Humana Press, Inc., Totowa, NJ

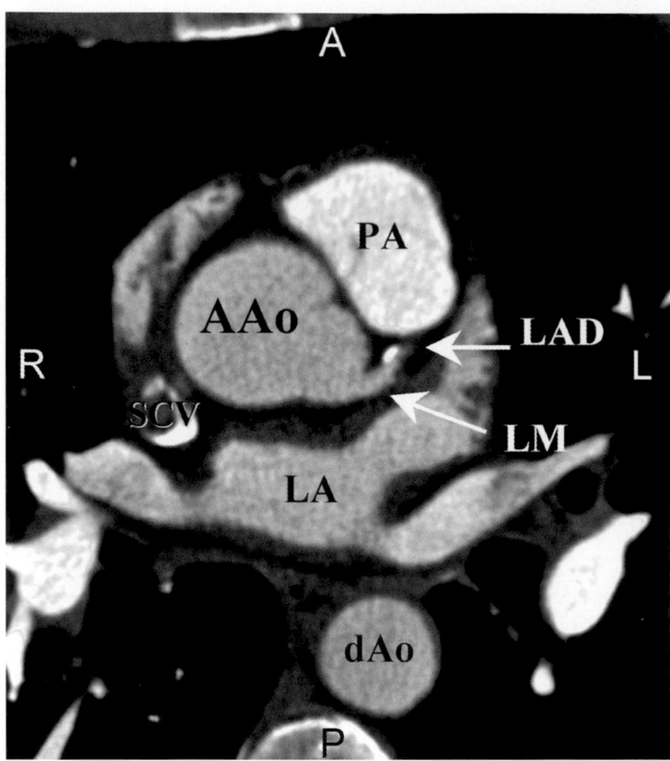

Fig. 1. Transverse slice through the aortic root. The left main coronary artery (LM) can clearly be seen, the proximal left anterior descending artery (LAD) turns around the pulmonary artery (PA) anteriorly. AAo, ascending aorta; SCV, superior caval vein; LA, left atrium; dAo, descending aorta; A, anterior thoracic wall; P, posterior (spine); L, left; R, right.

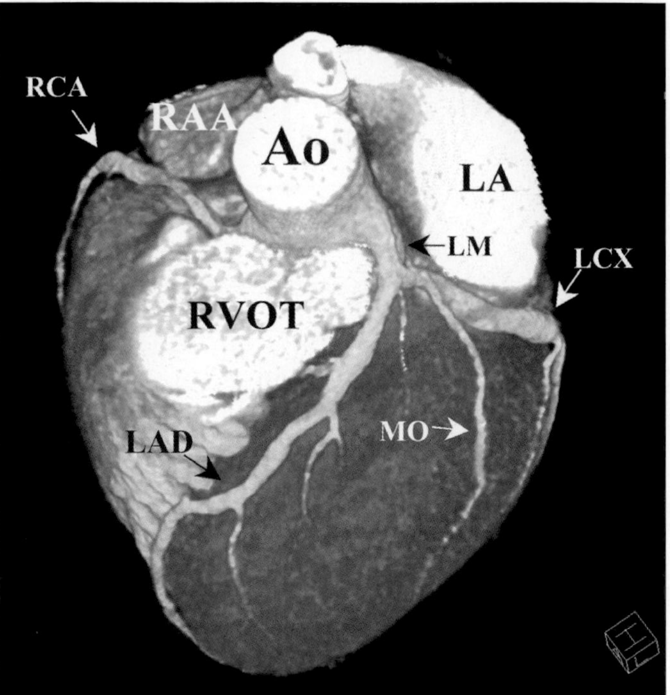

Fig. 2. Volume rendering of the left coronary artery after removal of the left atrial appendage and cranial part of the left atrium (LA) in the original topographic slices over 15 levels. Without this processing tool, the left atrial appendage normally overlaps the left main (LM) and proximal circumflex coronary artery (LCX). The right atrial appendage (RAA) may sometimes override the right coronary artery (RCA), but in this case manual removal was not necessary. LAD, left anterior descending coronary artery; RVOT, right-ventricular outflow tract; MO, margo obtusus of the circumflex coronary artery.

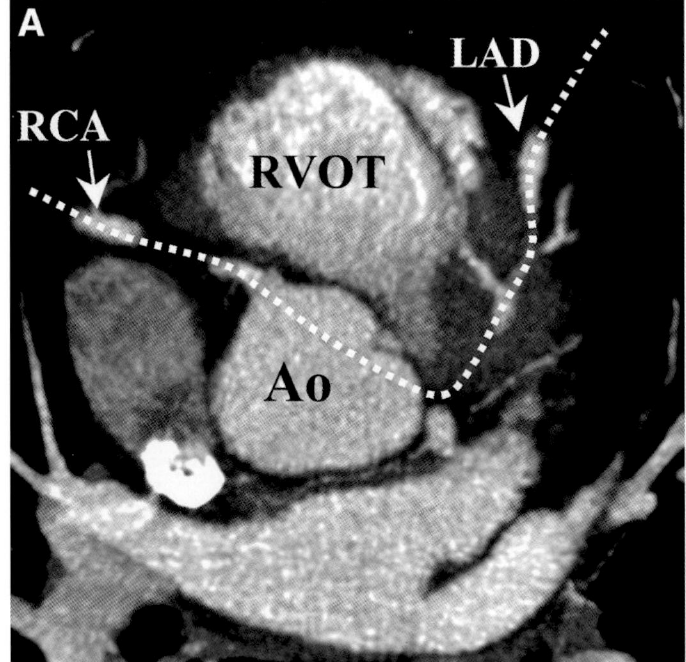

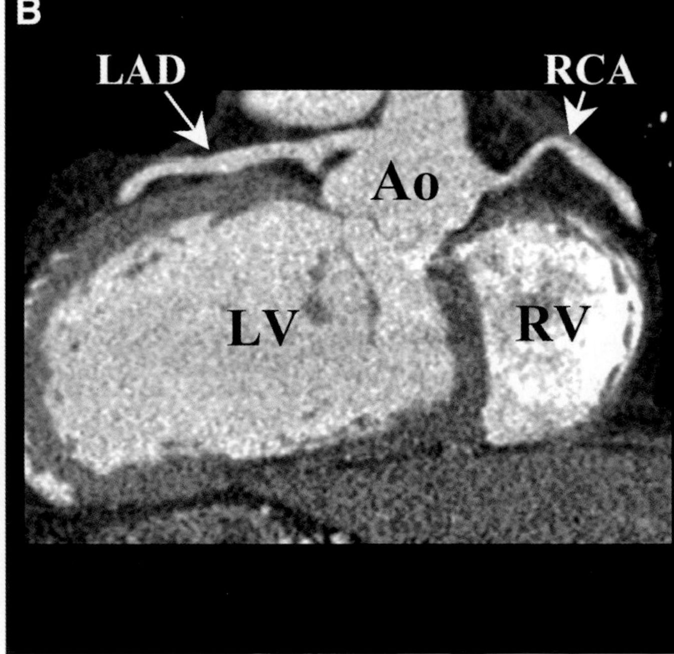

Fig. 3. Left anterior descending artery (LAD) and proximal right coronary artery (RCA) in a single plane. **(A)** Starting from a transverse plane through the middle of LAD, a curved reconstruction plane is selected through the proximal RCA, ascending aorta, left main and proximal LAD (dashed line). **(B)** Curved multiplanar reformation along LAD and RCA. The LAD follows a course over the anterior wall of the left ventricle to the apex of the heart. RVOT, right-ventricular outflow track; Ao, aorta; LV, left ventricle; RV, right ventricle.

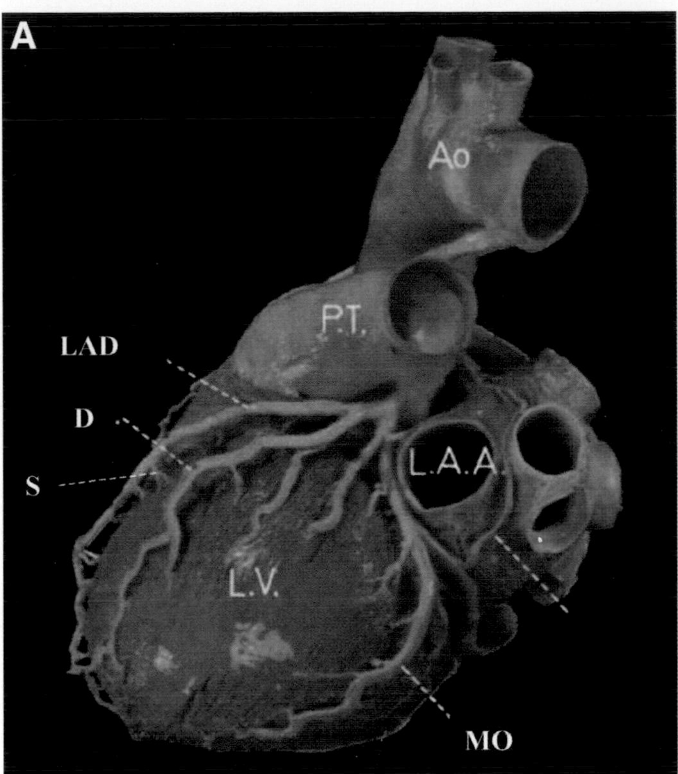

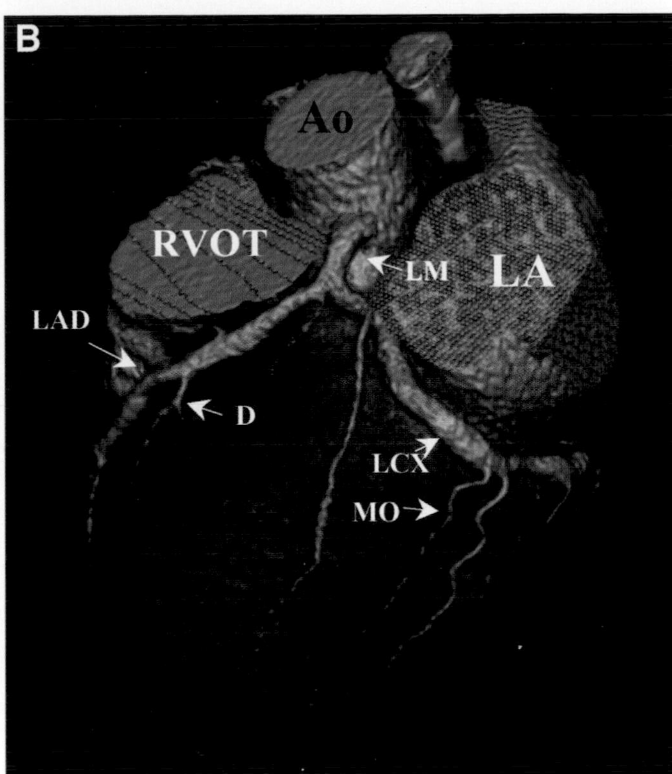

Fig. 4. **(A)** Anatomical view of the left coronary artery (reproduced with permission from *[13]*). The auricle of the left atrium (L.A.A.) overlapping the circumflex coronary artery is removed. The left main (LM) artery divides beneath the L.A.A. in the left anterior descending (LAD) and circumflex (LCX) coronary arteries. From the LAD artery diagonal branches (D) arise. The margo obtusus (MO) arises from the LCX artery. **(B)** A comparable noninvasive coronary angiogram with computed tomography. Ao, aorta; PT, pulmonary trunk; LA, left atrium, after removal of the auricle; LV, left ventricle; RVOT, right-ventricular outflow track.

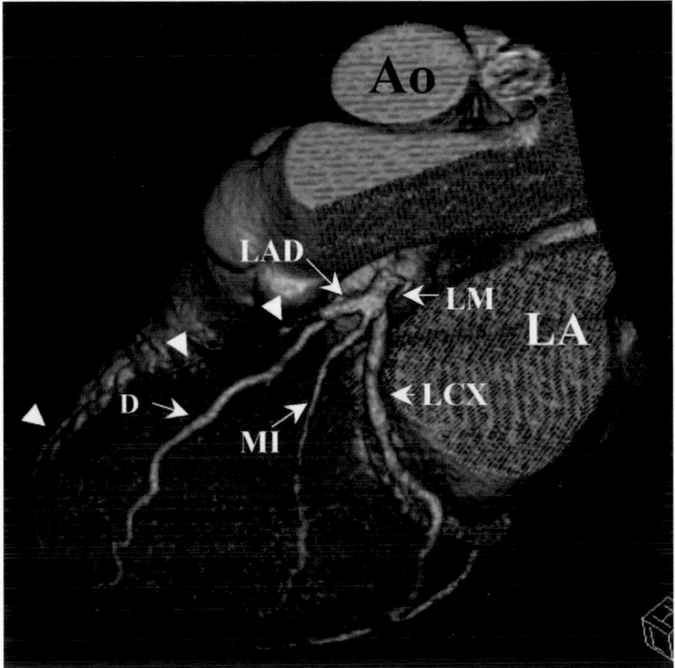

Fig. 5. Coronary CT angiography, trifurcation of the left main artery into left anterior descending (LAD), circumflex (LCX), and intermediate (MI) arteries. The LAD is occluded after the first diagonal branch (D) but shows some contrast filling through collateral vessels (arrowheads).

RIGHT CORONARY ARTERY

The RCA arises from the anterior aortic sinus, somewhat inferior to the origin of the LAD. It passes forward and then downward in the right atrioventricular groove (Fig. 6) and continues around the margin of the heart towards the crux, a point below where the atrioventricular groove and the posterior interventricular groove meet. Sometimes a single MPR image displays a long segment of the RCA if an imaging plane through the right atrioventricular groove is selected (Fig. 6). A longer part may be visible if this plane is tilted with the caudal side to the back of the patient. The first branch of the RCA is generally the conus artery that runs over the anterior surface of the right- ventricular outflow tract (Fig. 7). The second branch is usually the sinoatrial node artery; alternatively, the sinus node is supply by a proximal branch of the LCx, and in some cases both routes are available. In the majority (80%) of individuals, the RCA continues forwards from the crux along the posterior interventricular groove to become the posterior descending artery (PDA), running to the apex of the heart (Fig. 8). This is by convention called RCA dominance *(4)*. Septal branches supplying the posterior third of the septum arise from the PDA and can connect with the septal branches from the LAD and form a collateral circulation. The postero-lateral (PL) branch supplying the postero-inferior aspect of the left ventricle also arises from the RCA close to the crux. Shortly the PL is a continuation of the RCA in the left atrioventricular

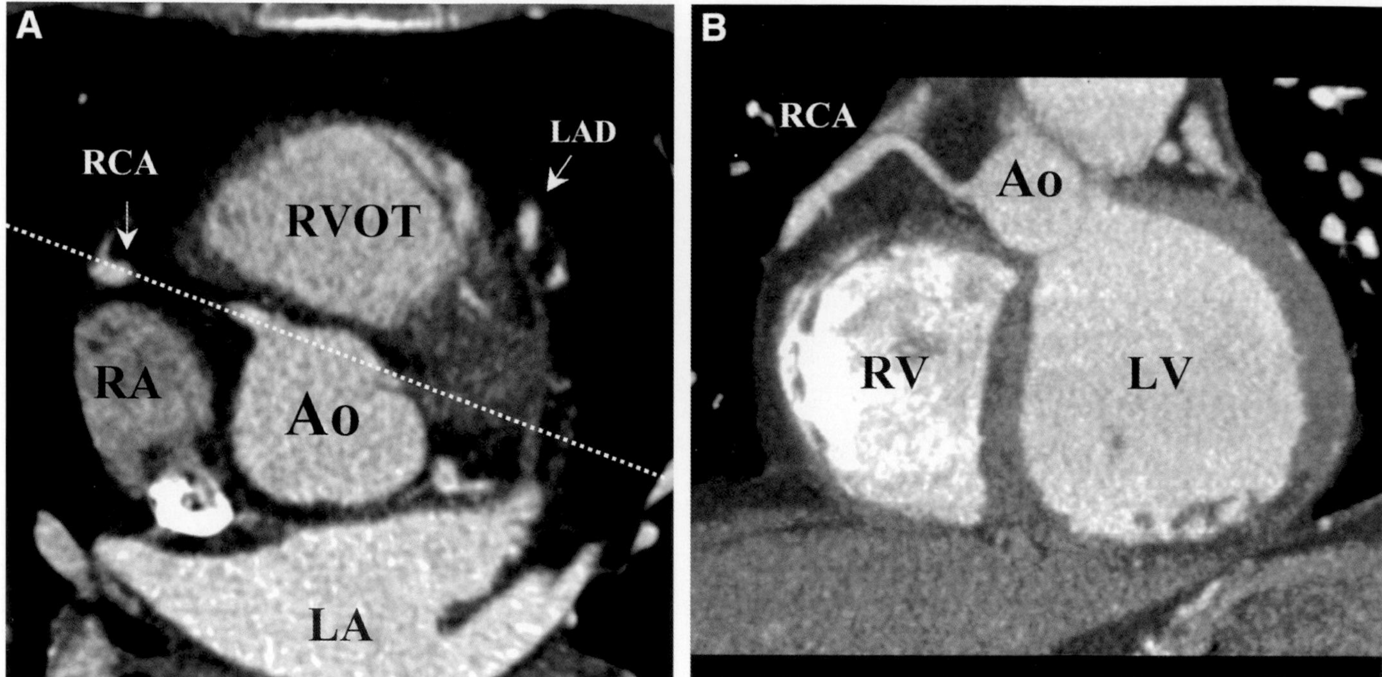

Fig. 6. Localization of the right coronary artery (RCA). **(A)** A transverse plane between the right ventricle outflow track (RVOT) and right atrium (RA) through the proximal RCA is selected (dashed line). **(B)** Image along the proximal and middle segment of the RCA. RV, right ventricle; LV, left ventricle.

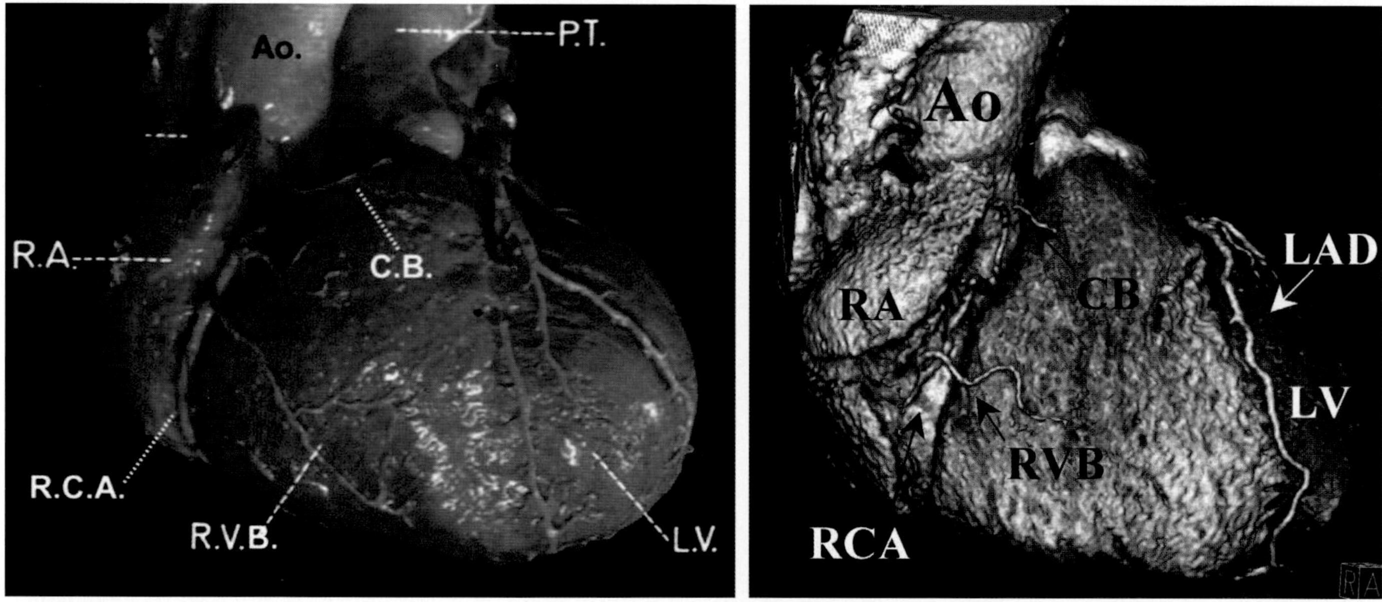

Fig. 7. (A) A pressure-fixed anatomical specimen showing the proximal and middle right coronary artery (RCA) with its side branches (conus branch [CB] and right-ventricular branch [RVB]). Reproduced from McAlpine *(13)* with permission of Springer-Verlag. **(B)** A 3D rendering of the right coronary artery. Because of the small size, only the proximal part of the conus branch can be seen. The RCA shows atherosclerotic disease over its full length. At the right side of the picture, the left anterior descending (LAD) coronary artery can be clearly seen. Ao, ascending aorta; PT, pulmonary trunk; LV, left ventricle; RV, right ventricle; RA, right atrium.

grove but within 1 or 2 cm the crux follows an epical course over the myocardium of the left ventricle parallel to the PDA. Here the RCA can serve as a collateral for an occluded LCx. Also close to the crux a small artery arises that passes upwards to the atrioventricular node of the conduction system. Left coronary dominance exists when the PDA arises from the circumflex artery (Fig. 9).

CORONARY VENOUS ANATOMY

With the growing possibilities in electrophysiology where ablation catheters or pacemaker leads are positioned in the coronary veins, there has been a renewed interest in the venous anatomy. There are two major systems of epicardial cardiac veins: tributaries of the coronary sinus and the anterior cardiac veins (Fig. 10). In principle, the veins run parallel to the arter-

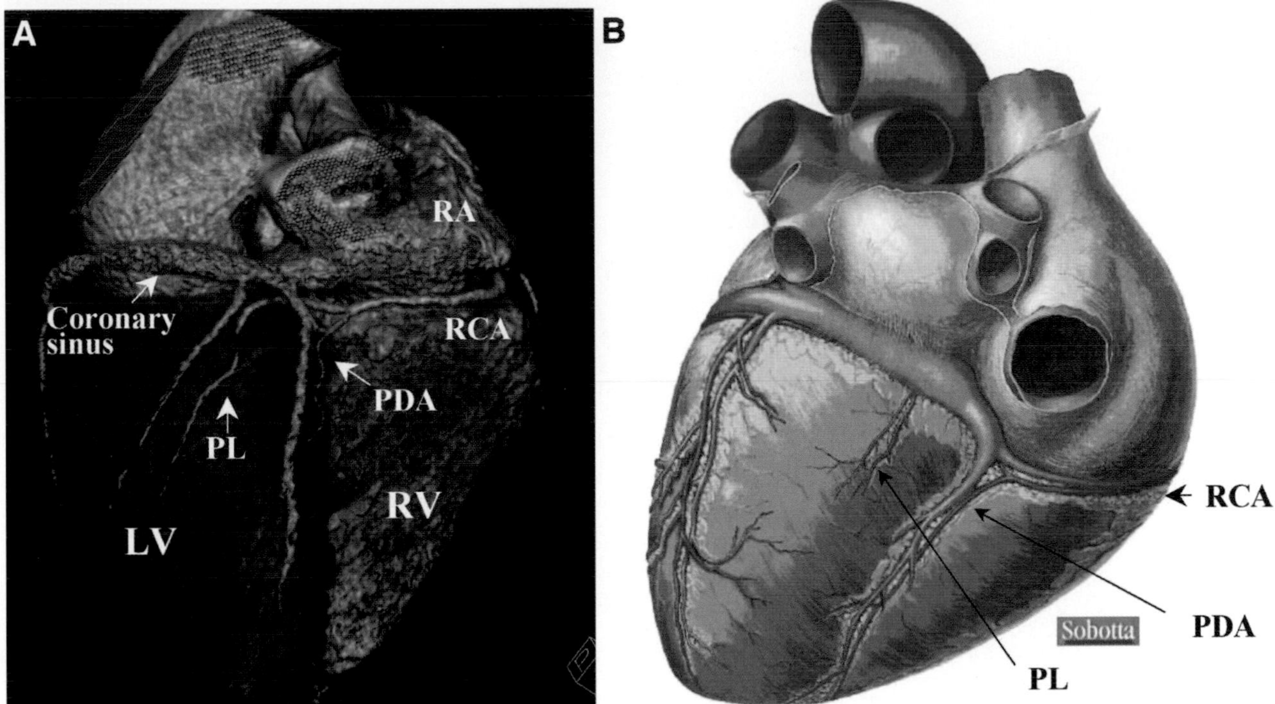

Fig. 8. Distal right coronary artery (RCA), diaphragmatic view. (**A**) Coronary CT angiography. At the crux the RCA divides into the postero-descending artery (PDA) and postero-lateral (PL) branch over the inferior wall of the left ventricle (LV). RV, right ventricle; RA, right atrium. (**B**) Anatomical view. (Reproduced with permission from *Sobotta Atlas der Anatomie des Menschen*, Elsevier GmbH, Munich.)

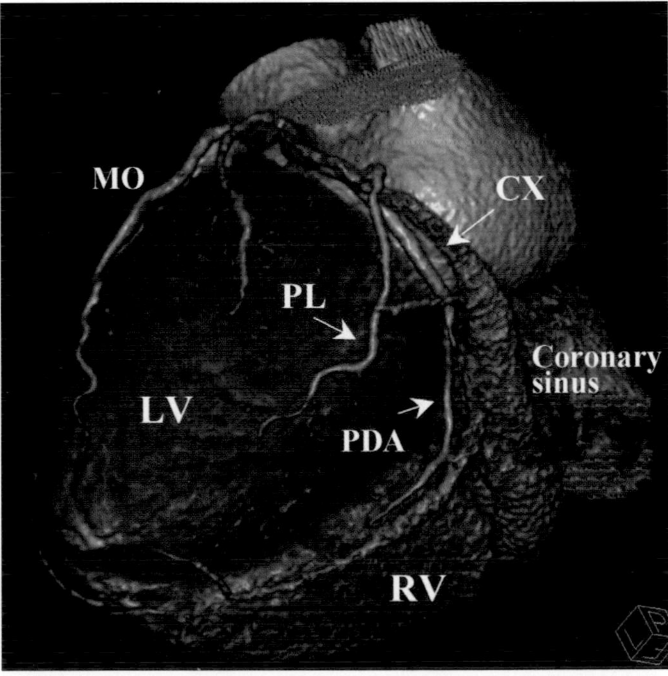

Fig. 9. Left coronary artery dominance. Posterior descending artery (PDA) and postero-lateral (PL) branch originate from the circumflex (CX) coronary artery. LV, left ventricle; RV, right ventricle.

ies. The great cardiac vein (GCV), receiving blood from the anterior two-thirds of the septum, runs parallel to the LAD in the anterior interventricular groove. At the origin of the LAD, the GCV turns into the left atrioventricular groove, running parallel to the circumflex artery, where it drains into the coronary sinus. The anatomical transition of the GCV into the coronary sinus is at the site of entrance of the oblique vein of the left atrium *(5)*. The coronary sinus continues parallel to the circumflex artery and drains into the right atrium. The ostium of the coronary sinus in the right atrium is most frequently covered by a thick valve (the valve of the coronary sinus or Thebesian valve) *(5)*.

The GCV and coronary sinus encircle most of the left atrioventricular connection and therefore are frequently used for location of assessorial electrical pathways that are present in the Wolff–Parkinson–White syndrome.

The middle cardiac vein (MCV), receiving blood from the posterior third of the septum, runs parallel to the PDA and enters the coronary sinus in 87% of the cases *(6)*. In only 36% of the cases is there a small cardiac vein, draining the blood of the right ventricle into the coronary sinus *(6)*. Additional coronary veins drain the lateral wall of the left ventricle and enter the coronary sinus between the GCV and MCV. The largest of these are used for implantation of the second lead of biventricular pacemakers. These lateral veins cover the area of the heart that is depolarized the latest in the presence of a left-ventricular bundle branch block, which makes it the most effective side for additional left-ventricular pacing.

The other epicardial venous system, that of the anterior veins, drains the blood from the right-ventricular wall into the right atrium via atrial sinuses *(7)*. Sometimes this so-called sinus coronarius atrii dextri is quite large *(6)* and can be confused with the RCA.

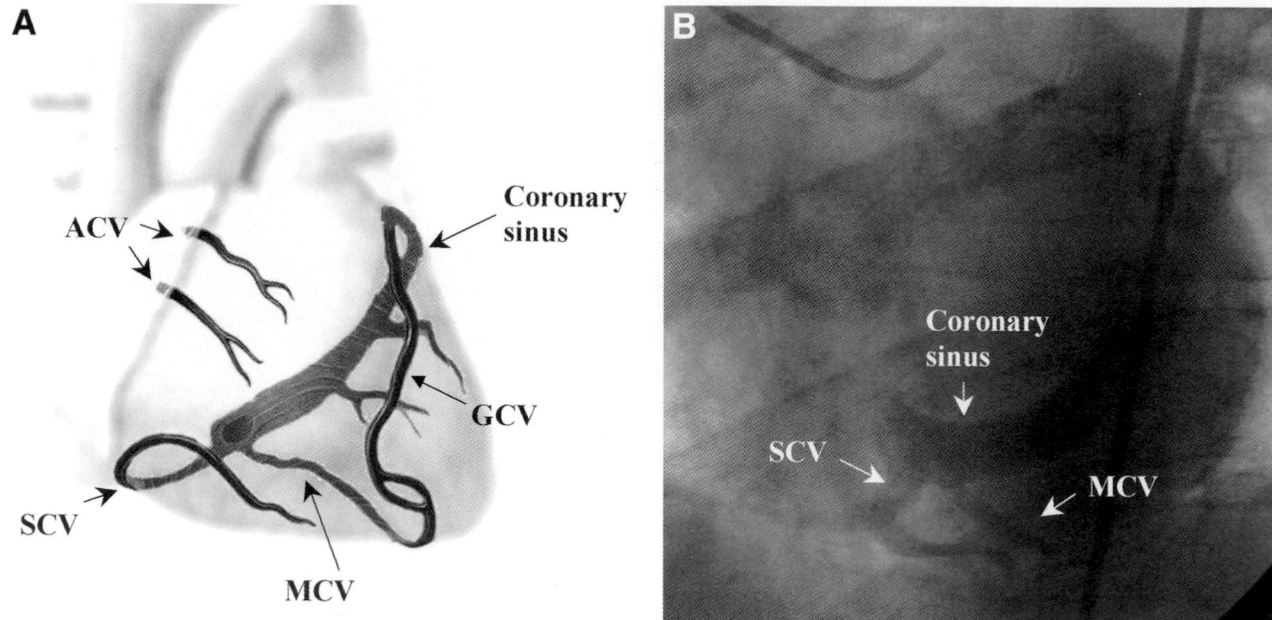

Fig. 10. Coronary veins. **(A)** Anatomical view. Two cardiac venous systems: anterior cardiac veins (ACV) and tributaries of the coronary sinus (great cardiac vein [GCV], middle cardiac vein [MCV], and small cardiac vein [SCV]). **(B)** Conventional coronary angiography, venous phase.

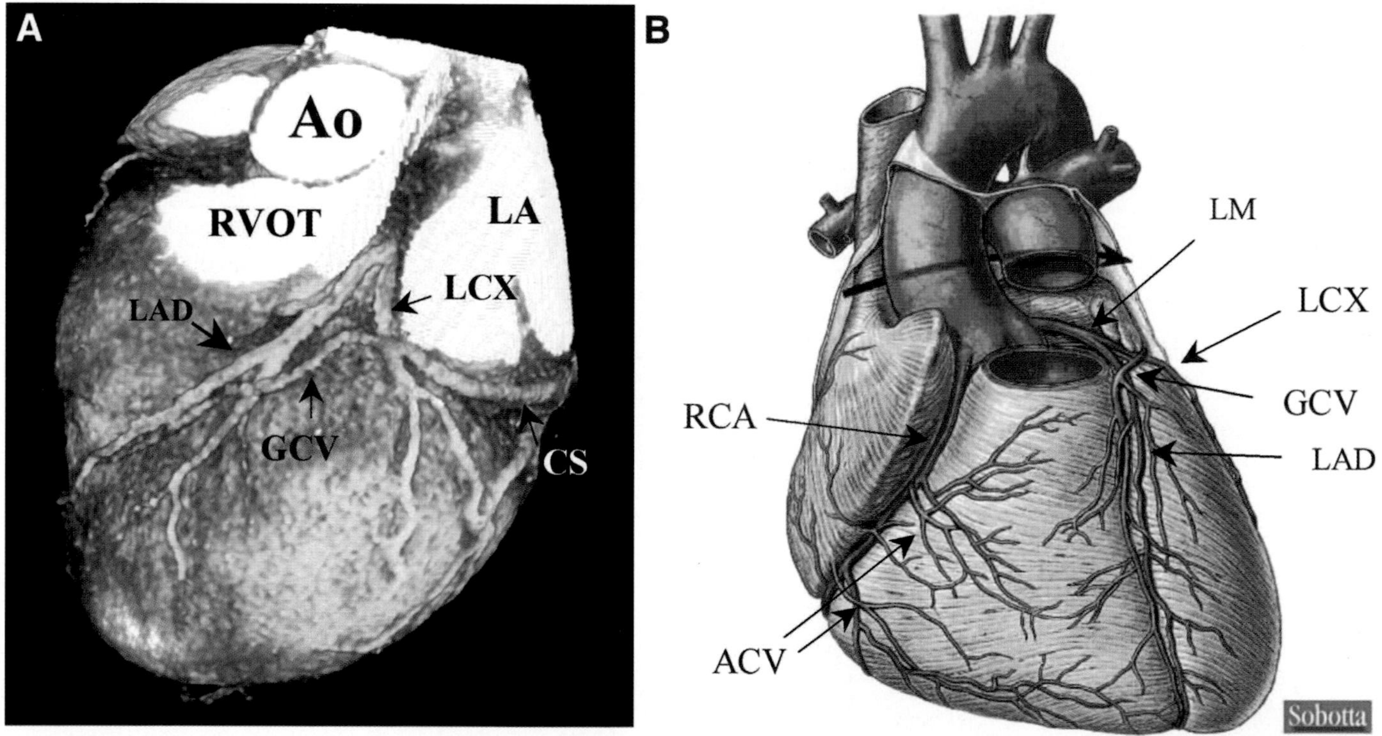

Fig. 11. The great cardiac vein (GCV) turns from the anterior interventricular groove into the atrioventricular groove, crossing all the branches of the left coronary artery and forming the triangle of Brocq and Mouchet together with the left anterior descending (LAD) and circumflex (LCX) coronary arteries. **(A)** CTA: the view at the LCX artery is obstructed by the GCV. **(B)** Comparative anatomical view. LM, left main artery; RCA, right coronary artery; ACV, anterior cardiac veins.

RELATION BETWEEN ARTERIES AND VEINS

LCA AND GCV

The GCV is the longest venous vessel of the heart. The vein originates at the anterior interventricular groove, near the apex of the heart, and it empties into the coronary sinus. In the lower and the middle parts of the interventricular groove, the GCV runs most often to the right of its related artery *(8)*. The GCV crosses over the LAD artery and all of it branches in 49% of the cases (Fig. 11). On reaching the atrioventricular groove, the GCV crosses the LAD and circumflex arteries,

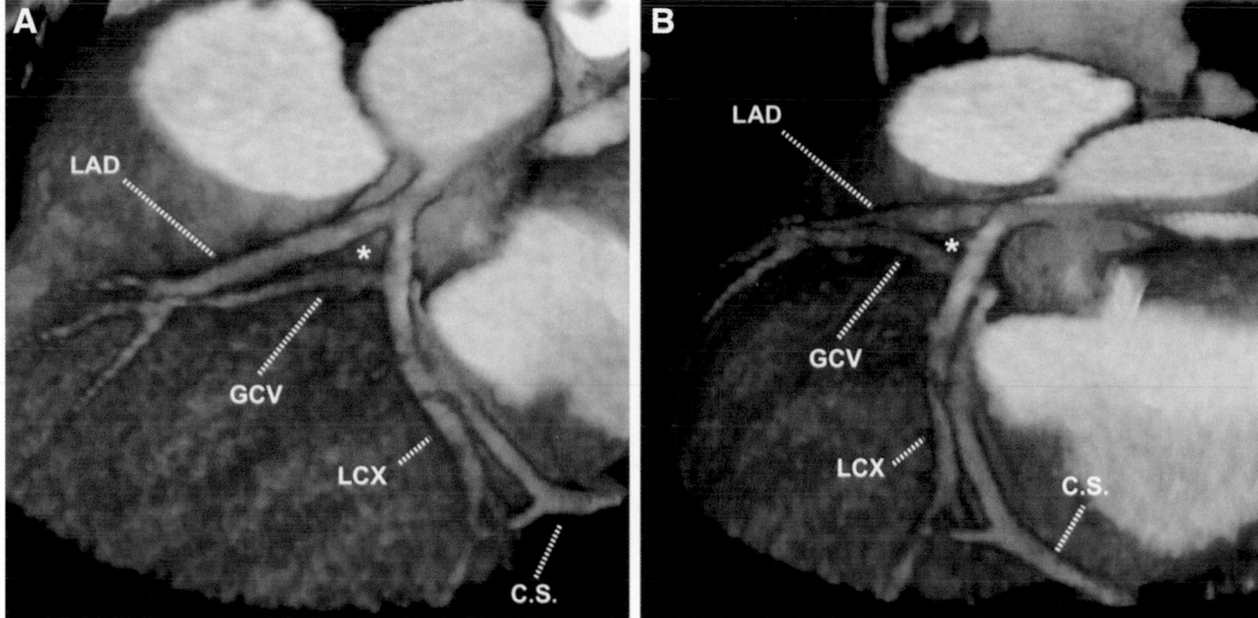

Fig. 12. Renderings of the left coronary arterial and venous systems. **(A)** Great cardiac vein (GCV) running parallel to the left anterior descending coronary artery (LAD), crossing under the circumflex artery (LCX) and entering the coronary sinus (CS). Triangle of Brocq and Mouchet formed by the proximal left anterior descending coronary artery, the proximal circumflex coronary artery, and the great cardiac vein crossing from the anterior interventricular groove to the atrioventricular groove. **(B)** 3D rendering of the same dataset, offering a more lateral and posterior view of the heart, arteries, and veins. This clearly shows the possibility of the 3D rendering technique to view the object from any angle. Reproduced with permission from *(14)*.

forming the base of the triangle of Brocq and Mouchet *(8)*. The distance from the GCV of the left main coronary artery is variable (0–7 mm *[8]*), and sometimes the GCV touches the left main coronary artery and turns with a very sharp angle to the left atrioventricular groove, crossing under the branches of the left main coronary artery (Fig. 12). The circumflex artery is covered by the GCV in 60% of the cases so that the underlying anatomy of circumflex artery is obscured or inadequately visualized.

RCA AND CORONARY SINUS

At the crux of the heart the RCA is, with very rare exceptions, inferior to the coronary sinus. The middle cardiac vein crosses over the postero-lateral branch of the RCA and stays left of the PDA when running in the posterior interventricular groove (Fig. 13). In cases of left circumflex artery dominance, veins draining blood from the inferior wall of the left ventricle cross over the artery before entering the coronary sinus.

CORONARY ARTERY ANOMALIES

A large number of coronary artery anomalies have been described in the literature *(2,9)*. Most extreme is the origin of one of the coronary arteries from the pulmonary artery; most frequently, this is the LAD, probably owing to its normal course underneath and around the pulmonary artery (Fig. 1). Because of the large amount of ischemia in such a case, symptoms are normally noticed the first 4 mo of life *(9,10)*. The most frequent anomalies are the different fistulae, which normally arise from the RCA; less frequently they arise from the LAD or LCx. Drainage usually occurs into the right ventricle,

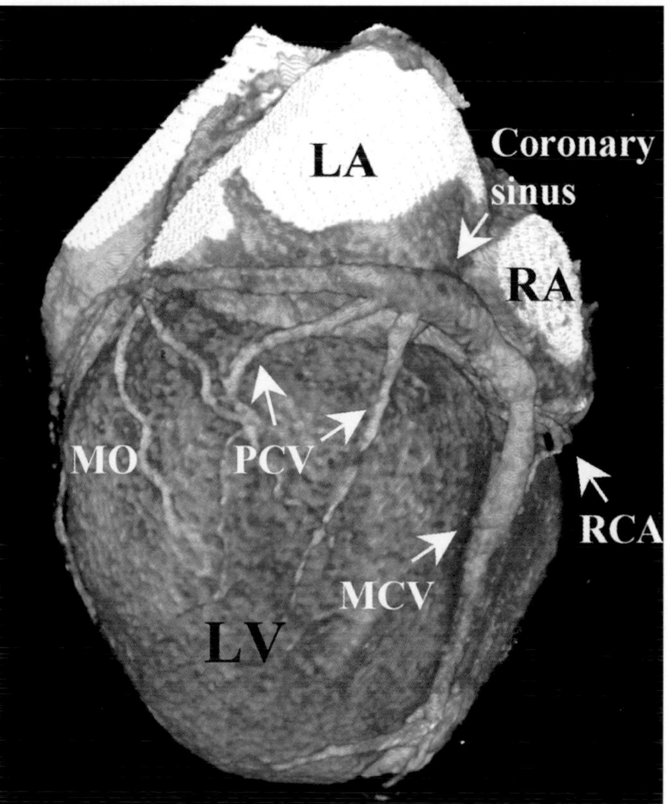

Fig. 13. Right coronary artery (RCA) in the inferior atrioventricular groove partly covered by the middle cardiac vein (MCV) and the coronary sinus. PCV, posterior cardiac vein; RA, right atrium; LV, left ventricle.

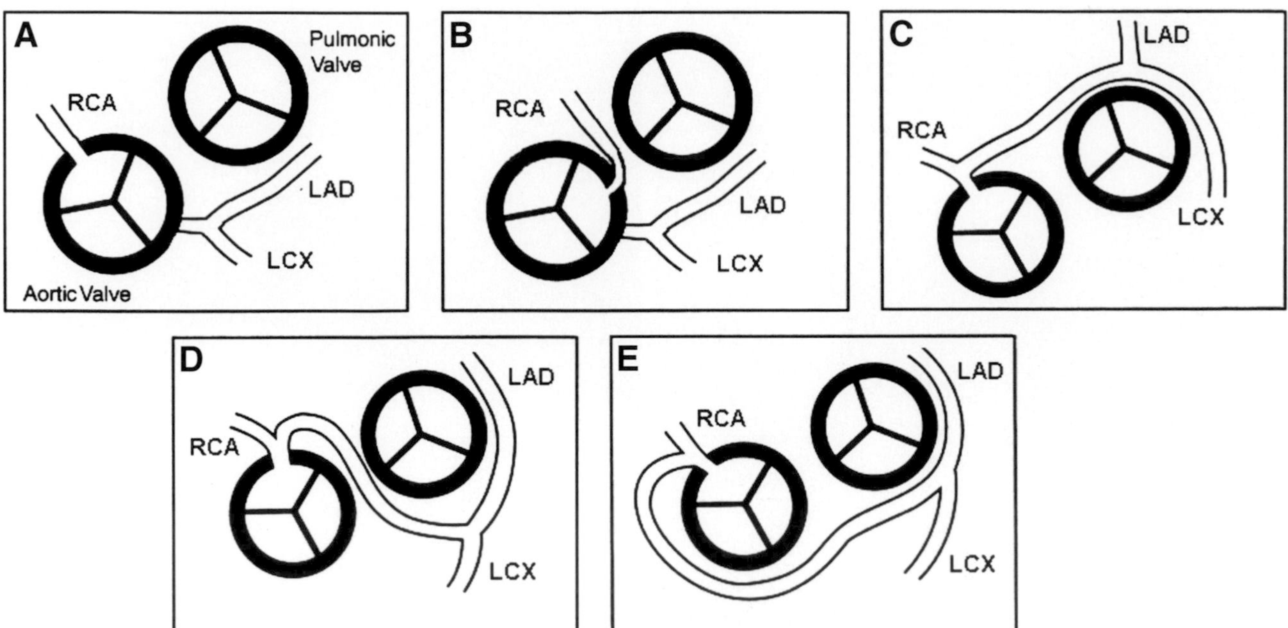

Fig. 14. Different pathway of aberrant origin of the coronary artery arteries. (**A**) Normal anatomy. Caudal view. (**B**) Right coronary artery (RCA) from left coronary cusp, inter-arterial course. (**C**) Left main (LM) from right coronary cusp, anterior course. (**D**) LM from right coronary cusp, inter-arterial course. (**E**) LM from right coronary cusp, posterior course.

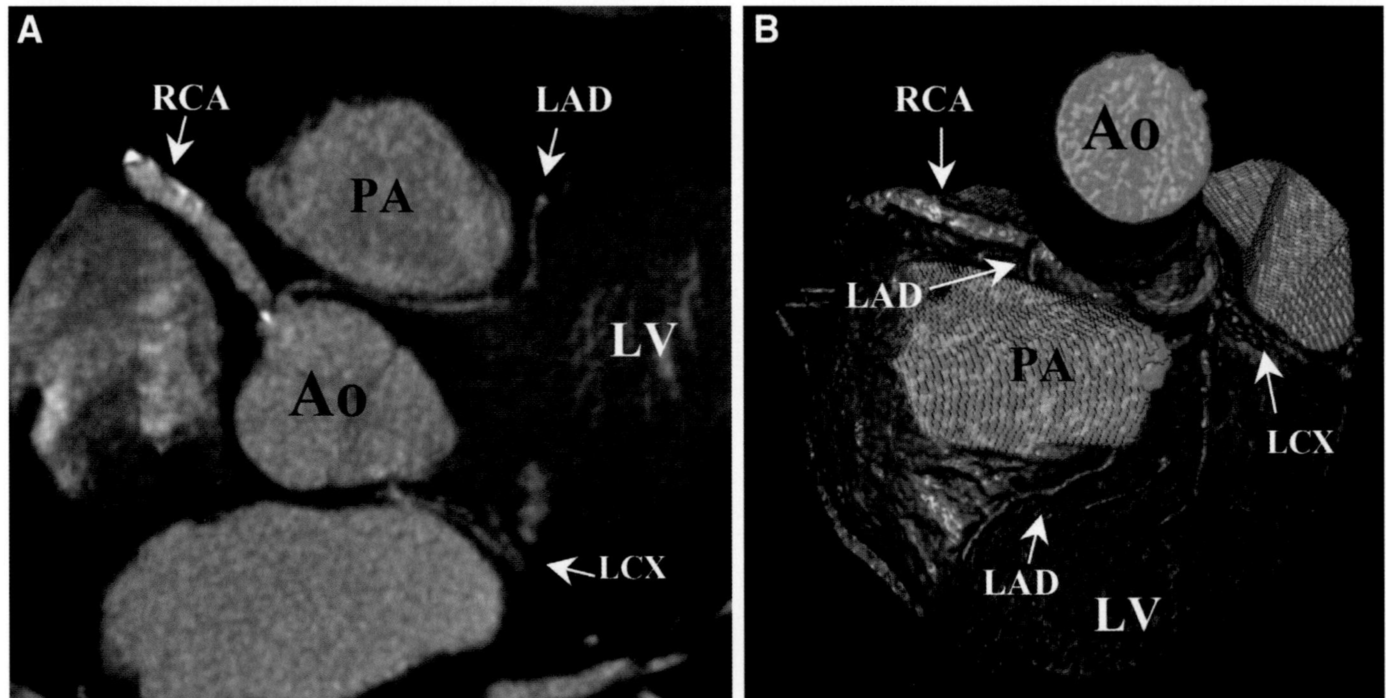

Fig. 15. Left anterior descending (LAD) coronary artery from right coronary cusp. (**A**) Curved axial MIP demonstrating the inter-arterial course of the LAD between the pulmonary artery (PA) and the aorta (Ao). (**B**) VRT image. The proximal and distal LAD are clearly visible; the inter-arterial course is covered by the PA. LCX, left circumflex coronary artery; RCA, right coronary artery; LV, left ventricle.

right atrium, or pulmonary artery. Occasionally, they drain in the left ventricle or superior caval vein. Symptoms of coronary artery fistulae are related to congestive heart failure as a result of left-to-right shunting, infective endocarditis, or myocardial ischemia.

Origin of a coronary artery from the contralateral sinus (Fig. 14) is normally detected only during selective coronary angiography for suspected coronary artery disease *(11,12)*. They are categorized into anomalies expected to cause myocardial ischemia or those unlikely to cause myocardial ischemia.

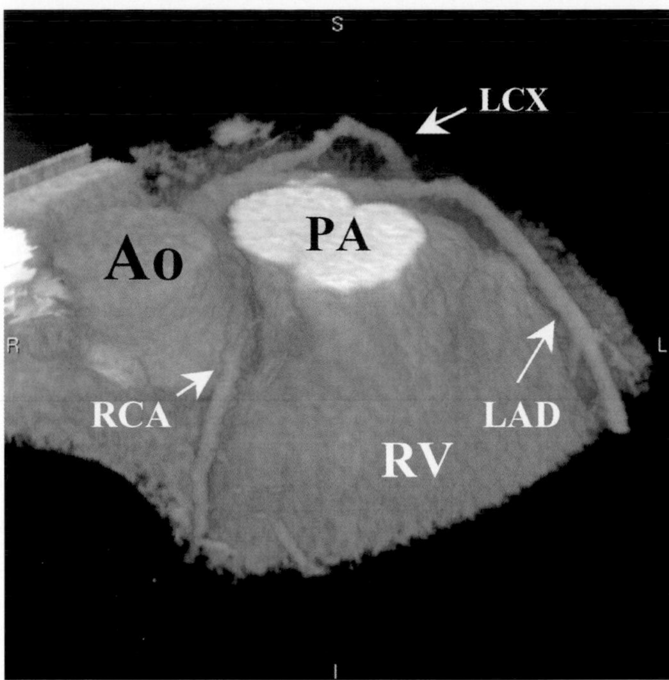

Fig. 16. Right coronary artery (RCA) from left coronary cusp with in inter-arterial course. Ao, aorta; PA, pulmonary artery; RV, right ventricle; LAD, left anterior descending artery; LCX, left circumflex coronary artery.

The latter have been associated with sudden death of young athletes during exercise. This category includes the interarterial course or septal course of the left main or left anterior descending coronary artery originating from the right coronary cusp and the interarterial course of a right coronary artery originating from the left coronary artery (Fig. 14B,D). The danger is explained by the slit-like ostium with a sharp angle between the coronary artery and aorta (Fig. 15). Another explanation is a possible compression of the vessel between the aorta and pulmonary artery or compression within the myocardium of the interventricular septum in such a course (Fig. 16). These abnormal vessels may be prone to earlier atherosclerosis and successive myocardial ischemia.

Coronary artery anomalies not related to ischemia follow a course anterior (Fig. 14C) to the pulmonary artery or a long trajectory posterior around the aorta (retroaortic course) (Fig. 14E).

CONCLUSION

Three-dimensional data sets from noninvasive 3D coronary imaging techniques such as CTA are displayed with MPR or VRT. This provides images of the coronary arteries and veins much like their real anatomy *(13)*, which are not always familiar to the practicing cardiologist. Knowledge of the course of the epicardial coronary arteries and veins is required for accurate analysis.

REFERENCES

1. James T. Anatomy of the coronary arteries in health and disease. Circulation 1965;32:1020–1033.
2. Yamanaka O, Hobbs R. Coronary artery anomalies in 126,595 patients undergoing coronary arteriography. Cathet Cardiovasc Diagn 1990;21:28–40.
3. Levin DC, Harrington DP, Bettmann MA, Garnic JD, Davidoff A, Lois J. Anatomic variations of the coronary arteries supplying the anterolateral aspect of the left ventricle: possible explanation for the "Unexplained" anterior aneurysm. Invest Radiol 1982; 17:458–462.
4. Braunwald E. Heart Disease. A Textbook of Cardiovascular Medicine. 4th ed. W.D. Saunders Company, Philadelphia: 1992.
5. Maric I, Bobinac D, Ostojic L, Petkovic M, Dujmovic M. Tributaries of the human and canine coronary sinus. Acta Anat (Basel) 1996;156:61–69.
6. von Ludinghausen M. Clinical anatomy of cardiac veins, Vv. cardiacae. Surg Radiol Anat 1987;9:159–168.
7. Pina JA. Morphological study on the human anterior cardiac veins, venae cordis anteriores. Acta Anat (Basel) 1975;92:145–159.
8. Pejkovic B, Bogdanovic D. The great cardiac vein. Surg Radiol Anat 1992;14:23–28.
9. Levin DC, Fellows KE, Abrams HL. Hemodynamically significant primary anomalies of the coronary arteries. Angiographic aspects. Circulation 1978;58:25–34.
10. Wilson CL, Dlabal PW, Holeyfield RW, Akins CW, Knauf DG. Anomalous origin of left coronary artery from pulmonary artery. Case report and review of literature concerning teen-agers and adults. J Thorac Cardiovasc Surg 1977;73:887–893.
11. Chaitman BR, Lesperance J, Saltiel J, Bourassa MG. Clinical, angiographic, and hemodynamic findings in patients with anomalous origin of the coronary arteries. Circulation 1976;53: 122- 131.
12. Kimbiris D, Iskandrian AS, Segal BL, Bemis CE. Anomalous aortic origin of coronary arteries. Circulation 1978;58:606–615.
13. McAlpine. Heart and Coronary Arteries. Springer-Verlag, Berlin: 1975.
14. Rensing BJ, Bongaerts AHH, van Geuns RJ, et al. In vivo assessment of three dimensional coronary anatomy using electron beam computed tomography after intravenous contrast administration. Heart 1999;82(4):523–525.

22 Techniques and Protocols for Acquisition and Display of Contrast-Enhanced CT Angiography

Christoph R. Becker, MD

INTRODUCTION

Contrast-enhanced computed tomography (CT) studies of the coronary arteries were performed first to visualize the vessel lumen and to achieve an angiographic-like presentation of the coronary arteries in combination with 3D postprocessing methods *(1)*. Because short exposure times are essential for coronary CT angiography (CTA), investigations initially were performed with electron beam CT (EBCT) scanners. These dedicated cardiac CT scanners were originally designed to measure myocardial perfusion *(2)*. For morphological assessment of cardiac structures, a restrictive scan protocol with EBCT allows for 100-ms exposure time, 3-mm slice thickness, and 130-kVp, 630-mA electron-gun power. The acquisition of every single slice is triggered prospectively by the electrocardiogram (ECG) signal at the end systolic phase of the cardiac cycle.

Multidetector-row CT (MDCT) scanners operate with a different acquisition mode called retrospective ECG gating. The combination of fast gantry rotation, slow table movement, and multislice helical acquisition allows for acquisition of a high number of X-ray projection data. The ECG trace is recorded simultaneously during the helical scan acquisition. The X-ray projections of the mid-diastolic phase are selected to reconstruct images from the slow-motion diastole phase of the heart. In MDCT the temporal resolution (approx 200 ms) is longer and the radiation exposure (approx 10 mSv) is higher than in EBCT. On the other hand, image quality is superior in MDCT compared to EBCT because of higher spatial resolution, lower image noise, and continuous volume acquisition.

In MDCT an attempt has been made to improve temporal resolution by multisector reconstruction. For this technique, X-ray projections of more than one heartbeat are used to reconstruct an image. This technique requires absolute consistent data from at least two consecutive heartbeats for successful image reconstruction. For multisector reconstruction, the table feed needs to be reduced to collect enough projections. This leads to longer scan times and higher radiation exposure compared to a partial scan reconstruction. However, the rhythm of the human heart may change rapidly, in particular under special conditions such as breath-holding and Valsalva maneuver. When multisector reconstruction is performed, the temporal resolution then depends on the actual heart rate and may vary during the acquisition. For this reason, this technique is of limited practical use under clinical conditions.

In general the redundant radiation exposure in the systole can substantially be reduced by a technique called prospective ECG tube current modulation. On the basis of the ECG signal, the X-ray tube current is switched to its nominal value during the diastole phase and is reduced significantly during the systole phase of the heart, respectively. This technique is most effective in patients with low heart rates. If the heart rate is lower that 60 beats per minute (bpm), the radiation exposure will be reduced by approx 50% *(3)*.

In addition, retrospective ECG gating allows for reconstruction of images at any time within the cardiac cycle. However, with the currently available temporal resolution in MDCT, the image quality is poor only if the images are reconstructed in any other than the mid-diastolic phase. The accuracy of the functional assessment by MDCT may be influenced if motion artifacts are present or if a β-blocker have been administered.

PATIENT PREPARATION

For a 16-row-detector CT scanner with 420 ms gantry rotation, an optimized partial scan view lasts about 200 ms. Reasonably good image quality with this temporal resolution can be achieved only in patients with low heart rates—e.g., <70 bpm *(4)*. Therefore, caffeine or any drug like atropine or nitroglycerin that increases the heart rate should be avoided prior to a cardiac CTA investigation. Instead the use of a β-blocker may become necessary for patient preparation aiming at a heart rate of 60 bpm or even less.

To consider β-blocker for patient preparation, contraindications (bronchial asthma, AV block, severe congestive heart failure, aortic stenosis, and so on *[5]*) have to be ruled out and informed consent must be obtained from the patient. In case the heart rate of a patient is significantly above 60 bpm, 50 to 200 mg of Metoprololtartrat can be administered orally 30–90 min prior to the investigation. Alternatively, 5–20 mg of Metoprololtartrat divided into 4 doses can be administered intravenously *(5)* immediately prior to scanning. Monitoring of vital functions (heart rate and blood pressure) is essential during this

From: *Contemporary Cardiology: CT of the Heart: Principles and Applications*
Edited by: U. Joseph Schoepf © Humana Press, Inc., Totowa, NJ

Table 1
Scan Parameters for 4- and 16-Detector-Row CT

	4-Detector CT	*16-Detector CT*
Slice thickness	1 mm	0.75
Tube current	400 mAs	500 mAs
Tube voltage	120 kVp	120 kVp
Gantry rotation	500 ms	420 ms
Table feed	3 mm/s	6 mm/s
Breath hold	40 s	20 s
Spatial resolution	8 linepairs (lp)/cm	8 lp/cm
Temporal resolution	250 ms	200 ms
Number of slices	200	240

approach. There are four positive effects of β-blocker on MDCT scanning: better patient compliance, less radiation exposure and cardiac motion artifacts, and higher vascular enhancement.

MDCT SCANNING

For retrospective ECG gating with MDCT, the pitch factor (detector collimation divided by table feed per gantry rotation) must not exceed 0.3 to allow for scanning the heart at any heart rate higher than 40 beats per minute. In a 4-detector-row CT with 1-mm slices and 500-ms gantry rotation, a typical scan range of 12 cm lasts approx 40 s. In a 16-detector-row CT with 0.75-mm slices and a gantry rotation time of 420 ms, the entire scan lasts about 20 s.

In 4- and 16-detector-row CT, tube current is set to 400 and 500 effective mAs, respectively. The higher tube current is needed to compensate for higher image noise caused by both thinner slices and the higher temporal resolution used with a 16- compared to 4-detector-row CT scanner. Higher temporal resolution equates to shorter exposure times and therefore does not necessarily translate into higher radiation exposure. The patient may either be exposed for a longer time with a lower tube current or for a shorter exposure time with higher tube current; however, the final amount of radiation for the same image noise remains the same.

The patients should be instructed not to press when taking a deep breath in, to avoid the Valsalva maneuver. During the Valsalva maneuver, the intraabdominal pressure increases with blood from the inferior vena cava entering the right atrium. With an increased pressure in the right atrium, blood mixed with contrast medium from the superior vena cava is prevented from entering the right atrium. Furthermore, as a reflex the increased blood volume in the right atrium leads to a decrease in heart rate.

The Valsalva maneuver may last several seconds under breath-hold conditions. After it releases, high-density contrast medium may enter the right atrium and the heart rate recovers to its original or even slightly higher frequency *(6)*. As a result, the CT may not be homogeneously enhanced and image quality may suffer from rapid changes of the heart rate.

After scan acquisition has been completed, reconstruction of the axial slices always begins with a careful analysis of the ECG trace recorded with the helical scan. The image reconstruction interval is best been placed in between the T and the P wave of the ECG, corresponding to the mid-diastole interval. The point of time for the least coronary motion may be different for every coronary artery. Minimal motion artifacts may result for reconstructing the right coronary artery (RCA), left anterior descending (LAD) artery, and left circumflex (LCx) artery at 50%, 55%, and 60% of the RR interval, respectively. Individual adaptation of the point of time for reconstruction seems to further improve image quality *(4)*. However, the lower the heart rate, the easier it is to find the best interval for all three major branches of the coronary artery tree. Images are reconstructed with spatial in-plane resolution of 8 linepairs (lp)/cm (0.6 mm). The slice thickness and reconstruction increment is 1.3 with 0.7 mm and 1 with 0.5 mm in 4- and 16-detector-row CT, respectively. Therefore, near-isotropic spatial resolution may be achieved only with the 16-detector-row CT.

Depending on the preparation, patient investigation time may last approx 10–15 min. Image reconstruction and post processing can be performed within approx 10 min. Because coronary CTA is performed with thin slices and low image noise, the radiation dose with tube current modulation is significantly higher (approx 5 mSv) that for coronary calcium screening (approx 1 mSv). However, the radiation of a CTA investigation is comparable to what is applied during a diagnostic coronary catheter procedure. Scan parameters are summarized in Table 1.

IMAGE POSTPROCESSING

The detection of coronary artery pathology in axial CT images is difficult since every slice displays only a small fragment of the entire coronary artery. Two- or three-dimensional postprocessing display such as multiplanar reformations and maximum intensity projections (MIP) or shaded surface display, virtual coronary endoscopy, and volume-rendering technique (VRT), respectively, may be helpful for a first glance at the course of the coronary arteries or for angiographic-like projections. It should be considered that any 2D or 3D reconstructions may come along with a loss of spatial resolution. Smaller side branches, for instance, which are visible in the axial source, may not be seen in volume-rendered images, and the presence of coronary artery stenosis may be overestimated. In particular, motion and ECG trigger artifacts in 2D and 3D images may appear as pathologies or even stenoses that do not exist. In addition, the primary axial slices are superior to any postprocessing method to rule out coronary artery disease (CAD) and atherosclerosis. Therefore, none of the available

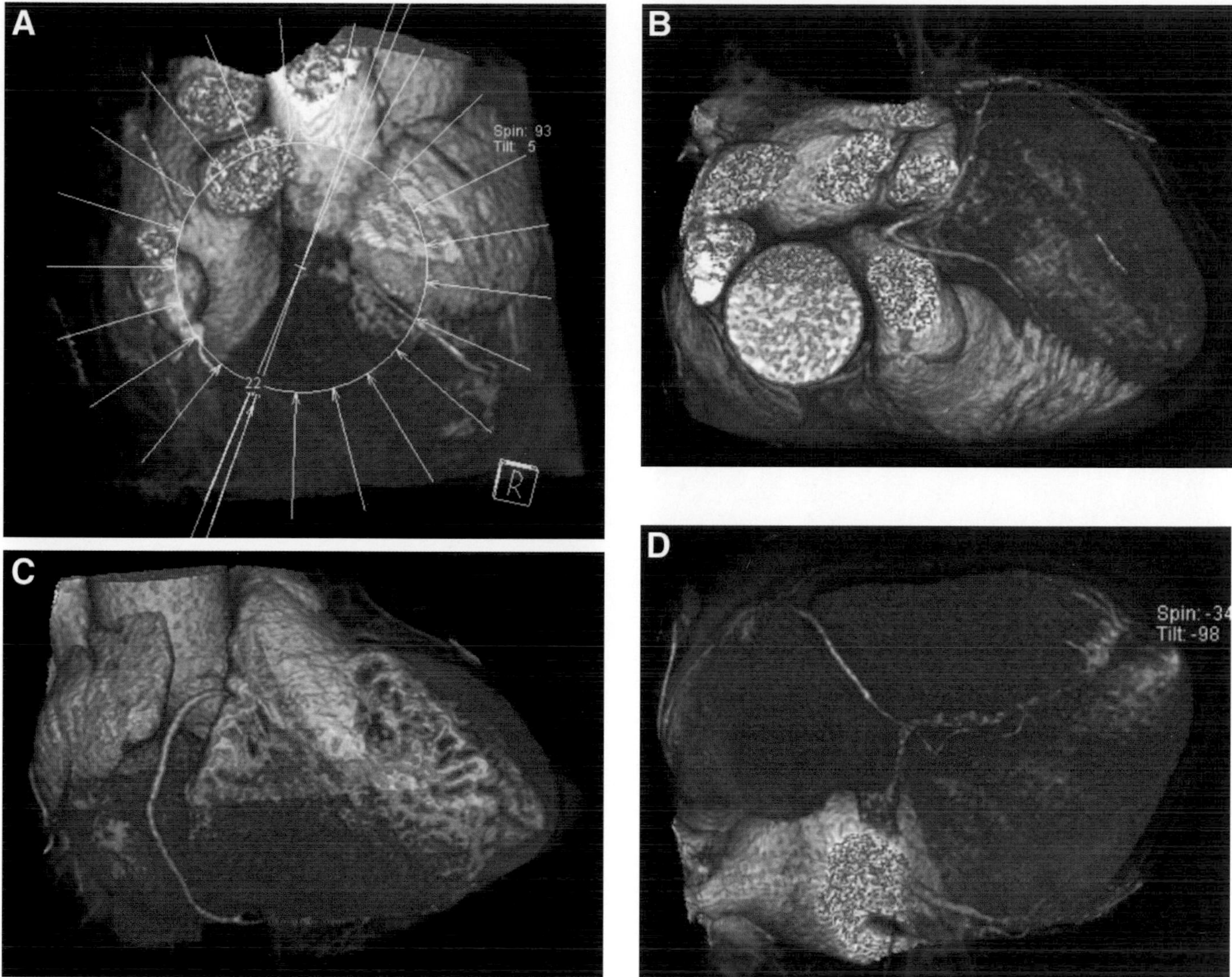

Fig. 1. Volume-rendering technique after segmentation of the bones and auricle performed along the long axis of the heart (**A**). Selective images display the course of the left anterior descending and circumflex coronary artery (**B**) as well as the proximal and middle right coronary artery (**C**). At the base of the heart, the distal right and posterior descending coronary artery can be seen (**D**).

postprocessing tools is better than the axial slices to detect coronary artery stenosis *(7)*.

VRT requires the segmentation of the sternum, the rips, and the vertebral column. The auricle of the left atrium may also be segmented to gain access to the left main coronary artery. Standardized projection views around the long axis of the heart allow for display of the superficial course of all three major coronary arteries (Fig. 1).

Standardized thin (3 mm) MIP slices with 1.5-mm increment between the slices may be reconstructed in three different planes, similar to standard cardiac catheter projections *(8)*. MIP along the interventricular groove creates images in the right anterior oblique plane that best displays the course of the LAD (Fig. 2). MIP along the atrioventricular groove in the left anterior oblique plane displays best the course of the right and circumflex coronary artery (Fig. 3). In addition, a left anterior oblique projection can be reconstructed following the course of the left anterior descending coronary artery in the lateral view. This projection plane spreads the branches of the LAD and is therefore called the "spider view." The spider view is well suited to demonstrate the proximal part of all three major coronary arteries (Fig. 4).

ANALYSIS OF AXIAL CT IMAGES

All findings from postprocessed images have to be confirmed in the original axial CT slices. The primary axial slices are superior to any postprocessing method to rule out CAD. Image analysis begins with identification of the coronary artery segments in the axial CT slices. Coronary segments can be numbered (Fig. 5) according to the model suggested by the American Heart Association *(9)*.

In patients with acute or chronic myocardial infarctions, a lack of contrast uptake in the myocardium or thinning of the myocardial wall may be detected only in the axial slices *(10)*. Depending on the coronary vessel affected, different anatomic regions may be involved (Fig. 6). In case of an involvement of

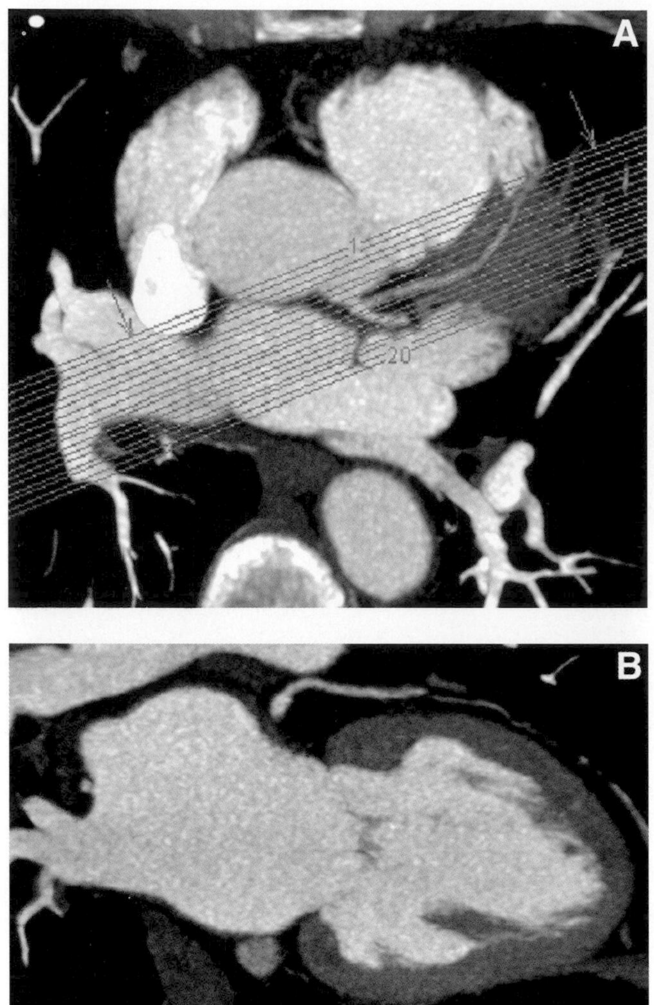

Fig. 2. The right anterior oblique (RAO) view reconstructed along the septum **(A)** is designed to display the course of the left anterior descending coronary artery **(B)**.

the left anterior descending, a myocardial infarction may be identified in the anterior left-ventricular wall, the roof of the left ventricle, the apex, the superior part of the septum, or in the anterior papillary muscle. The posterior left-ventricular wall and the posterior papillary muscle are supplied by the circumflex coronary artery. The inferior left-ventricular wall and the inferior part of the septum finally are supplied by the right coronary artery.

With later development, a subendocardial or transmural myocardial infarction may result in an aneurysm. As a result of hypokinesia in the aneurysm, thrombus formation is likely to develop in the cardiac chamber and can be detected by CTA even better than by transthoracic ultrasound *(11)*.

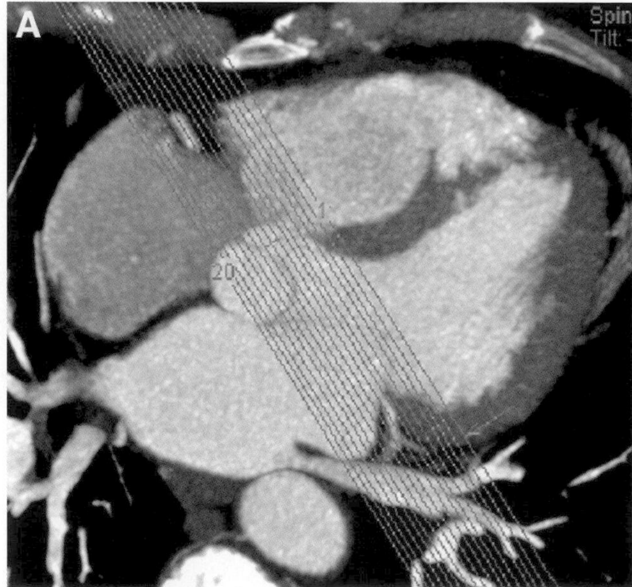

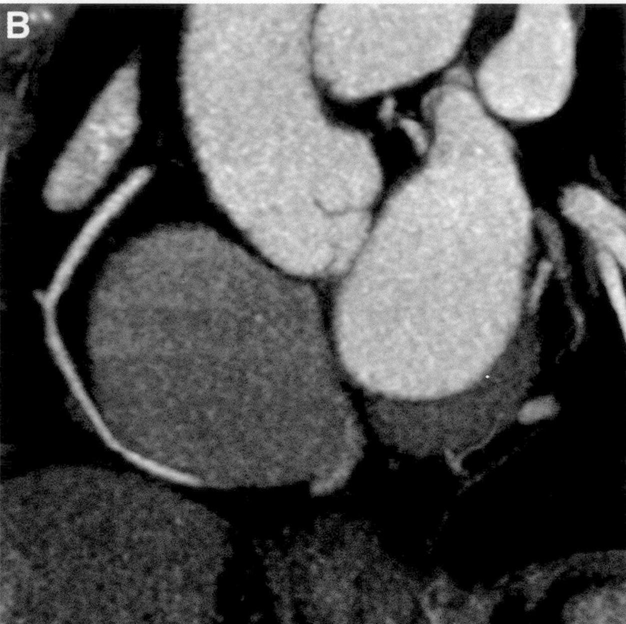

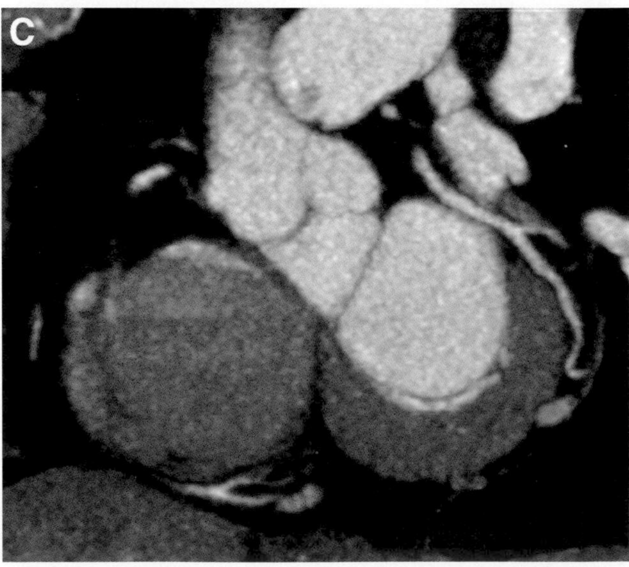

Fig. 3. *(right)* The left anterior oblique (LAO) view **(A)** reconstructed along the atrio-venticular groove is best suited to display the right **(B)** and circumflex coronary artery **(C)**.

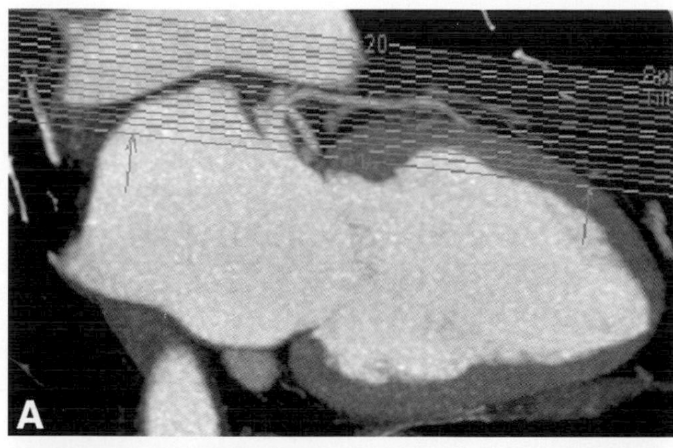

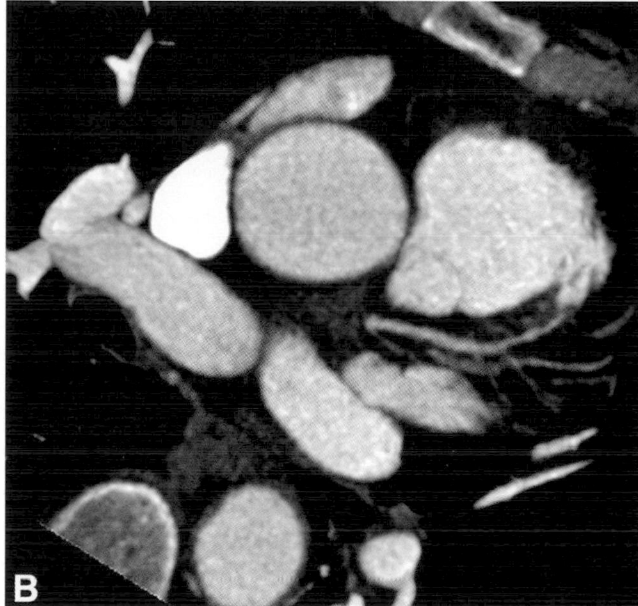

Fig. 4. Left anterior oblique (Spider) views are reconstructed along the plane of the left anterior descending coronary artery (**A**) for displaying this vessel and its major diagonal branches (**B**).

A late uptake of contrast media after first pass in the myocardium of patients after infarction was observed in CT about 17 yr ago *(11)*. It is rather likely that this kind of myocardial enhancement may correspond to nonviable myocardium due to interstitial uptake of contrast media within necrotic myocytes, 6 wk to 3 mo after onset. To allow for superior detection of the late myocardial enhancement with the new generation MDCT scanners, images should be acquired with thick slices, high signal-to-noise ratio, and reconstructed with a very soft tissue kernel. The optimal point of time for scanning may be between 10 and 40 min after first pass *(12)*.

with a larger field of view, or a more dedicated (CT) investigation should then be recommended.

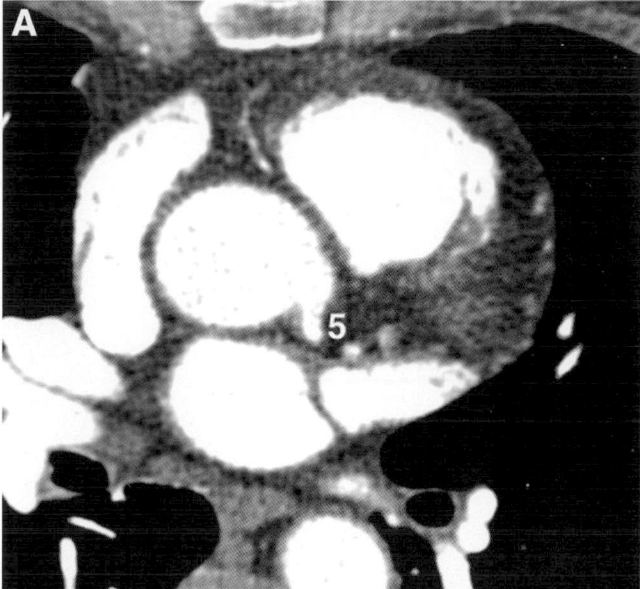

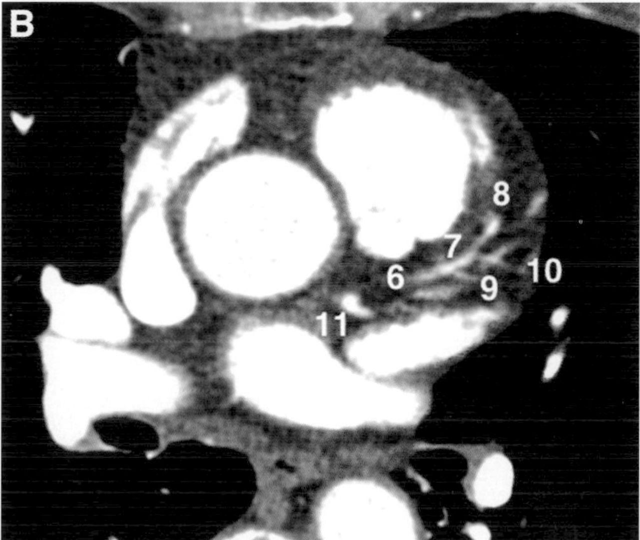

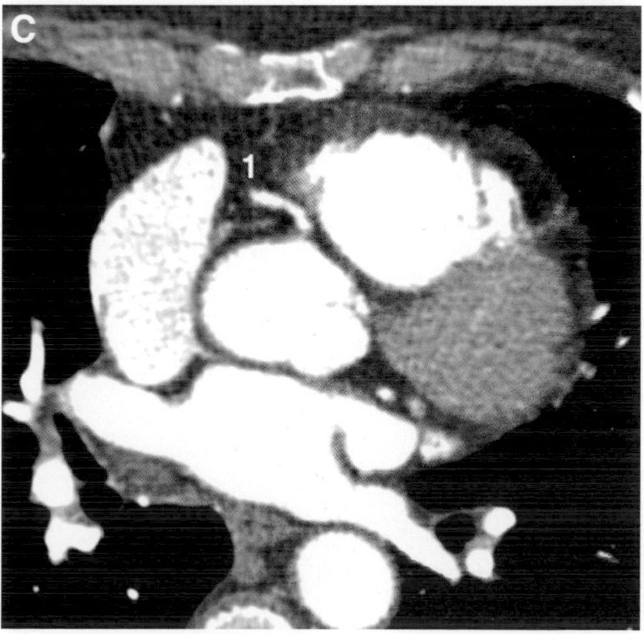

Fig. 5A–G. (*right and page 224*) In the axial slices, the coronary artery segments are identified and numbered according the American Heart Association model.

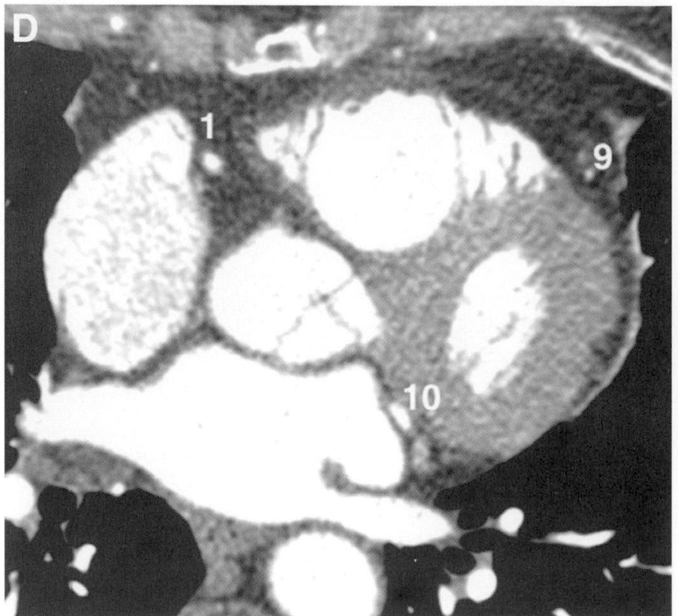

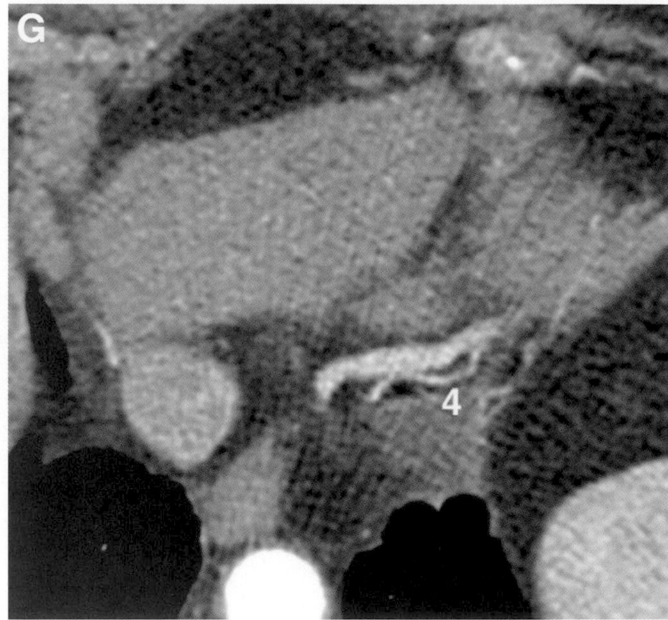

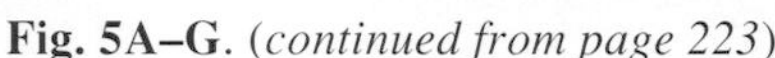

Fig. 5A–G. (*continued from page 223*)

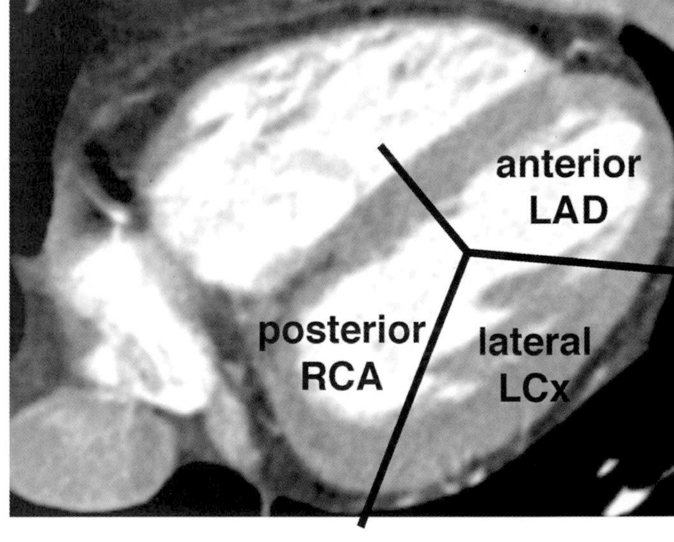

Fig. 6. The myocardium can be divided into three different territories: the anterior, inferior, and posterior wall, supplied by the left anterior, right, and circumflex coronary artery. In this particular image, an infarction scan can be seen in the posterior wall.

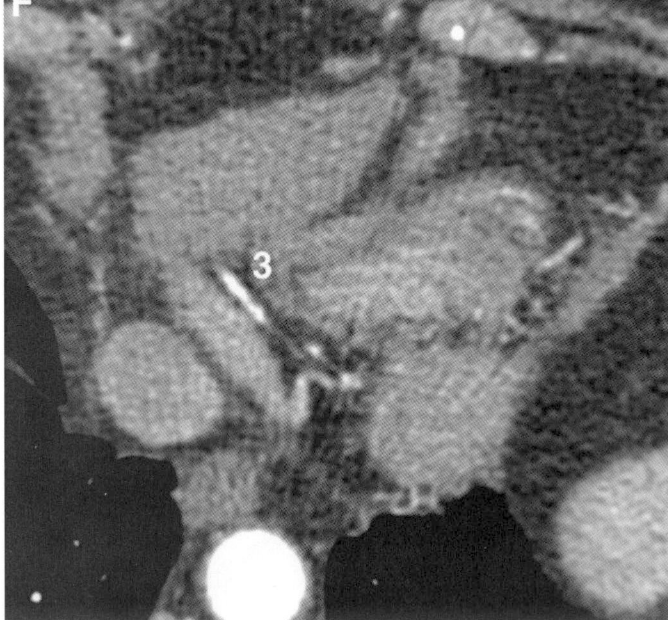

CONCLUSION

With 16-detector-row scanners, investigation of the coronary arteries and the myocardium becomes a feasible and practical CT application. Patient preparation and instruction is mandatory to acquire diagnostic image quality for the coronary arteries. Under these conditions, postprocessing in a standardized fashion may help to identify the pathology. However, any finding needs to be confirmed by the source images to identify artifacts that may arise from motion. Pathologies arising from the peri- and myocardium may be assessable only in the axial slices.

REFERENCES

1. Moshage WE, Achenbach S, Seese B, Bachmann K, Kirchgeorg M. Coronary artery stenoses: three-dimensional imaging with electrocardiographically triggered, contrast agent-enhanced, electron-beam CT. Radiology 1995;196(3):707–714.
2. Boyd D. Computerized transmission tomography of the heart using scanning electron beams. In: Higgins C (ed), CT of the Heart and the Great Vessels: Experimental Evaluation and Clinical Application. Futura, Mount Kisco, New York: 1983.
3. Jakobs TF, Becker CR, Ohnesorge B, et al. Multislice helical CT of the heart with retrospective ECG gating: reduction of radiation exposure by ECG-controlled tube current modulation. Eur Radiol 2002;12(5):1081–1086.
4. Hong C, Becker CR, Huber A, et al. ECG-gated reconstructed multidetector row CT coronary angiography: effect of varying trigger delay on image quality. Radiology 2001;220(3):712–717.
5. Ryan T, Anderson J, Antman E, et al. ACC/AHA guidelines for the management of patients with acute myocardial infarction. A report of the American College of Cardiology/American Heart Association Task Force on Practice Guidelines (Committee on Management of Acute Myocardial Infarction). J Am Coll Cardiol 1996;28: 1328–1428.
6. Mao SS, Oudiz RJ, Bakhsheshi H, Wang SJ, Brundage BH. Variation of heart rate and electrocardiograph trigger interval during ultrafast computed tomography. Am J Card Imaging 1996;10:239–243.
7. Vogl TJ, Abolmaali ND, Diebold T, et al. Techniques for the detection of coronary atherosclerosis: multi-detector row CT coronary angiography. Radiology 2002;223(1):212–220.
8. Johnson M. Principles and practice of coronary angiography. In: Skorton D, Schelbert H, Wolf G, Brundage B (eds), Marcus Cardiac Imaging: A Companion to Braunwald's Heart Disease. 2nd ed. WB Sanders Company, Philadelphia: 1996;220–250.
9. Austen WG, Edwards JE, Frye RL, et al. A reporting system on patients evaluated for coronary artery disease. Report of the Ad Hoc Committee for Grading of Coronary Artery Disease, Council on Cardiovascular Surgery, American Heart Association. Circulation 1975;51(4 Suppl):5–40.
10. Paul JF, Dambrin G, Caussin C, Lancelin B, Angel C. Sixteen-slice computed tomography after acute myocardial infarction: from perfusion defect to the culprit lesion. Circulation 2003;108(3): 373–374.
11. Masuda Y, Yoshida H, Morooka N, Watanabe S, Inagaki Y. The usefulness of x-ray computed tomography for the diagnosis of myocardial infarction. Circulation 1984;70:217–225.
12. Huber D, Lapray J, Hessel S. In vivo evaluation of experimental myocardial infarcts by ungated computed tomography. AJR 1981; 136:469–473.
13. Horton KM, Post WS, Blumenthal RS, Fishman EK. Prevalence of significant noncardiac findings on electron-beam computed tomography coronary artery calcium screening examinations. Circulation 2002;106(5):532–534.

23 Contrast Material Injection Techniques for CT Angiography of the Coronary Arteries

FILIPPO CADEMARTIRI, MD AND KOEN NIEMAN, MD

INTRODUCTION

Conventional catheter angiography is based on capturing X-ray images of the iodinated contrast material (CM) while it flows into the vessels. Computed tomography angiography (CTA) is based on the same concept, scanning the patient and his/her heart while a high concentration of iodinated CM flows through the coronary arteries *(1)*. The CM inside the vessels increases the density of the vessel lumen compared to the surrounding tissues, and allows us to distinguish between lumen and soft tissues.

Because the CM is administered intravenously in CTA, the optimal phase to scan coronary arteries will be the arterial one. In fact, during the delayed phase, several tissues enhance due to the CM perfusion, and the CM itself dilutes into the extracellular fluid, reducing the intravascular attenuation. Then vessels are no longer easily visualized as in the arterial phase *(1)*.

Spiral computed tomography technology was limited by low speed and spatial resolution. Multislice computed tomography (MSCT) technology provides better image quality because of thinner slice thickness, and faster acquisition time because of reduced scan rotation time and multiple detector rows. The advantages of MSCT technology related to CM use are: (1) use of less CM (30–50%); (2) the injection rate can be increased with a concomitant better enhancement of the vessels; and (3) most of the data can be acquired during a defined phase (e.g., arterial phase for CTA) *(1)*.

The latest generation of spiral computed tomography (CT) scanner, featuring up to 16-row MSCT technology, provides fast data acquisition, increasing the need for an accurate optimization of CM administration and synchronization techniques.

Scanning during the arterial phase in CTA, with low or no venous enhancement, enables optimal analysis of the acquired images and is critical for postprocessing techniques. Although axial images are commonly used for other conventional CT applications such as thoracic and abdominal imaging, for visualization and diagnosis of cardiac CT data sets, 2D multiplanar reformations (MPR) with standard and multiple intensity projection (MIP) algorithms, curved planar reformations (CPR), and 3D reconstructions are more important. Those techniques need a high vascular contrast in order to provide diagnostic images.

For all of these reasons, CM volume, concentration, rate, and ultimately the synchronization between CM material passage and data acquisition, need to be optimized in order to exploit the potential of MSCT technique.

The bolus timing can be based on the knowledge of bolus geometry (e.g., demographics-based delay or fixed delay), but can better rely on synchronization techniques. An optimal timing is achieved by predicting the veno-arterial transit time (e.g., test bolus), or synchronizing data acquisition with CM passage (e.g., bolus tracking).

BASICS OF BOLUS GEOMETRY

Bolus geometry is the pattern of enhancement plotted on a time(s)/attenuation (Hounsfield units—HU) curve, after intravascular injection of contrast material, and measured in a region of interest (ROI) *(1)*. The value of enhancement is extracted by subtracting the attenuation value in an unenhanced baseline scan from the attenuation values in the enhanced scans *(1)*. Optimal bolus geometry, for the purpose of CTA, corresponds to an immediate rise to the maximum value of enhancement (high attenuation—HU) just before the start of the acquisition of CT data, and a steady state in which the enhancement does not alter during data acquisition (Fig. 1A). Actual bolus geometry is different. After intravascular injection of CM, there is a steady increase in enhancement; the peak of the curve will be reached after the end of contrast injection, followed by a steady decline in the enhancement. Normally, CTA will be performed during the upslope and downslope of the enhancement curve, and the peak of maximum enhancement (PME) will be inside the scan period (Fig. 1B).

The actual bolus geometry can be defined by the peak of maximum enhancement in HU (PME) and the time to reach that peak in seconds (tPME) *(1)*.

PARAMETERS INFLUENCING BOLUS GEOMETRY

Demographics

The time to peak (tPME) is not affected by age *(2–4)*, weight *(2–5)*, height *(3,4)*, body surface *(3,4)*, blood pressure *(3)*, heart rate *(3,5)*, and gender *(2,3)*, and PME is not affected by age or gender *(2)*. A heavier body weight is associated with a higher

From: *Contemporary Cardiology: CT of the Heart: Principles and Applications*
Edited by: U. Joseph Schoepf © Humana Press, Inc., Totowa, NJ

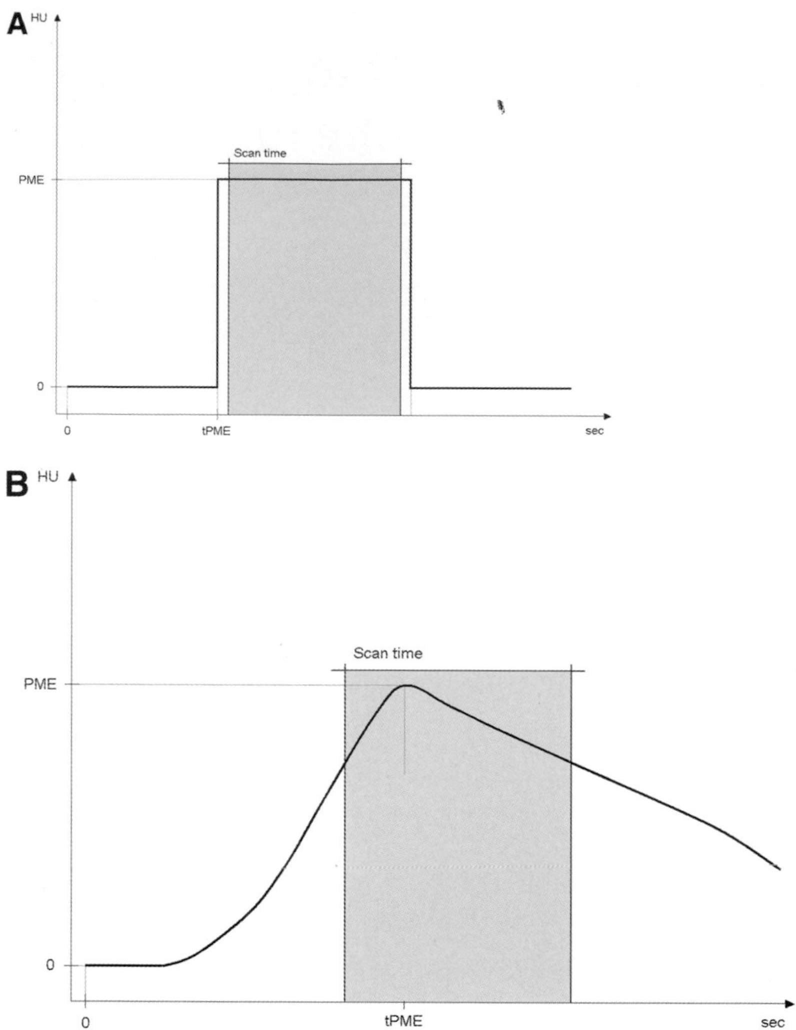

Fig. 1. Optimal and actual bolus geometry in CT angiography (CTA). **(A)** Optimal bolus geometry. The abrupt rise and the steady plateau of attenuation characterize the optimal pattern of bolus geometry. Ideally, the scan time tightly overlaps with the length of the plateau of enhancement in order to use the entire volume of contrast material (CM) administered for the acquisition. **(B)** Actual bolus geometry. The pattern of actual bolus geometry is quite different from the ideal one. Before and after the peak of maximum enhancement there are slopes of enhancement. Generally the up-slope is steeper than the down-slope, especially with CM administration protocols for CTA characterized by a high injection rate.

extracellular intravascular fluid volume. This results in a dilution of CM with a lower iodine concentration in blood, and therefore a reduced PME.

Diseases

A reduced cardiac output produces a proportionally higher PME and longer tPME in the aortic bolus geometry *(6)*. This is a result of the increase in circulation time and CM "pooling," which occur during reduced cardiac output conditions *(6)*.

Injection Volume

A higher volume of CM shifts the time/attenuation curve upwards and rightwards (Fig. 2A) *(1)*. This determines a higher PME and a longer tPME. The relation is independent of injection rate and iodine concentration *(7–9)*.

Injection Rate

Increasing the injection rate produces a proportionally higher PME and earlier tPME with a shift of the time/attenuation curve upwards and leftwards (Fig. 2B) *(1)*. The relationship is independent of iodine concentration and CM injection volume *(2,6–8,10,11)*.

Iodine Concentration

Higher iodine concentration produces a higher PME (Fig. 2C) *(18,12)*. Different iodine concentrations with constant rate and volume, do not affect the injection duration, and this means that the tPME remains unchanged.

Fig. 2. *(right and page 240)* Parameters affecting bolus geometry. **(A)** The influence of contrast material (CM) volume. Increasing the volume of injected CM produces an increase in peak of maxiumum enhancement (PME), and a delayed time to peak (tPME). **(B)** The influence of CM injection rate. Increasing the rate of injected CM produces an increase in PME, and an earlier tPME. **(C)** The influence of CM iodine concentration. Increasing the iodine concentration of the injected CM produces an increase in PME, without any influence on tPME.

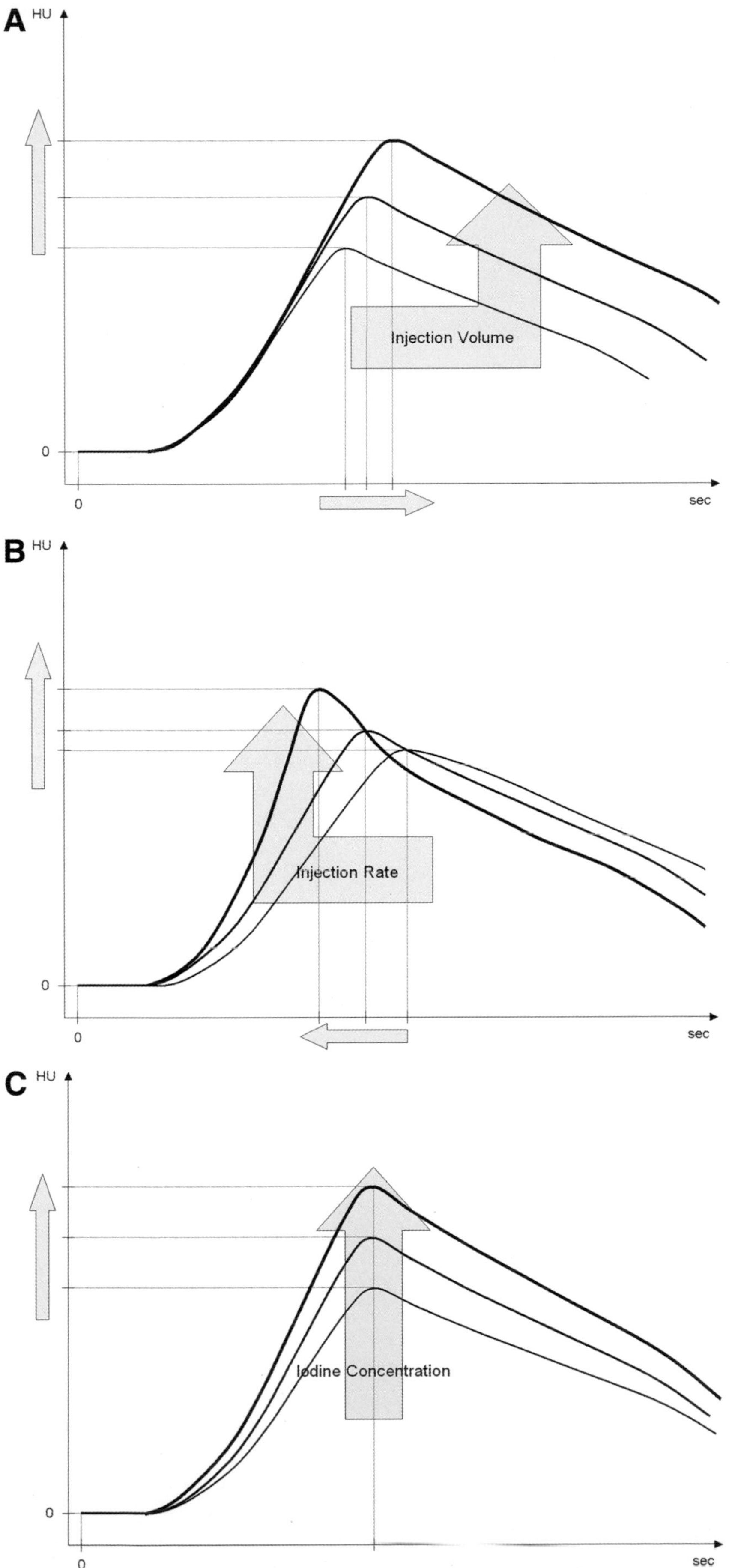
A
HU
Injection Volume
0
0
sec
B
HU
Injection Rate
0
0
sec
C
HU
Iodine Concentration
0
0
sec

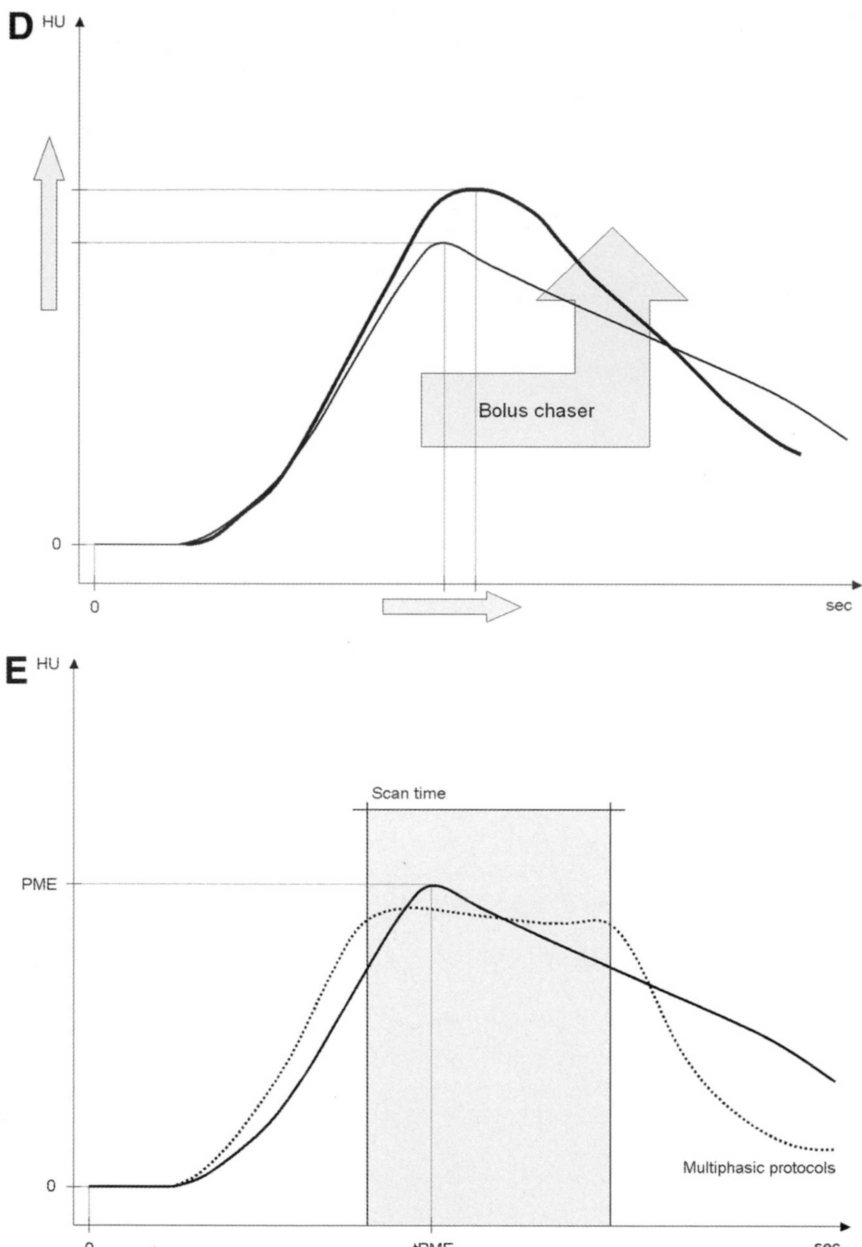

Fig. 2. *(continued from page 238)* **(D)** The influence of saline chaser. The saline chaser pushes the injected contrast medium through the veins of the forearm, providing a result similar to the injection of a larger contrast volume. The example shows the effect of a 50-mL saline chaser (thicker curve), using a bolus with the same volume, rate, and iodine concentration. Moreover, the saline chaser prevents the decrease of the CM in the arm veins, which may normally cause an increase in the CM concentration after the end of the contrast injection. **(E)** The influence of multiphasic protocols. Multiphasic protocols allow producing a longer plateau of enhancement. If the scan time is long (approx 30–35 s), then advantages are consistent, but with a shorter scan time, as with 16-row multislice CT, the importance of a long plateau of enhancement is reduced if compared to the impact of a very high PME.

Bolus Chaser

A bolus chaser is a saline solution pushed through the injection line immediately after the injection of the main bolus *(1)*. Advantages are reported from this technique applied in CT *(13–15)*. Bolus chaser is generally administered by a double-head power injector system *(13)*. With bolus chaser, less contrast medium volume (up to 40% less) can be used for a CTA scan, without affecting arterial enhancement and diagnostic accuracy *(15)*. The PME is higher and the tPME is longer when a bolus chaser is added to the CM injection *(16)*, while no increase in PME and tPME are expected if a bolus chaser is added to the injected volume with a concomitant decrease in the contrast volume, resulting in an unchanged total injection volume (Fig. 2D).

Multiphasic Protocols

Multiphasic protocols are characterized by a decreasing of the injection rate during CM administration *(6,17–20)*. The aim of multiphasic protocols is to create a steady plateau of enhancement during the scan by means of a higher injection rate at the beginning of the injection and a lower rate in the second part (Fig. 2E) *(17)*. The introduction of the last generation of MSCT scanners with shorter scan times reduced the importance of multiphasic protocols. A higher PME can be far more important for the qualitative outcome of the CTA scan.

Injection Site

Contrast material can be administered through an antecubital vein that drains directly into the deep venous circulation of the arm (basilic vein), or a forearm vein that drains into the deep venous circulation of the forearm and subsequently in the deep venous circulation at the elbow joint or into the subclavian vein through the cephalic vein. Larger veins allow higher rates and more safety.

PREDICTION AND SYNCHRONIZATION OF BOLUS GEOMETRY

Patient Demographics

No or poor correlation was reported between a calculated tPME and the actual tPME *(3,21)*. Nevertheless, it is not possible to exclude that in the future a relationship between demographics and bolus timing parameters will be found.

Fixed Delay

Fixed delay is a routinely applied technique for CTA. The increased scan speed of MSCT scanners needs a more careful CM administration. The risks of a fixed-delay technique are related to the fact that, in a percentage of patients, circulation time is quite different from the protocol applied. In those cases the scan could be successful if the circulation time is shorter than that fixed delay, even if a prominent venous enhancement can be observed; but when the circulation time is longer than fixed delay, the scan fails because of the lack of proper attenuation inside the coronary arteries (Fig. 3A).

Test Bolus

Test bolus technique entails that a ROI is plotted inside the lumen of an artery close to the region that needs to be studied. A small amount of CM (10–15 mL, or around 10% of the main bolus) is injected at the same rate as the main bolus while a single level dynamic scan (e.g., monitoring scan) is performed at short intervals (approx 1–2 s). When CM arrives in the lumen of the artery at the level of the ROI, test bolus geometry is assessed and the time between the start of the test bolus injection and a determined point of the time/attenuation curve of the test bolus is used as delay time for the injection of the main bolus (Fig. 3B) *(1)*.

The use of test bolus is based on a relationship between the geometry of the test bolus and that of the main bolus. There is no or poor correlation between test bolus tPME and main bolus tPME *(2,5,22)*, while there is a strong correlation between test bolus tPME and time to reach determined attenuation thresholds like T50, T100, T150, and T200 *(2,5)* (i.e., the time from the beginning of the injection to reach 50/100/150/200 HU in the ROI) in main bolus (Fig. 3B). The result of this is that with conventional test bolus technique the scan is safe but can be too early, especially if the vessels of interest are located at the beginning of the scan range.

Bolus Tracking

Bolus tracking technique is real-time bolus triggering technique. It is based on an ROI that is plotted inside the lumen of an artery close to the region which has to be studied, and a trigger attenuation value (threshold) that is arbitrarily chosen before starting the CTA data acquisition *(1)*. A single level dynamic scan (e.g., monitoring scan) is performed at short intervals (1–2 s) during the injection of CM. When the CM arrives at the level of the ROI, the change in attenuation is detected and a CT scan is started after reaching the triggering threshold (Fig. 3C) *(1)*.

Bolus tracking provides a better timing and allows the use of less CM with a higher injection rate. A pitfall of this technique occurs when the threshold is not reached. Even though it is a very rare event when the protocol is optimized, it is always possible to start the scan manually. In this case it is difficult to obtain a high-quality CTA because of the later start of the scan, the decreased amount of contrast medium inside the vessels, and the prominent venous enhancement.

PATTERNS OF ENHANCEMENT OF CORONARY ARTERIES

Coronary arteries originate at the root of the ascending aorta, and the intravenous CM arrives at that level already diluted, after pulmonary circulation and left-ventricle contraction. Therefore, it can be assumed that the characteristics and the dynamics of bolus geometry inside coronary arteries are the same as in the ascending aorta. Differences in attenuation between ascending aorta and coronary arteries can be determined by stenosis or occlusions. In this case, in fact, there can be various degrees of attenuation inside coronary arteries and their branches depending on the flow through the stenotic vessel or on the backflow provided by collateral circulation. In a patent coronary artery, the flow speed guarantees an optimal enhancement in a few seconds. With stenosis and occlusions, the flow speed can be reduced. The MSCT scanners with 16 slices and approx 0.4-s rotation time provide a scan time of less than 20 s. With a good synchronization technique, the heart has at least 4–6 s before the smaller branches (diagonal and marginal) of the coronary arteries are acquired with a scan performed in the cranio-caudal direction. This time span is generally enough to allow an arterial perfusion and even the collateral circulation to fill in the case of stenosis or occlusion of one or more vessels.

BOLUS TIMING TECHNIQUES WITH 16-ROW MSCT

For cardiac and coronary MSCT imaging, fixed delay, test bolus, and bolus tracking techniques have been applied *(23–28)*. There are no published data comparing bolus timing techniques applied to coronary imaging in the 4-slice era. In fact, the modalities applied for bolus timing have been severely influenced by the speed of acquisition and by the hyperventilation performed just before the scan to allow a longer apnea. In some cases, the use of oxygen to increase the apnea has been reported. For these reasons, bolus tracking was not possible with 4-row MSCT scanners.

With scanners that have 6 or more rows, the scan time can be reduced significantly, especially if there is a parallel reduction in gantry rotation time (<500 ms). With those features, scan time can be reduced below 30 s. Apnea becomes more "affordable" for a larger number of patients without prescan hyperventilation or oxygen administration.

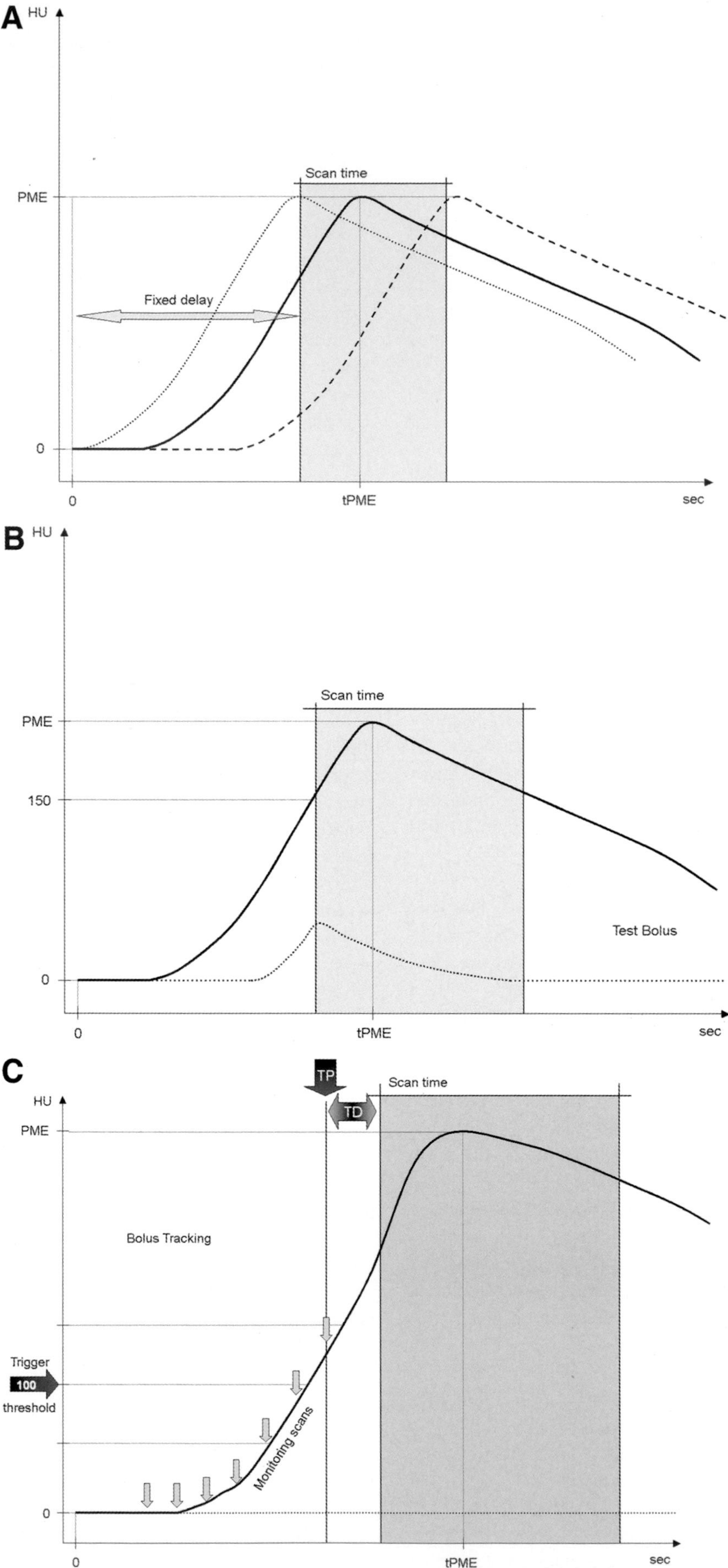
A
HU
Scan time
PME
Fixed delay
0
0
tPME
sec
B
HU
Scan time
PME
150
Test Bolus
0
0
tPME
sec
C
TP
TD
Scan time
HU
PME
Bolus Tracking
Trigger
100
threshold
Monitoring scans
0
0
tPME
sec

Fig. 3. *(left)* Timing and synchronization techniques. (**A**) Fixed delay technique. The image shows the main pitfall of fixed delay technique. The continuous curve shows the ideal situation when the fixed delay and bolus geometry correspond. In some cases the bolus geometry of the patient can be different from the expected one. If actual bolus geometry is faster than fixed delay (dotted curve), the enhancement of vascular structures will be still present but reduced, and prominent venous enhancement can be evident. If actual bolus geometry is slower than fixed delay (tittled curve), the risk is to scan the passage of contrast material (CM) only in the distal portion of the scan range with poor contrast enhancement of arteries. (**B**) Test bolus technique. The correlation between test bolus time to peak of maximum enhancement (tPME) and main bolus tPME is displayed. In this case, the test bolus tPME correlates with the time to reach 150 HU in main bolus. A main scan based on this information will be successful, even though not optimal as a CT angiography (CTA). In fact the vascular attenuation of 150 HU at the beginning of the scan is too low for optimal CTA. Worse results are obtained when the correlation is with the time to reach 50 HU or 100 HU. Test bolus actually has a different geometry than main bolus. The lack of injection power after the end of the injection of test bolus determines a pooling of the test bolus in the venous system without any *vis a tergo*. In other words, test bolus is left alone in the venous system of the arm, without the help of saline solution (bolus chaser) or adjunctive contrast media (main bolus) that pushes it forward. (**C**) Bolus tracking technique. The sequence for real-time bolus tracking is displayed. After the topogram is acquired, the monitoring scan is set at the level of aortic root and the region of interest (ROI) inside the lumen of ascending aorta. The trigger threshold is set at 100 HU. Then, CM administration and monitoring sequence are started at the same time, and when the attenuation in the ROI reaches a value greater than 100 HU at the triggering point (TP), a transition delay (TD—generally 4 s are enough for this procedure) starts while the table reaches its starting position and the patient receives breath-holding instructions.

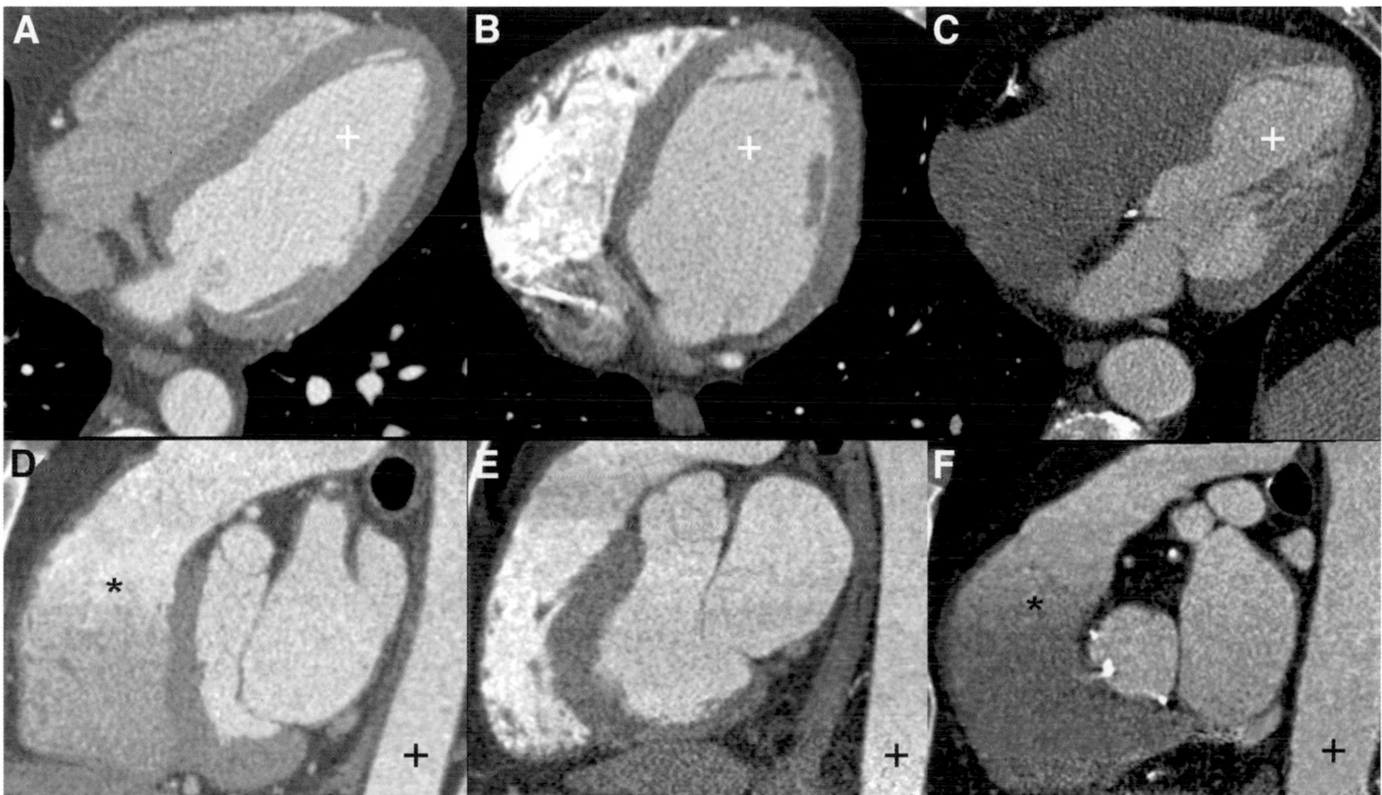

Fig. 4. Examples of different contrast material administration protocols in 16-row multislice coronary CT angiography. Axial (**A**, **B**, and **C**) and sagittal (**D**, **E**, and **F**) multiplanar reformations of three different protocols of CM administration are displayed: 100 mL of 320 mgI/mL CM at 4 mL/s (**A** and **D**); 140 mL of 320 mgI/mL CM at 4 mL/s (B and E); 100 mL of 320 mgI/mL CM + 40 mL of saline chase at 4 mL/s (**C** and **F**). The images from the protocol with 100 mL and the images with 100 mL + 40 mL are similar, as expected, and show a decreasing cranio-caudal gradient of attenuation inside the pulmonary artery (**D** and **F**; black asterisks), that is not present in the protocol with 140 mL (**E**). The enhancement in the descending aorta is preserved in every protocol (**D**, **E**, and **F**; black +), as well as the enhancement in the left ventricle (**A**, **B**, and **C**; white +).

Bolus tracking is an optimal method for CM synchronization in noninvasive CTA (Fig. 4). Bolus tracking, in fact, is less time consuming than test bolus techniques (because of the calculation needed with test bolus), allows the use of less CM (the larger bolus needed to have a wider enhancement plateau with fixed delay, or the 20 mL needed for test bolus), and prevents suboptimal synchronization (determined by inter-individual veno-arterial circulation time with fixed delay, and by the lack of reliable relationship between the tPME of test bolus and main bolus). No significant differences are observed regarding the attenuation reached at the level of aortic root, whether an injection volume of 100 mL or 140 mL is used.

Therefore, a volume of 100 mL, especially if followed by a saline chaser, provides optimal enhancement with reduced volume and renal toxicity for the patient. A rate of injection of 4 mL/s is optimal because it is feasible in almost every patient through a 18-gauge venflon (green), with a very low risk of CM extravasation. Iodine concentration is proportional to the attenuation value obtained, and concentrations of 320–350 mgI/mL are optimal for coronary angiography purposes. Bolus chaser is always recommended because it allows using a reduced volume of CM more effectively.

GUIDELINES FOR CONTRAST MATERIAL ADMINISTRATION

CM administration technique for the purpose of noninvasive CTA with multislice scanners can be summarized as follows:

Choice of CM: use nonionic iodinated CM. Higher iodine concentrations will provide higher attenuation, and different molecules will not affect the final result significantly. The iodine concentration ranges between 300 mgI/mL and 400 mgI/mL.

Site of administration: start with the right antecubital access and then use the left one if there are difficulties. Use forearm or hand only if the antecubital accesses are not available. When using central IV lines, reduce the rate of infusion slightly to 2.5–3.0 mL/s.

Administration device: an 18-gage venflon (green) is suitable in all patients. In women or younger patients, the access could be easier with a 20-gage venflon (pink), even though a reduced rate is recommended in this case (3.0 mL/s).

Volume: with the 16-row generation scanners, 100 mL of CM provides optimal enhancement if a bolus tracking technique is properly applied. With a lower number of detector rows, an increased volume is needed, down to 150 mL of CM with 4-row generation scanners.

Rate: a 4 mL/s rate provides optimal results. Reduced injection rates (3.0 mL/s) are needed with smaller venflons and/or in patients with small or fragile veins.

Bolus chaser: the use of bolus chaser, when possible, is strongly recommended to increase the amount of CM used during the scan and/or to reduce the overall amount of CM administered.

TIMING AND SYNCHRONIZATION TECHNIQUES

Fixed delay technique: a delay of 18 s allows a good scan in most of the patients. In patients with mildly or severely impaired cardiac function, a delay of 25 s is recommended.

Test bolus technique: calculate the tPME of the test bolus and then add 4 s for an optimal scan delay.

Bolus tracking technique: is safe and allows a tailored scan synchronization. The trigger threshold is set at 100 HU with a transition delay of 4 s needed to give breath-hold instructions to the patient. It requires proper training of the patient, and of the technician.

REFERENCES

1. Cademartiri F, van der Lugt A, Luccichenti G, Pavone P, Krestin GP. Parameters affecting bolus geometry in CTA: a review. J Comput Assist Tomogr 2002;26:596–607.
2. Platt JF, Reige KA, Ellis JH. Aortic enhancement during abdominal CT angiography: correlation with test injections, flow rates, and patient demographics. AJR Am J Roentgenol 1999;172:53–56.
3. Puskas Z, Schuierer G. [Determination of blood circulation time for optimizing contrast medium administration in CT angiography] Kreislaufzeitbestimmung zur Optimierung der Kontrastmittelapplikation bei der CT-Angiographie. Radiologe 1996;36: 750–757.
4. Kirchner J, Kickuth R, Laufer U, Noack M, Liermann D. Optimized enhancement in helical CT: experiences with a real-time bolus tracking system in 628 patients. Clin Radiol 2000;55:368–373.
5. van Hoe L, Marchal G, Baert AL, Gryspeerdt S, Mertens L. Determination of scan delay time in spiral CT-angiography: utility of a test bolus injection. J Comput Assist Tomogr 1995;19:216–220.
6. Bae KT, Heiken JP, Brink JA. Aortic and hepatic contrast medium enhancement at CT. Part II. Effect of reduced cardiac output in a porcine model. Radiology 1998;207:657–662.
7. Garcia P, Genin G, Bret PM, Bonaldi VM, Reinhold C, Atri M. Hepatic CT enhancement: effect of the rate and volume of contrast medium injection in an animal model. Abdom Imaging 1999;24: 597–603.
8. Han JK, Kim AY, Lee KY, et al. Factors influencing vascular and hepatic enhancement at CT: experimental study on injection protocol using a canine model. J Comput Assist Tomogr 2000;24: 400–406.
9. Nakayama M, Yamashita Y, Oyama Y, Ando M, Kadota M, Takahashi M. Hand exercise during contrast medium delivery at thoracic helical CT: a simple method to minimize perivenous artifact. J Comput Assist Tomogr 2000;24:432–436.
10. Coche EE, Muller NL, Kim KI, Wiggs BR, Mayo JR. Acute pulmonary embolism: ancillary findings at spiral CT. Radiology 1998; 207:753–758.
11. Luboldt W, Straub J, Seemann M, Helmberger T, Reiser M. Effective contrast use in CT angiography and dual-phase hepatic CT performed with a subsecond scanner. Invest Radiol 1999;34:751–760.
12. Bluemke DA, Fishman EK, Anderson JH. Effect of contrast concentration on abdominal enhancement in the rabbit: spiral computed tomography evaluation. Acad Radiol 1995;2:226–231.
13. Haage P, Schmitz-Rode T, Hubner D, Piroth W, Gunther RW. Reduction of contrast material dose and artifacts by a saline flush using a double power injector in helical CT of the thorax. AJR Am J Roentgenol 2000;174:1049–1053.
14. Hopper KD, Mosher TJ, Kasales CJ, TenHave TR, Tully DA, Weaver JS. Thoracic spiral CT: delivery of contrast material pushed with injectable saline solution in a power injector. Radiology 1997; 205:269–271.
15. Bader TR, Prokesch RW, Grabenwoger F. Timing of the hepatic arterial phase during contrast-enhanced computed tomography of the liver: assessment of normal values in 25 volunteers. Invest Radiol 2000;35:486–492.
16. Sadick M, Lehmann KJ, Diehl SJ, Wild J, Georgi M. [Bolus tracking and NaCl bolus in biphasic spiral CT of the abdomen] Bolustriggerung und NaCl-Bolus bei der biphasischen Spiral-CT des Abdomens. Rofo Fortschr Geb Rontgenstr Neuen Bildgeb Verfahr 1997; 167:371–376.
17. Fleischmann D, Rubin GD, Bankier AA, Hittmair K. Improved uniformity of aortic enhancement with customized contrast medium injection protocols at CT angiography. Radiology 2000; 214:363–371.
18. Hittmair K, Fleischmann D. Accuracy of predicting and controlling time-dependent aortic enhancement from a test bolus injection. J Comput Assist Tomogr 2001;25:287–294.
19. Fleischmann D, Hittmair K. Mathematical analysis of arterial enhancement and optimization of bolus geometry for CT angiography using the discrete Fourier transform. J Comput Assist Tomogr 1999;23:474–484.
20. Bae KT, Tran HQ, Heiken JP. Multiphasic injection method for uniform prolonged vascular enhancement at CT angiography: pharmacokinetic analysis and experimental porcine model. Radiology 2000;216:872–880.

21. Nakajima Y, Yoshimine T, Yoshida H, et al. Computerized tomography angiography of ruptured cerebral aneurysms: factors affecting time to maximum contrast concentration. J Neurosurg 1998; 88: 663–669.
22. Kaatee R, Van Leeuwen MS, De Lange EE, et al. Spiral CT angiography of the renal arteries: should a scan delay based on a test bolus injection or a fixed scan delay be used to obtain maximum enhancement of the vessels? J Comput Assist Tomogr 1998;22:541–547.
23. Nieman K, Oudkerk M, Rensig BJ, et al. Coronary angiography with multislice computed tomography. Lancet 2001;357:599–603.
24. Achenbach S, Ulzheimer S, Baum U, et al. Noninvasive coronary angiography by retrospectively ECG-gated multislice spiral CT. Circulation 2000;102:2823–2828.
25. Knez A, Becker CR, Leber A, et al. Usefulness of multislice spiral computed tomography angiography for determination of coronary artery stenoses. Am J Cardiol 2001;88:1191–1194.
26. Nieman K, Rensing BJ, van Geuns RJ, et al. Usefulness of multislice computed tomography for detecting obstructive coronary artery disease. Am J Cardiol 2002;89:913–918.
27. Vogl TJ, Abolmaali ND, Diebold T, et al. Techniques for the detection of coronary atherosclerosis: multi-detector row CT coronary angiography. Radiology 2002;223:212–220.
28. Nieman K, Cademartiri F, Lemos PA, Raaijmakers R, Pattynama PM, de Feyter PJ. Reliable noninvasive coronary angiography with fast submillimeter multislice spiral computed tomography. Circulation 2002;106:2051–2054.

24 Visualization Techniques for Contrast-Enhanced CT Angiography of Coronary Arteries

Jean-Louis Sablayrolles, MD and Pascal Giat, PhD

INTRODUCTION

One of the critical components for effective cardiac computed tomography (CT) application is a fully integrated and optimized image visualization, postprocessing, and analysis tool. Study of native axial images is not enough to assess all cardiac structures, especially coronary arteries (Fig. 1). Postprocessing is critical to visualize the arterial system and heart chambers. Specific tools have been designed and are still under development. They require a powerful postprocessing workstation. A complete study of coronary arteries needs to follow a systematic protocol including various postprocessing tools.

STUDY OF CORONARY ARTERIES

SELECTION OF OPTIMUM PHASE WITH MULTIPHASE REVIEW OF REFORMATTED IMAGES

Acquisition synchronized with the electrocardiogram (ECG) makes it possible to eliminate motion blur caused by the heartbeats. After acquisition, the data are collected and processed along with the ECG recording. Slice thickness, increment, and reconstruction window can be varied with respect to the duration of the cardiac cycle. In general, diastole is centered at 80% of the cycle time when the coronaries and chambers show less motion and best coronary filling. For coronary artery examination, it is sometimes necessary to reconstruct several stages of the cardiac cycle to obtain optimum image quality without motion artifacts (Fig. 2). It is possible to reconstruct images of other phases in the cardiac cycle and to produce dynamic sequences not only with the basic axial images but also using reconstructed images.

This is a first step in cardiac CT imaging that is crucial prior to any image postprocessing. In practice, data are reconstructed at different cardiac phases, typically every 10% of the RR cycle interval using 0.6-mm slice thickness every 0.6 mm. All slices of all phases are loaded on the workstation (Advantage Windows, GE Medical Systems) simultaneously, using specific postprocessing tools (CardIQ Analysis). The selection of the best phase is performed on 2D reformatted images using three planes: (1) short axis plane to check the regularity of both ventricles; (2) double oblique coronal plane with multiplanar volume reformation (MPVR) (4–5 mm) of the right coronary artery; and (3) double oblique axial plane with MPVR of left common artery, left anterior descending (LAD) artery, and left circumflex artery. Each phase is displayed successively and the best phase is selected. Figure 3, taken from a study done on 87 exams, shows that the best phase, which depends on the patient, is usually between 75 and 80%.

IDENTIFICATION OF RIGHT AND LEFT CORONARY ARTERIES TOGETHER WITH COLLATERAL BRANCHES IN VOLUME DATA SETS

Locating the coronary arteries is based on a 3D image process fully dedicated to heart assessment. This 3D image processing enables mapping of the coronary arteries network with respect to other cardiac structures and mediastinal vessels. It allows the user to localize coronary artery lesions, and to diagnose and map an occlusion or an aneurysm.

For the coronary artery study, only the best phase is used. For the same patient, cycle times may be different for the study of the right coronary artery, the circumflex, and the left anterior descending artery. When misregistration occurs due to a varying heart rate, images are produced in different cardiac phases and combined using phase registration to improve image quality. In addition, the use of all phases together allows a morphological study in diastole and systole of the left ventricle walls.

Volume Rendering

This 3D study is used to visualize and to identify the coronary arteries. Special software is required to automatically remove bone structures and some mediastinal structures, notably the pulmonary trunk and left atrium, by using the Autoselect tool. This allows better visualization of the coronary ostia and branches in any plane by erasing the left atrium and pulmonary trunk (Fig. 4).

One can also rotate the 3D heart view by selecting a one-touch catheterization protocol that orientates the image to a typical cath lab view. Cine mode imaging of all predefined projections can be achieved on all axes. This 3D image process provides detail on the localization of coronary arteries with respect to other cardiac structures, especially in the case of the anomalous origin of coronary arteries and coronary bypasses.

From: *Contemporary Cardiology: CT of the Heart: Principles and Applications*
Edited by: U. Joseph Schoepf © Humana Press, Inc., Totowa, NJ

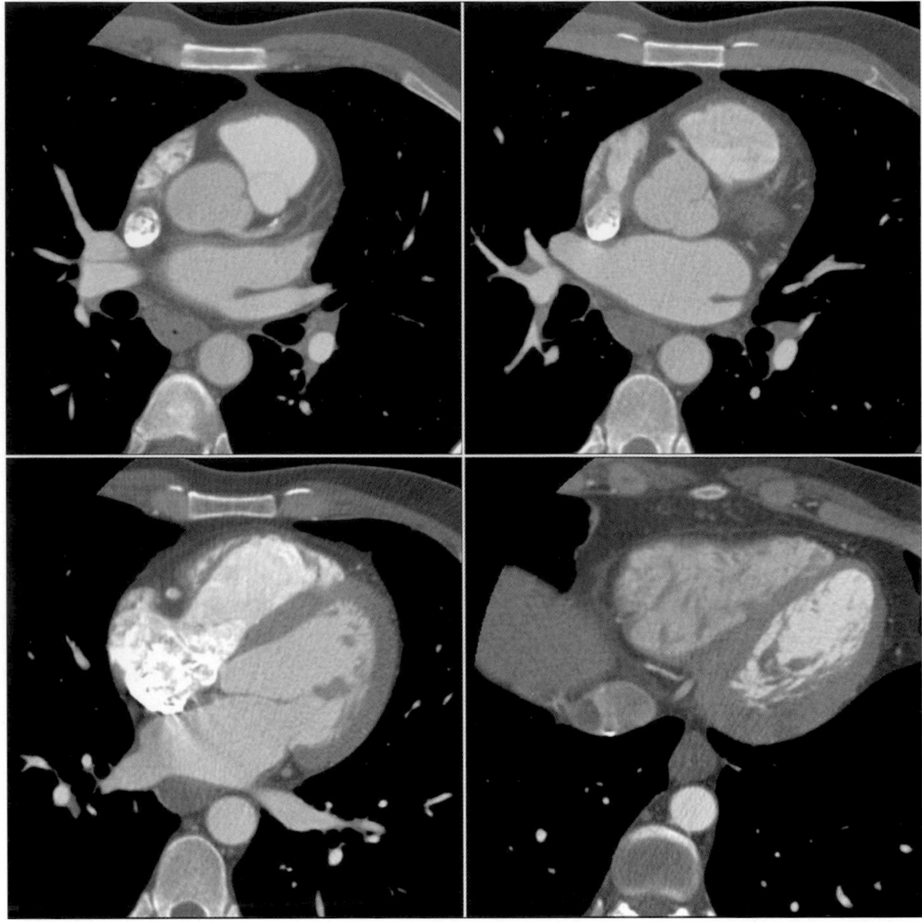

Fig. 1. Axial: Axial sections—ECG-synchronized volumetric acquisition with 0.6-mm sections.

3D Maximum Intensity Projection

Three-dimensional maximum intensity projection (MIP) gives a MIP projection of coronary arteries with automatic fading of contrasted cardiac chambers. Images obtained can be aligned in right anterior oblique view, left anterior oblique view, spider view, or any view routinely used for conventional X-ray coronary angiography (Fig. 5). Three-dimensional MIP is used to study the different branches of the right and left coronary arteries in all projections and to isolate a given artery in order to determine the potential area of lesions. This can be easily done when the stenosis is caused by soft plaque. However, this is more complex for stenosis caused by calcified plaque, which requires a 2D study to clearly separate the lumen from the calcifications of the artery wall.

Three-dimensional MIP that leads to real coronary artery mapping supports MPVR to 2D reformat.

Both 3D techniques show advantages and disadvantages. Three-dimensional MIP enables good visualization of the lumen and parietal wall calcifications. Three-dimensional volume rendering is more appropriate to specify the mapping of each coronary artery and its position relative to the surrounding structures (Fig. 6).

Coronary Vessel Tree

A coronary vessel tree can be generated and displayed in a semi-automatic process (from a single point in the ascending aorta), to give users a qualitative overview of coronary vessel structures in MIP or volume rendering.

STUDY OF BIFURCATIONS WITHIN DIFFERENT PROJECTIONS

MPVR is an MIP with a thickness =5 mm. The different seg-ments of the coronary arteries can be differentiated. The system makes use of the low contrast level of the fatty tissue surrounding the vessels. Each coronary artery can be displayed, in its entirety or segment by segment, using cine MPVR (Fig. 7). For example, this can be used to study arterial bifurcations, which require special attention because the risk of stenosis or thrombosis is even greater where the bifurcation can be divided into at least two branches of the same size, and show an increasingly sharp angle between the artery and its branches (Fig. 8).

STUDY OF VESSEL WALLS WITH CARDIQ ANALYSIS IN 2D, MPVR, OR VIRTUAL ENDOSCOPY

Three-dimensional images allow the user to localize coronary artery lesions but are insufficient to enable precise study of lesions. Two-dimensional reformatting is necessary for the study and the quantification of stenosis, atheromatous plaques, and intra-stent lumen in both the short and long axis of the vessel.

MPVR With Autobone

Based on 3D MIP reconstructed images with automatic fading of contrasted cardiac cavities, all collaterals are analyzed

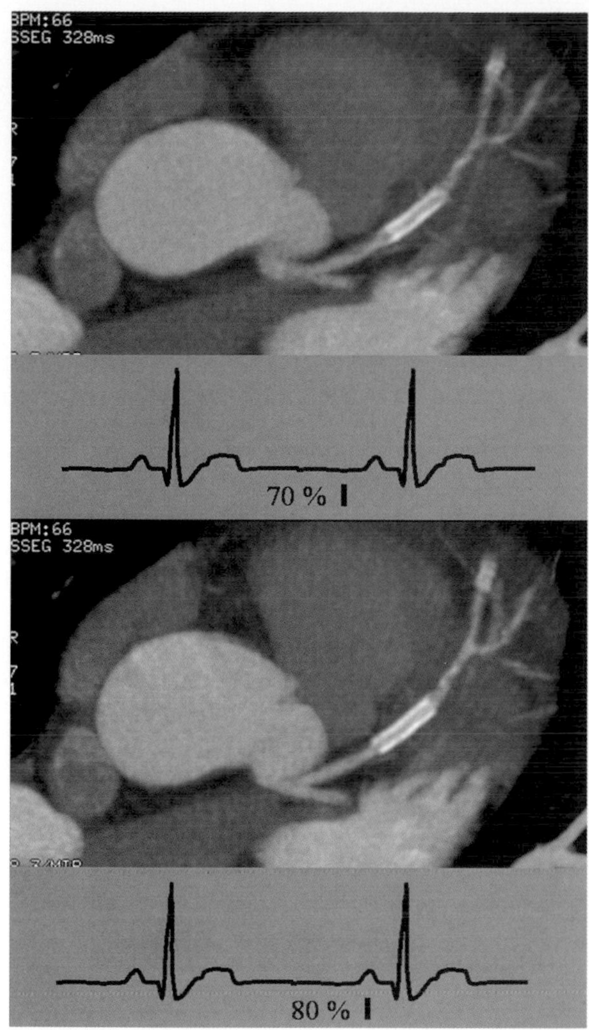

Fig. 2. Phase selection: Reconstruction of data in several phases. Optimal phase = 80%.

65%	70%	75%	80%	85%	90%
2	12	33	32	7	1

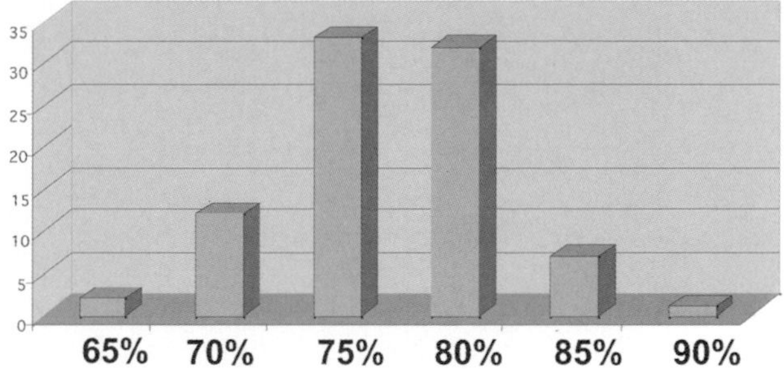

Fig. 3. Table and graph of cardiac phases. Optimal motion suppression typically occurs at 75% and 80% RR.

together with their distal branches without being hidden by the other opacified structures (e.g., pulmonary artery and veins, left atrium, and so on) (Fig. 9).

Curved 2D Reformatting

Curved 2D reformatting preserves the characteristics of the basic axial slices; the lumen and the wall can be dissociated (soft plaque, calcification, stent). This study can easily be made using cardiac vessel analyzing (CVA), a dedicated postprocessing procedure that automatically tracks, extracts, and measures coronary artery vessels. This allows rapid and consistent imaging and analysis of cardiac vessel pathologies. With single-point deposit on each vessel, it automatically identifies and tracks the vessel centerline of each branch. CVA automatically produces vessel lumen view, MPVR, and 2D curved reformation (Fig. 10). It is then possible:

To analyze each branch in MPVR and 2D in different projections (Fig. 11).

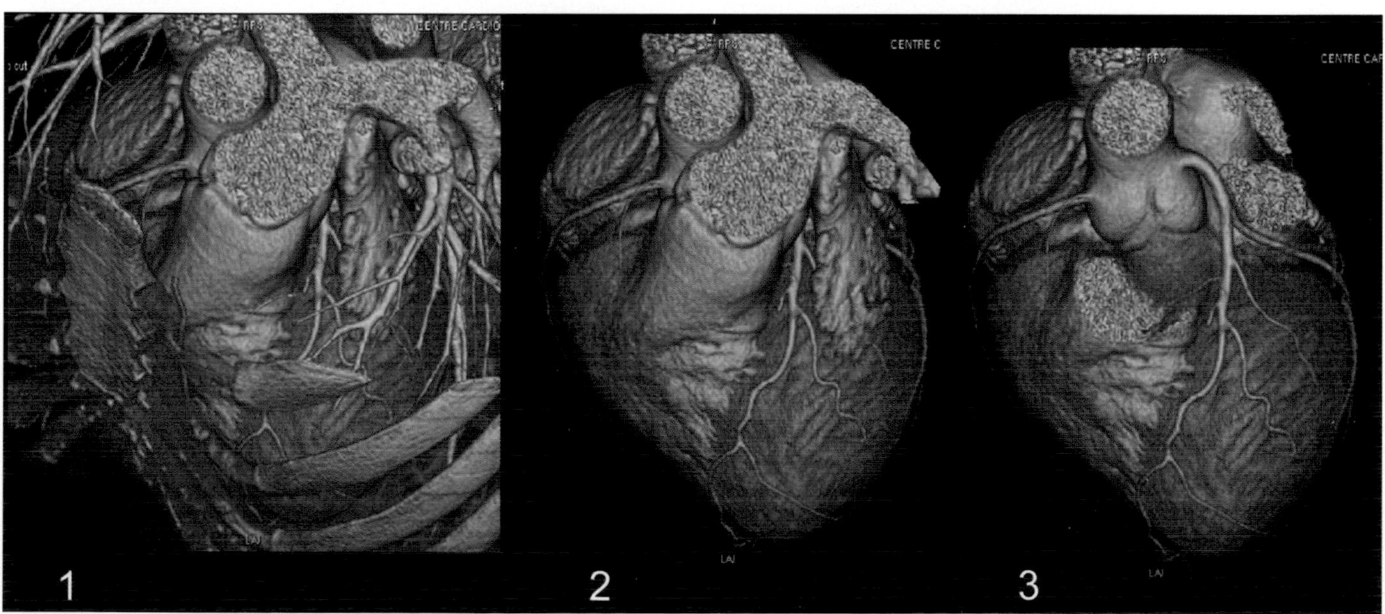

Fig. 4. Volume-rendering technique (VRT) shows entire thorax (1). VRT after automatic suppression of thoracic structures (2). VRT after suppression of pulmonary vessels and of left atrium by Autoselect (3).

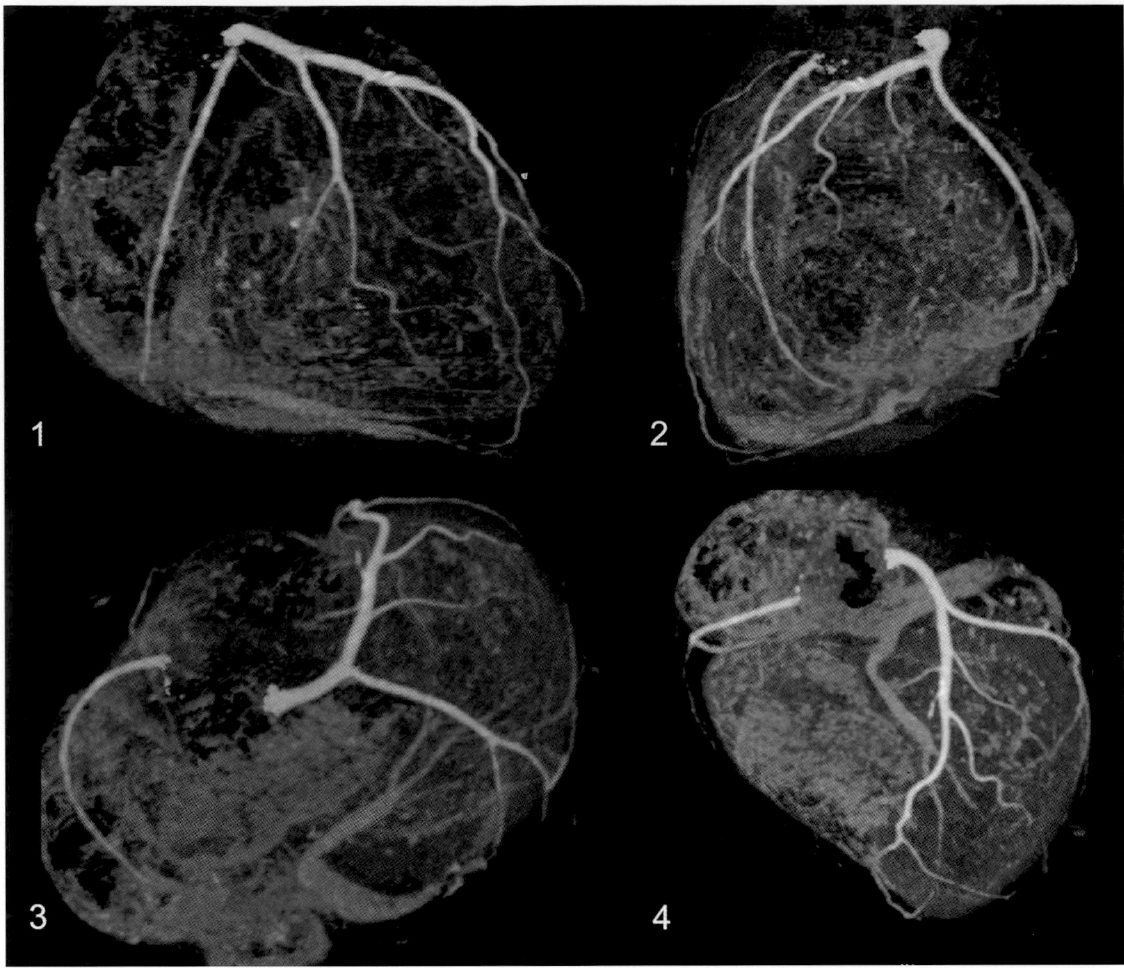

Fig. 5. Maximum intensity projection with automatic suppression of opacified cavities. Routine projections in X-ray corony catheter: frontal view (**1**), lateral view (**2**), spider view (**3**), left anterior oblique view with cranial angulation (**4**).

To assess and quantify a stenosis. CVA enables quantitative analysis of the stenosis. The lumen view is an automatic unfolded view of the true lumen of the vessel with quantification of the mean diameter and the surface area at each point along the centerline (Fig. 12).

Plaque Study With Curved 2D Reformatting

Two-dimensional reformatting is the only reconstruction technique that is able to differentiate the vessel lumen from the atheromatous plaque that causes the stenosis, and to specify its nature. This approach could provide information for the identification of vulnerable plaque. At present, it is possible to define soft, combined, or calcified plaque and to characterize plaque composition and rupture-prone soft coronary lesions.

Based on mean CT attenuation, predominantly lipid-rich plaque can be differentiated from predominantly fibrous-rich plaque.

- The noncalcified lipid-rich plaque (mean density 20 HU) shows a hypodense structure whose density value is greater than the density of perivascular fat. At the present time, the current spatial and density resolution of a CT scanner does not allow a precise study of the plaque's lipidic component, ulceration, or dissection (Figs. 13 and 14).
- The fibrous-rich or atheromatous plaque is a well-defined, homogenous plaque with intermediate density (50 HU) (Fig. 15).
- The eccentric combined plaque shows an internal component that is hypodense together with a peripheral calcified component (Fig. 16).
- Calcified plaque (density >130 HU) shows a density greater than the density of the lumen at the stenosis level with a blooming component that exaggerates its size. Calcified plaque generates an irregular increase in the size of the artery owing to its external development.
- The intimal hyperplasia of an intrastent restenosis is expressed by an intrastent hypodensity compared with the wall of the hyperdense stent, which causes a small irregular lumen diameter (Fig. 17).

Stenosis Quantification

The measurements of diameters and surfaces allows the automatic quantification of the degree of stenosis. The accuracy of the contour detection allows the differentiation of the calcified plaques from contrasted lumen. An objective estimation of the degree of stenosis can be achieved. Those measures depend on the quality of the acquisition, especially with respect to the spatial resolution (Fig. 18).

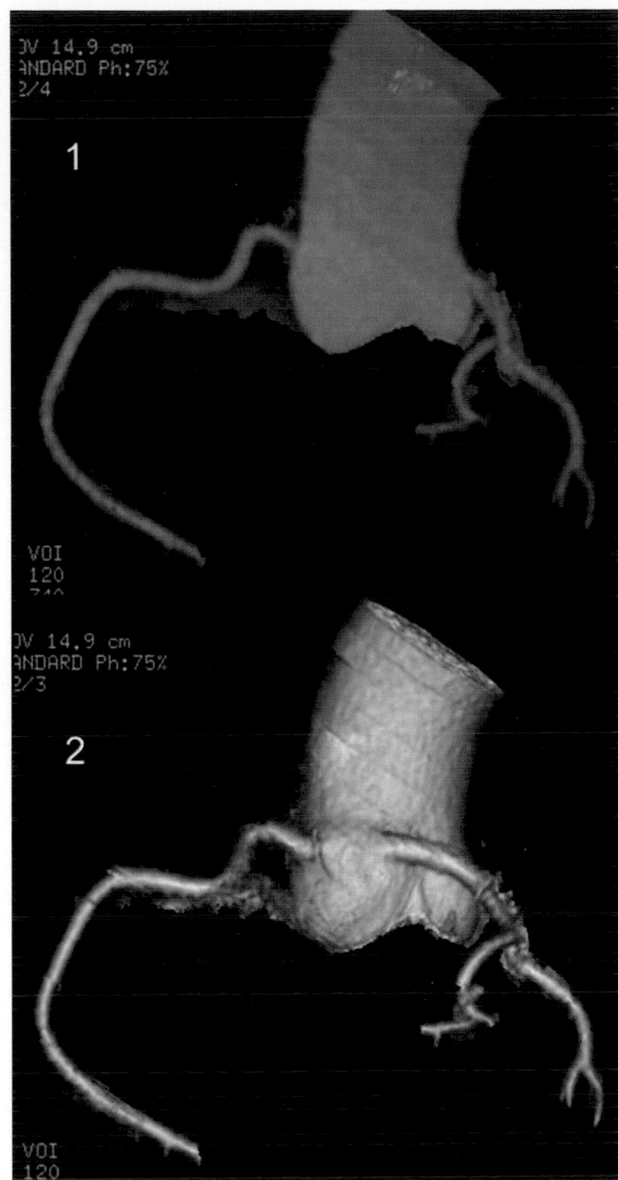

Fig. 6. Maximum intensity projection (**1**) and volume rendering (VR) (**2**) of coronary ostia. In VR, improved visualization of anomalous origin of left coronary artery: ostium in right sinus, main trunk passes ventral to the aorta.

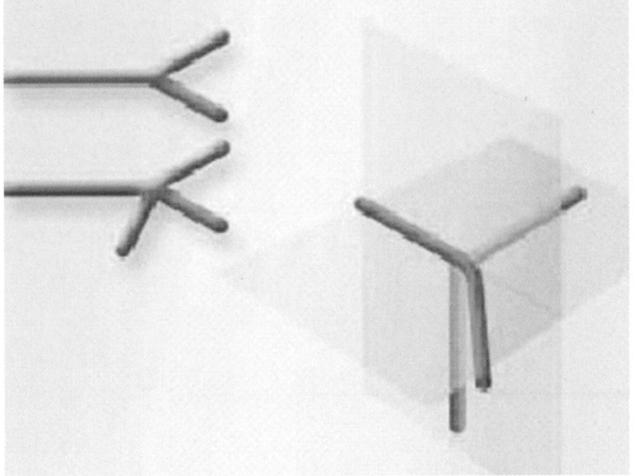

Fig. 8. Bifurcations: areas at risk for stenosis.

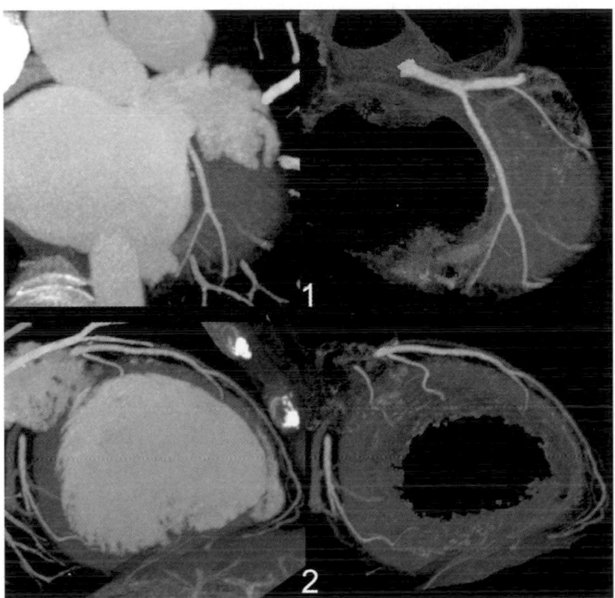

Fig. 9. Multiplanar volume reformation with Autobone from maximum intensity projection reconstructions: Good visualization of main trunk, left circumflex (**1**), and left anterior descending (**2**) with excellent display of their distal branches.

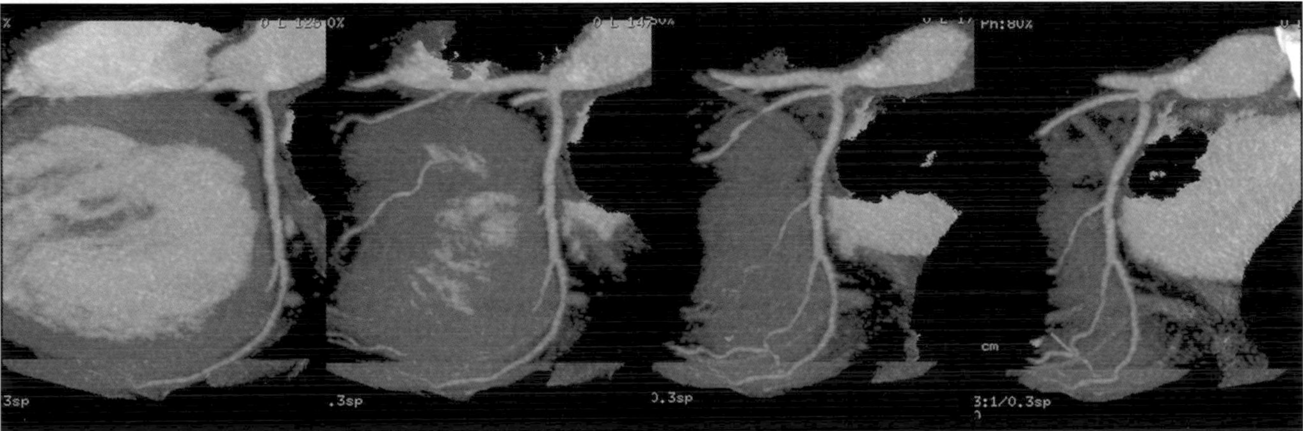

Fig. 7. A cine multiplanar volume reformation centered on the left circumflex artery is used to visualize the ostia of each collateral.

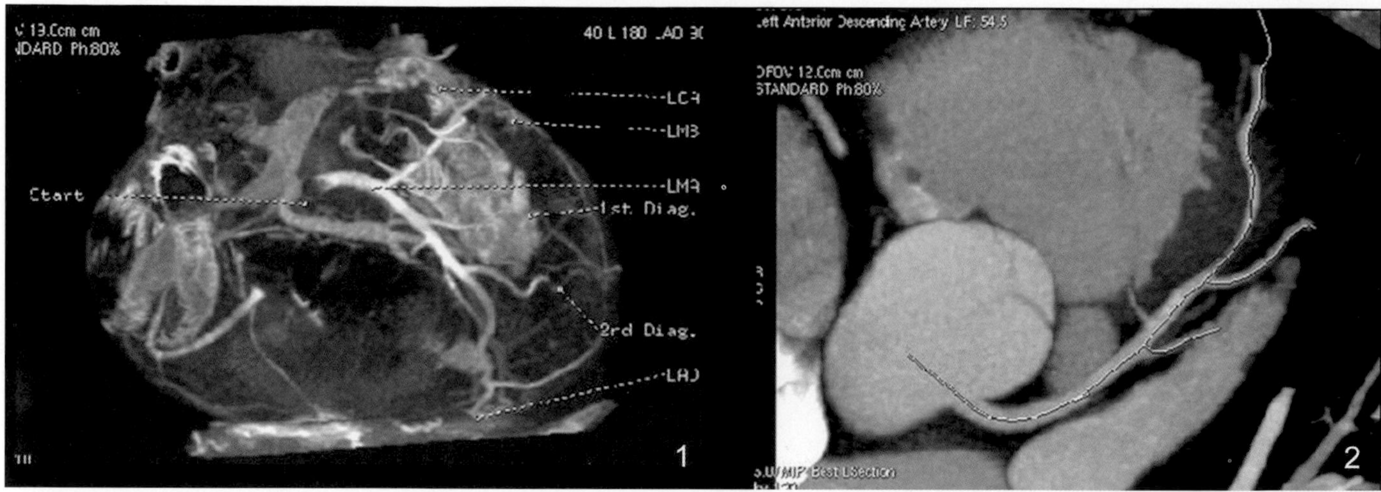

Fig. 10. Coronary vessel analysis: automatic location (**1**) and identification (**2**) of the lumen of each left coronary artery branch.

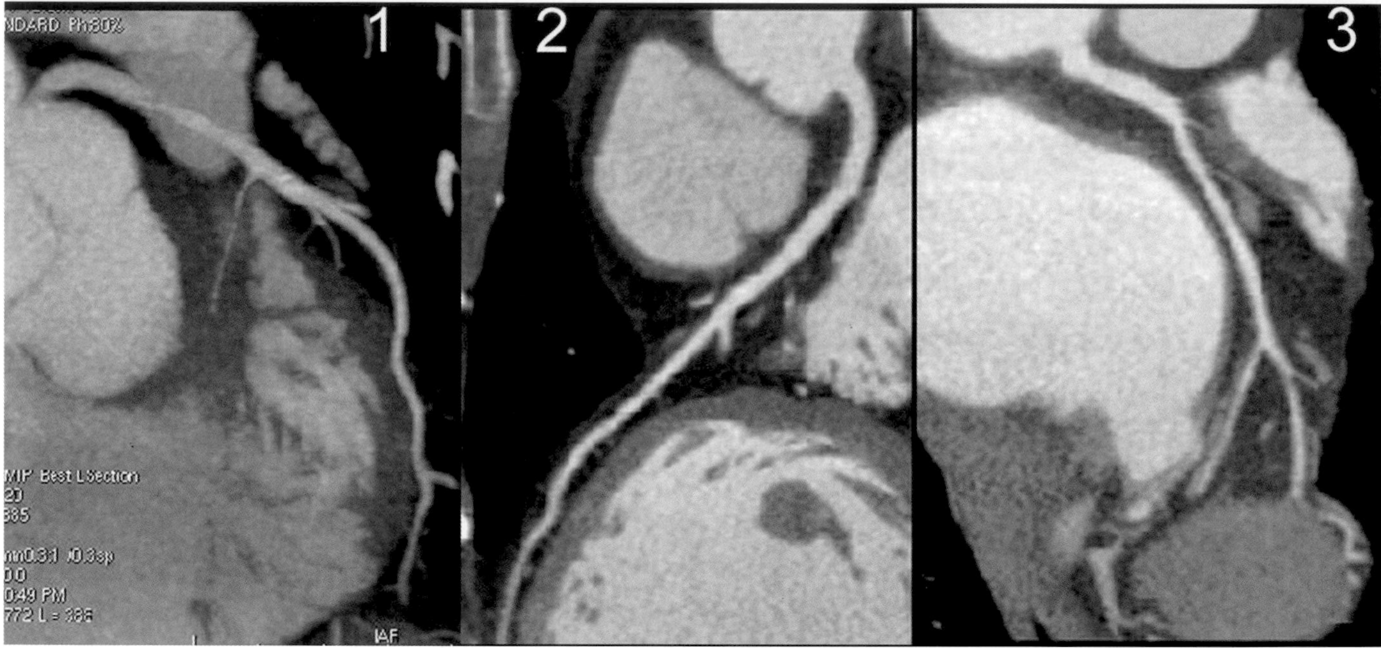

Fig. 11. Coronary vessel analysis: study in multiplanar volume reformation (**1**) and in 2D (**2**) of left anterior descending and in 2D (**3**) of left circumflex.

Navigator/Virtual Endoscopy

The navigator or virtual endoscopy performs an endoluminal exploration of all arterial segments, particularly in the case of anomalous origin of coronary arteries or bifurcations, where stenosis or occlusions often occur (Fig. 19).

STUDY OF MYOCARDIUM WALL AND HEART CHAMBERS

MORPHOLOGIC IMAGING WITH SINGLE OR MULTIPHASE 2D REFORMATTING

With the same data, volume acquisition allows excellent assessment of the cardiac chambers, the myocardium, pericardium, and heart valves on 2D reconstructions in different planes adapted to their anatomy. For evaluation of the myocardium wall, cardiac images may be reformatted in various orientations, such as short-axis and long-axis chamber views, using integrated batch-processing tools. The reformatted images can be saved as separate image series for further processing, such as cardiac cine review and functional analysis.

As with other cross-sectional techniques such as echocardiography or magnetic resonance imaging (MRI), the cardiac chambers can be studied according to the following views. Compared to previous techniques mentioned above, 2D images obtained by CT are reconstructed retrospectively using post-processing based on volume acquisition, and are not directly generated during the acquisition.

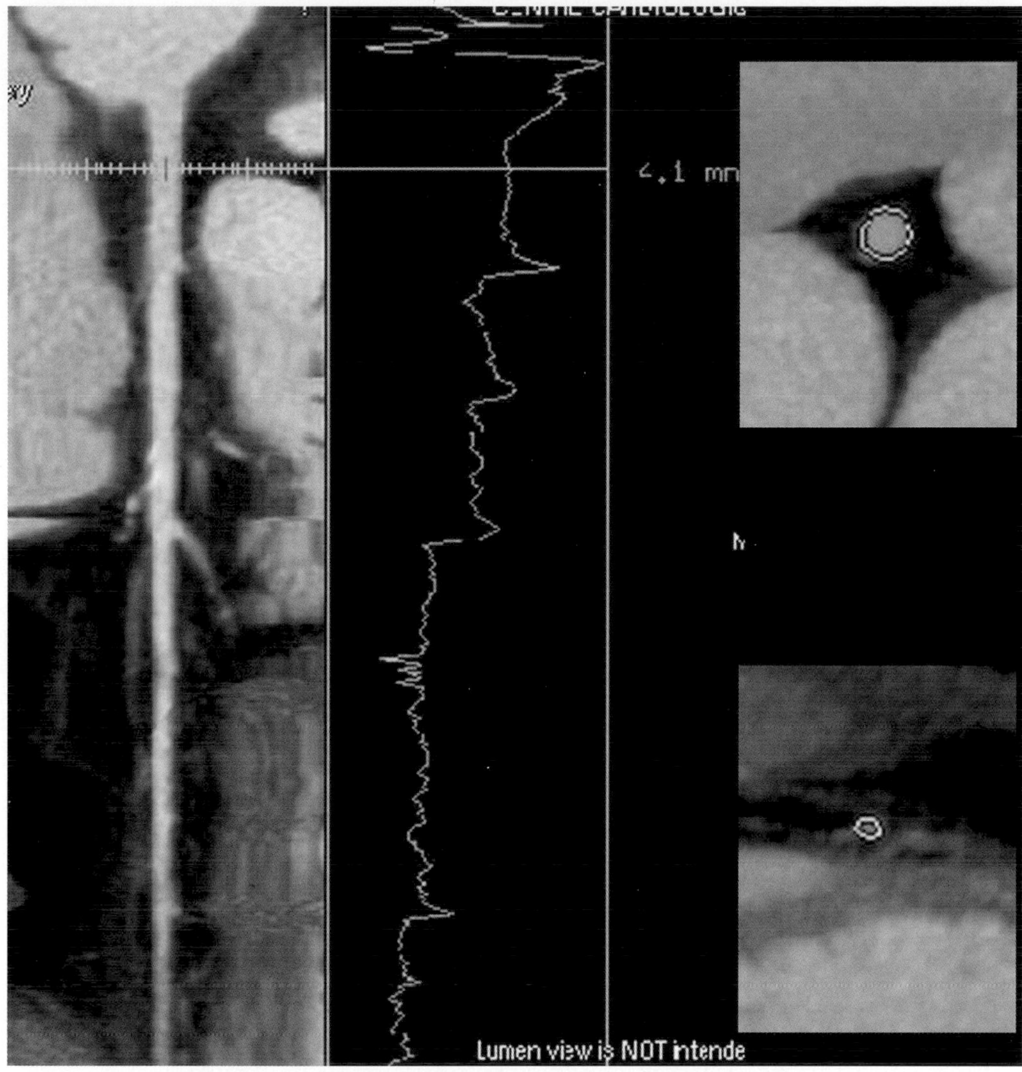

Fig. 12. Coronary vessel analysis: automatic measurements of lumen diameter and area.

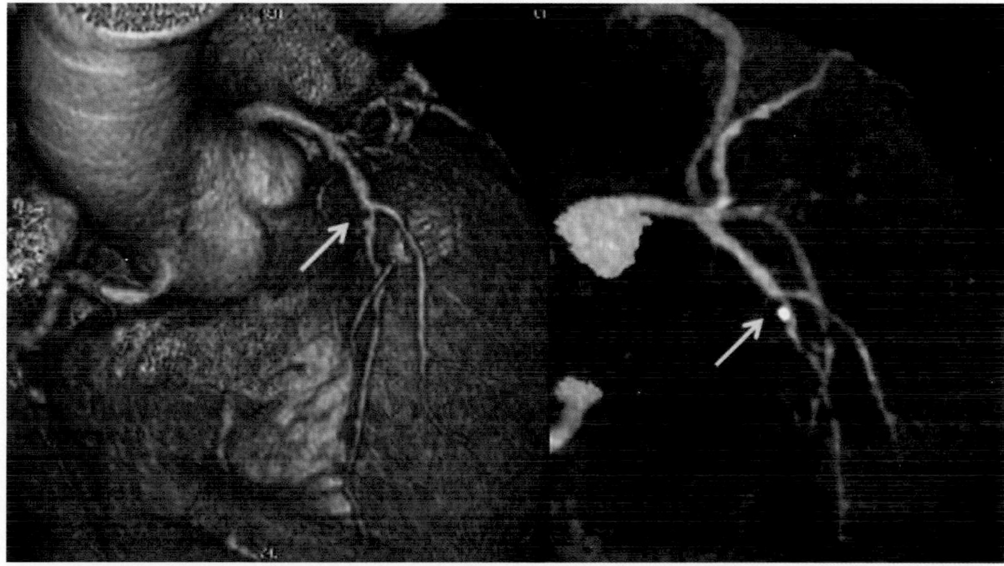

Fig. 13. Coronary vessel analysis: maximum intensity projection and volume rendering: left anterior descending stenosis.

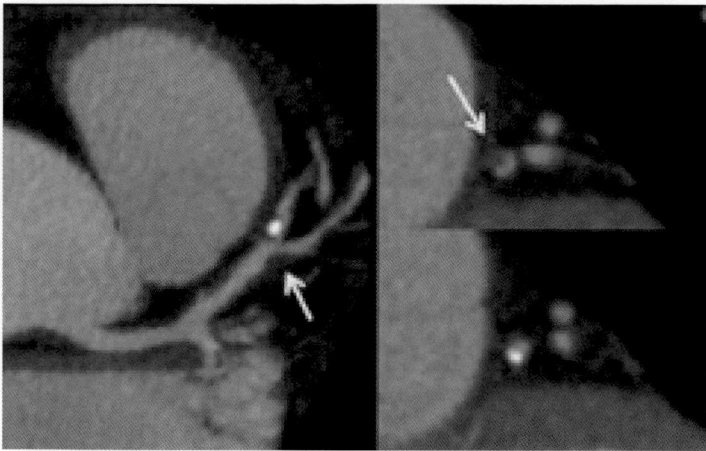

Fig. 14. Coronary vessel analysis: left anterior descending stenosis in 2D long axis and short axis–soft plaque.

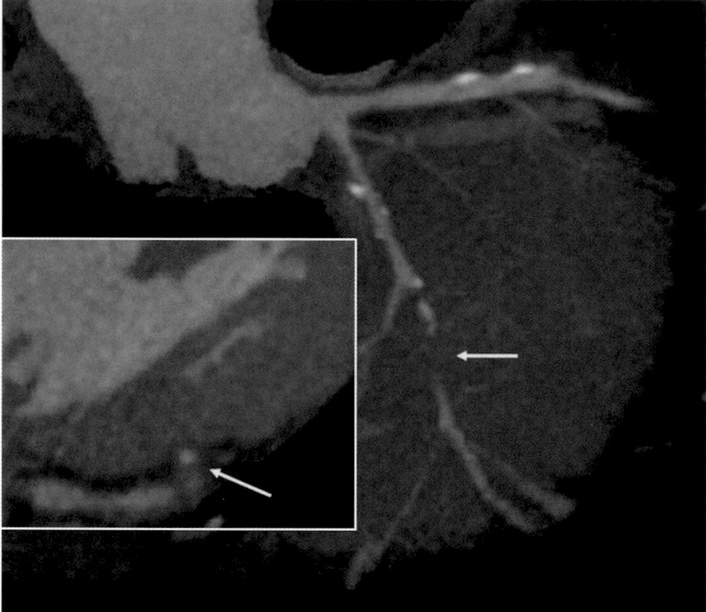

Fig. 15. Coronary vessel analysis: left circumflex stenosis on fibrous plaque in 2D long axis and short axis.

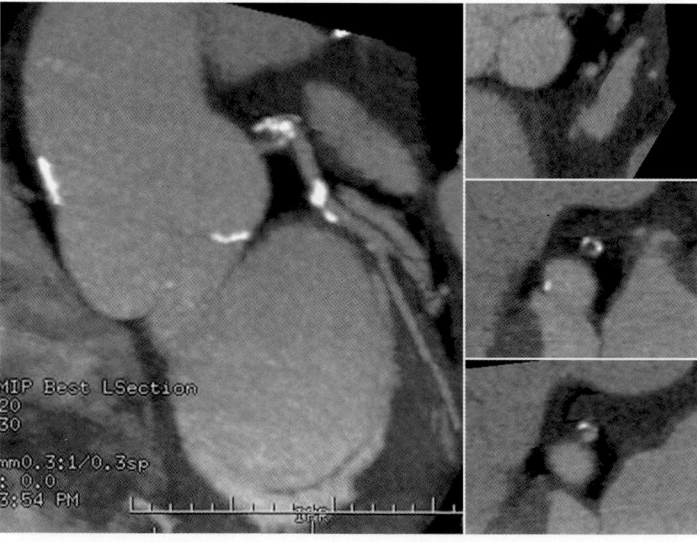

Fig. 16. Coronary vessel analysis: main trunk stenosis on mixed plaque in 2D long axis and short axis.

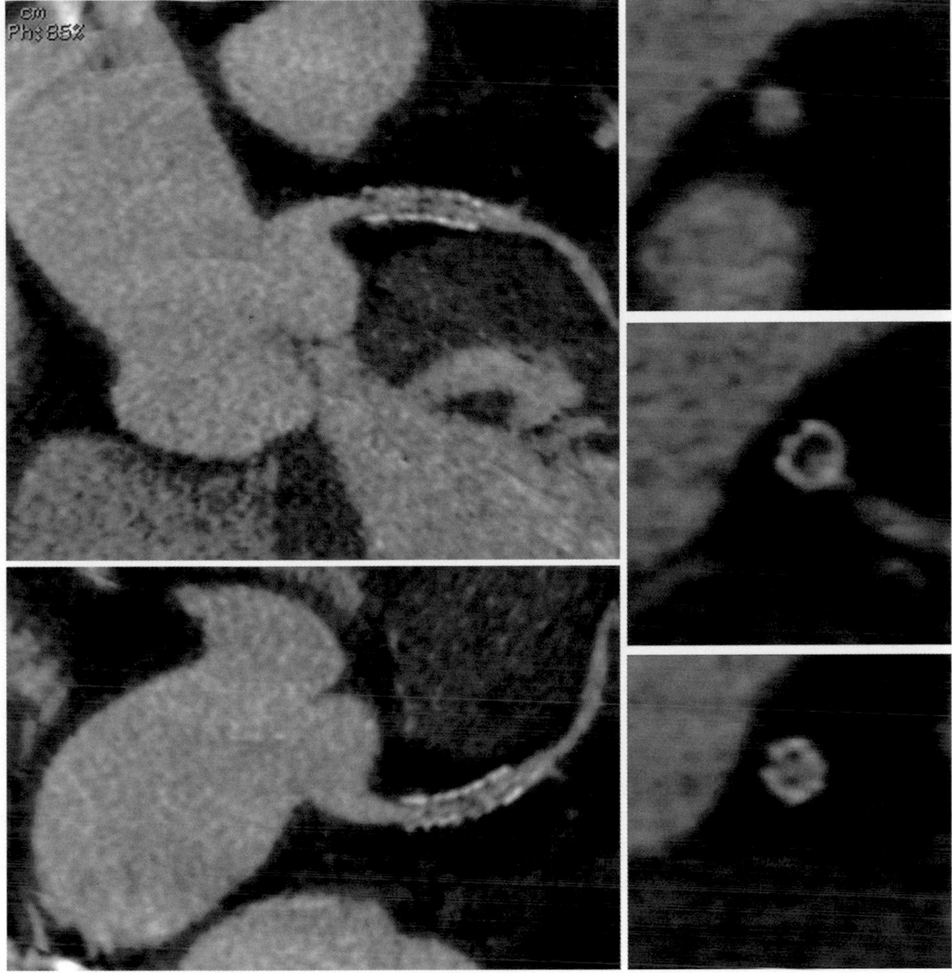

Fig. 17. Coronary vessel analysis: LAD stent restenosis in 2D LA and SA.

- Two-chamber view in diastole and systole: the reference plane is perpendicular to the septum and runs through the middle of the mitral valve plane and the apex of the left ventricle.
- Four-chamber view in diastole and systole: the reference plane of the long axis view runs through the middle of the mitral valve plane and the apex of the left ventricle.
- Short-axis view in diastole and systole: cuts run perpendicular to the reference plane of the major axis view (Fig. 20).

It is possible to perform automatic measurement of volumes, ejection fraction, total or segmental myocardial mass, and perfusion, with imaging of the surface of the lesion.

LEFT-VENTRICULAR WALL MOTION AND FUNCTION ANALYSIS

The CardIQ function allows the user to display multiphase cardiac CT images and calculate heart function parameters. CardIQ function measures, graphically plots, and tabulates a number of left- and right-ventricular (LV and RV) functions and wall motion parameters derived from reformatted short-axis data sets. Function analysis comprises several steps:

1. Automatic detection of endocardial and epicardial contours of LV on short-axis reformated images. Automatic contour detection can be modified manually. Automatic detection of endocardium contours can be easily detected automatically due to the difference in density between opacified cavities and myocardium. On the other hand, automatic detection of epicardium needs more time and should be performed manually.
2. Calculation of LV and RV end-diastolic and systolic volume, stroke volume, ejection fraction (EF), and myocardial mass at end diastole. These 3D measurements are currently being validated with comparison to conventional techniques (Fig. 21).
3. Generation of a volumetric 3D movie with the cardiac contours (Fig. 21).
4. Left-ventricular wall motion, thickness, and thickening are available in either a graphic or a bull's-eye format to aid in the detection of heart abnormalities (Fig. 22).

Practical experience and technological progress have made it possible to overcome the problems of acquisition and reconstruction, with the aim of developing a simple method of noninvasive examination, on an out-patient basis, for patients suffering from ischemic heart disease. This method would provide not only precise diagnostic possibilities but also information that is essential for the therapeutic decision.

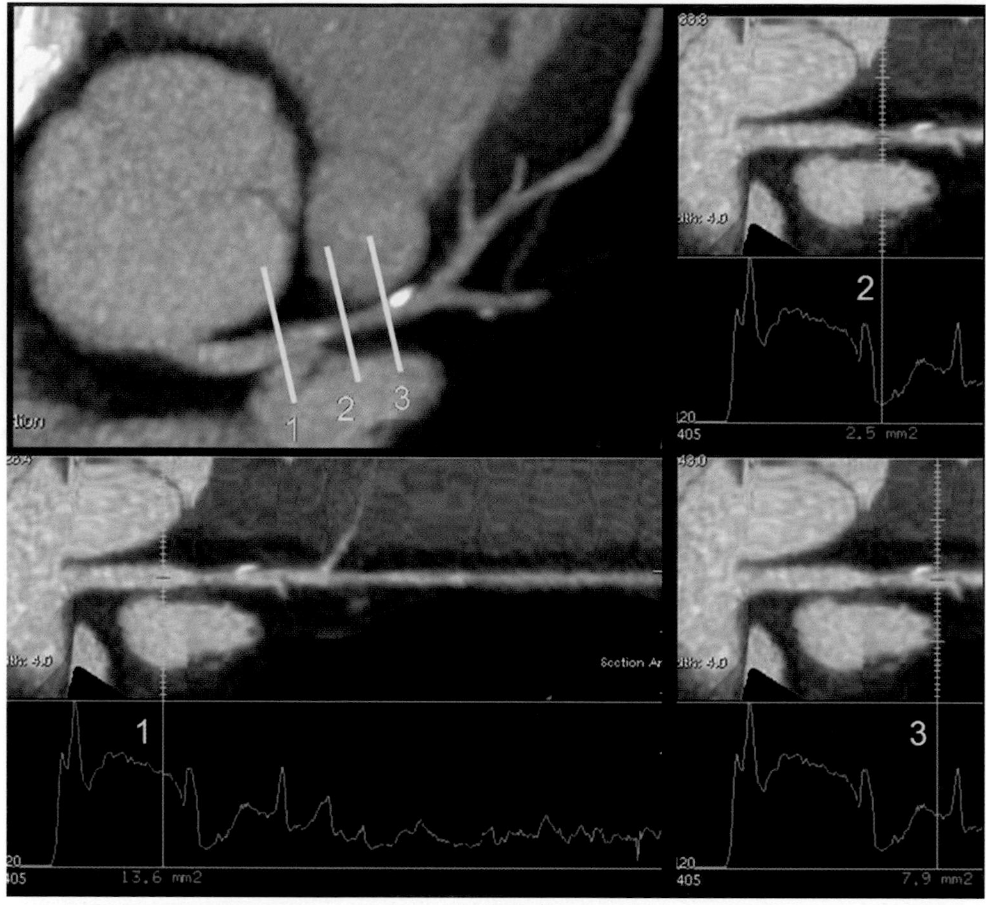

Fig. 18. Coronary vessel analysis: quantification of a segment 1 left anterior descending (LAD) stenosis—surfacic measurements: main trunk = 13.6 mm, LAD stenosis = 2.5 mm, LAD downstream from the stenosis = 7.9 mm.

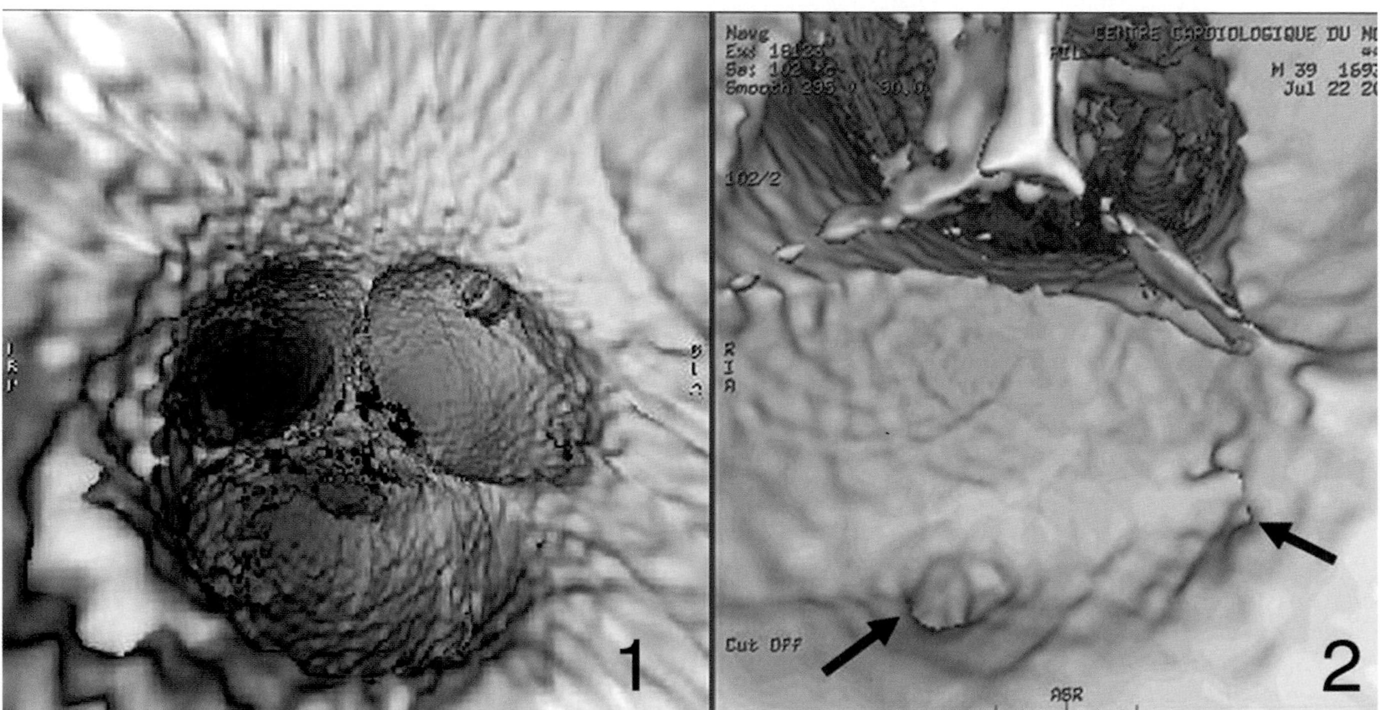

Fig. 19. Coronary vessel analysis: virtual endoscopy 1: main trunk stent for ostium stenosis. Near part of stent extends into aorta lumen 2: anomalous origin of right and left coronary artery ostia in right sinus (arrows).

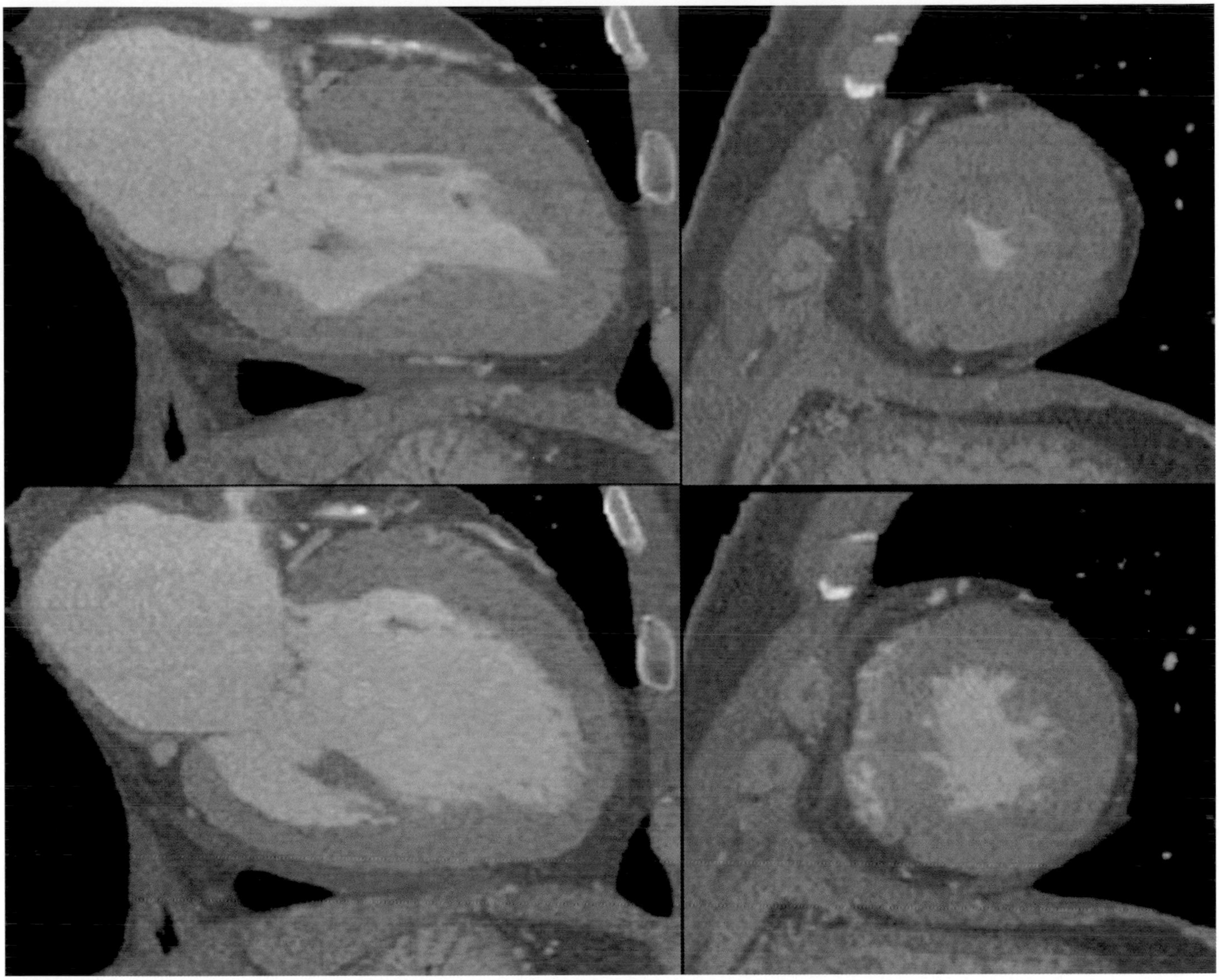

Fig. 20. Ventriculography: 2-chamber 2D slices and SA in systole and diastole.

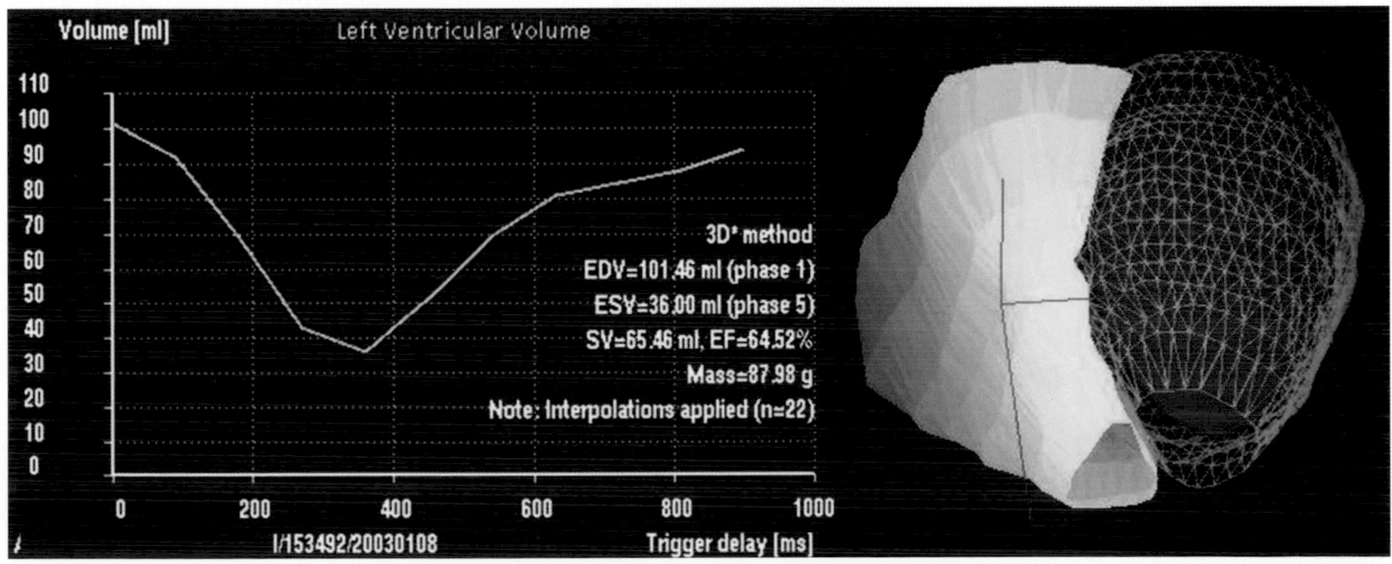

Fig. 21. Function: function analysis and 3D movie.

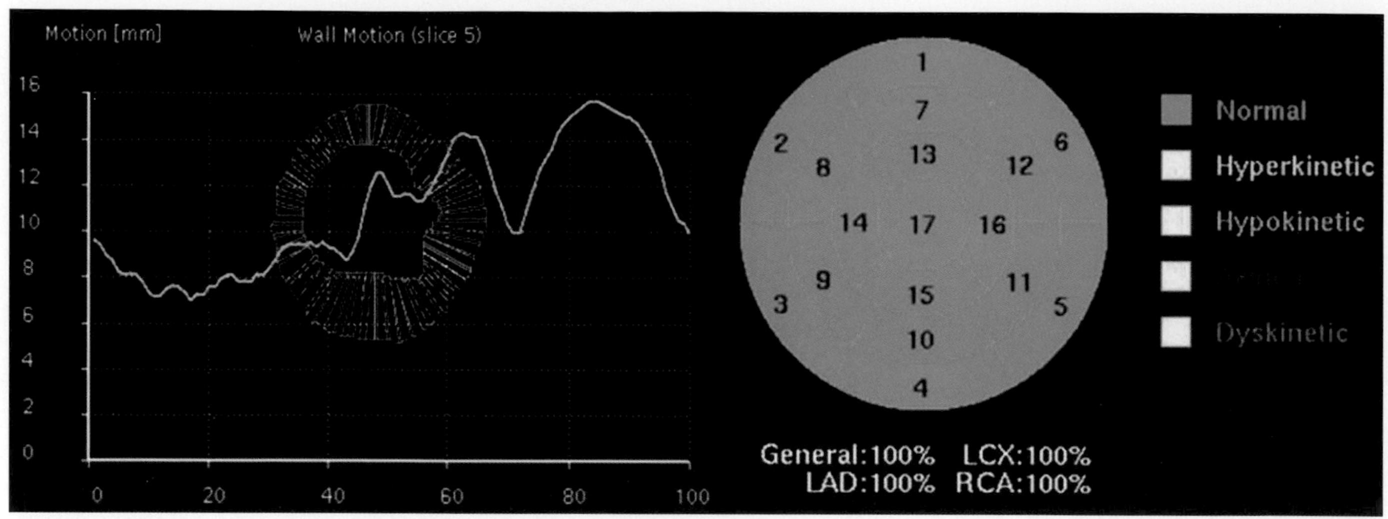

Fig. 22. Function: left-ventricular wall motion, thickness, and thickening.

25 CT Angiography for Assessment of Coronary Artery Anomalies

Steffen C. Froehner, md, Matthias Wagner, md, Juergen Brunn, md, and Rainer R. Schmitt, md

INTRODUCTION

In Summer 2002, a 21-yr-old man was found dead one early morning in his apartment. He had been a healthy sportsman, but sometimes he felt an atypical pressure in the left side of his chest, independent of body stress. In all former medical examinations (i.e., electrocardiogram [ECG], stress ECG, and echocardiography), particularly in the armed forces, no pathological diagnosis had been found. The gross specimen showed an anomaly of his coronary arteries: the right coronary artery (RCA) had its origin out of the left sinus of Valsalva and showed a so-called interarterial course, between aorta and pulmonary artery.

This type of coronary artery anomaly is considered to run a higher risk of myocardial ischemia or sudden death, especially in younger patients under the age of 35 yr *(1,2)*.

Such coronary anomalies are identified only incidentally during life, often because of insufficient clinical suspicion. However, because abnormal coronary artery origin is now amenable to surgical treatment, early clinical identification is crucial. With regard to congenital coronary artery anomalies in young competitive athletes, standard testing with ECG under resting or exercise conditions is rather unlikely to provide clinical evidence of myocardial ischemia, and would not be reliable as a screening test in large athletic populations. Premonitory cardiac symptoms often occur shortly before sudden death. Therefore, it appears wise to exclude such an anomaly after a history of exertional syncope or chest pain. These observations also have important implications for the preparticipation screening of competitive athletes *(3)*.

Under certain conditions, anomalies of the coronary arteries may lead to severe complications in valve and bypass surgery, by accidental injury of the aberrant vessels during an operation *(4)*. There are also reports describing a compression of an aberrant left circumflex coronary artery (LCx) following bioprosthetic valve ring implantation *(5)*. Coronary artery fistulae can be subject to such injuries as well, not to mention the often hemodynamically significant shunt volume they show.

Although sudden infant death syndrome (SIDS) is a cause for sudden infant death, other causes should be ruled out before diagnosing SIDS. Cardiac causes for sudden infant death include anomalies of the coronary arteries in many cases. The Bland–White–Garland syndrome has to be mentioned in the first place.

Anomalies of the coronary arteries found in children may be associated with other congenital anomalies of the heart like Fallot's syndrome, transposition of the great arteries, "Taussig–Bing" heart (double outlet right ventricle), or common arterial trunk *(6)*.

Beside the hemodynamic effects, anomalies of coronary arteries are thought to be associated with a higher risk of arteriosclerosis, particularly in vessels with aberrant courses *(7)*.

In catheter angiography as a 2D imaging method, the depiction of coronary artery anomalies may be very difficult. The accurate course of these anomalous vessels often is not clearly displayed. In many cases a selective angiography of the aberrant vessels is impossible.

As a noninvasive method which has proved its higher sensitivity, multislice computed tomography (MSCT) of the coronary arteries, with its 3D approach, may well become the method of choice for the detection and characterization of coronary artery anomalies and related syndromes.

This chapter describes the value of MSCT in detection of anomalies of the coronary arteries; it also characterizes the different types of coronary artery anomalies, including their clinical relevance. Finally, diagnostic aspects and capabilities of MSCT in this clinical setting are discussed.

Congenital anomalies of the coronary arteries are a very heterogeneous group of lesions, which can produce severe clinical symptoms or be clinically silent, leading only incidentally to a correct diagnosis. There may be "malignant" or "nonmalignant" forms, depending on their course. For that reason it is of high prognostic and sometimes therapeutic importance to define the correct origin and course of the aberrant artery and to describe its course accurately.

From: *Contemporary Cardiology: CT of the Heart: Principles and Applications*
Edited by: U. Joseph Schoepf © Humana Press, Inc., Totowa, NJ

EXAMINATION AND RECONSTRUCTION TECHNIQUES FOR ASSESSMENT OF CORONARY ARTERY ANOMALIES WITH MSCT

MSCT, in particular the now available 16- and 64-row scanners, with their ability to generate approximately isotropic voxels, represent a new and highly promising tool to visualize coronary arteries with respect to their origin and course. Specifically, the manifold reconstruction potentials—multiplanar reformations (MPR), multiplanar volume reformations (MPVR), surface shading (SSD), vessel tracking, and volume rendering (VR)—enable accurate visualization of coronary arteries. Using these 3D complementary capabilities, the detection and characterization of anomalies of the coronary artery system is feasible with high precision and detail.

Examination protocols to depict anomalies of the coronary arteries with MSCT do not differ from those presented in previous chapters to evaluate coronary artery disease. In special cases, such as anomalies with ectopic origin of coronary arteries (*see* subheading "Anomalies of Ectopic Origin and Course of Coronary Arteries"), it is important to use a wider scan field to cover the whole course of these vessels. MPRs and 3D volume rendering may be very helpful to demonstrate these anomalies and to provide an accurate depiction of the special vascular anatomy.

The disadvantage of this method is the time-consuming reconstruction of the data sets by an experienced physician. In particular, complex vessel anomalies have to be reconstructed accurately with full use of software and anatomic knowledge.

SYNOPSIS OF CORONARY ARTERY ANOMALIES

CORONARY ARTERY ANOMALIES OF ORIGIN AND COURSE

Prevalence and Etiology

Coronary artery anomalies constitute 1–3% of all congenital malformations of the heart, but in approx 0.46 to 1% *(8)* of the normal population, anomalies of the coronary arteries are reported to be found incidentally during catheter angiography, echocardiography, or autopsy *(9,10)*.

The etiology of coronary artery anomalies is still uncertain. A possibility of maternal transmission of some varieties is suggested, particularly for a single coronary artery *(11)*. Familial clustering is also reported for anomalies of an LCx originating from the right sinus of Valsalva, one of the most common anomalies *(12)*.

Anomalies of the coronary arteries may also be combined with Klinefelter's syndrome, although both entities are very rare *(13)*. In trisomy 18 (i.e., Edwards syndrome), coronary artery anomalies rarely can be found as well *(14)*.

A raised plasma phenylalanine as in phenylketonuria of pregnant women may induce several congenital pathological changes of the heart, including coronary artery anomalies, sometimes in combination with mental and physical retardation. Maternal phenylketonuria may be responsible for these malformations, which may be prevented by dietary treatment *(15)*.

Although all these syndromes and predispositions may lead to coronary artery anomalies, most of the patients with anomalies of the coronary arteries do not present any of them. The etiology of coronary anomalies in primarily healthy persons is still not known and requires further embryological and genetic research.

Clinical Importance of Coronary Artery Anomalies

Anomalies of the course of coronary arteries can be categorized into"malignant" and "nonmalignant" forms. Malignant forms are combined with an increased risk of myocardial ischemia or sudden death *(1,16,17)*.

These forms mostly show a course between pulmonary artery and aorta (interarterial). The most common case is an origin of the right coronary artery from the left sinus of Valsalva, coursing between aorta and pulmonary artery. But anomalies of the left main artery (LM) or the left anterior descending artery (LAD) arising from the right sinus of Valsalva with this course are also associated with higher risk. It has been suggested that myocardial ischemia and sudden death result from transient occlusion of the aberrant coronary artery, caused by an increase of blood flow through the aorta and pulmonary artery during exercise or body stress. The reason is either a kink at the sharp leftward or rightward bend at the vessel's ostium or a pinchcock mechanism between aorta and pulmonary artery. Up to 30% of these patients are at risk for sudden death *(18)*. Long courses of anomalous coronary arteries ventral to the pulmonary artery may sometimes be associated with a higher risk of myocardial ischemia. Dilatation of the pulmonary trunk—for example, as a result of pulmonary hypertension—can lead to a stretching of the aberrant vessel, which causes lumen reduction and consequent myocardial ischemia.

An origin of either the left or right coronary artery from the pulmonary artery (Bland–White–Garland syndrome for the left coronary artery) also must be considered as malignant. This anomaly is frequently associated with myocardial ischemia and sudden death in early childhood. A surgical intervention is absolutely required.

Other courses do not lead to any clinical symptoms. They are rather incidental findings in catheter angiography, CT of the coronary arteries, or autopsy, without any clinical relevance. In case of planned cardiac surgery, these anomalies nevertheless take on an increasing importance, because the risk of accidental surgical injuries, in particular because congenital anomalies of the heart (e.g., Fallot's syndrome, transposition of the great arteries, Taussig–Bing heart, or common arterial trunk) are often combined with anomalies of the coronary arteries *(19)*.

Therefore, every anomaly of origin and course of the coronary arteries should be described accurately prior to cardiac surgery. If the catheter angiography cannot provide detailed information *(20)* (which it usually does not), MSCT has to be performed to describe the exact courses of aberrant vessels.

Finally, aberrant coronary arteries seem to run a higher risk of arteriosclerosis. In patients with anomalies of the coronary arteries, the aberrant vessels where found to be more diseased than the vessels with normal course *(21)*. So it is necessary to pay attention to these vessels in case of atypical chest pain or pathological ECG findings.

Classification of Coronary Artery Anomalies of Origin and Course

The most frequent and clinically significant anomalies are detailed in Table 1. In the following subheadings, the different types of coronary artery anomalies are presented and the clinical relevance is discussed.

Origin of the RCA From the Left Sinus of Valsalva

Anatomy: this anomaly of the RCA may present different appearances. There may be a common ostium or two different ostia. The right coronary artery can take three different courses. First, ventral to the pulmonary artery; second, between pulmonary artery and the aorta (interarterial); and third, dorsal to the aorta. These aberrant vessels lead to the right atrioventricular groove, where the RCA takes its normal course. Fig. 1A–D demonstrates an origin of the right coronary artery from the left sinus of Valsalva and an interarterial course. The decrease of the lumen in the proximal part and the sharp kink are clearly depicted.

Clinical relevance: according to the literature *(22)*, the most common type of anomalous coronary arteries in our data was an origin of the right coronary artery from the left sinus of Valsalva or the left main artery. Approximately 34% of the anomalies detected showed this particular appearance.

An interarterial course has to be considered malignant as a result of the possible pinchcock mechanism and the sharp rightward kink of the vessel directly distal to the ostium. A higher risk of myocardial ischemia and sudden death is likely.

Origin of the RCA From Branches of the Left Coronary Artery

Anatomy: rarely, the right coronary artery can have its origin from branches of the left coronary artery system, particularly from the LAD with a course ventral to the pulmonary artery, or from the LCx with a course dorsal to the aorta.

Clinical relevance: no clinical relevance; these anomalies are only incidental findings.

Origin of the Right Coronary Artery Fromthe Posterior Sinus of Valsalva

Anatomy: a very rare anomaly of the coronary arteries is an origin of the right coronary artery from the posterior sinus of Valsalva. This anomaly is detected only incidentally by catheter angiography or autopsy.

Clinical relevance: no clinical relevance.

Separate Origins of Right Coronary Artery and Conus Artery

Anatomy: the conus artery may arise from a separate ostium in the right sinus of Valsalva, either as a small conus artery providing only the conus area (Fig. 2A,B), or as a large conus artery supplying a wide area of the genuine RCA area with a consecutive hypoplastic RCA.

Clinical relevance: this aberrant conus artery is particularly at risk to be injured by ventriculotomy or other maneuvers in heart surgery.

Origin of the Right Coronary Artery From the Pulmonary Trunk

Anatomy: analogous to the Bland–White–Garland syndrome with an origin of the left coronary artery from the pulmonary trunk, the right coronary artery also can originate from this. We may call it a "reversed" Bland–White–Garland syndrome.

Clinical relevance: these patients suffer from myocardial ischemia or sudden death in early childhood. A surgical intervention is recommended as soon as possible.

Origin of the RCA From the LCx

Anatomy: a very rare but often described anomaly of the right coronary artery is the agenesis of the right coronary ostium with a continuation of the LCx as a right coronary artery and a retrograde perfusion of the RCA's supply area *(23)*.

Clinical relevance: this type of anomaly may lead to early and severe myocardial ischemia resulting from already moderate stenosis of the LCx.

Anomalies of Origin and Course of the Left Main Coronary Artery

Separate Ostia or Common Ostium of LAD and LCx

Anatomy: the most common anomaly of the left coronary vessel system is the absence of the left main coronary artery. LAD and LCx have separate ostia in the left coronary cusp without an anomaly of the course (Fig. 3A–B). LAD and LCx may also originate from one common ostium (Fig. 4A–B).

Clinical relevance: no clinical relevance, but selective contrast injection during catheter angiography may be difficult, causing insufficient angiographic.

Origin of the Left Main Coronary Artery From the Right Sinus of Valsalva

Anatomy: the most common and important anomaly of origin of the left main coronary artery is an origin from the right sinus of Valsalva. There may be a common ostium or an origin from the right coronary artery. Three different courses are possible: a course of the left main coronary artery between aorta and pulmonary artery (Fig. 5), a course ventral to the pulmonary artery (Fig. 6A–E), and a course dorsal to the aorta to the left side.

Clinical relevance: depending on their course, these anomalies can be malignant or nonmalignant. The first one has an increased risk of myocardial ischemia or sudden death caused by a sharp kink at the ostium and a possible compression of the vessel between aorta and pulmonary artery in case of higher blood flow under exercise. The detailed description can be found under the subheading "Clinical Importance of Coronary Artery Anomalies."

Origin of the Left Main Coronary Artery From the Right Sinus of Valsalva and Different Courses of Left Anterior Descending and Left Circumflex

Anatomy: another possibility of a left main artery's anomaly with an origin from the right sinus of Valsalva is an early division in LAD and LCx. The LAD then shows a course ventral to the pulmonary artery, the LCx an interarterial course between aorta and pulmonary trunk.

Clinical relevance: the interarterial course of the LCx is also combined with a higher risk of myocardial ischemia.

Transseptal Course of the Aberrant Left Main Artery

Anatomy: a very rare anomaly of the left main coronary artery is a transseptal course to the left side after originating from the right sinus of Valsalva.

Clinical relevance: the clinical relevance of these anomalies is still not known. In case of myocardial hypertrophy or volume overload of the ventricles, there may be a higher risk of myocardial ischemia.

Table 1
Most Frequent and Clinically Significant Anomalies of the Coronary Arteries

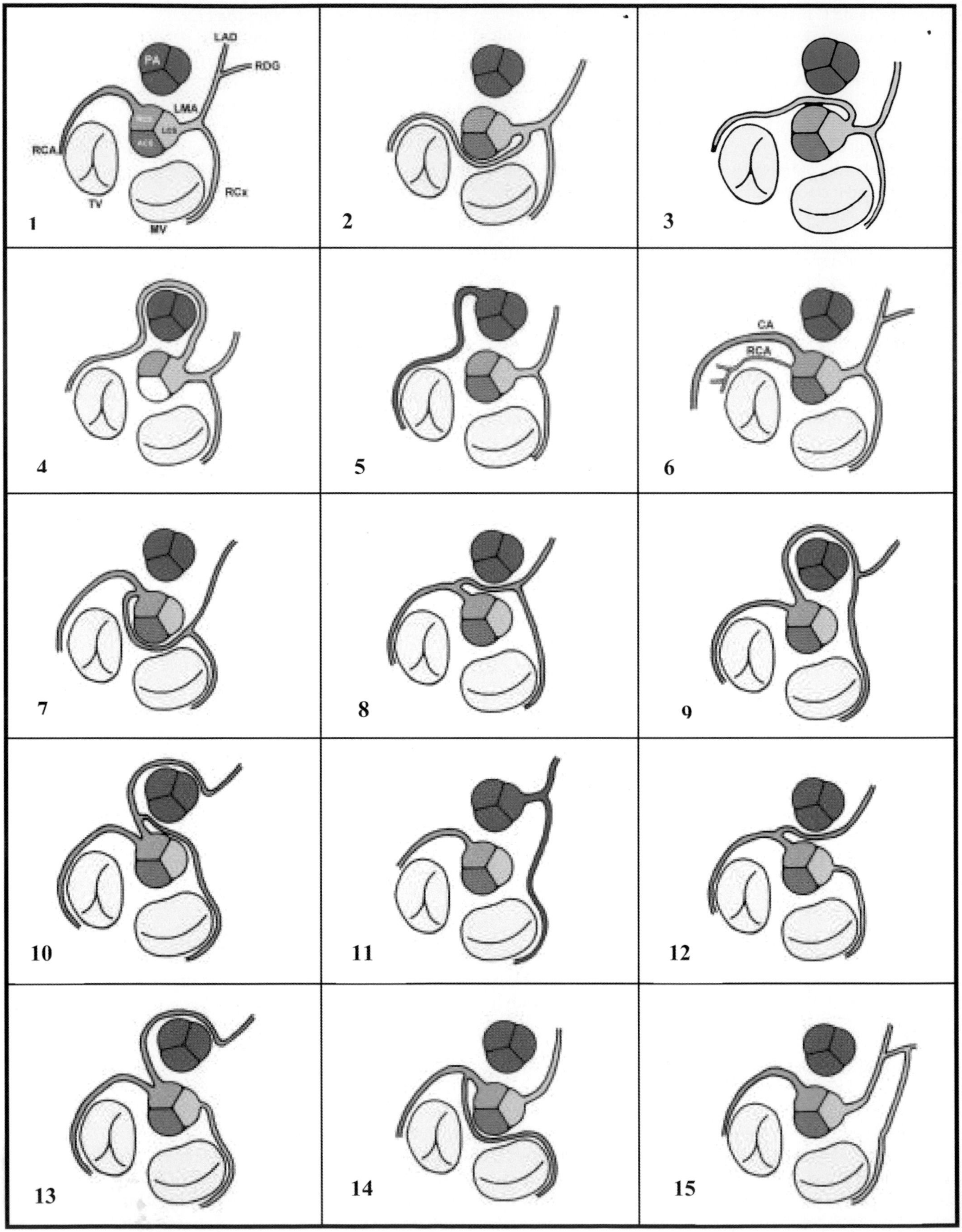

1 LAD RDG PA LMA RCA TV RCx MV	2	3
4	5	6 CA RCA
7	8	9
10	11	12
13	14	15

Table 1 *(Continued)*
Most Frequent and Clinically Significant Anomalies of the Coronary Arteries

1: Normal anatomy of the coronary arteries.

2: Origin of the right coronary artery (RCA) from the left main artery, course dorsal to the aorta.

3: Origin of the right coronary artery from the left sinus of Valsalva, course between aorta and pulmonary artery (interarterial course).

4: Origin of the right coronary artery from the left sinus of Valsalva, course ventral to the pulmonary artery.

5: Origin of the right coronary artery from the pulmonary artery ("reversed" Bland–White–Garland syndrome).

6: Dominant conus artery (CA) with a separate ostium, which supplies the main area of the RCA. The RCA is a small vessel, with early division. A reverse case is also possible: separate ostia of conus artery and RCA, but the conus artery is the smaller vessel.

7: Origin of the left main artery from the right coronary artery, course dorsal to the aorta.

8: Origin of the left main artery from the right coronary artery, course between aorta and pulmonary artery (interarterial course).

9: Origin of the left main artery from the right sinus of Valsalva, course ventral to the pulmonary artery.

10: Origin of the left main artery from the right sinus of Valsalva, the left descending coronary artery (LAD) courses ventral to the aorta, the left circumflex shows a course interarterial between aorta and pulmonary artery.

11: Origin of the left main artery from the pulmonary artery (Bland–White–Garland syndrome).

12: Origin of the LAD from the RCA, course between aorta and pulmonary artery (interarterial course).

13: Origin of the LAD from the right sinus of Valsalva, course ventral to the pulmonary artery.

14: Origin of the circumflex branch from the right coronary artery, course dorsal to the aorta.

15: Origin of the circumflex branch from the first diagonal branch of the LAD.

Anomalies of origin of the left main coronary artery in the right sinus of Valsalva are frequently found in patients with other congenital anomalies of the heart, particularly in cases of Fallot's syndrome.

Origin of The Left Main Coronary Artery From the Pulmonary Artery (Bland–White–Garland Syndrome)

Anatomy: one of the most important anomalies of coronary arteries in children is an origin of the left coronary artery from the pulmonary trunk, known as Bland–White–Garland syndrome.

Clnical relevance: clinical symptoms result from myocardial ischemia caused by an arterio-venous shunt owing to reversed flow in the left main coronary artery to the pulmonary artery. The childhood type of this anomaly presents high mortality from heart failure. The adult type develops myocardial infarction, arrhythmias, sudden cardiac death, or signs of congestive heart failure. These patients can generally be prevented from myocardial ischemia or heart failure only by a surgical intervention*(24)*. The risk of fatality from a congenital coronary abnormality far outweighs the smaller risk of a surgical intervention. Nevertheless, cases of a Bland–White–Garland syndrome have been reported in which the patient survived to middle age with minimal cardiovascular problems. Good exercise tolerance and long-term survival may occasionally be possible even without surgery for patients with this anomaly *(25)*. Some patients show only ECG alterations, without any clinical symptoms such as angina, atypical chest pain, or abnormal shortness of breath during or after exercise *(26)*.

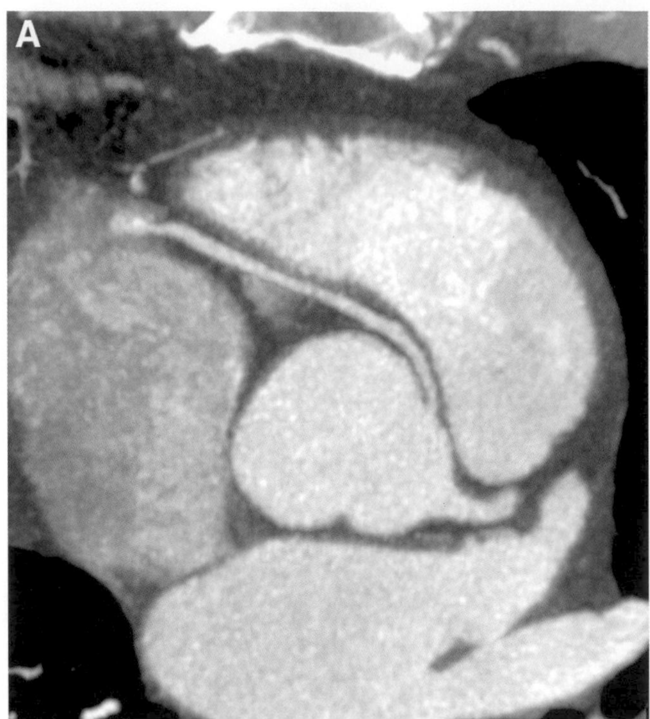

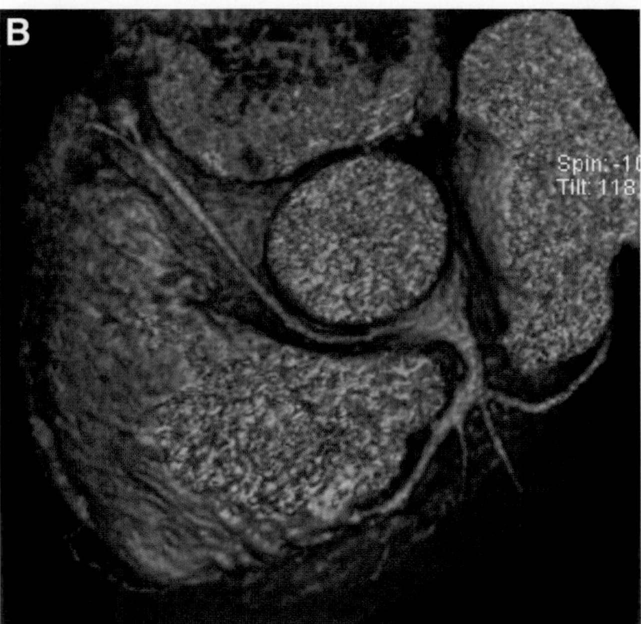

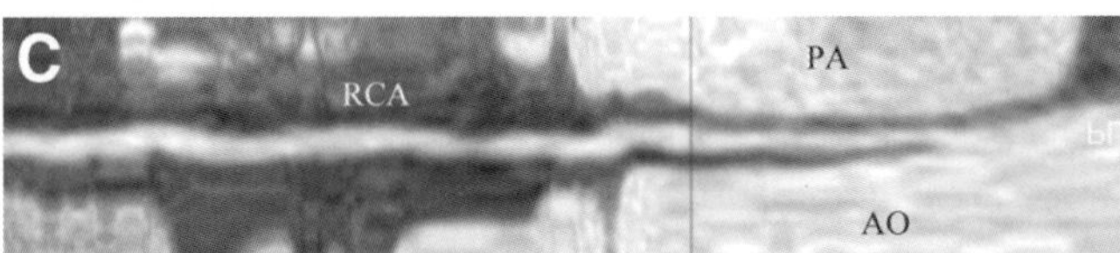

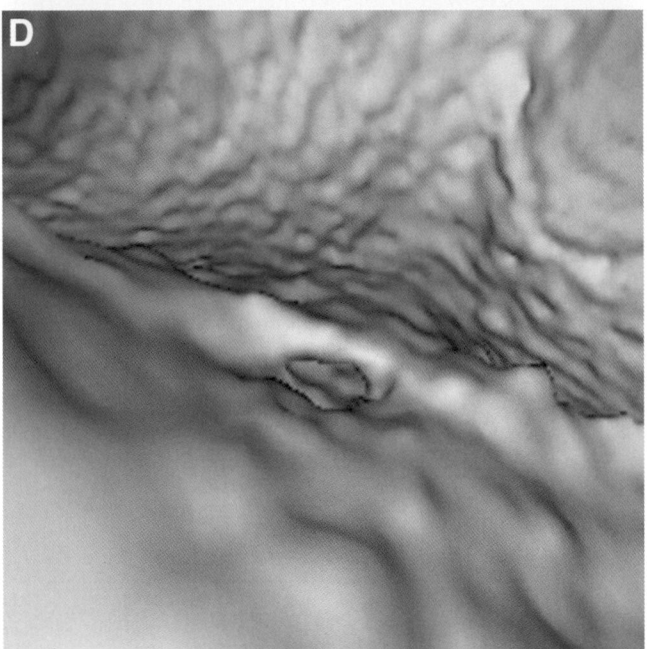

Fig. 1. Origin of the right coronary artery (RCA) from the left sinus of Valsalva, showing a course between aorta and pulmonary artery. The proximal part of the RCA shows a decrease of the lumen and a sharp kink directly after the ostium. **(A)** "Thin maximum intensity projection" reconstruction. **(B)** Volume rendering. **(C)** "Vessel view" reconstruction, showing the vessel stretched longitudinally. The decrease of the vessel's lumen is also demonstrated in this reconstruction method. PA, pulmonary artery; AO, aorta. **(D)** Virtual angioscopy of the ostium of the RCA. View from aortic root into the ostium of the RCA.

Anomalies of Origin and Course of the Left Anterior Descending Artery

The LAD can show similar anomalies of origin and course like the left main artery.

ORIGIN OF THE LEFT ANTERIOR DESCENDING ARTERY FROM THE RIGHT SINUS OF VALSALVA

Anatomy: the LAD may originate from the right sinus of Valsalva either with a common ostium together with the RCA or separate ostia, or from the RCA itself. Two different courses are possible: ventral to the pulmonary artery or between aorta and pulmonary trunk.

Clinical relevance: the latter course is combined with a higher risk of myocardial ischemia.

ORIGIN OF THE LEFT ANTERIOR DESCENDING FROM THE LEFT CIRCUMFLEX

Anatomy: a rare coronary artery anomaly is an origin of the LAD from the LCx and a course leading to the anterior interventricular groove.

Clinical relevance: clinical symptoms are not known.

ORIGIN OF THE LEFT ANTERIOR DESCENDING FROM THE PULMONARY ARTERY

Anatomy: similar to the Bland–White–Garland syndrome, the LAD can arise out of the pulmonary trunk.

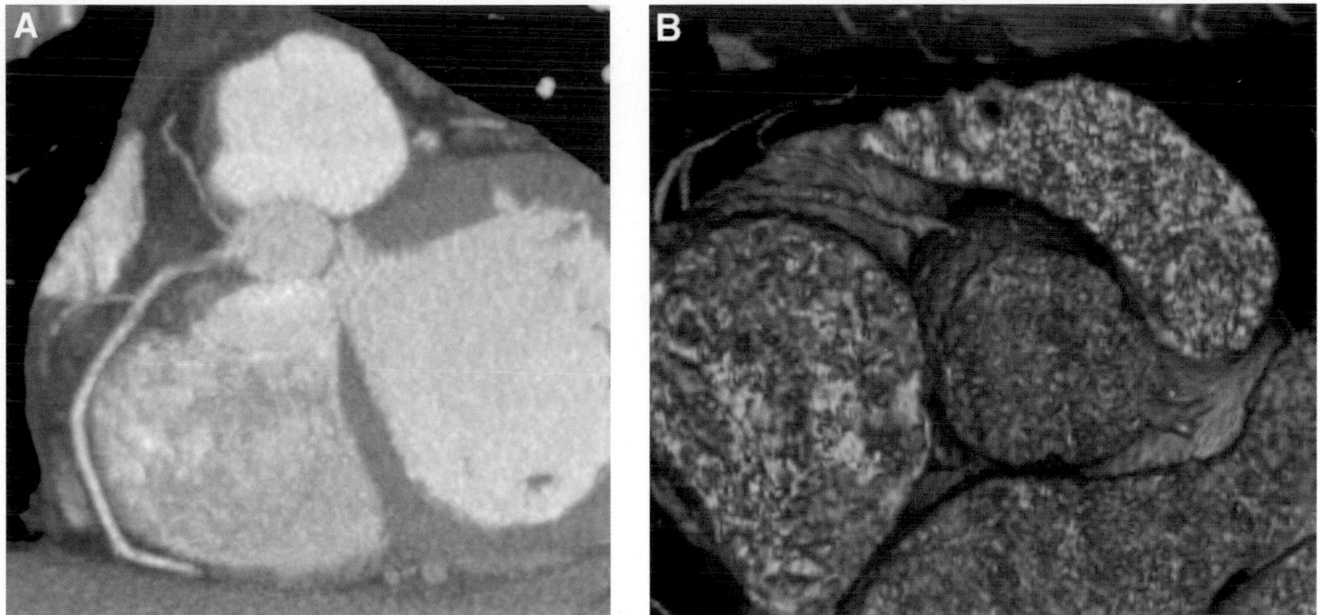

Fig. 2. Aberrant conus artery with an origin from the right sinus of Valsalva. **(A)** "Thin maximum intensity projection" reconstruction. **(B)** Volume-rendering.

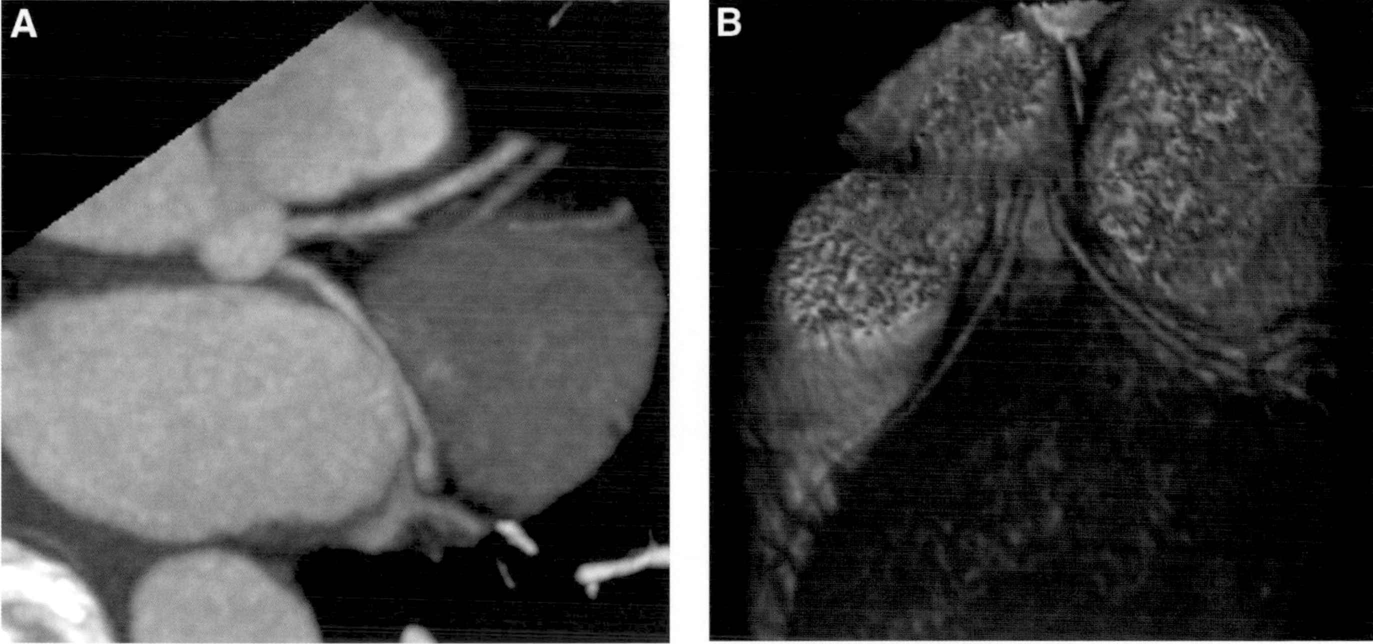

Fig. 3. Separate ostia of left anterior descending and left circumflex arteries in the left sinus of Valsalva. **(A)** "Thin maximum intensity projection" reconstruction. **(B)** Volume-rendering.

Clinical relevance: the symptoms and clinical relevance for this particular anomaly are similar to those mentioned for the Bland–White–Garland syndrome.

DOUBLE LEFT ANTERIOR DESCENDING CORONARY ARTERY

Anatomy: a very rare anomaly is a double left anterior descending coronary artery arising either from the left main artery and the RCA or right sinus of Valsalva. The branch originating from the RCA or the right aortic cusp may course interarterial or ventral to the pulmonary artery.

Clinical relevance: this anomaly may be combined with an isolated transposition of the great arteries *(27)*. An interarterial course is accompanied by a higher risk of myocardial ischemia.

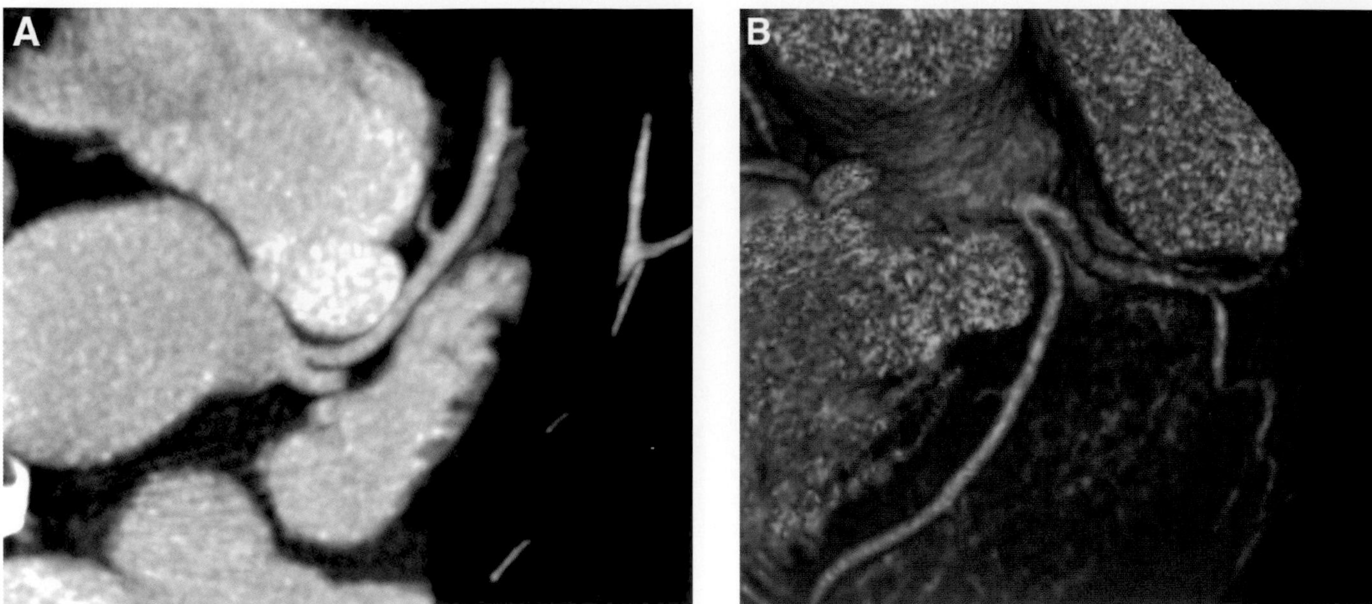

Fig. 4. Common ostium of left anterior descending and left circumflex arteries out of the right sinus of Valsalva. (**A**) "Thin maximum intensity projection" reconstruction. (**B**) Volume rendering.

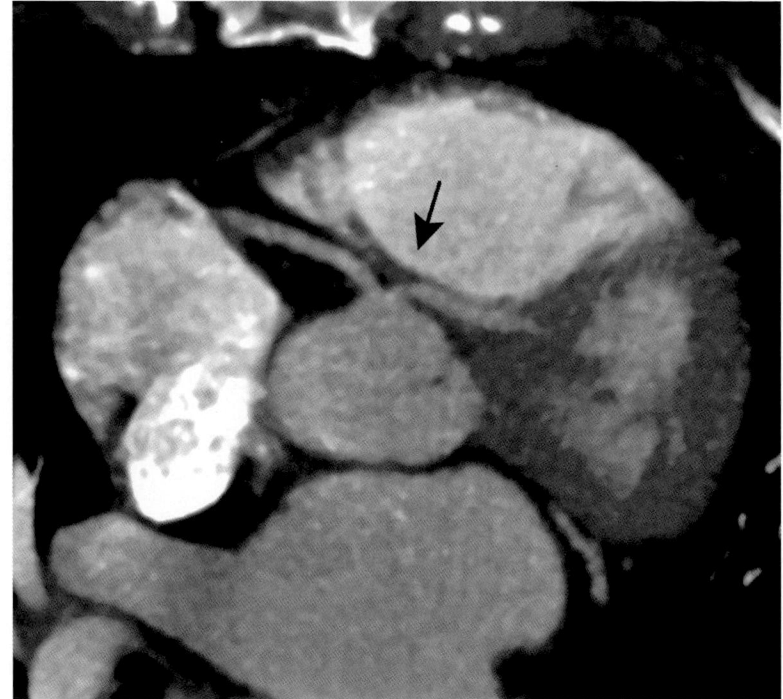

Fig. 5. Origin of the left main coronary artery out of the right sinus of Valsalva, course between aorta and pulmonary artery—"thin maximum intensity projection" reconstruction. Note the sharp kink of the left main coronary artery (arrow).

Fig. 6. (*right*) Origin of the left main artery out of the right sinus of Valsalva with a common ostium together with the right coronary artery (RCA), course ventral of the pulmonary artery. (**A**) "Thin maximum intensity projection (MIP)" reconstruction. (**B**) "Thin MIP" reconstruction of the long left main coronary artery. A first diagonal branch leaves the left main coronary artery (LMA) before left anterior descending (LAD) and left circumflex (LCx) arise. (**C**) The volume rendering shows the common ostium and the early division. (**D**) The long course of the left main coronary artery ventral of the pulmonary artery and the late division into LAD and LCx. Note the origin of the first diagonal branch before the division into LAD and LCx. (**E**) Virtual angioscopy of the common ostium of left main coronary artery and RCA. The small ostium of the sinus node artery (SNA) out of the proximal RCA is depicted clearly.

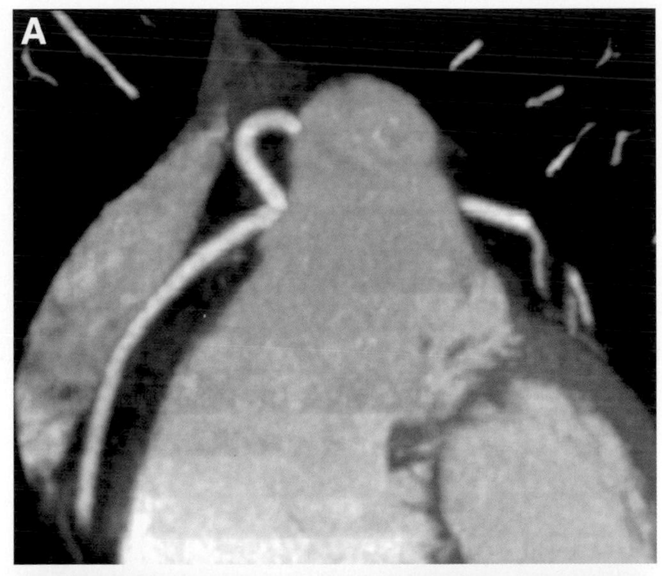
A

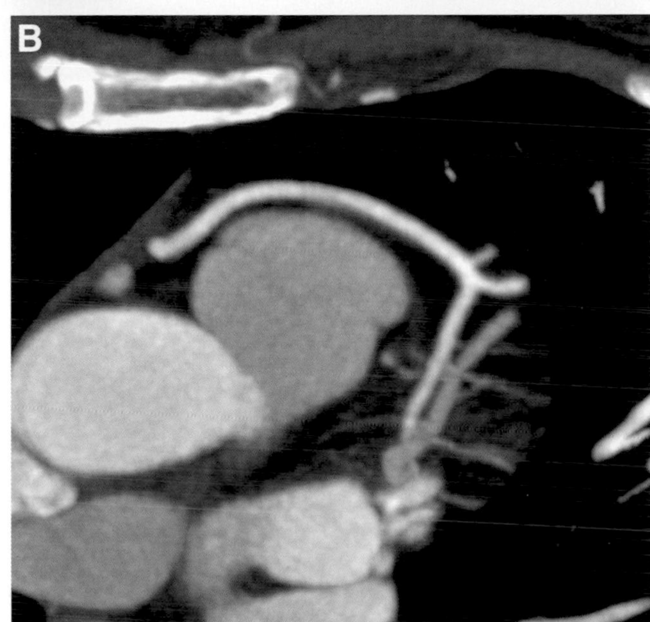
B

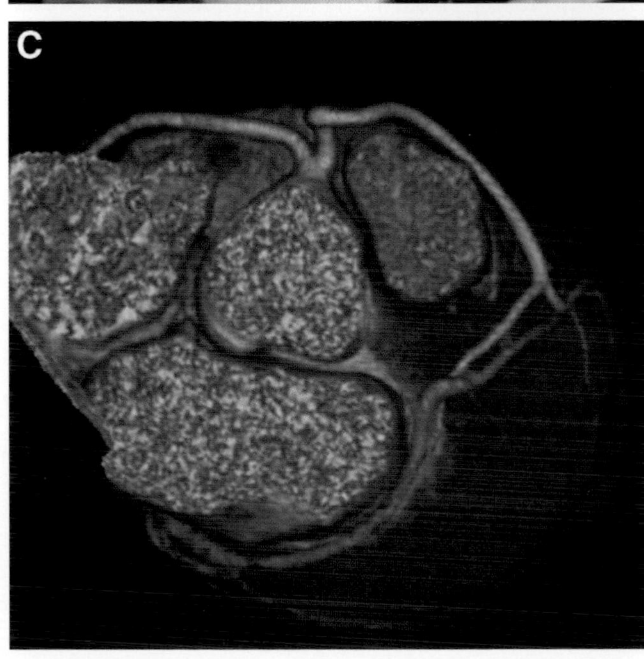
C

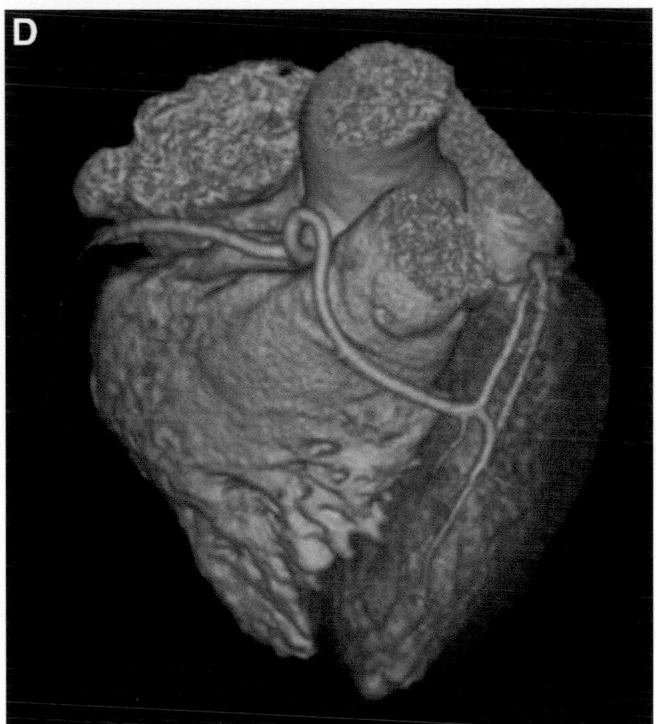
D

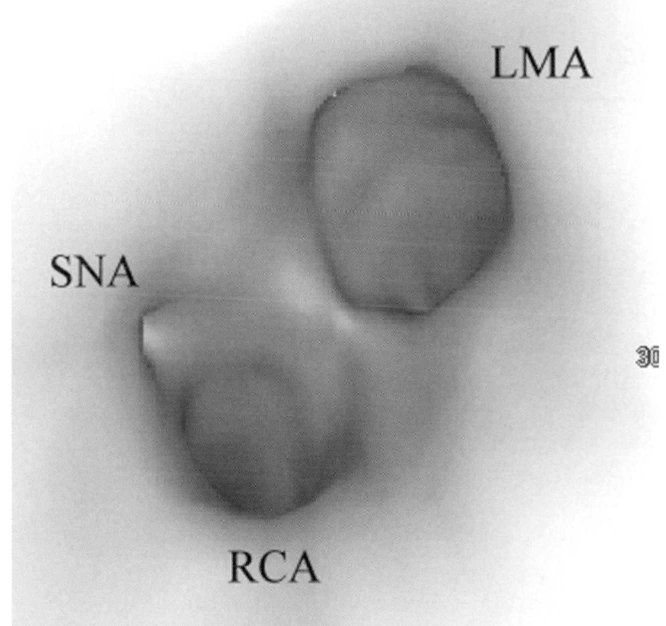
E
LMA
SNA
RCA

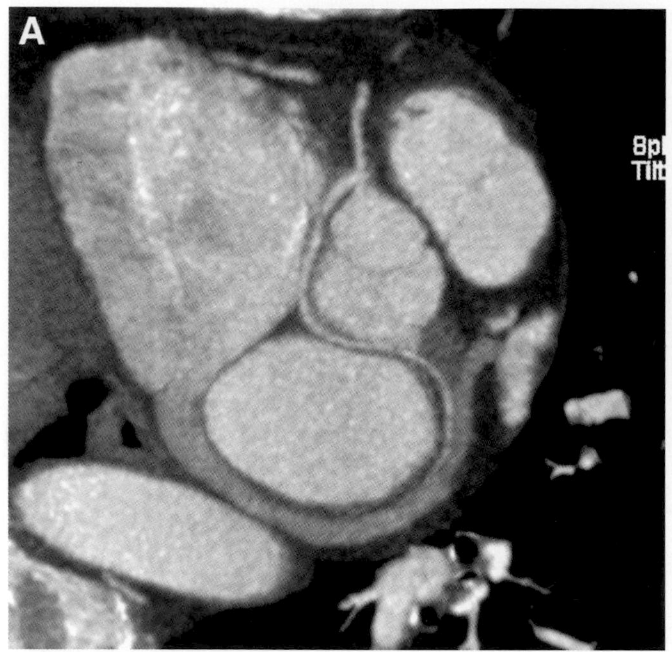

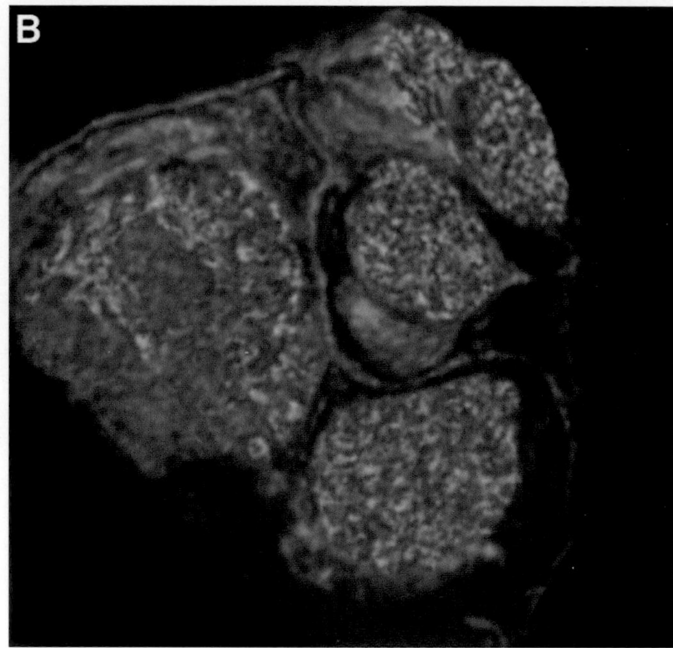

Fig. 7. Origin of the left circumflex out of the right sinus of Valsalva, course dorsal of the aorta. **(A)** "Thin maximum intensity projection" reconstruction. **(B)** Volume rendering.

Transseptal Course of the Aberrant Left Anterior Descending

Anatomy: a transseptal course of the LAD originating from the right sinus of Valsalva is also possible but extremely rare *(28)*.

Clinical relevance: as described under subheading "Transseptal Course of the Aberrating Left Main Artery," such courses of coronary arteries are believed to be malignant.

Anomalies of Origin and Course of the Left Circumflex Coronary Artery

In general, anomalies of the origin of the LCx are generally considered nonmalignant. However, a few reports of myocardial ischemia exist also in these anomalies *(29)*. These anomalies are mostly identified incidentally in catheter angiography or autopsy, without causing any clinical symptoms.

A comparison with Thallium-201 myocardial imaging in patients with angina pectoris and anomalous origin of the LCx concluded that an anomalous origin of the circumflex coronary artery did not cause impairment of myocardial perfusion unless it is the site of significant coronary arterial stenosis *(30)*.

Origin of the Left Circumflex Coronary Artery From the Right Sinus of Valsalva

Anatomy: the most common anomaly of the LCx is an origin from the right sinus of Valsalva or the RCA and a course dorsal to the aorta leading to the left atrioventricular groove (Fig. 7A–B).

Clinical relevance: this anomaly is found in 0.7% of angiographies. It is considered to be more frequent in patients with congenital stenosis of the aortic valve *(31)*. There is no higher risk of myocardial ischemia or sudden death.

Origin of the Left Circumflex Coronary Artery From Branches of the Left Anterior Descending

Anatomy: another appearance of anomalies of the LCx is an origin out of the first diagonal branch of the LAD or others of its branches leading likewise to the left atrioventricular groove.

Clinical relevance: a clinical relevance is not given; these anomalies are only detected incidentally.

Origin of the Left Circumflex Coronary Artery From the Pulmonary Artery

Anatomy: a rare anomaly of the LCx is an origin from the pulmonary trunk or the right pulmonary artery. There may be a large LCx arising from the right or left pulmonary artery or the pulmonary trunk which is filled in a retrograde way from a dominant LAD *(32)*.

Clinical relevance: this type of anomaly leads to myocardial ischemia in the same manner as the Bland–White–Garland syndrome and is reported occasionally *(33)*. A surgical correction is always required in early childhood to prevent myocardial ischemia and consequent heart failure.

Origin of the Left Circumflex Coronary Artery From the Distal Right Coronary Artery

Anatomy: another possibility of anomalies of the LCx is an origin of this vessel as a terminal extension of the RCA, leading to the left atrioventricular sulcus *(34)*.

Clinical relevance: this type of anomaly may lead to early and severe myocardial ischemia due to preexisting moderate stenosis of the RCA.

Complex and Combined Anomalies of Origin and Course of the Coronary Arteries

Among the numerous variations of anomalies of the coronary arteries, combined and complex appearances also can be detected.

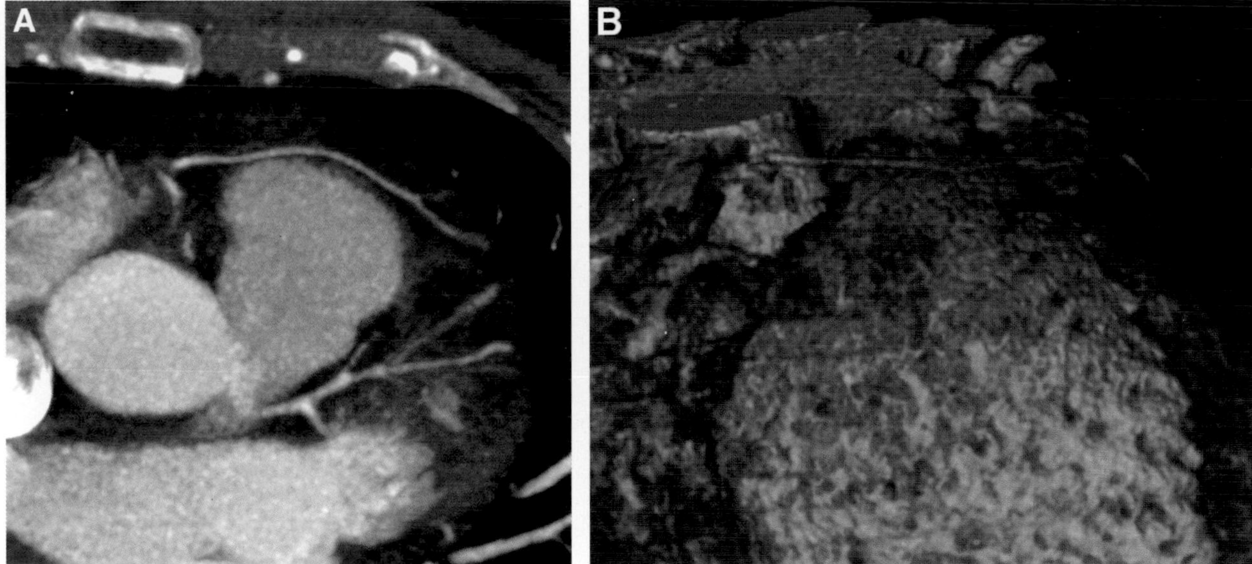

Fig. 8. An aberrant vessel originating from the right coronary artery runs ventral to the pulmonary artery to the left side and feeds the middle and distal part of the left anterior myocardium. The left anterior descending artery turns into a very thin vessel after 3 cm. **(A)** "Thin maximum intensity projection" reconstruction. **(B)** Volume rendering.

ORIGIN OF ALL CORONARY ARTERIES FROM ONE SINUS OF VALSALVA

Anatomy: all of the three main coronary arteries can arise either out of the right, left, or posterior sinus of Valsalva, presenting common or separated ostia with all the courses delineated above. Combinations of the different anomalies described before are also possible. There may be several appearances possible which have not been reported yet.

Clinical relevance: the clinical relevance of these anomalies depends on the course of the vessel. Interarterial courses are considered to be malignant, with a higher risk of myocardial ischemia.

INTRACAVITARY COURSE OF THE RIGHT CORONARY ARTERY

Anatomy: another complex course of coronary arteries concerns the RCA. It can take an intracavitary course in the right atrium after a primarily epicardial course. Also, muscular branches of the RCA are rarely found to run subendocardially into the right atrium *(35)*.

Clinical relevance: the clinical relevance of this particular anomaly is still not known; further investigation is needed. A higher pressure in the right atrium, for instance due to pulmanary embolism or tricuspid valve insufficiency, may lead to compression of the coronary artery.

ABERRANT ARTERY ORIGINATING FROM THE RIGHT CORONARY ARTERY SUPPLYING THE LEFT ANTERIOR MYOCARDIUM

Anatomy: a special case is shown in Fig. 8A–B—the LAD turns into a very thin vessel after the first 3 cm. In that case, an aberrant vessel originating from the RCA passes ventral to the pulmonary artery to the left side and feeds the middle and distal parts of the anterior left myocardium.

Clinical relevance: in case of pulmonary hypertension, the dilatation of the pulmonary artery may lead to a stretching of this aberrant vessel and subsequent myocardial ischemia.

Anomalies of Origin and Course of Individual Branches of the Coronary Arteries

Variations of the normal anatomy as a ramus intermedius are often seen in catheter angiography, MSCT, or autopsy. The branches of the coronary artery system can present multiple nonpathological variations. Because of its 2D projectional display, catheter angiography may sometimes be unable to depict the accurate course of the variations. Therefore, some of these aberrations may mimic coronary artery fistulae in catheter angiography.

ABERRANT SINUS NODE ARTERY

Anatomy: A frequent anomaly is an aberrant sinus node artery, originating from the LCx, finding its way dorsal to the aorta and leading to the right side. This anomaly is one of the most common (Fig. 9A–B).

Clinical relevance: this particular anomaly of the coronary arteries has no clinical relevance and has therefore to be considered nonmalignant. In catheter angiography, this anomaly is considered a normal finding, but it can mimic a coronary artery fistula. Another possible anomaly of branches of the coronary arteries is an aberrant conus artery.

Anomalies of Ectopic Origin and Course of Coronary Arteries

These extremely rare anomalies of the coronary arteries are mostly of no hemodynamic relevance. However, they are important for the angiographer and the surgeon—the angiographer may have difficulty visualizing the coronary artery course by selective coronary angiography or aortography; the surgeon may injure an ectopic vessel during an operation.

ECTOPIC ORIGIN OF CORONARY ARTERIES ABOVE THE AORTIC CUSP

Anatomy: most common is an origin of coronary arteries from the ascending aorta above the particular aortic cusp.

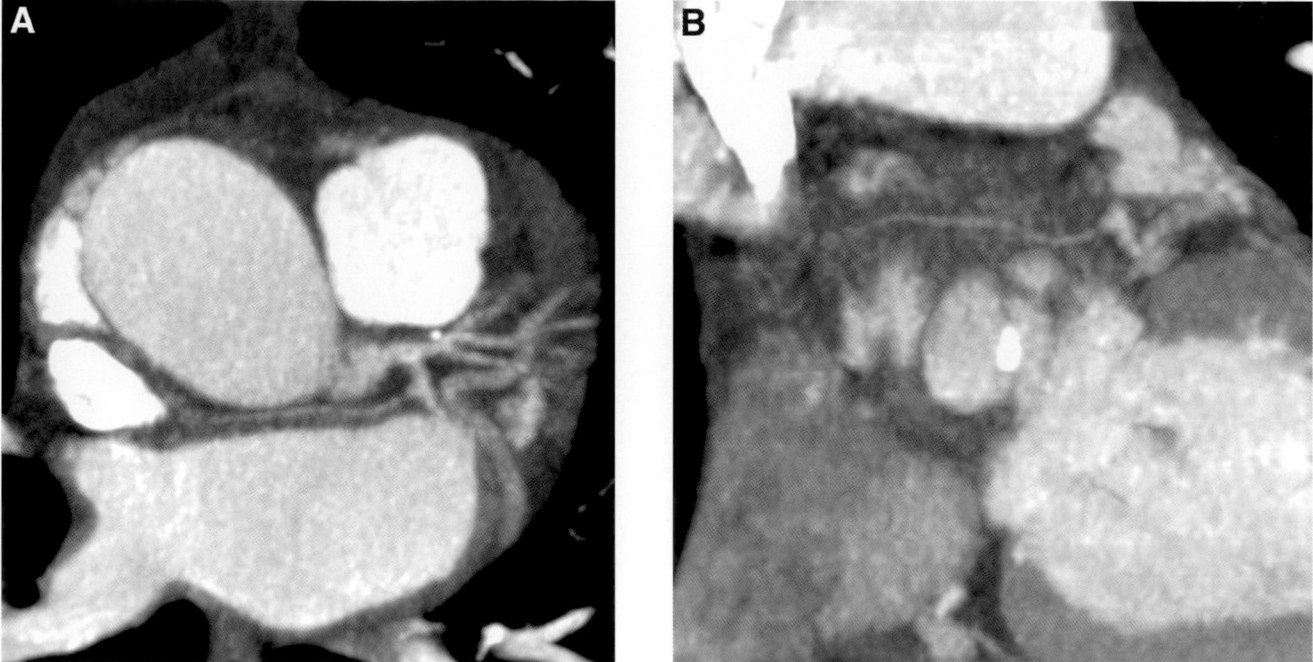

Fig. 9. Aberrant sinus node artery originating from the left circumflex with a course dorsal to the aorta. **(A)** "Thin maximum intensity projection" reconstruction. The dorsal pathway of the aberrant vessel is seen clearly. **(B)** Multiplanar reformation.

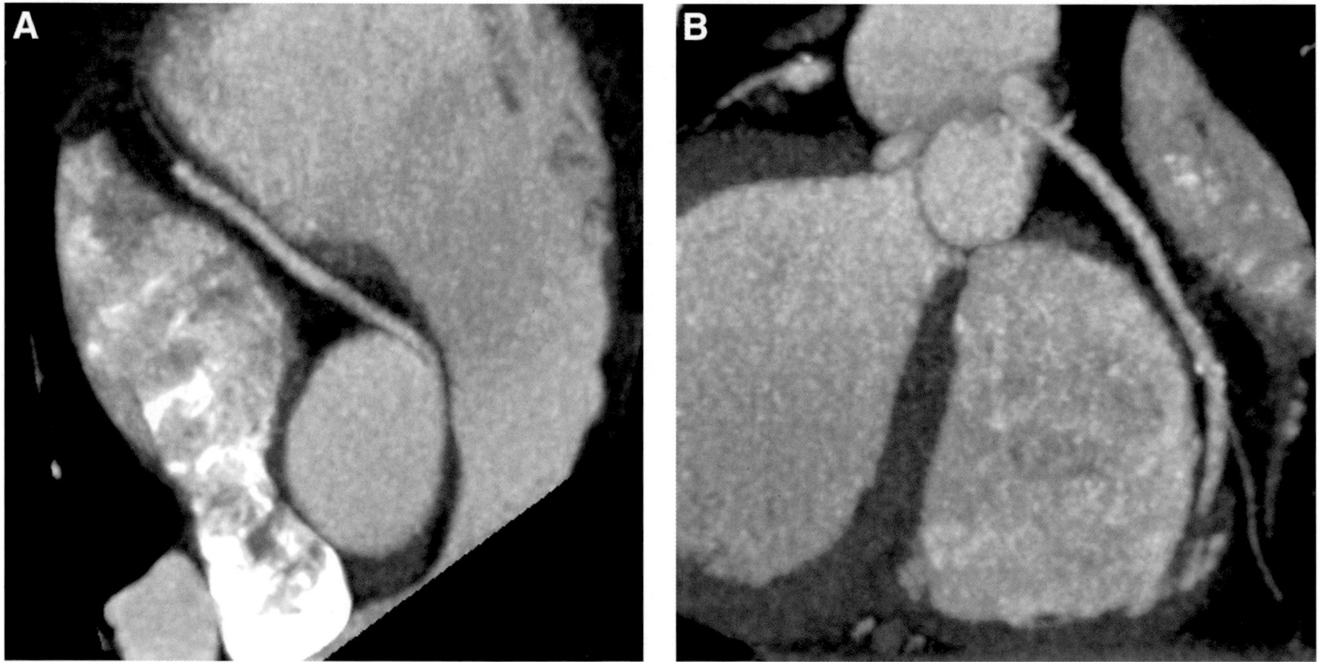

Fig. 10. *(above and on next page)*Aberrant right coronary artery (RCA) with a ventral origin from the aorta above the right sinus of Valsalva and an inter-arterial course between aorta and pulmonary artery. **(A,B)** "Thin maximum intensity projection" reconstruction. The sharp kink of the aberrant vessel and the decrease of the lumen near the origin are clearly visible . The RCA originates leftwards above the right sinus of Valsalva. **(C,D)** Volume rendering. The origin of the RCA leftwards above the right sinus of Valsalva is accurately shown. **(E)** Virtual angioscopy of the ostia of left main coronary artery (LMA) out of the left aortic cusp (LC) and the aberrant origin of the RCA out of the ascendant aorta above the right aortic cusp (RC).

Depending on the origin and course, these anomalies may produce clinical symptoms as well. Fig. 10A–E shows an origin of the RCA out of the ascending aorta slightly above the right aortic cusp with a sharp kink to the right and a partial course between aorta and pulmonary artery.

Clinical relevance: as a result of the partial interarterial course this anomaly has to be considered malignant. Without any evidence of coronary heart disease in CT angiography (CTA), this particular patient had atypical angina symptoms with exercise.

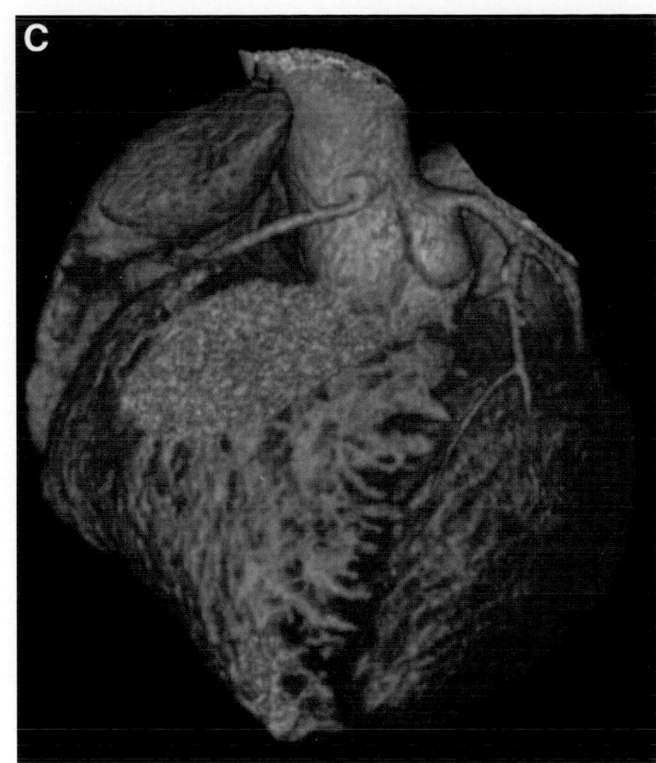

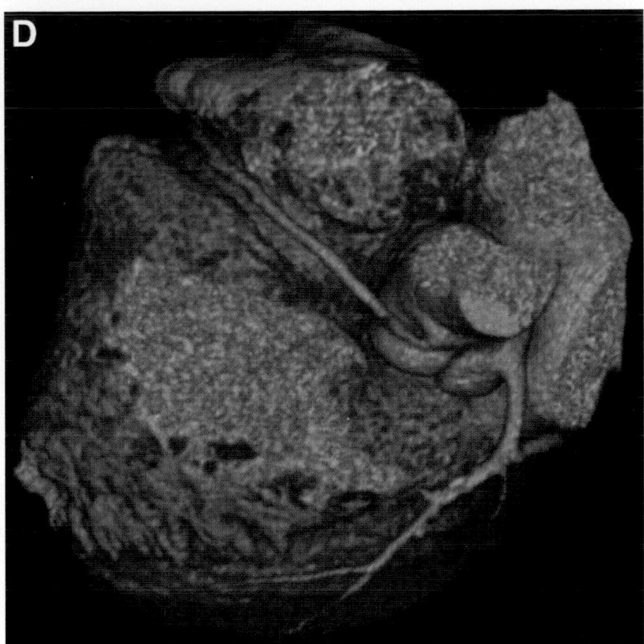

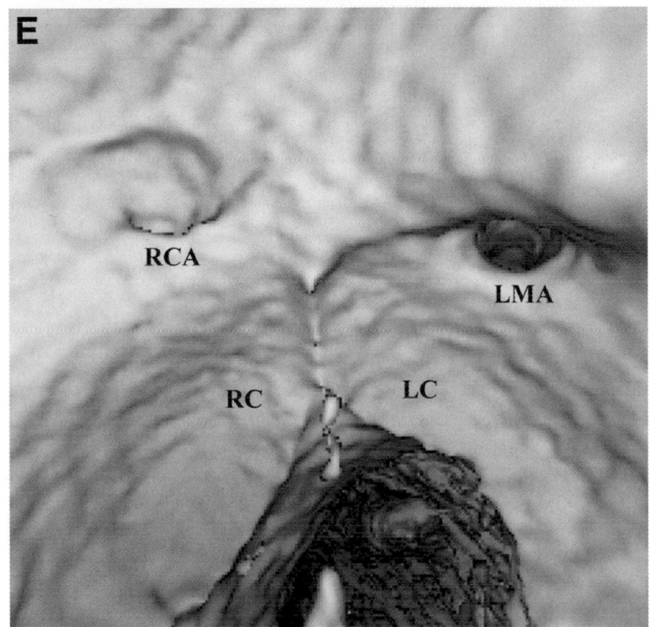

Aberrant coronary arteries with an origin above the particular aortic cusp may also present a kink at the sharp downward bend, which implies a higher risk of myocardial ischemia.

Ectopic Origin of Coronary Arteries Above the Aortic Cusp in Combination With a Malrotation of the Aortic Root

Anatomy: another complex anomaly is shown in Fig. 11A–E. The aortic root is rotated 90° clockwise. The RCA originating from the right sinus of Valsalva arises ventrally and follows a short pathway between aorta and pulmonary artery. The left main coronary artery originates above the left sinus of Valsalva with a sharp leftward kink.

Clinical relevance: this anomaly is thought to be malignant.

Single Coronary Artery

Anatomy: a single coronary artery may arise ectopically from the innominate or the right carotid artery. Ectopic origin of a coronary artery from the internal mammary artery, the left subclavian artery, or from bronchial branches is extremely rare.

Clinical relevance: the clinical relevance of these extremely rare anomalies depends on their course. Their significance is not known. In such cases of long-distance aberrations, an additional scan with a larger scan field is necessary in MSCT to depict the whole course of the special vascular anatomy.

CORONARY ARTERY FISTULAE

Prevalence and Etiology

Coronary fistula are repeatedly described in case reports. The general prevalence is still not known. In our study of more than 1100 patients, two coronary artery fistula where found.

Kawasaki disease (*see* Chapter 26) as an acute vasculitis of unknown cause often affects children, and in 20–25% of cases it can cause coronary artery anomalies like coronary fistulae. In spite of an early therapy consisting of intravenous gamma globulin and aspirin, coronary involvement may develop during the first years after diagnosis, even if an early regression of the main underlying disease is found *(36)*.

Anatomy and Pathophysiology of Coronary Artery Fistulae

Coronary artery fistula is a rare condition in which a communication exists between one or two coronary arteries and a cardiac chamber or a systemic vein. It causes a shunt from the high-pressure coronary artery to a lower-pressure cardiac chamber or vein in 90% of cases *(37)*. Coronary artery fistulae resemble other aortic runoff lesions in which blood leaves the aorta through the fistula during diastole, in this instance entering one of the cardiac chambers. This causes an obligatory

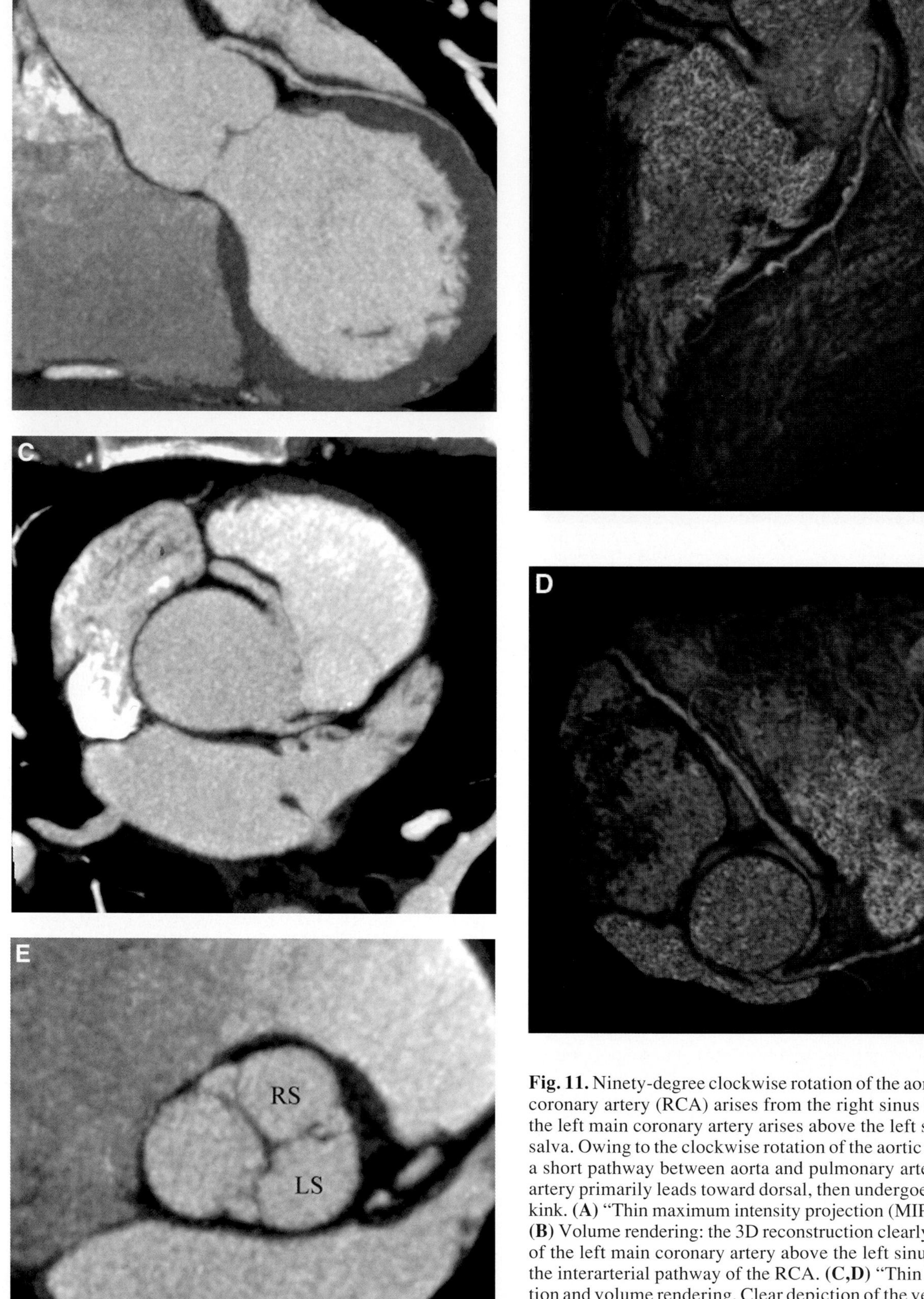

Fig. 11. Ninety-degree clockwise rotation of the aortic root. The right coronary artery (RCA) arises from the right sinus (RS) of Valsalva; the left main coronary artery arises above the left sinus (LS) of Valsalva. Owing to the clockwise rotation of the aortic root, the RCA has a short pathway between aorta and pulmonary artery. The left main artery primarily leads toward dorsal, then undergoes a sharp leftward kink. **(A)** "Thin maximum intensity projection (MIP)" reconstruction. **(B)** Volume rendering: the 3D reconstruction clearly shows the origin of the left main coronary artery above the left sinus of Valsalva and the interarterial pathway of the RCA. **(C,D)** "Thin MIP" reconstruction and volume rendering. Clear depiction of the ventral origin of the RCA and the dorsal origin of the left coronary artery resulting from the clockwise rotation of the aortic root. **(E)** "Thin MIP" reconstruction of the aortic root with aortic valve showing the 90° clockwise rotation.

shunt, because it connects the high-pressure aorta with the low-pressure cardiac chamber. When the shunt leads into a right-sided cardiac chamber, the hemodynamics resemble those of an extracardiac left-to-right shunt. Shunt flow occurs during systole and diastole except with fistulae to the left ventricle, which have largely diastolic flow. When the connection is to a left-sided cardiac chamber, the hemodynamics mimic those of an aortic insufficiency. Usually the volume of blood through the fistula is small, but it may occasionally be as large as twice the cardiac output. When it is large, a wide aortic pulse pressure is found. Myocardial perfusion may be diminished for that portion of the myocardium supplied by the abnormally connecting coronary artery. This represents a hemodynamic steal phenomenon, and may lead to myocardial ischemia *(38,39)*.

Because of the increased blood flow, the involved coronary artery is dilated and often tortuous. In some instances, the left-to-right shunt through the fistula may be small, but the afferent coronary arteries may be greatly dilated. Focal saccular aneurysms may develop, which eventually can calcify.

Because the fistulae allow increased blood flow from the aorta into the cardiac chambers, the involved chambers may be dilated in proportion to the volume of shunt.

The fistulae more commonly terminate in the right side of the heart and occasionally in the superior or inferior vena cava, right atrium *(40)*, coronary sinus, right ventricle (65%), or pulmonary artery (17%). However, they also may terminate in the left side of the heart, either to the left atrium or the left ventricle. Communications to either peripheral pulmonary artery branches, pulmonary vein, or mediastinal veins are extremely rare. Up to 50% of the fistulae arise from the right coronary artery.

Coronary artery fistulae can occasionally show abstruse courses up to a spider-like configuration and arise from more than one coronary artery *(41)* (Fig. 12 A–D). Numerous communications between the coronary artery and the terminating localization can rule out surgical correction.

Clinical Relevance

Most of the patients with this condition are eventually recognized by the appearance of a continuous and usually loud murmur. On physical examination, there may be evidence of cardiac enlargement and increased cardiac activity. The first and second heart sounds may be normal or slightly increased if the flow through the heart is moderately increased.

Whether chest pain can be caused by small coronary artery fistulae is uncertain. Larger communications represent a hemodynamic burden and may cause myocardial ischemia. Particularly pediatric patients tend to be symptomatic, showing atypical and typical chest pain and myocardial ischemia associated with ECG alterations *(42)*. Almost all coronary artery fistulae can be repaired by surgery *(43)* or embolization and stenting *(44)*, except for diffuse angiomatous communications. To prevent further progression and complications such as aneurysms, even small fistulae with a hemodynamically low significant shunt should be closed *(45)*. A spontaneous closure of an coronary artery fistula is extremely rare, but has been reported *(46)*.

MYOCARDIAL BRIDGES

Prevalence and Etiology

Myocardial bridging also appears to be a congenital anomaly, due to failure of externalization of the primitive coronary intratrabecular arterial network. A systolic coronary artery nar-rowing is observed in 0.5–12% of patients undergoing coronary arteriography. Although this entity is mostly benign, cases of acute myocardial ischemia, cardiogenic shock, and sudden death are reported *(47,48)*. Myocardial bridges are a common finding in autopsy. The incidence at postmortem examination is about 30–55% *(49)*. In catheter angiography, they are detected in less than 10% of the patients on very careful review of high-quality angiograms.

Anatomy

Any left coronary branch may be involved. The midsegment of the LAD is by far the most common localization. There is a higher prevalence in males (70%). Myocardial bridges are also more common in patients with idiopathic left-ventricular hypertrophy.

Normally the coronary arteries and their major branches course in the epicardial fat, but occasionally they course beneath the myocardium for some distance.

Myocardial bridges usually cross the LAD and less frequently involve other left-ventricular muscular branches. Myocardial bridges affecting the right coronary artery system should not cause systolic compression, because the right-ventricular systolic pressure is lower than the aortic pressure.

Clinical Relevance

The clinical significance of myocardial bridges is still unknown. The coronary artery is compressed during systole. This event can be demonstrated angiographically. Although coronary blood flow occurs primarily during diastole, blood flow may be significantly hampered by the bridges during tachycardia.

Most of the patients do not have typical symptoms of angina and have negative exercise stress test results, suggesting that the myocardial bridge is normally not physiologically significant. The risk of myocardial ischemia, vasospasm *(50)*, malignant arrhythmia, and sudden cardiac death is nevertheless increased *(51–54)*. Occasionally, typical findings of myocardial ischemia are found in patients with a myocardial bridge. Such a patient may benefit from either stenting the vessel under the bridge *(55,56)*, operative division of the bridging muscle band *(57)*, or coronary artery bypass grafting. Nowadays, minimally invasive methods should be the first choice *(58)*.

The presence of myocardial bridging distal to coronary lesions should be considered seriously in preprocedural evaluation of the lesions as a potential risk factor for intracoronary thrombus formation. Although pathologists had long recognized that the epicardial coronary artery might on occasion course directly through a segment of cardiac muscle, the physiological significance of this phenomenon was considered benign. This is partly based in traditional teaching that coronary blood flow delivery to the left-ventricular myocardium occurs primarily during the diastolic phase of the cardiac cycle.

Unlike coronary angiography, MSCT is capable of depicting vessels as well as muscle. Using thin perpendicular MPR reconstructions or volume rendering, myocardial bridges and their intramyocardial pathway can be depicted accurately. Also, thin MIP reconstructions are very useful to show these alterations (Fig. 13A–C) . In comparison to catheter angiography, even in diastole a lumen decrease sometimes is found. Whether

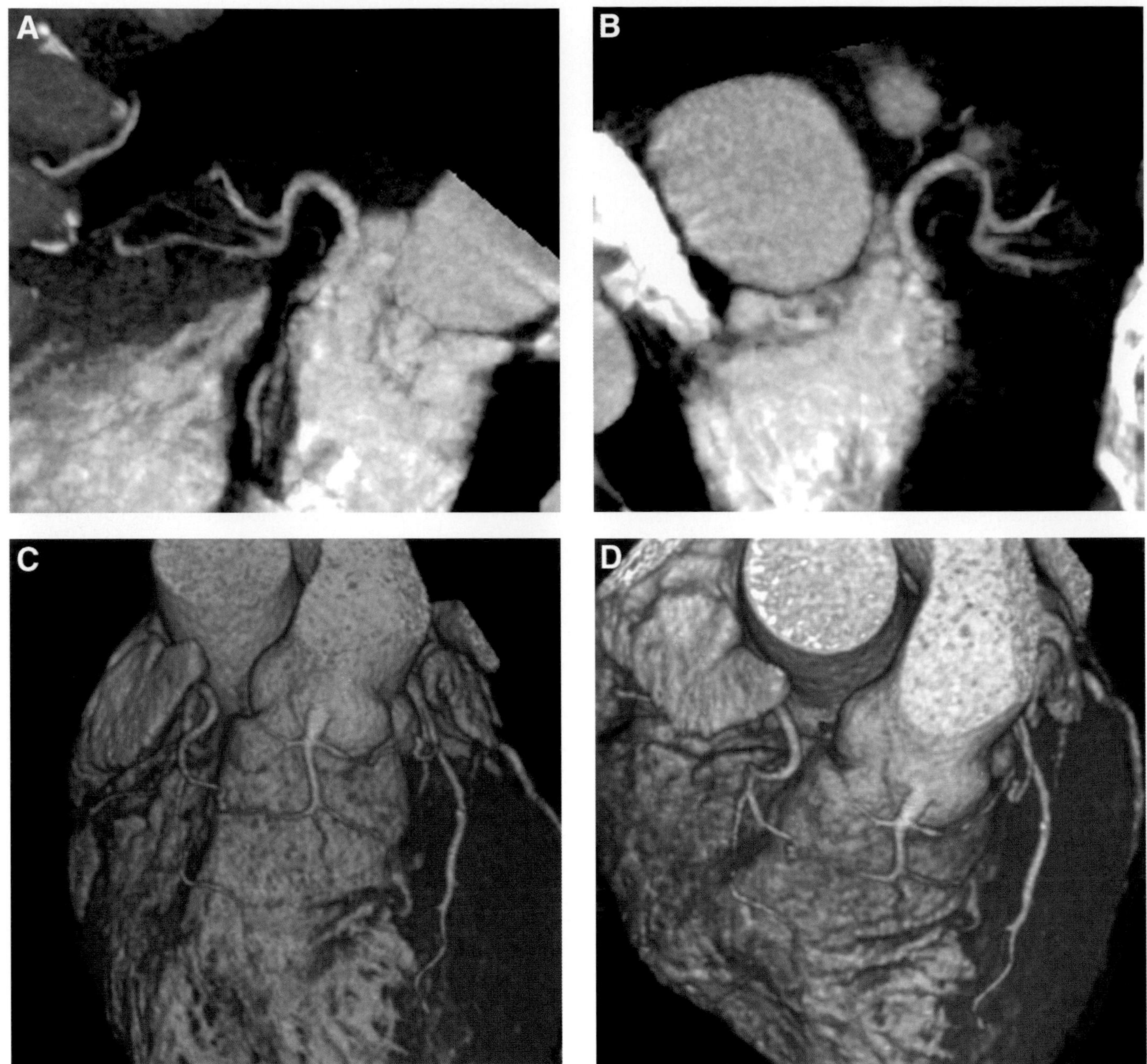

Fig. 12. Multiple spider-like fistulae from left anterior descending (LAD) artery and right coronary artery (RCA) to the pulmonary artery. **(A,B)** "Thin maximum intensity projection" reconstruction. From RCA **(A)** and LAD **(B)**, multiple fistulae lead to the pulmonary artery. **(C,D)** Volume rendering. The spider-like fistulae are clearly depicted. There is a common confluence to the pulmonary artery.

this means a higher risk of myocardial ischemia or not has to be evaluated in future studies. A statistical survey about the sensitivity and specificity of MSCT detecting myocardial bridges still does not exist, but it promises to become a potent tool in investigations of myocardial bridges. Especially, reconstructions in systole open a new approach to this entity.

SUMMARY

Anomalies of origin and course of the coronary arteries and coronary artery fistulae are often difficult to detect on catheter angiography. In addition, selective visualization may be impossible in many cases.

The prevalence of coronary artery anomalies is reported to be under 1%. These statistical data are based on catheter angiographic examinations. In our cohort of more than 1100 MSCT examinations of the coronary arteries, the prevalence was 2.6%. The reason for this discrepancy may be that coronary artery anomalies are very difficult to depict in catheter angio-graphy, and if they are visualized, their course is likely to be described inaccurately. In our studies, only 36% of the anomalies found in computed tomography could be displayed selectively in catheter angiography (Table 2). Based on our experience, it is not surprising that a high number of coronary artery anomalies was not detected angiographically before.

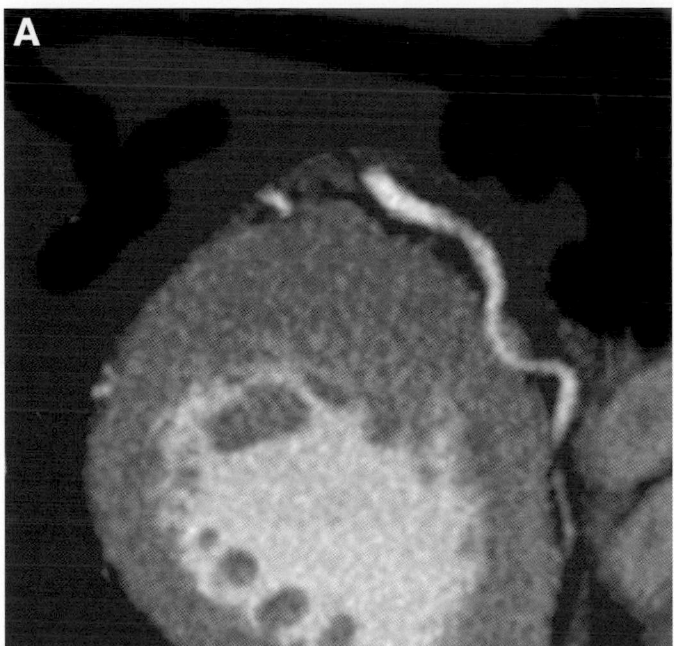

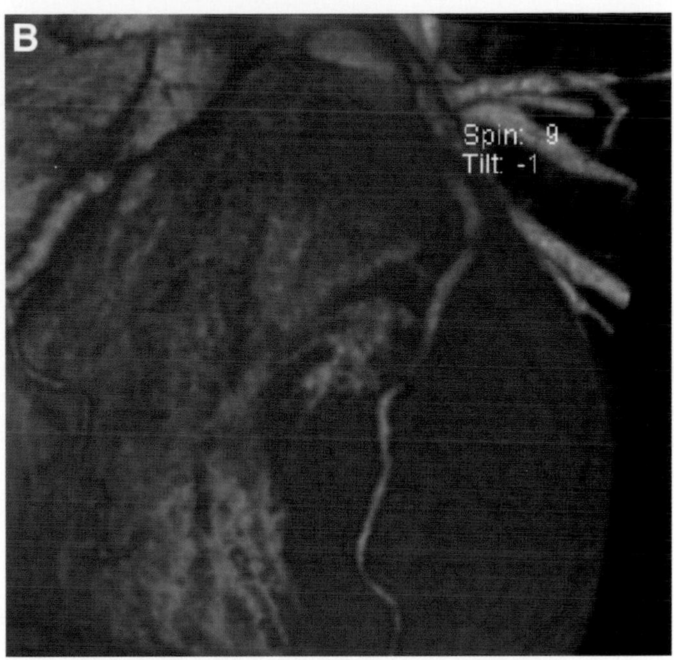

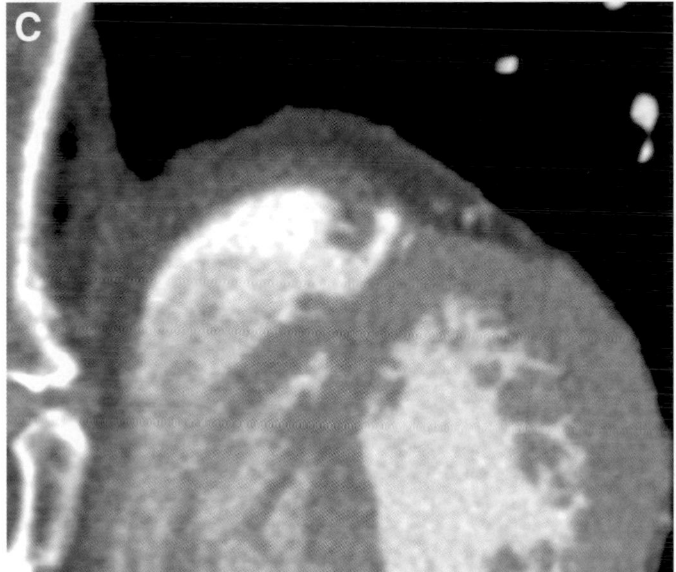

Fig. 13. Myocardial bridge in the middle segment of the left anterior descending (LAD) artery. **(A)** "Thin maximum intensity projection" reconstruction. **(B)** Volume rendering. The LAD immerses into myocardium and emerges after one and a half centimeters without lumen reduction. **(C)** Multiplanar reconstruction: the LAD shows an intramuscular pathway.

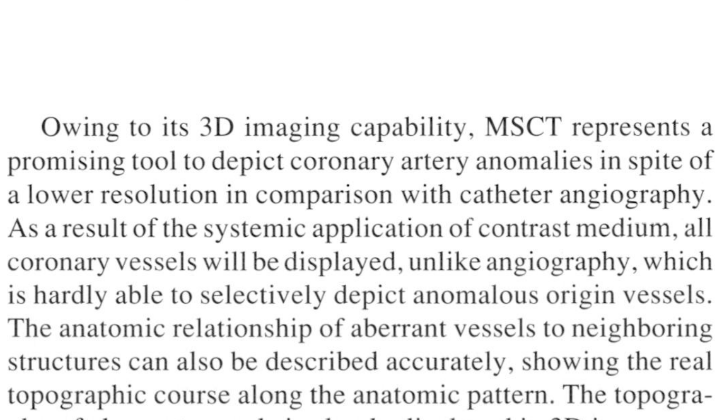

Owing to its 3D imaging capability, MSCT represents a promising tool to depict coronary artery anomalies in spite of a lower resolution in comparison with catheter angiography. As a result of the systemic application of contrast medium, all coronary vessels will be displayed, unlike angiography, which is hardly able to selectively depict anomalous origin vessels. The anatomic relationship of aberrant vessels to neighboring structures can also be described accurately, showing the real topographic course along the anatomic pattern. The topography of aberrant vessels is clearly displayed in 3D images, as opposed to the 2D catheter angiography projection.

MSCT furthermore provides clear visualization of coronary artery fistulae. The courses can be delineated accurately and their origin can be determined exactly. Unlike catheter angiography, where the configuration of fistulae often is difficult to depict, MSCT is able to show the individual feeders, and particularly the confluence, which is essential for the planning of surgical interventions. Most of the fistulae have more than one feeder but only a single outlet into the cardiac chamber or vein. For visualization of coronary artery fistulae, volume rendering has proved to be the best reconstruction method, showing the entire complexity of this anomaly in a 3D format.

The value of MSCT in depiction of myocardial bridges still has to be evaluated; however, the first experiences look very promising.

MSCT angiography of the coronary arteries is emerging as an essential imaging tool and the method of choice to detect and characterize anomalies of the coronary arteries with high resolution and significance. In comparison with catheter angiography, the capability to detect coronary artery anomalies is much higher. In conclusion, any suggested anomaly of the coronary arteries should be assessed with CTA to determinate its accurate course and origin.

REFERENCES

1. Virmani R, Burke AP, Farb A. Sudden cardiac death. Cardiovasc Pathol 2001;10(6):275–282.
2. Fornes P, Lecomte D. [Sudden death and physical activity and sports]. Rev Prat 2001;51(12 Suppl):S31–S35.

Table 2
Overview of the Coronary Anomalies Found in 1100 Multislice CT Studies, Their Courses, and the Number Seen at Selective Catheterization

Type of anomaly		*CT*	*Coronary angiography*	
Origin	*Course*	*Cases found*	*Angiography performed*	*Selective angiography possible*
RCA from LSV	interarterial	10	7	2
LCA from RSV	ventral	2	1	1
	interarterial	2	2	1
LAD from RSV	ventral	1	1	0
LCx from RSV	dorsal	3	2	2
LAD, LCx separately from LSV	normal	4	1	1
"Single coronary artery" from RSV	ventral	1	1	0
Sinus node artery from LCx	dorsal	1	1	0
Conus artery from RSV	normal	1	0	0
Malrotation of aortic root	interarterial	1	0	0
Ectopic origin of RCA	interarterial	1	1	0
Coronary artery fistula	ventral	2	2	0
Totals		29	19	7 (=36%)

LAD, left anterior descending artery; LCA, left coronary artery; LCx, left circumflex artery; LSV, left sinus of Valsalva; RCA, right coronary artery; RSV, right sinus of Valsalva.

3. Basso C, Maron BJ, Corrado D, Thiene G. Clinical profile of congenital coronary artery anomalies with origin from the wrong aortic sinus leading to sudden death in young competitive athletes. J Am Coll Cardiol 2000;35(6):1493–1501.
4. Mikaeloff P, Loire R, Amiel M, et al. [Anomaly of the origin of the circumflex artery. Effects on the risk of mitral and mitro-aortic valve replacement]. Arch Mal Coeur Vaiss 1979;72(8):895–898.
5. de Marchena EJ, Russo CD, Wozniak PM, Kessler KM. Compression of an anomalous left circumflex coronary artery by a bioprosthetic valve ring. J Cardiovasc Surg (Torino) 1990;31(1):52–54.
6. Felmeden D, Singh SP, Lip GY. Anomalous coronary arteries of aortic origin. Int J Clin Pract 2000;54(6):390–394.
7. Samarendra P, Kumari S, Hafeez M, Vasavada BC, Sacchi TJ. Anomalous circumflex coronary artery: benign or predisposed to selective atherosclerosis. Angiology 2001;52(8):521–526.
8. Harikrishnan S, Jacob SP, Tharakan J, et al. Congenital coronary anomalies of origin and distribution in adults: a coronary arteriographic study. Indian Heart J 2002;54(3):271–275.
9. Click RL, Holmes DR, Jr., Vlietstra RE, Kosinski AS, Kronmal RA. Anomalous coronary arteries: location, degree of atherosclerosis and effect on survival—a report from the Coronary Artery Surgery Study. J Am Coll Cardiol 1989;13(3):531–537.
10. Garg N, Tewari S, Kapoor A, Gupta DK, Sinha N. Primary congenital anomalies of the coronary arteries: a coronary arteriographic study. Int J Cardiol 2000;74(1):39–46.
11. Ohshima T, Lin Z, Sato Y. Unexpected sudden death of a 12-year-old male with congenital single coronary artery. Forensic Sci Int 1996;82(2):177–181.
12. Rowe L, Carmody TJ, Askenazi J. Anomalous origin of the left circumflex coronary artery from the right aortic sinus: a familial clustering. Cathet Cardiovasc Diagn 1993;29(4):277–278.
13. Albazzaz SJ. Klinefelter's syndrome with anomalous origin of left main coronary artery. Cathet Cardiovasc Diagn 1990;20(4):241–243.
14. Arizawa M, Nakayama M, Suehara N. [Clinical spectrum and congenital anomalies in trisomy 18]. Nippon Sanka Fujinka Gakkai Zasshi 1989;41(10):1545–1550.
15. Henglein D, Niederhoff H, Bode H. Origin of the left coronary artery from the right pulmonary artery and ventricular septal defect in a child of a mother with raised plasma phenylalanine concentrations throughout pregnancy. Br Heart J 1990;63(3):180–182.
16. Cox ID, Bunce N, Fluck DS. Failed sudden cardiac death in a patient with an anomalous origin of the right coronary artery. Circulation 2000;102(12):1461–1462.
17. Le T, Laskey WK, McLaughin J, White C. Utility of magnetic resonance imaging in a patient with anomalous origin of the right coronary artery, acute myocardial infarction, and near-sudden cardiac death. Cathet Cardiovasc Diagn 1997;42(2):205–207.
18. Page HL, Engel HJ, Campbell WB, et al. Anomalous origin of the left circumflex coronary artery. Recognition, angiographic demonstration and clinical significance. Circulation 1974;50:768–773.
19. Brown JW, Park HJ, Turrentine MW. Arterial switch operation: factors impacting survival in the current era. Ann Thorac Surg 2001;71(6):1978–1984.
20. Felmeden D, Singh SP, Lip GY. Anomalous coronary arteries of aortic origin. Int J Clin Pract 2000;54(6):390–394
21. Samarendra P, Kumari S, Hafeez M, Vasavada BC, Sacchi TJ. Anomalous circumflex coronary artery: benign or predisposed to selective atherosclerosis. Angiology 2001;52(8):521–526.
22. Garg N, Tewari S, Kapoor A, Gupta DK, Sinha N. Primary congenital anomalies of the coronary arteries: a coronary arteriographic study. Int J Cardiol 2000;74(1):39–46.
23. Shammas RL, Miller MJ, Babb JD. Single left coronary artery with origin of the right coronary artery from distal circumflex. Clin Cardiol 2001;24(1):90–92.
24. Cherian KM, Bharati S, Rao SG. Surgical correction of anomalous origin of the left coronary artery from the pulmonary artery. J Card Surg 1994;9(4):386–391.
25. Nightingale AK, Burrell CJ, Marshall AJ. Anomalous origin of the left coronary artery from the pulmonary artery: natural history and normal pregnancies. Heart 1998;80(6):629–631.
26. Flamm MD, Stinson EB, Hultgren HN, Shumway NE, Hancock EW. Anomalous origin of the left coronary artery from the pulmonary artery. Surgical treatment by ostial occlusion through pulmonary arteriotomy. Circulation 1968;38(1):113–123.
27. Salachas A, Achenbach K, Liberatos G, Hatzioannidis V, Goudevenos I, Sideris D. Isolated corrected transposition of great arteries and double left anterior descending artery originating from the left and right coronary artery. A rate combination of coronary artery anomaly and congenital heart disease. Angiology 1996;47(1):67–72.

28. Roberts WC, Dicicco BS, Waller BF, et al. Origin of the left main from the right coronary artery or from the right aortic sinus with intramyocardial tunneling to the left side of the heart via the ventricular septum. The case against clinical significance of myocardial bridge or coronary tunnel. Am Heart J 1982;104(2 Pt 1): 303–305.
29. Silverman KJ, Bulkley BH, Hutchins GM. Anomalous left circumflex coronary artery: "normal" variant of uncertain clinical and pathologic significance. Am J Cardiol 1978;41(7):1311–1314.
30. Molajo AO, Bray CL, Prescott MC, Testa HJ. Thallium-201 myocardial imaging in patients with angina pectoris and anomalous aortic origin of the circumflex coronary artery. Int J Cardiol 1988;18(3): 371–381.
31. Levin DC, Fellows KE, Abrams HL. Hemodynamically significant primary anomalies of the coronary arteries. Angiographic aspects. Circulation 1978;58(1):25–34.
32. Ott DA, Cooley DA, Angelini P, Leachman RD. Successful surgical correction of symptomatic cor triatriatum dexter. J Thorac Cardiovasc Surg 1979;78(4):573–575.
33. Hernando JP, Oliva MJ, Zarauza MJ, et al. [Anomalous origin of the circumflex artery from the pulmonary artery in a patient with rheumatic mitral stenosis]. Rev Esp Cardiol 1995;48(5):359–361.
34. Sagkan O, Ornek E, Yesildag O. Left circumflex coronary artery arising as a terminal extension of right coronary artery. A case report. Angiology 1994;45(5):405–408.
35. Kolodziej AW, Lobo FV, Walley VM. Intra-atrial course of the right coronary artery and its branches. Can J Cardiol 1994;10(2): 263–267.
36. Sciacca P, Falsaperla R, Barone P, et al. [Cardiac involvement in Kawasaki disease. Our experience]. Minerva Pediatr 2001;53(2): 87–93.
37. Braunwald E, Zipes D, Libby P, eds. Heart Disease, 6th ed. Saunders, Philadelphia: 2001.
38. Rubini G, Ettorre GC, Sebastiani M, Bovenzi F. [Evaluation of hemodynamic significance of arteriovenous coronary fistulas: diagnostic integration of coronary angiography and stress/rest myocardial scintigraphy]. Radiol Med (Torino) 2000;100(6):453–458.
39. Brigui M, Remadi F, Belkhiria N, Zemni J, Chabrak S, Gargouri R. [Angina and myocardial ischemia related to a fistula between the anterior interventricular artery and the pulmonary artery in a 56-year old man]. Ann Cardiol Angeiol (Paris) 1995;44(2):86–90.
40. Goldberg L, Mekel J. Congenital aneurysm of the left main coronary artery with fistulous communication to the right atrium and coronary "steal" phenomenon. Cardiovasc J S Afr 2001;12(1): 48–51.
41. Lai MC, Chen WJ, Chiang CW, Ko YL. An unusual case of dual coronary artery fistulas to main pulmonary artery. Chang Gung Med J 2002;25(1):51–55.
42. Wang NK, Hsieh LY, Shen CT, Lin YM. Coronary arteriovenous fistula in pediatric patients: a 17-year institutional experience. J Formos Med Assoc 2002;101(3):177–182.
43. Kamiya H, Yasuda T, Nagamine H, et al. Surgical treatment of congenital coronary artery fistulas: 27 years' experience and a review of the literature. J Card Surg 2002;17(2):173–177.
44. Atmaca Y, Altin T, Ozdol C, Pamir G, Caglar N, Oral D. Coronary-pulmonary artery fistula associated with right heart failure: successful closure of fistula with a graft stent. Angiology 2002;53(5): 613–616.
45. Bauer M, Bauer U, Alexi-Meskishvili V, et al. [Congenital coronary fistulas: the most frequent congenital coronary anomaly]. Z Kardiol 2001;90(8):535–541.
46. Muhler E, Keutel J, von Bernuth G. [Spontaneous occlusion of a congenital coronary artery fistula]. Z Kardiol 1984;73(8):538–540.
47. Nayar PG, Nyamu P, Venkitachalam L, Ajit SM. Myocardial infarction due to myocardial bridging. Indian Heart J 2002;54(6): 711–712.
48. Arnau Vives MA, Martinez Dolz LV, Almenar BL, Lalaguna LA, Ten Morro F, Palencia PM. [Myocardial bridging as a cause of acute ischemia. Description of a case and review of the literature]. Rev Esp Cardiol 1999;52(6):441.
49. Ferreira AG, Jr., Trotter SE, Konig B, Jr., Decourt LV, Fox K, Olsen EG. Myocardial bridges: morphological and functional aspects. Br Heart J 1991;66(5):364–367.
50. Kodama K, Morioka N, Hara Y, Shigematsu Y, Hamada M, Hiwada K. Coronary vasospasm at the site of myocardial bridge—report of two cases. Angiology 1998;49(8):659–663.
51. Fornes P, Lecomte D. [Sudden death and physical activity and sports]. Rev Prat 2001;51(12 Suppl):S31–S35.
52. Arnau Vives MA, Martinez Dolz LV, Almenar BL, Lalaguna LA, Ten Morro F, Palencia PM. [Myocardial bridging as a cause of acute ischemia. Description of a case and review of the literature]. Rev Esp Cardiol 1999;52(6):441.
53. Agirbasli M, Hillegass WB, Jr., Chapman GD, Brott BC. Stent procedure complicated by thrombus formation distal to the lesion within a muscle bridge. Cathet Cardiovasc Diagn 1998;43(1):73–76.
54. Agirbasli M, Martin GS, Stout JB, Jennings HS, III, Lea JW, Dixon JH, Jr. Myocardial bridge as a cause of thrombus formation and myocardial infarction in a young athlete. Clin Cardiol 1997;20(12): 1032–1036.
55. Prendergast BD, Kerr F, Starkey IR. Normalisation of abnormal coronary fractional flow rcscrvc associated with myocardial bridging using an intracoronary stent. Heart 2000;83(6):705–707.
56. Jeremias A, Haude M, Ge J, et al. [Emergency stent implantation in the area of extensive muscle bridging of the anterior interventricular ramus after post-interventional dissection]. Z Kardiol 1997;86(5): 367–372.
57. Furniss SS, Williams DO, McGregor CG. Systolic coronary occlusion due to myocardial bridging—a rare cause of ischaemia. Int J Cardiol 1990;26(1):116–117.
58. Pratt JW, Michler RE, Pala J, Brown DA. Minimally invasive coronary artery bypass grafting for myocardial muscle bridging. Heart Surg Forum 1999;2(3):250–253.

26 Multidetector-Row CT for Assessment of Kawasaki Disease

Toru Sakuma, MD and Kunihiko Fukuda, MD

KAWASAKI DISEASE

GENERAL

Kawasaki disease is an acute febrile illness, causing mucosal inflammation, skin rash, and cervical lymphadenopathy, recognized most often in children younger than 4 yr of age. It was first described by Dr. Tomisaku Kawasaki in Japanese literature in 1967 *(1)*, and then in English in 1974 *(2)*. The disease is of unknown etiology that produces a systemic vasculitis, which is most severe in the medium-sized arteries, and especially prominent in the coronary arteries. This can be associated with considerable morbidity and mortality, mostly the result of myocardial involvement and coronary artery complications such as aneurysm, calcification, and stenosis. In Japan as well as in North America, Kawasaki disease is presently a leading cause of acquired heart disease in children *(3)*.

DIAGNOSTIC CRITERIA

The diagnosis of Kawasaki disease is made according to the guidelines prepared by the Committee on Rheumatic Fever, Endocarditis, and Kawasaki Disease, Council on Cardiovascular Disease in the Young, American Heart Association (Table 1) *(4)*, and the Japan Kawasaki Disease Research Committee *(5)*, because of the absence of a specific laboratory test. The principal diagnostic criteria of Kawasaki disease are persistent fever, conjunctival injection, inflamed oropharyngeal mucosa, changes in the peripheral extremities, erythematous rash, and cervical lymphadenopathy. At least five of these six principal diagnostic criteria should be satisfied to establish a diagnosis of Kawasaki disease. Where coronary aneurysms are recognized by transthoracic echocardiography or coronary angiography (CAG), patients with four of the above diagnostic criteria can also be diagnosed with Kawasaki disease.

TREATMENT AND MANAGEMENT

Standard initial treatment involves intravenous administration of high-dose γ globulin and oral administration of aspirin. Treatment is started preferably within the first 10 d from the onset of illness *(6–8)*. Two mg/kg intravenous γ globulin (IVGG) combined with at least 30 to 50 mg/kg/d aspirin provides maximum protection against development of coronary abnormalities after Kawasaki disease. Gamma globulin helps to prevent coronary artery complications, and aspirin clears acute inflammatory symptoms *(9)*. IVGG therapy has reduced both the morbidity of Kawasaki disease and the apparent incidence of coronary artery abnormalities from approx 20–25% to less than 5% at 6–8 wk after initiation of therapy *(6)*. In the pre-IVGG treatment stage, the incidence of coronary aneurysm in acute Kawasaki disease was 25%, 55% of which showed regression on follow-up angiography. This is a characteristic phenomenon in Kawasaki disease. Regression is likely to occur within 1 or 2 yr after onset, and it is unlikely to occur more than several years after onset *(10–12)*. During follow-up, ischemic heart disease developed in 4.7% and myocardial infarction in 1.9%. Death occurred in 0.8% *(13)*. The standardized mortality ratio of Kawasaki disease was 1.25, but for the male group with cardiac sequelae was 2.35. So the mortality rate among male patients with cardiac sequelae due to Kawasaki disease seemed higher than that in the general population *(14)*. The number of patients with cardiac lesions 1 mo after onset has decreased year by year, and that is possibly attributable to the increase in the proportion of patients treated with IVGG and an increase in the dosage *(15)*.

Long-term management of Kawasaki disease, which is based on risk stratification, is also shown by the research committee, and risk level categories are summarized *(3)*. Patients with a normal coronary artery, evaluated by echocardiography or CAG during the acute stage of Kawasaki disease, have little morbidity in childhood, and no strict follow-up is usually required.

ASSESSMENT OF CORONARY ARTERY

ECHOCARDIOGARPHY

The initial evaluation and follow-up of the coronary arterial lesions in Kawasaki disease are done by echocardiography, because it is considered to be the most useful and essential method to evaluate coronary aneurysms. Evaluation of coronary artery morphology should include quantitative and qualitative assessment of the inner diameter of the vessels. When the coronary artery diameter is larger than normal but a segmental aneurysm is not apparent, the vessel is described as ectatic. Aneurysms are classified as small (less than 5 mm in internal diameter), medium (5 to 8 mm in internal diameter), or giant (more than 8 mm in internal diameter). Many publications have demonstrated the high efficacy and accuracy of echocardio-

From: *Contemporary Cardiology: CT of the Heart: Principles and Applications*
Edited by: U. Joseph Schoepf © Humana Press, Inc., Totowa, NJ

Table 1
Diagnostic Criteria

Principal Clinical Findings [a]

Fever persisting at least 5 d [b] and the present of at least four of the following five principal features:

1. Changes in extremities:
   a. Acute: erythema and edema of hands and feet
   b. Convalescent: membranous desquamation of fingertips
2. Polymorphous exanthema
3. Bilateral, painless bulbar conjunctival injection without exudates
4. Changes in lips and oral cavity: erythema and cracking of lips, strawberry tongue, diffuse injection of oral and pharyngeal mucosae
5. Cervical lymphadenopathy (=1.5 cm in diameter), usually unilateral

[a] Patients with fever and fewer than four principal symptoms can be diagnosed as having Kawasaki disease when coronary artery disease is detected by 2D echocardiography or coronary angiography. Other diagnoses should be excluded. The physician should be aware that some children with illness not fulfilling these criteria have developed coronary artery aneurysms.

[b] Many experts believe that in the presence of classic features, the diagnosis of Kawasaki disease can be made by experienced observers before d 5 of fever.

Adapted from ref. *4*.

graphy in detecting and characterizing coronary artery diseases *(16,17)*. It has been reported that echocardiography has 98% sensitivity and 95% specificity in the diagnosis of left main coronary artery aneurysms in comparison with CAG. However, echocardiography is less sensitive in detecting right coronary artery (RCA) lesions, as the middle part of the RCA is located behind the sternum and the distal part of RCA is the furthest away from the chest wall. In addition, it is impossible to evaluate small aneurysms in the peripheral branches and the lumens of calcified aneurysms by echocardiography. There is also a limitation in the accurate evaluation of the degree of stenosis and the size of intramural thrombosis within aneurysms. Furthermore, visualization and characterization of the coronary arteries through transthoracic echocardiography become progressively more difficult as the child grows.

CORONARY ANGIOGRAPHY

CAG offers complete images of coronary arteries and more detailed definition of coronary artery anatomy than echocardiography, making it possible to detect coronary artery stenosis or thrombotic occlusion and to determine the extent of collateral artery formation. However, there are certain risks associated with this procedure as a result of its invasive nature and the exposure to ionizing radiation, as well as its being more expensive. Whether to use CAG should be determined on a risk-vs-benefit balance, including abnormal findings on echocardiography, symptoms or signs of ischemia, auscultatory evidence of valvular regurgitation, evidence of cardiac dysfunction, and the need for intracoronary thrombolytic treatment *(3)*.

Whether or not regression may reverse and eventually develop into stenosis is uncertain at the present time. However, postmortem examinations of some patients with angiographically documented regression of coronary artery aneurysm have revealed intimal proliferation and fibrosis not apparent on the angiogram *(18)*. On intravascular ultrasound imaging (IVUS), the regressed coronary aneurysms also demonstrated a marked thickening of the intima with or without calcification, which bore a striking resemblance to early atherosclerotic lesions *(19,20)*. The coronary artery wall, at the site of the regressed aneurysm, had poor distensibility and was stiff on examination with intracoronary isosorbide dinitrate *(21)*. These findings suggest that regressed ectasia and aneurysm has potential risk for later complications, even in cases of normal CAG. Therefore, long-term follow-up is recommended in cases of asymptomatic transient aneurysm, to screen for development of premature coronary artery atherosclerosis in adulthood.

MAGNETIC RESONANCE IMAGING

Electrocardiogram (ECG)-gated magnetic resonance imaging (MRI) has also been used for the noninvasive evaluation of the aortic root and the major proximal portion of the coronary arteries *(22)*. Recent development of magnetic resonance (MR) hardware and rapid acquisition pulse sequences enables high resolution MR angiography (MRA) of the coronary arteries. Sensitivity, specificity, accuracy, and negative predictive value for patients with coronary artery disease by coronary MRA were 94%, 45%, 75%, and 82% respectively, compared with CAG *(23)*. Free-breathing 3D coronary MRA also accurately defines coronary artery aneurysms in patients with Kawasaki disease *(24)*. However, several data acquisitions are needed along the major axis of the arteries because of the limitation in the volume coverage of the scans. The scanning time of approx 30 min is a relatively long time for young children and adolescents. In addition, voxel size of 0.7 × 1.0 × 1.5 mm is not adequate for 3D imaging in comparison with the isotropic data obtained with multidetector-row CT (MDCT).

ASSESSMENT OF CORONARY ARTERIES BY MDCT

INTRODUCTION

Single-slice helical CT has a limited role in the management of Kawasaki disease because of cardiac motion artifacts due to long acquisition times and lack of ECG gating, although there has been one report presenting two cases of Kawasaki disease with unrecognized coronary artery aneurysms detected by single-slice helical CT *(25)*.

Electron beam CT (EBCT) is an effective, noninvasive method of identifying coronary artery aneurysms. Frey et al. reported in their series that 9 of 10 coronary artery aneurysms in Kawasaki disease were visualized with EBCT. In one false

Table 2
Scan Protocol

	SOMATOM Volume Zoom	*SOMATOM Sensation 16*
Collimation	4 × 1 mm	12 × 0.75 mm
Gantry rotation time (ms)	500	420
Temporal resolution (ms)	125–250	105–210
Spacial resolution	0.7 × 0.7 × 1.25	0.7 × 0.7 × 0.8
Table feed (mm/rotation)	1.5	2.8
Tube voltage (kV)	150	120
Maximum tube current (mA)	500	500
Contrast agent (mL)	2.0 × body weight (BW)	2.0 × BW
Scan delay time (s)	20	bolus tracking
Scan time (s)	35	10

case, two contiguous aneurysms were mistaken for a single aneurysm. The inability to resolve the aneurysms as separate structures was probably due to 8-mm section thickness in this case *(26)*. Spatial resolution of EBCT is suboptimal for the evaluation of coronary arteries compared with that of MDCT. Z-axis collimation of EBCT is up to 3 mm, while in 16-row MDCT it is 0.75 mm. Another problem with EBCT is that the prospectively ECG-triggered sequential method cannot obtain phase-constant cardiac volume imaging during the scan, which results in potential image degradation.

MDCT with retrospective ECG gating is considered a well-suited modality for noninvasive diagnosis of the coronary arteries, as it can optimize temporal resolution, spatial resolution, and volume coverage.

METHOD

Three-dimensional volume data were obtained with MDCT (SOMATOM Volume Zoom and SOMATOM Sensation 16, Siemens AG, Medical Solutions) (Table 2). Average scan range was 100 mm. All image acquisitions were performed in deep inspiratory breath-hold among patients who were able to do so, and those patients who could not do so were allowed to breath freely under sedation with chloral hydrate to achieve an adequate study. The injection of 2 mL/kg of 370-mgI/mL nonionic contrast medium (iopamidol) was performed via a peripheral intravenous route during one breath-hold, with simultaneous registration of the ECG signal also being performed. The injection speed ranged from 1 to 3 mL/s, depending on the patient's age and size. The ECG signal was used to reconstruct the images at identical time points, about 400 ms before the next R wave. For 3D reconstruction and visualization of the coronary arteries, curved multiplanar reformation (MPR) and maximum intensity projection (MIP) techniques were applied (Heart View CT, Siemens AG, Medical Solutions). Curved MPR images were rendered along the course of each coronary artery from the axial data set, while MIP images were produced in the same way with 3-mm thickness.

DETECTABILITY BY MDCT

MDCT findings in 70 cases with Kawasaki disease were analyzed, where the coronary arteries were subdivided into proximal and distal parts. The area within reach of echocardiography was defined as the proximal part and the region beyond the reach of echocardiography as the distal part. The visibility of coronary arteries was 93.6% in the proximal part and 62.9% in the distal part. In the proximal part, 18 calcifications, 24 aneurysms, 19 both calcification and aneurysms and one stenosis were found. The sensitivity of MDCT was 94.3% in the detection of abnormalities within the proximal segments of the coronary arteries, and the specificity was 100% when echocardiography was used as the gold standard. In the distal part, where echocardiography cannot reach, 16 calcifications, 2 aneurysms, 8 both calcifications and aneurysms, and 4 stenoses were detected.

REPRESENTATIVE CASE STUDIES

Case 1: 19-Yr-Old Male

This patient presented with continuous fever, conjunctival injection, erythema and edema of hands and feet, and polymorphous exanthema. He was diagnosed with Kawasaki disease at 20 mo from birth. The patient was treated with aspirin and dipyridamole, recovering within 25 d. Echocardiography revealed coronary aneurysms in the proximal part of the RCA and left coronary artery (LCA). The initial CAG was performed 2 mo after the onset, because of abnormal Q wave and arrhythmias, and revealed a coronary aneurysm with stenosis and thrombus in the RCA and an aneurysm with stenosis in the LCA. Repeat coronary angiographies were performed at the ages of 5, 8, 11, 14, and 19 yr. At the age of 19, left circumflex (LCx) obstruction was discovered, and thallium-201 myocardial perfusion scintigraphy revealed ischemia in the lateral wall of the left ventricle. There were multiple calcified aneurysms in the proximal part of the coronary arteries, which were all detected on 4-row MDCT (Fig. 1A,B). Although these aneurysms were followed up by echocardiography, intraluminal patency was impossible to evaluate because of heavy mural calcification. MDCT showed large thrombosis within the giant calcified aneurysm of the coronary arteries. One of the advantages of MDCT over echocardiography is that MDCT can depict intraluminal information within the calcified wall.

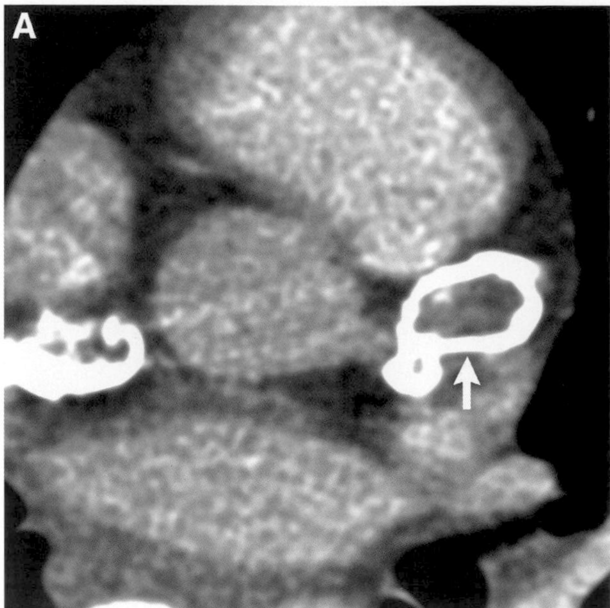

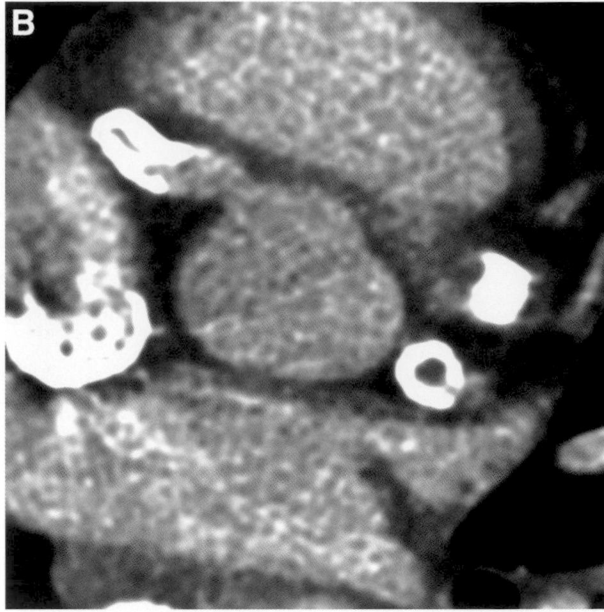

Fig. 1. Thin-slice maximum intensity projection images of proximal right coronary artery and left coronary artery reveal multiple calcified aneurysms, which were successfully followed up by echocardiography. However, large thrombosis (arrow) within the giant aneurysm was not depicted by echocardiography because of heavy calcification.

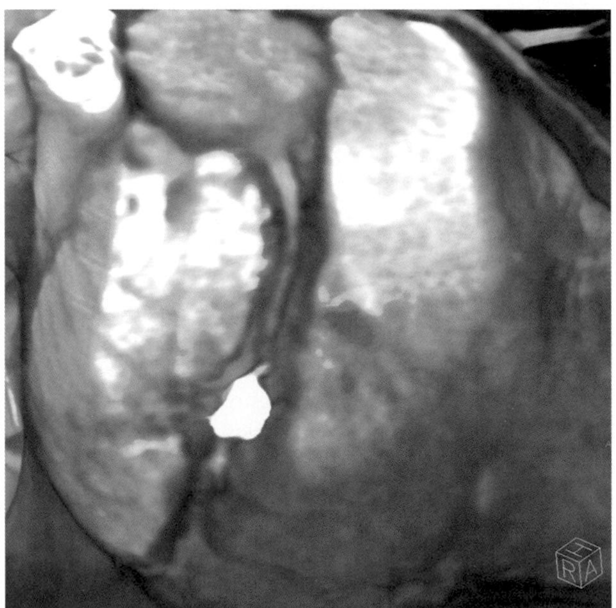

Fig. 2. Volume-rendered image of multidetector-row CT delineates heavily calcified aneurysm in segment 2, which was beyond the scope of ultrasound.

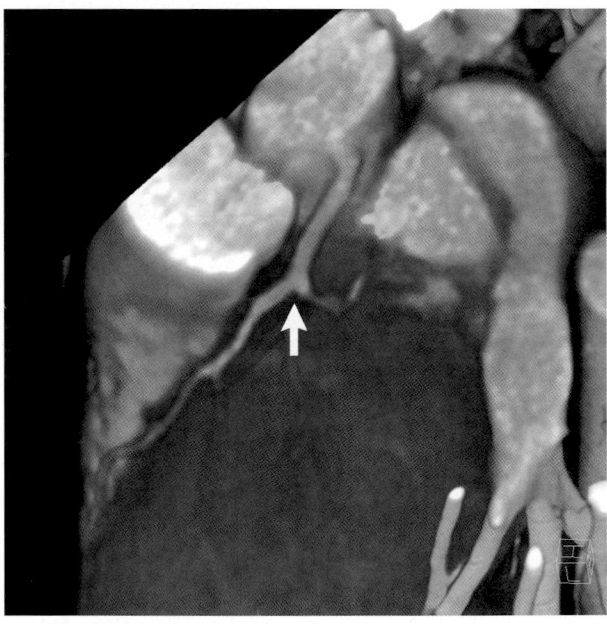

Fig. 3. Volume-rendered image shows obstruction in left circumflex coronary artery (arrow).

Case 2: 20-Yr-Old Male

The disease was diagnosed when the patient was admitted to our hospital suffering a high temperature at 6 yr of age. He was treated with aspirin and dipyridamole, being discharged from hospital after 38 d. CAG, performed at the age of 14, showed LCx stenosis and calcification of the RCA. The patient was followed up with treatment of aspirin and dipyridamole. At the age of 18, he underwent further angiography, which showed LCx stenosis and RCA segment 2 calcified aneurysm. Sixteen-row cardiac MDCT was performed on an out-patient basis in order to evaluate the potential lesions in the coronary arteries. Cardiac CT confirmed all the abnormalities detected by CAG and verified no new development (Figs. 2 and 3).

Case 3: 21-Yr-Old Female

The disease was diagnosed when the patient was 2 yr of age, when she was admitted to our hospital with a high temperature. She was discharged from the hospital after 48 d treatment with aspirin and dipyridamole. Echocardiography delineated RCA

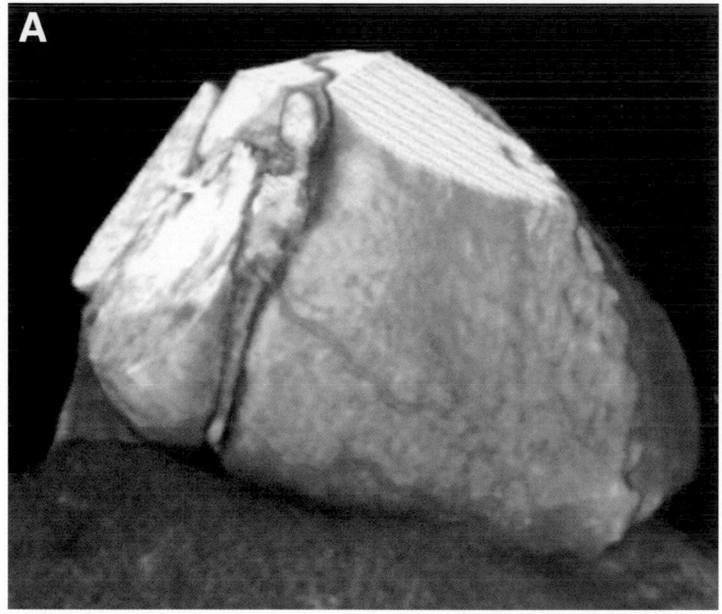

Fig. 4. Volume-rendered images of multidetector-row CT clearly delineate giant aneurysm in segment 1, calcified giant aneurysm in segments 2 and 6.

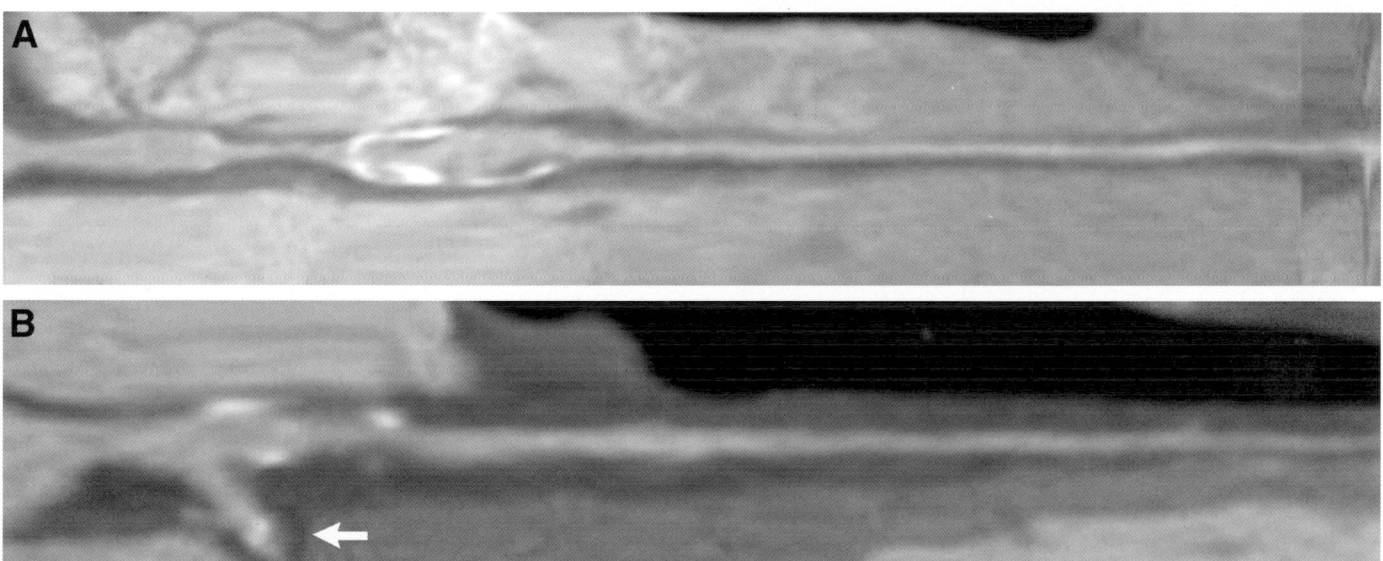

Fig. 5. Automated segmentations of right coronary (**A**) and left anterior descending artery (**B**) show mural calcification and intraluminal thrombosis in giant aneurysm, which are suitable for quantitative assessment of vessel diameters and stenosis degree. There is a focal area of calcification in the proximal left circumflex, which is in normal caliber (arrow). Findings are in keeping with regressed aneurysm. Such lesions carry the potential risk to develop luminal stenosis, and therefore careful and close follow-up is required. Multidetector-row CT is able to detect small calcifications, which cannot be shown by coronary angiography.

and LCA aneurysms, which were also detected in CAG performed at the ages of 3, 4, 6, and 7. At the age of 10, she underwent further angiography, which showed giant aneurysms in segment 1, segments 2–3, and segments 5–6, small aneurysm in segment 11, and calcification in segments 2–3 and segment 5. The patient was followed up with treatment of aspirin, dipyridamole, ticlopidine HCl, and ubidecarenone. At the age of 19, pharmacological stress electrocardiography showed ST-T changes in II, III, aVF, but no ischemia detected on thallium-201 myocardial perfusion scintigraphy. Echocardiography revealed a giant aneurysm of the distal RCA and calcification of the left main trunk. Cardiac CT on 16-row MDCT was performed on an out-patient basis in order to evaluate the potential lesions in the coronary arteries. Cardiac CT confirmed all the abnormalities detected by CAG (Fig. 4A). Furthermore, intramural thrombosis in calcified giant aneurysms and small calcifications in LCx, which were not evaluated by CAG, were also clearly delineated (Figs. 5A,B and 6A).

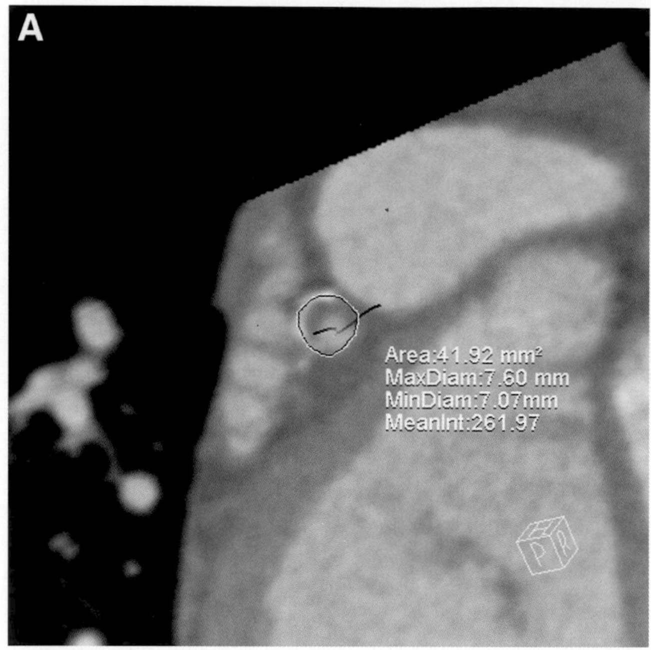

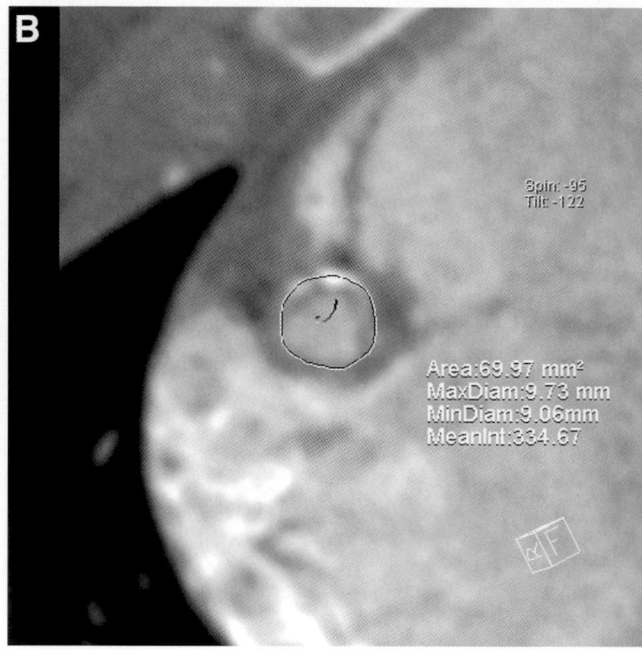

Fig. 6. Quantitative analysis of short-axis multiplanar reformation images of large calcified aneurysms, using Vessel-View soft ware (Siemens AG, Medical Solutions), shows accurate diameter of aneurysms.

SUMMARY

MDCT enables evaluation of coronary arteries, which cannot be reached by echocardiography, such as areas behind calcification and the distal part of coronary arteries. MDCT is considered to be highly efficient in the delineation of abnormalities in coronary arteries with Kawasaki disease.

Coronary artery bypass grafting using internal thoracic and gastroepiploic arteries is increasing in Japan and the United States, because of the long patency of arterial grafts. The actuarial graft patency rate for arterial grafts has been reported as 77.1% ± 1.1% *(27)*. Several types of catheter intervention have also been performed in the management of coronary stenosis caused by Kawasaki disease *(28,29)*. Therefore, MDCT is also thought to be a promising non-invasive modality for the assessment of the patency of bypass grafts or coronary stenosis after interventional treatment instead of conventional CAG.

REFERENCES

1. Kawasaki T. Acute febrile mucocutaneous syndrome with lymphoid involvement with specific desquamation of the fingers and toes in children.(in Japanese) Jpn J Allergy 1967;16:178–222.
2. Kawasaki T, Kosaki F, Okawa S, Shigematsu I, Yanagawa H. A new infantile acute febrile mucocutaneous lymph node syndrome (MLNS) prevailing in Japan. Pediatrics 1974;54:271–276.
3. Dajani AS, Taubert KA, Takahashi M, et al. Guidelines for long-term management of patients with Kawasaki disease: report from the Committee on Rheumatic Fever, Endocarditis, and Kawasaki Disease, Council on Cardiovascular Disease in the Young, American Heart Association. Circulation 1994;89:916–922.
4. Council on Cardiovascular Disease in the Young, Committee on Rheumatic Fever, Endocarditis, and Kawasaki Disease, American Heart Association. Diagnostic Guidelines for Kawasaki Disease. Circulation 2001;103:335–336.
5. The Japan Kawasaki Disease Research Committee. Diagnostic Guidelines of Kawasaki Disease (in Japanese). The 5th Revised Edition, February 2002.
6. Newburger JW, Takahashi M, Burns JC, et al. The treatment of Kawasaki syndrome with intravenous gamma globulin. N Engl J Med 1986;315:341–347.
7. Newburger JW, Takahashi M, Beiser AS, et al. A single intravenous infusion of gamma globulin as compared with four infusions in the treatment of acute Kawasaki syndrome. N Engl J Med 1991;324: 1633–1639.
8. Dajani AS, Taubert KA, Gerber MA, et al. Diagnosis and therapy of Kawasaki disease in children. Circulation 1993;87:1776–1780.
9. Terai M, Shulman ST. Prevalence of coronary artery abnormalities in Kawasaki disease is highly dependent on gamma globulin dose but independent of salicylate dose. J Pediatr 1997;131:888–893.
10. Nakano H, Ueda K, Saito A, Nojima K. Repeated quantitative angiograms in coronary arterial aneurysm in Kawasaki disease. Am J Cardiol 1985;56:846–851.
11. Takahashi M, Mason W, Lewis AB. Regression of coronary aneurysms in patients with Kawasaki syndrome. Circulation 1987;75: 387–394.
12. Akagi T, Rose V, Benson LN, Newman A, Freedom RM. Outcome of coronary artery aneurysms after Kawasaki disease. J Pediatr 1992; 121:689–694.
13. Kato H, Inoue O, Kawasaki T, Fujiwara H, Watanabe T, Toshima H. Long-term consequences of Kawasaki disease. Circulation 1996;94: 1379–1385.
14. Nakamura Y, Yanagawa H, Harada K, Kato H, Kawasaki T. Mortality among persons with a history of Kawasaki disease in Japan: the fifth look. Arch Pediatr Adolesc Med 2002;156:162–165.
15. Yanagawa H, Nakamura Y, Yashiro M, et al. Incidence survey of Kawasaki disease in 1997 and 1998 in Japan. Pediatrics 2001; 107:e33.
16. Capannari TE, Daniels SR, Meyer RA, Schwartz DC, Kaplan S. Sensitivity, Specificity and predictive value of two-dimensional

echocardiography in detecting coronary artery aneurysms in patients with Kawasaki disease. J Am Coll of Cardiol 1986;7: 335–60.

17. Hiraishi S, Misawa N, Takeda N, Horiguchi Y. Transthoracic ultrasonic visualisation of coronary aneurysm, stenosis, and occlusion in Kawasaki disease. Heart 2000;83:400–405.
18. Naoe S, Takahashi K, Masuda H, Tanaka N. Coronary findings post Kawasaki disease in children who died of other causes. Prog Clin Biol Res 1987;250:341–346.
19. Suzuki A, Yamagishi M, Kimura K, et al. Functional behavior and morphology of the coronary artery wall in patients with Kawasaki disease assessed by intravascular ultrasound. J Am Coll Cardiol 1996; 27:291–296.
20. Sugimura T, Kato H, Inoue O, Takagi J, Fukuda T, Sato N. Vasodilatory response of the coronary arteries after Kawasaki disease: evaluation by intracoronary injection of isosorbide dinitrate.J Pediatr 1992;121:684–688.
21. Sugimura T, Kato H, Inoue O, et al. Congenital heart disease: intravascular ultrasound of coronary arteries in children: assessment of the wall morphology and the lumen after Kawasaki disease. Circulation 1994;89:258–265.
22. Bisset III GS, Strife JL, KcCloskey J. MR imaging of coronary artery aneurysms in a child with Kawasaki disease. AJR 1989;152: 805–807.
23. Kim WY, Danias PG, Stuber M, et al. Coronary magnetic resonance angiography for the detection of coronary stenosis. N Engl J Med 2001;345:1863–1869.
24. Greil GF, Stuber M, Botnar RM, et al. Coronary magnetic resonance angiography in adolescents and young adults with Kawasaki disease. Circulation 2002;105:908–911.
25. Hamada R, Yano I, Fujiwara M, et al. CT screening for unrecognized coronary sequel of Kawasaki disease. Acta Paediatr Jpn 1995; 37:416–418.
26. Frey EE, Matherne GP, Mahoney LT, Sato Y, Stanford W, Smith WL. Coronary artery aneurysms due to Kawasaki disease: diagnosis with ultrafast CT. Radiology 1998;167:725–726.
27. Kitamura S, Kameda Y, Seki T, et al. Long-term outcome of myocardial revascularization in patients with Kawasaki coronary artery disease. A multicenter cooperative study. J Thorac Cardiovasc Surg 1994;107:663–673.
28. Akagi T, Ogawa S, Ino T, et al. Catheter interventional treatment in Kawasaki disease: a report from the Japanese Pediatric Interventional Cardiology Investigation Group. J Pediatr 2000;137: 181–186.
29. Ishii M, Ueno T, Ikeda H, et al. Sequential follow-up results of catheter intervention for coronary artery lesions after Kawasaki disease: quantitative coronary artery angiography and intravas-cular ultrasound imaging study. Circulation 2002;105:3004–3010.

27 Multidetector-Row CT of the Coronary Arteries for Planning of Minimally Invasive Bypass Surgery

Christopher Herzog, MD, Selami Dogan, MD, and Thomas J. Vogl, MD

INTRODUCTION

Minimally invasive coronary artery bypass surgery is gaining increasing clinical importance as an alternative procedure to conventional open-chest techniques *(1,2)*. Recent technical developments in the field of computer-enhanced technology have markedly reduced surgical access, now enabling the clinical use of entirely closed-chest procedures such as totally endoscopic coronary artery bypass grafting (TECABG) *(3)*.

However, one of the technical drawbacks in TECABG procedures is the lack of tactile feedback. The dissection and exposition of intramural coronary arteries or vessels hidden deep inside the epicardiac fatty tissue relies mainly on visual information and thus is technically much more challenging than conventional surgery *(3,4)*. Unfortunately, preoperative coronary angiography (CAG) often does not provide all relevant visual information for these minimally invasive surgical procedures. Thus, if collateral circulation is absent, the coronary territory distal to a total vascular occlusion often cannot be displayed properly, consequently rendering impossible a sufficient evaluation of wall quality, plaque composition, and vascular diameter of the target anastomotic site. In addition, even if visualization of the diseased vessel and its distal segments is possible, angiograms often lack other important morphological information, such as the vessel's position relative to the surrounding cardiac fatty tissue or its exact cardiac course *(5)*. The latest developments in TECABG procedures, such as interventions on the beating heart *(6)* or the introduction of a fourth swivel arm, even more necessarily require exact preoperative analysis of the target site. Thus, in beating-heart procedures, the distal anastomosis can only be performed on coronary arteries that are temporarily pinched off. Suture and exploration times therefore have to be as short as possible in order to avoid any ischemic damage to the mycardiac tissue distal to this ligature. A fourth swivel arm distinctly aggravates correct placement, since any intraoperative collision of the arms must strictly be avoided. The main task of preoperative multidetector-row CT (MDCT) examinations, therefore, is to provide additional morphologic information of the surgical target site and to portray the exact topographic relationship between the heart and the surrounding tissue.

From: *Contemporary Cardiology: CT of the Heart: Principles and Applications*
Edited by: U. Joseph Schoepf © Humana Press, Inc., Totowa, NJ

MINIMALLY INVASIVE BYPASS SURGERY

OVERVIEW OF MINIMALLY INVASIVE SURGICAL TECHNIQUES

The philosophy behind all types of "keyhole" procedures is to perform cardiac surgery without cardio-pulmonary bypass (CPB) in order to avoid inflammatory whole-body responses or intra-/postoperative embolic infarction *(7)*. In addition, the surgical trauma is reduced, thus distinctly improving the cosmetic and functional postoperative outcome. Until recently, this was mainly achieved through an antero-lateral minithoracotomy, a surgical approach that combined the advantages of reduced surgical trauma with the benefits of off-pump surgery *(8–10)*. However, minimally invasive direct coronary artery bypass grafting (MIDCABG), as this technique is called, in general is limited to the revascularization of a maximum of two target vessels owing to restricted access to the surgical target site.

For a multivessel revascularization, CPB still is mandatory, nowadays performed by using new but less biocompatible technologies such as the Port Access System® (Heartport Inc.) *(11–13)*. This CPB system consists of a femoro-femoral cardiopulmonary bypass and an endoaortic balloon clamp.

With the recent advent of robotically enhanced telemanipulation, a new, powerful tool has been created to further minimize surgical access, for the first time allowing true closed chest totally endoscopic procedures (Figs. 1, 2) *(2,14–16)*. TECABG surgery initially also was restricted to the use of Port Access systems for CPB. However, the latest developments in surgical techniques render possible TECABG procedures on the beating heart and therefore help to avoid undesirable side effects of extracorporeal circulation *(7)*, refine procedural flow, and shorten the operative time.

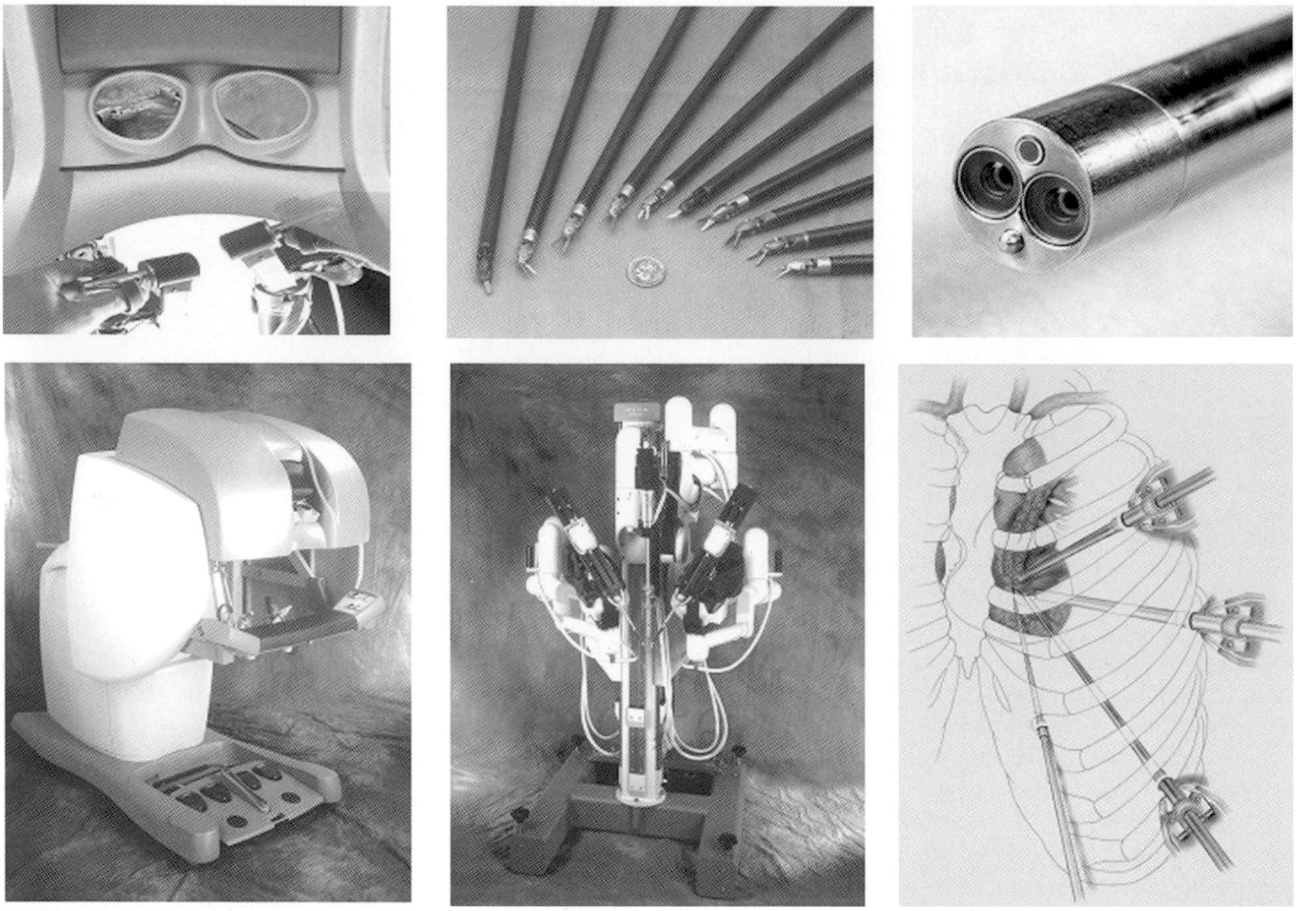

Fig. 1. Equipment for totally endoscopic coronary artery bypass grafting procedures. On the left, the main console (lower row), consisting of binoculars that allow three-dimensional endoscopic visualization of the surgical field and scissors-like handles that allow telemanipulation of the robot's swivel arms (upper row). In the middle, the "slave unit," with its swivel arms, fixing the endoscopic camera and all surgical instruments (upper row) within the patient's body and directly transferring even the slightest movements of the scissor-like handles. On the right is a schematic drawing of the endoscopic instruments, ports position respectively, within the patient's thorax (lower row) and a picture of the endoscopic camera for 3D visualization of the surgical field (upper row).

OPERATIVE TECHNIQUE FOR TECABG PROCEDURES

For a typical left-sided approach for left internal mammary artery (LIMA) to LCA bypass grafting, the patient is placed on the operating table in a supine position with the left chest elevated by about 30–40°. Usually the fifth intercostal space (ICS) close to the anterior axillary line is identified, and after deflation of the left lung a camera port is placed bluntly to

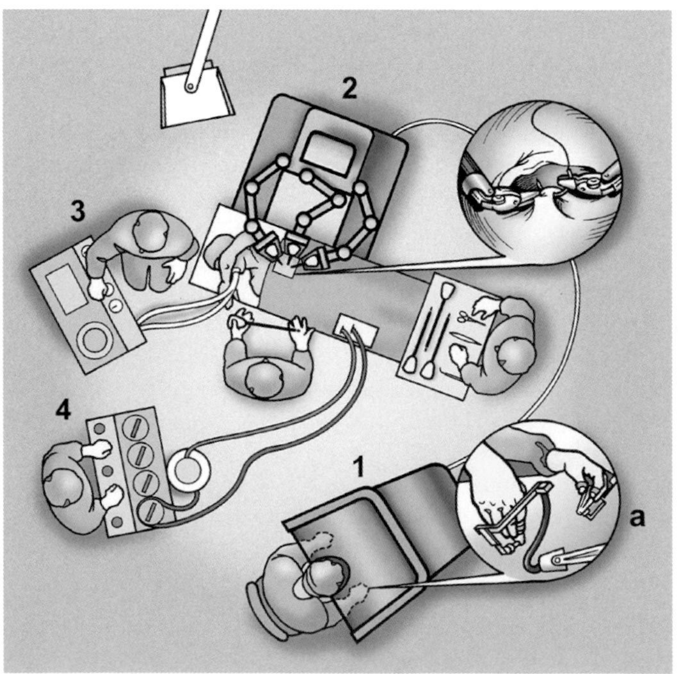

Fig. 2. Schematic drawing, view from above, showing the intraoperative setting of a totally endoscopic coronary artery bypass grafting (TECABG) procedure. The surgeon is sitting in front of the console (**1**) allowing 3D endoscopic visualization of the intraoperative field, and telemanipulates the robot (**2**) with scissors-like handles (a). The robot itself consists of three swivel arms, one carrying the camera, two holding the surgical instruments (newest prototypes now consist of four swivel arms). Perioperative monitoring is provided through the anesthesiologist (**3**). Though many TECABG procedures still are performed with assistance of a heart-lung machine (**4**), latest technical developments such as the Port Access System® also render possible procedures on the beating heart. Reprinted from ref. *35*, with permission from the Radiological Society of North America.

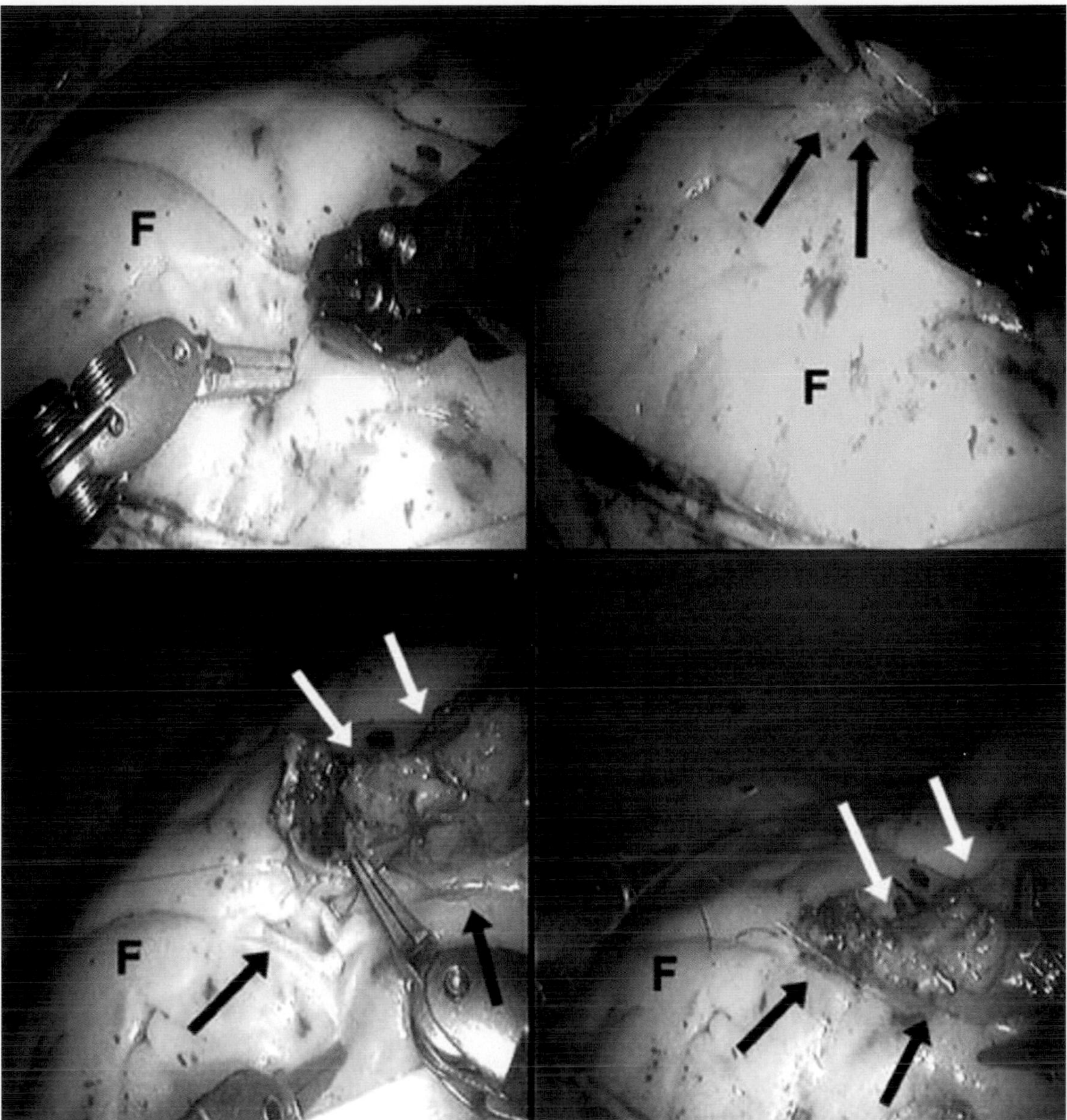

Fig. 3. Four steps of a totally endoscopic coronary artery bypass grafting procedure, left anterior oblique projection. The black arrows point to the coronary artery, the white arrows mark the bypass. After dissection of the epicardium, the surgeon first has to identify the relevant cardiac structures. As shown in this case, epicardiac fatty tissue (F) very often prevents a direct visualization of the target vessel (upper row left). Without further morphological information, only careful dissection of the fatty tissue allows exact localization of the vessel's position (upper row right). The target vessel then is incised over a distance of 6 to 7 mm (lower row left) and subsequently grafted in an end-to-side technique with the left internal mammary artery, which previously has been mobilized from the chest wall (lower row right). Reprinted from ref. *35*, with permission from the Radiological Society of North America.

avoid left-ventricular injury. The chest is insufflated with warm CO_2 (37°C). After insertion of the endoscope, two ports are placed under visual control to accommodate the two robot arms usually in the third and seventh ICS (Fig. 1). The LIMA is mobilized from the subclavian artery down to the distal bifurcation using a 30-degree endoscope angled upwards. The distal end of the LIMA is skeletonized for grafting, and a soft bulldog clamp (Scanlan Int.) is placed *(2,3)*.

The left femoral artery and vein are dissected with a 3-cm oblique incision in the groin. After heparinization, CPB is instituted by femoro-femoral perfusion using the Port Access System. After initiation of CPB and venting the right ventricle via the pulmonary artery, the heart is decompressed and endoscopic pericardiotomy is performed safely. Identification of the target vessel is performed prior to cardiac arrest using direct endoscopic visualization. Infusion of antegrade cristalloid St. Thomas cardioplegia delivered to the aortic root via the Port Access endoclamp provides reliable cardiac arrest. A 6–7-mm arteriotomy is carried out, and the left anterior descending artery (LAD) is grafted with the LIMA in an end-to-side technique (Fig. 3) with a running 7.0 prolene suture (7.5 cm length, Fumalene, Fumedica Medizintechnik).

Table 1
Scanning and Image Reconstruction Parameters.
Comparison Between 4- and 16-Row Multidetector-Row CT (MDCT)

		4-Row MDCT	*16-Row MDCT*
Plain Series			
Scanning Parameters			
	Rotation time (ms)	420	500
	Temp. Resolution min	105	125
	Temp. Resolution max	210	250
	kV	120	120
	mAs	300	300
	Collimation	4 × 2.5	16 × 1.5
	Table feed/rotation	3.8	5.7
	Image Reconstruction		
	FOV (mm)	220	220
	Kernel	B 35	B 35
	Slice Tickness (mm)	3	2
	Increment (mm)	1.5	1
Contrast enhanced series			
Scanning Parameters			
	Rotation time (ms)	420	500
	Temp. Resolution min	105	125
	Temp. Resolution max	210	250
	kV	120	120
	mAs	300	300
	Collimation	4 × 1	16 × 0.75
	Table feed /rotation	1.5	2.8
	Contrast medium (mL)	150 (+ 30 /Test Bolus)	120
	Flow Rate (mL/s)	3.5	4
Image Reconstruction			
	FOV (mm)	220	220
	Kernel	B 35	B 35
	Slice Tickness (mm)	1.25	0.75
	Increment (mm)	0.6	0.3

FOV, field of view.

After completion of the anastomosis, the aortic endoclamp is deflated and the patient is weaned from CPB. Venous and arterial cannulae are removed and two chest tubes are placed through the camera port and an instrument port incision *(2,3)*.

MDCT EVALUATION

SCANNING PARAMETERS

All MDCT examinations should be performed using ECG-gating. In our studies we used both 4-row (SOMATOM Plus 4 VolumeZoom, Siemens) and 16-row (SOMATOM Sensation 16, Siemens) CT scanners. Sixteen-row technology allowed sufficient evaluation even of small vessels (>1 mm) and resulted in less motion artifacts at elevated heart rates (>75 beats per minute [bpm]) as compared to four-row scanners, thus in general leading to better image quality. In addition, as a result of the favorable combination of high contrast media flow rates and fast scan times, streak artifacts caused through undiluted contrast medium flowing into the right atrium are distinctly reduced.

Patients with heart rates higher than 65 bpm should previously receive a short-lasting β-blocker (Brevibloc®, 100 mg, 1 mL/10 kg BW) in order to obtain rates of 60 bpm or less. For proper assessment of calcified plaques, both contrast-enhanced and plain examinations are mandatory. Scanning is done on both scanners with 120 kV and 300 mAs. For the 4-row scanners, scanning parameters were 500 ms rotation time, 4 × 2.5 collimation and 3.8-mm table feed per rotation for the plain series, 4 × 1 mm slice collimation and 1.5-mm table feed per rotation for the contrast-enhanced series respectively (Table 1). All patients receive 150 mL of a nonionic contrast medium (Ultravist®, Schering Inc.) through an 18G intravenous antecubital catheter infused with a flow rate of 3.5 mL/s. Start delay is calculated using Test Bolus Technique® with a region of interest (ROI) placed in the ascending aorta (30 mL contrast medium at a flow rate of 3.5 mL/s) (Table 1).

For the 16-row scanner, scanning parameters are 420 ms rotation time, 16 × 1.5-mm collimation and 5.7-mm table feed per rotation for the plain series, 16 × 0.75 mm slice collimation and 2.8-mm table feed per rotation for the contrast-enhanced series, respectively (Table 1). In these patients, only 120 mL of a nonionic contrast medium is infused with a flow rate of 4.0 mL/s. Using Care Bolus Technique®, no additional contrast medium is necessary to determine the start delay. After contrast medium injection scanning starts automatically as soon as a certain trigger point is reached (usually 160 Hounsfield units [HU]) in a ROI that is placed in the ascending aorta (Table 1).

IMAGE RECONSTRUCTION

Image reconstruction is performed using retrospective ECG gating, a technique that allows continuous image reconstruction from volume data sets during any phase of the cardiac cycle *(17,18)*. Reconstruction parameters for 4-row and 16-row examinations are 220-mm FOV, kernel B35, a medium soft-tissue kernel, 3-mm effective slice thickness, and 1.5-mm increment for the plain series (Table 1). For the contrast-enhanced series, image reconstruction is done on the 4-row scanner with 1.25-mm effective slice thickness and 0.6-mm increment, with 1.0-mm effective slice thickness and 0.5-mm increment on the 16-row scanner respectively (Table 1).

For image reconstruction on both scanners, the adaptive cardiac volume reconstruction algorithm (ACV) is used, which is provided with the software *(19)*. Taking into account basic cardiac physiology, sufficient image reconstruction seems to be feasible solely if performed between the late systole (i.e., ascending t wave) and the late diastole (i.e., beginning of p wave) *(20,21)*. Each data set is consequently reconstructed at multiple time points within this interval, differing from each other by 50 ms. Owing to a decrease in the length of the t wave–p wave interval at increasing heart rates (HRs), the number of possible reconstruction time points per patient ranges between 10 (low HR) and 6 (elevated HR). It is favorable at each time point to perform an antegrade and absolute (i.e., in milliseconds) image reconstruction in relation to the R peak *(21)*. Subsequently for each patient and each main coronary artery (RCA, LCA, LCx) separately, one specific reconstruction should be determined showing the least motion artifacts, therefore allowing proper image interpretation *(22–25)*.

IMAGE REFORMATION AND EVALUATION

MDCT image evaluation usually is done on both transverse scans and secondary reformations, i.e., MPR and 3D reformations. We analyze transverse scans, MPR, and 3D reformations on a separate workstation (VZ Leonardo, Siemens). Three-dimensional reformations are produced using volume-rendering technique. Transverse scans and MPR are displayed on a 512 × 512 matrix, three-dimensional reformations on a 256 × 256 matrix.

Criteria that need to be analyzed are: (a) the atherosclerotic plaque load of each single coronary artery segment; (b) the composition of the individual plaques; and (c) the epicardial/intramural course of the vessel.

Plaque load and plaque composition are best determined on transverse scans and MPR. The cardiac course of the coronary vessels can be additionally assessed on 3D reformations, which also serve for surgical morning-round demonstrations and intra-operative orientation for the surgeon.

To grade the segmental plaque load, we use the classifications of the American Heart Association (AHA), which subdivide the coronary artery territory into 15 segments and distinguish between six different degrees of atherosclerosis *(26)*: (I) irregular wall outline with <25% stenosis; (II) slight stenosis (25–50%); (III) moderate stenosis (51–74%); (IV) hemodynamically relevant stenosis (75–89%); subtotal stenosis (90–99%) and (V) vascular occlusion (100%). The prevailing degree of occlusion is ascertained by using an automated distance-measuring tool (Plus4VZ Wizzard, Siemens).

Regarding the composition of the plaque, it is classified as calcified and non-calcified plaques. Plaques with a mean attenuation >130 HU are graded as calcified, while plaques with a mean attenuation <130 HU are graded as noncalcified *(27)*. Calcified plaques were identified on plain scans, noncalcified plaques on contrast-enhanced scans.

The cardiac course of each coronary artery is assessed by distinguishing a possible epicardiac or intramural course of the prevailing arterial segment (AHA 1–15).

Finally, taking into consideration the results of all three reformation techniques, a conclusive recommendation is given regarding which coronary segment is best suited for allocation of the distal bypass-anastomosis, and the coronary diameter in this region is calculated. In general only segments showing no calcified plaques and a rather near-surface course are regarded as suited for distal bypass touchdown.

RESULTS OF ACTUAL STUDIES

Regarding the value of 4- and 16-row MDCT before TECABG, until now only two studies have been performed. Both are briefly described in the following.

4-ROW MDCT

Methods

In a comparative study performed between July 2000 and January 2002, 36 consecutive patients (22 males and 14 females) scheduled for TECABG underwent both invasive CAG and four-row MDCT before surgery. CAG was performed in a routine manner to identify potential candidates for surgery, followed by an additional MDCT examination less than 48 h before the operation. The mean time between CAG and MDCT amounted to 17 d (range 7 to 23 d). The patients' average age was 60.1 yr (range 41 to 78 yr), their mean heart rate amounted to 62.9 bpm (range 47 to 86 bpm). All patients presented with single-vessel coronary heart disease. Thirty-two patients had a hemodynamically relevant (>75%) stenosis of the proximal LCA, one patient presented with a >75% stenosis of both the proximal LCA and the first diagonal branch, and four with a total occlusion of the proximal RCA. Thirty-four operations were performed on the arrested heart using a heart-lung machine *(1)*; in two patients, surgery was performed on the beating heart in total off-pump coronary artery bypass (TOPCAB) technique *(2)*. Assessment criteria for CAG and 4-row MDCT were: visibility and cardiac course of coronary arteries, localization and degree of stenoses, composition of atherosclerotic plaques, and vascular diameter at the site of anastomosis. Finally, both techniques were used separately to recommend an appropriate site for distal bypass anastomosis. All MDCT evaluations were performed according to the criteria described in detail (*see* "Preoperative MDCT Evaluation") and were analyzed by two independent observers. All results were calculated relative to the prevailing results from CAG and surgery.

Coronary angiograms had been performed in different technical systems using the Judkins technique. At least four views of the left and two views of the right coronary artery system were analyzed by two observers in consensus, who were both trained in this technique. In order to avoid recall bias, neither of them had any knowledge of the CT results, and evaluation was undertaken only on data sets that had previously been blinded.

On angiograms, plaque composition and visibility of coronary artery segments on CAG was described as either calcified or noncalcified, visible or nonvisible, respectively. Calcified plaques were searched for on both plain and contrast-enhanced series.

The prevailing degree of stenosis and the segmental diameter at the planned site of distal anastomosis was determined using a stenosis grading tool with automatic distance and scale calibration (Osiris, Digital Imaging Unit—UHGE).

As with MDCT, finally a conclusive recommendation was given regarding the optimal place for distal bypass-anastomosis, and the segmental diameter in this region was calculated.

All results were intraoperatively evaluated by one of the surgeons, using 3D reformations and angiograms for comparison. As a result of a restricted field of vision, only those segments were compared that could be visualized through the operation microscope, i.e., the stenotic/occluded segment itself, the segments before and behind this occlusion/stenosis, any surrounding side branches, and possible crossing veins. All differences as well as conformities were noted and additionally documented on videotape, thus allowing a second inspection after the operation.

The number of coronary segments that could be evaluated on MDCT scans and coronary angiograms was determined in proportion to both the total number of segments and the segments that could be visualized during surgery. Agreement between investigators for this evaluation was calculated by means of the κ statistic, interpreting the results according to the κ value as poor (<0.20), fair (0.21–0.40), moderate (0.41–0.60), good (0.61–0.80), very good (0.81–0.90), or excellent (0.91–1.00). A 95% confidence interval (CI), calculated by a standard method, was assigned to the calculated κ value. Possible differences between both methods were tested for significance using a comparison of Poisson frequencies.

Regarding the detection and grading of atherosclerosis and with reference to all 15 AHA segments, a coefficient of agreement for both techniques was calculated by means of a binominal confidence interval for ϑ. The agreement between the methods and investigators was interpreted according to the ϑ value or κ value respectively, as poor (<0.20), fair (0.21–0.40), moderate (0.41–0.60), good (0.61–0.80), very good (0.81–0.90), or excellent (0.91–1.00). A 95% CI, calculated by a standard method, was assigned to each calculated ϑ and κ value.

Sensitivity, specificity, positive and negative predictive value of MDCT and coronary angiography in the detection of hemodynamically relevant stenoses was determined by subdivision of AHA groups I–VI into two different groups: (1) patients without hemodynamically relevant stenoses (< 75%), i.e. AHA groups I, II, and III; and (2) patients with hemodynamically relevant stenoses (>75%), i.e., AHA groups IV, V, and VI. Values for MDCT were calculated relative to all 15 AHA segments (reference standard: coronary angiograms) as well as relative to those segments that were intraoperatively explored (reference standard: surgery). Values for invasive angiograms were calculated only with surgery serving as the reference standard.

Sensitivity and specificity as well as positive and negative predictive values in the detection of calcified plaques were calculated for MDCT and CAG relative to the surgical findings. The agreement between investigators for this evaluation was assessed by means of the κ statistic as described above. A 95% CI, calculated by a standard method, was assigned to the calculated κ value.

The validity of both imaging methods in the correct identification of a segment's cardiac course—on the epicardiac surface, deep within the fatty tissue, or within the myocardium—was calculated as proportional to the actual surgical findings.

The correspondence rate of MDCT and coronary angiography regarding the allocation of distal bypass-anastomosis and the segmental diameter at the site of anastomosis was also calculated proportional to the surgical results. A segmental diameter was regarded to be of equal size if the measured difference amounted to less than 1 mm. Bypass allocation was rated as correct if segmental allocation corresponded to surgery. Results concerning the segment's cardiac course, the allocation of bypass-anastomosis, and the segmental diameter at the site of anastomosis were obtained by both observers in consensus.

Results

On 4-row MDCT scans, 80.4% (434/540) of all coronary segments could be evaluated by observer 1 and 78.3% (423/540) by observer 2. The κ value between investigators amounted to 0.870 (CI: 0.786, 0.954), thus showing a very good agreement.

On the average, 100% (108/108) of all proximal segments (1, 5, and 11), 94.5% (68/72) of the medial RCA (segments 2, 3), 90.3% (65/72) of the medial LCA (segments 6, 7), 83.3% (30/36) of the medial LCx (13), 91.7% (33/36) of the distal RCA (segment 4), 80.6% (29/36) of the distal LCA (segment 8), and 55.6% (20/36) of the distal LCx (segment 15) were classified as visible. Side branches of the LCA (segments 9, 10) were regarded as visible in 70.8 (51/72), those of the LCx (segments 12, 14) in 41.7% (30/72) (Table 2).

Table 2
Average Visibility of Coronary Arteries (%):
Correlation Among 4-Row Multidetector-Row CT (MDCT), 16-Row MDCT Coronary Angiography, and Surgical Findings

			4-row MDCT		*16-row MDCT*		*Angiography*		*4-row MDCT/Surgery*		*16-row MDCT/surgery*		*Angiography/surgery*	
			%	*absolute*	*%*	*absolute*	*%*	*absolute*	*%*	*absolute*	*%*	*absolute*	*%*	*absolute*
RCA	proximal	(S 1)1	100	(36/36)	100	(12/12)	100	(36/36)	100	(5/5)			100	(5/5)
	medial	(S 2–3)	94.5	(68/72)	83.3	(10/12)	97.2	(70/72)		50	(5/10)		60	(6/10)
	distal	(S 4)	91.7	(33/36)	83.3	(10/12)	94.4	(34/36)						
LCA	proximal	(S 5)	100	(36/36)	100	(12/12)	100	(36/36)	100	(22/22)	100	(10/10)	100	(22/22)
	medial	(S 6–7)	90.3	(65/72)	100	(24/24)	90.3	(65/72)	88.5	(54/61)	100	(24/24)	90.2	(55/61)
	distal	(S 8)	80.6	(29/36)	87.5	(21/24)	91.7	(33/36)	78.1	(25/32)	91.7	(11/12)	90.6	(29/32)
	diagonal2	(S 9–10)	70.8	(51/72)	83.3	(20/24)	80.6	(58/72)	67.2	(43/64)	91.4	(10/14)	85.9	(55/64)
LCx	proximal	(S 11)	100	(36/36)	100	(12/12)	100	(36/36)						
	medial	(S 13)	83.3	(30/36)	83.3	(10/12)	100	(36/36)						
	distal	(S 15)	55.6	(20/36)	58.3	(7/12)	100	(36/36)						
	marginal[c]	(S 12/14)	41.7	(30/72)	66.7	(8/12)	98.6	(71/72)						
	total		80.4	(434/540)	87.7	(158/180)	94.6	(511/540)	79.4	(154/194)	91.7	(55/60)	88.7	(172/194)

RCA, right coronary artery; LCA, left coronary artery; LCx, left circumflex artery.
[a]Brackets indicate AHA segments (S 1–15).
[b]Diagonal branches.
[c]Marginal branches.

On coronary angiograms, 94.6% (511/540) of all segments could be evaluated (Table 2). Segments which were not displayed properly were all located behind total vascular occlusions.

Considering only segments that were intraoperatively explored (194/540), on 4-row MDCT scans, 79.4% (154/194) could be evaluated by observer 1 and 76.8% (149/194) by observer 2. The κ value between investigators amounted to 0.925 (CI: 0.784, 1.000), thus representing an excellent agreement. On angiograms, 88.7% (172/194) were visible to the observer (Table 2). Both methods showed no significant differences in overall visualization, either for observer 1 ($p = 0.346$) or for observer 2 ($p = 0.219$).

The coefficient of agreement (ϑ) for both techniques regarding detection and grading of atherosclerosis (AHA I–VI) amounted to 0.759 (CI: 0.721, 0.795) for observer 1 and 0.731 (CI: 0.691, 0.768) for observer 2, thus showing a good agreement for both. On the average, 4-row MDCT overestimated 17.6% (29/165) and underestimated 6.5% (11/165) of all stenoses.

Considering all 15 AHA segments, sensitivity and specificity for MDCT and observer 1 in the identification of hemodynamically relevant stenoses (>75%) amounted to 76.4% (CI: 62.9%, 86.7%) (42/55) and 99.6% (CI: 98.5%, 99.9%) (483/485). For observer 2 a sensitivity of 70.9% (CI: 57.1%, 82.4%) (39/55) and a specificity of 98.4% (CI: 96.8%, 99.3%) (477/485) was obtained. Positive predictive value (PPV) was 95.5% (CI: 84.5, 99.4) (42/44) for observer 1 and 82.9% (CI: 69.2%, 92.4%) (39/47) for observer 2. Negative predictive value (NPV) amounted to 97.4% (CI: 95.6%, 98.6%) (483/496) for observer 1 and to 96.8% (CI: 94.8%, 98.1%) (477/493) for observer 2 (Table 3). The κ value between investigators was 0.9518 (CI: 1.000, 0.867), thus equivalent to an excellent agreement.

Considering only those segments that were intraoperatively explored from the endoluminal side ($n = 37$), hemodynamically relevant stenoses (>75%) were identified on 4-row MDCT scans with 91.9% sensitivity (34/37) (CI: 78.1, 98.0) by observer 1 and with 89.2% sensitivity (33/37) (CI: 74.6, 97.0) by observer 2. Sensitivity for coronary angiograms amounted to 100% (37/37) (Table 3). Specificity, PPV, NPV, and κ were not calculated because of a lack of negative controls.

Both observers detected calcified plaques on 4-row MDCT scans with 100% sensitivity (CI: 84.7%, 100%) (18/18). For CAGs, sensitivity was 83.3% (CI: 58.6%, 96.4%) (15/18) (Fig. 4, Table 3). Specificity was 100% (CI: 85.4, 100%) (19/19) for both techniques and both MDCT observers respectively. For 4-row MDCT, PPV (18/18) (CI: 84.7%, 100%) and NPV (19/19) (CI: 85.4%, 100%) amounted to 100% for each. For coronary angiography, PPV was 100% (CI: 81.9%, 100%) (15/15) and NPV 86.4% (CI: 65.1%, 97.1%) (19/22) (Table 3). The κ value between MDCT investigators was 1.00, thus showing an excellent agreement.

The appropriate allocation for distal bypass anastomosis was correctly identified on 4-row MDCT scans in 75.1% (28/37), on coronary angiograms in 70.3% (26/37) (Table 4, Fig. 5). 4-row MDCT led to nine wrong preoperative bypass allocations: two due to a low experience curve at the beginning of the investigation, three because the intraoperative situation required a different bypass technique (switch to jump-graft technique in one case, venous bypass instead of IMA-bypass grafting in two cases), and four because of incorrect identification of either fatty tissue (1×), an intramural course (e.g., myocardial bridging) (1×) or the vascular segments themselves (2×) (Table 4).

CAG resulted in 11 wrong allocations: two owing to a low experience curve at the beginning, three because intraoperative findings required a different surgical approach, and six because the target vessel intraoperatively either was hidden deep inside the epicardial fatty tissue (3×) or showed an intramural course (3×) (Fig. 5).

Bridging of coronary artery segments through either myocardium or epicardial fatty tissue thus was identified more reliably on MDCT scans than on angiograms (Fig. 5): 80% (4/5) as compared to 20% (1/5) for myocardial bridging, 66.7% (2/3) as compared to 0% (0/3), respectively, for bridging through epicardial fatty tissue (Table 4).

The segmental diameter at the site of distal anastomosis was measured correctly on MDCT scans in 72.0% (18/25), on angiograms in 80.0% (20/25) (Table 4). Measurements were undertaken only in the last 25 patients.

On MDCT scans, seven segments were not assessed properly: three due to moving artifacts, three because of missing contrast media enhancement due to a proximal total vascular occlusion, and one because of underestimation of the actual diameter.

On angiograms, all five segments that were not visualized adequately were located behind a total vascular occlusion.

16-ROW MDCT

This study is still in progress, and concentrates on the potential benefit of 16-row MDCT in patients scheduled for TECABG procedures on the beating heart *(2)* and being operated on with assistance of a newly introduced, fourth swivel arm. In these procedures, bypass anastomosis can be achieved only through short-time ligature of the prevailing coronary artery. Since exploration and suture time must not exceed 20 min in order to prevent any ischemic damage to the myocardium, fast and correct identification of both the prevailing vessel and the suited region for anastomosis—i.e., a rather superficially located segment which is definitively free of calcified plaques—is highly important for the postoperative outcome. In addition, a fourth swivel arm distinctly aggravates correct planning of the port placement for the endoscopic instruments: not only must each patient's anatomy be considered individually, but also any intraoperative collision of the arms must be avoided.

Methods

The study was initiated in September 2002. Until now, 12 consecutive patients (9 males and 3 females) were included, undergoing both invasive coronary angiography (CA) and 16-row MDCT. The mean time between CA and MDCT amounted to 21 d (range 9 to 30 d). The patients' average age was 58.1 yr (range 52 to 69 yr), their mean heart rate amounted to 68.3 bpm (range 56 to 112 bpm). Eight patients presented

Table 3
4-row Multidetector-Row CT (MDCT) Correlated to Coronary Angiography and Surgery
(sensitivities, specificities, positive [PPV], and negative [NPV] predictive values for both MDCT observers listed separately)

			Sensitivity		*Specificity*		*PPV*		*NPV*	
			%	*absolute*	%	*absolute*	%	*absolute*	%	*absolute*
4-row MDCT	high grade stenoses (>75%) (considering AHA segments 1–15 / reference standard: angiography)	Observer 1	76.4	(42/55)	99.6	(483/485)	95.5	(42/44)	97.4	(467/496)
		Observer 2	70.9	(39/55)	98.4	(477/485)	82.9	(39/47)	96.8	(477/493)
	high grade stenoses (>75%) (considering only segments explored intraop. / reference standard:surgery)	Observer 1	91.9	(34/37)	n.c.	n.c.	n.c.	n.c.	n.c.	n.c.
		Observer 2	89.2	(33/37)	n.c.	n.c.	n.c.	n.c.	n.c.	n.c.
	calcified plaques (>130 HU) (considering only segments explored intraop. / reference standard: surgery)	Observer 1	100	(18/18)	100	(19/19)	100	(18/18)	100	(19/19)
		Observer 2	100	(18/18)	100	(19/19)	100	(18/18)	100	(19/19)
16-row MDCT	high grade stenoses (>75%) (considering AHA segments 1–15 / reference standard: angiography)	Observer 1	80.0	(12/15)	96.8	(153/158)	70.6	(12/17)	98.1	(153/156)
		Observer 2	73.3	(11/15)	94.9	(150/158)	61.9	(11/19)	98.7	(150/154)
	high grade stenoses (>75%) (considering only segments explored intraop. / reference standard:surgery)	Observer 1	91.7	(11/12)	n.c.	n.c.	n.c.	n.c.	n.c.	n.c.
		Observer 2	91.7	(11/12)	n.c.	n.c.	n.c.	n.c.	n.c.	n.c.
	calcified plaques (>130 HU) (considering only segments explored intraop. / reference standard: surgery)	Observer 1	100	(13/13)	100	(5/5)	100	(13/13)	100	(5/5)
		Observer 2	100	(13/13)	100	(5/5)	100	(13/13)	100	(5/5)
Angiography										
	high grade stenoses (>75%) (considering only segments explored intraop. / reference standard: surgery)		100	(37/37)	n.c.	n.c.	n.c.	n.c.	n.c.	n.c.
	calcified plaques (>130 HU) (considering only segments explored intraop./ reference standard: surgery)		61.5	(8/13)	100	(5/5)	100	(8/8)	50	(5/10)

n.c., Not calculated owing to lack of negative controls.

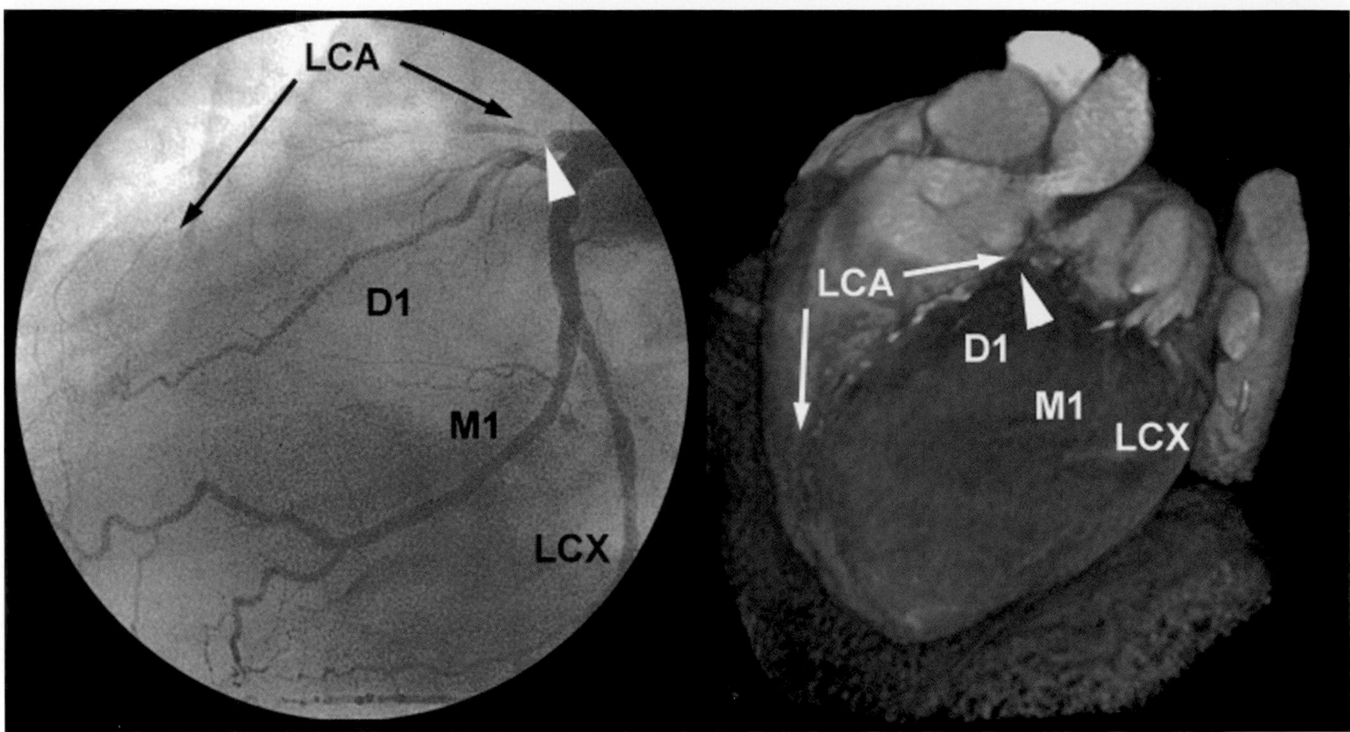

Fig. 4. Comparison between invasive angiography (left), mirror-inverted 15° right anterior oblique projection and multidetector-row CT (MDCT) (right), left anterior oblique. Both techniques correctly identified the 100% stenosis (white arrowhead) within segment 6 of the left coronary artery (LCA), but only MDCT revealed the marked calcifications of segment 7 of the LCA (delineated by white arrows), rendering bypass grafting in this region rather difficult. Based upon this information the surgical access was adapted in order to reach the more distal segment 8 and bypass grafting was performed successfully. D1 designates the first diagonal branch, M1 the first marginal branch, and LCX the left circumflex artery. reprinted from ref. *35*, with permission from the Radiological Society of North America.

Table 4
Preoperative Assessment of Segmental Diameter, Allocation of Distal Bypass, and Detection of Morphological Traps (comparison between 4- and 16-row multidetector-row CT [MDCT] and invasive angiography)

		Correct rating	
		%	*absolute*
4-row MDCT			
	segmental diameter (reference standard: surgery)	72.0	(18/25)
	bypass allocation (reference standard: surgery)	75.1	(28/37)
	myocardial bridging (reference standard: surgery)	80	(4/5)
	epicardiac fatty tissue (reference standard: surgery)	66.7	(2/3)
16-row MDCT			
	bypass allocation (reference standard: surgery)	91.7	(11/12)
	myocardial bridging (reference standard: surgery)	100	(2/2)
	epicardiac fatty tissue (reference standard: surgery)	100	(3/3)
Coronary angiography			
	segmental diameter (reference standard: surgery)	80.0	(20/25)

(*continued*)

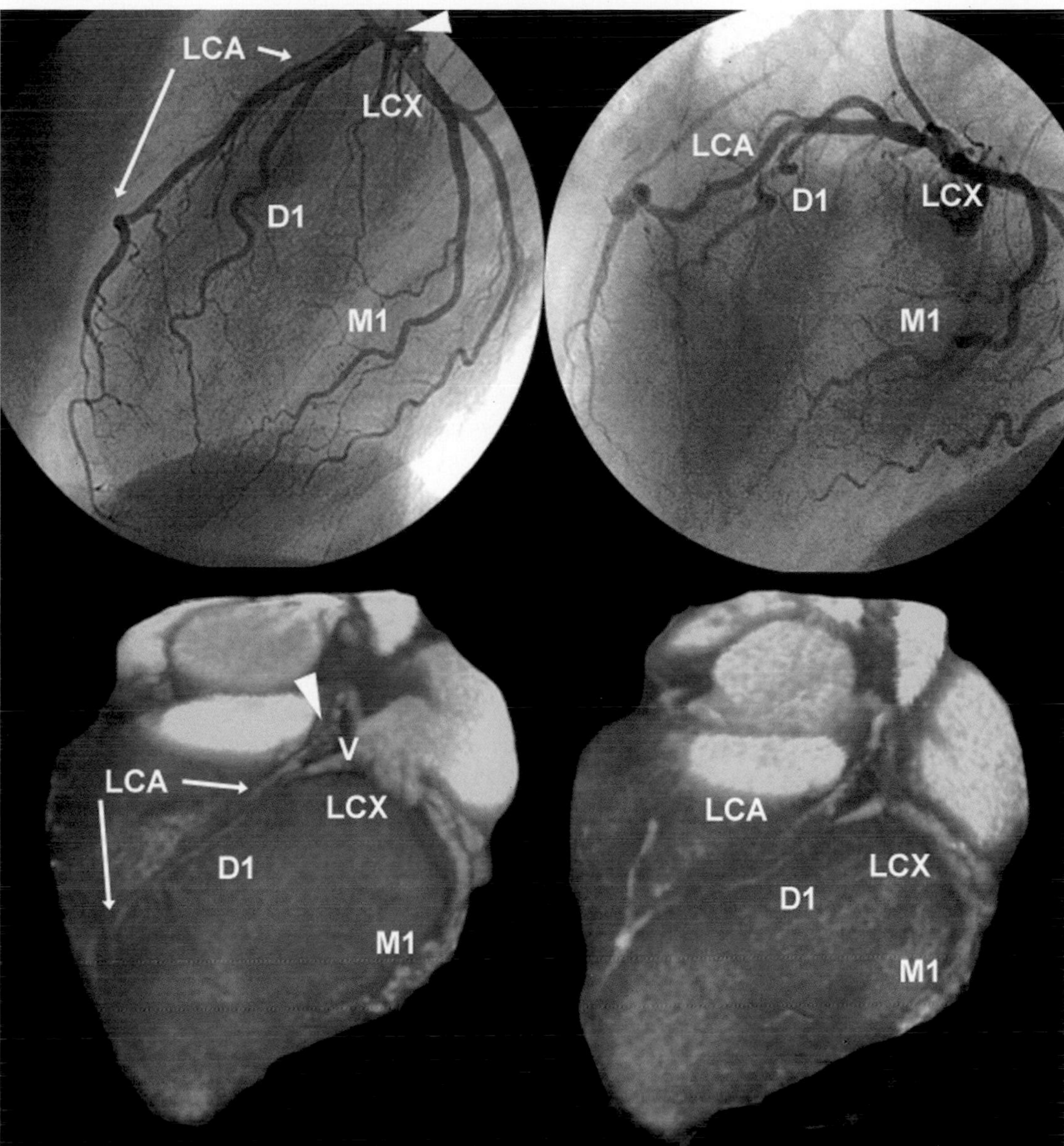

Fig. 5. Comparison between invasive angiography (upper row), mirror-inverted 15° right anterior oblique projection and multidetector-row CT (MDCT) (lower row), left anterior oblique. Both techniques correctly identified the 80% stenosis (white arrowhead) within segment 6 of the left coronary artery (LCA), but only MDCT revealed the intramural course of segment 7 of the LCA (delineated by the white arrows). Based upon this information, the surgical access was altered in order to reach the more distal segment 8 and bypass grafting was performed successfully. Note the vein (V) that accompanies the intramural course of the LCA on the myocardial surface. D1 designates the first diagonal branch, M1 the first marginal branch, and LCX the left circumflex artery. Reprinted from ref. *35*, with permission from the Radiological Society of North America.

Table 4 ***(Continued)***
Preoperative Assessment of Segmental Diameter, Allocation of Distal Bypass, and Detection of Morphological Traps (comparison between 4- and 16-row multidetector-row CT [MDCT] and invasive angiography)

	Correct rating	
	%	*absolute*
bypass allocation (reference standard: surgery)	70.3	(26/37)
myocardial bridging (reference standard: surgery)	20	(2/5)
epicardiac fatty tissue (reference standard: surgery)	0	(0/3)

with a hemodynamically relevant (>75%) stenosis of the proximal LCA, three with an additional stenosis of the first diagonal branch, and one with a stenosis of the LCA, the first diagonal, and the first obtuse marginal branch. Assessment criteria for CAG and 16-row MDCT were visibility and cardiac course of coronary arteries, localization and degree of stenoses, composition of atherosclerotic plaques, and vascular diameter at the site of anastomosis. Finally, both techniques were interpreted separately to recommend an appropriate site for distal bypass anastomosis. All 16-row MDCT examinations and evaluations were performed according to the methods in detail described above under the heading "MDCT Evaluation." All results were calculated relative to the prevailing results from CAG and surgery, which were obtained from the same observers and in the same manner as described under the subheading "Four-Row MDCT: Methods." Statistical calculations were also done following the approach used for 4-row MDCT.

Results

Preliminary results show that 16-row MDCT properly displayed 87.7% (158/150) of all coronary segments. 100% (36/36) of all proximal segments (1, 5, and 11), between 83.3% (segments 2, 3, and 13) and 100 % (segments 6, 7) of all medial segments, between 58.3% (segment 15) and 87.5% (segment 8) of all distal segments, 83.3% of all diagonal (segment 9, 10), and 66.7% of all marginal branches (segment 12, 14) were classified as visible (Table 2).

The κ value between investigators amounted to 0.79 (CI: 0.723, 1.000). The coefficient of agreement (ϑ) for 16-row MDCT and CA regarding detection and grading of atherosclerosis (AHA I–VI) amounted to 0.793 (CI: 0.762, 0.813) for observer 1 and to 0.752 (CI: 0.736, 0.775) for observer 2, thus showing a good agreement for both. On the average, MDCT underestimated 24.1% (7/29) and overestimated 13.8% (4/29) of all stenoses.

Hemodynamically relevant stenoses were identified with 16-row MDCT with 80.0% (CI: 51.9%, 95.7%) (12/15) sensitivity by observer 1, 73.3% (CI: 44.9%, 92.2%) (11/15) sensitivity respectively by observer 2 (Table 3). PPV was 70.6% (CI: 44.0, 89.7) (12/17) for observer 1 and 61.9% (CI: 38.4%, 81.9%) (11/19) for observer 2. NPV amounted to 98.1% (CI: 94.5%, 99.6%) (153/156) for observer 1 and to 98.7% (CI: 95.3%, 99.8%) (150/154) for observer 2 (Table 3). The κ value between investigators was 0.831 (CI: 1.000, 0.782), thus equivalent to a good agreement.

Considering only those segments that were intraoperatively explored from the endoluminal side ($n = 12$), hemodynamically relevant stenoses (>75%) were identified on 16-row MDCT scans with 91.7% sensitivity (11/12) (CI: 61.5, 99.8) by both observers.

Both observers detected calcified plaques on 16-row MDCT scans with 100% sensitivity (CI: 79.4%, 100%) (13/13) (Table 3) and 100% specificity (CI: 54.9, 100%)(5/5). PPV (13/13) (CI: 79.4%, 100%), and NPV (5/5) (CI: 54.9%, 100%) for both observers also amounted to 100% (Table 3). The κ value between MDCT investigators was 1.00, thus showing an excellent agreement.

Sixteen-row MDCT identified bridging of coronary segments through either myocardium (2/2) or epicardial fat (3/3) in all cases and correctly determined the distal site for bypass touchdown in 91.6% (11/12).

CONCLUSION AND FUTURE DIRECTIONS

TECABG is a new method for coronary artery bypass grafting, which can be used in selected patients to achieve single or double arterial bypass grafting with internal thoracic arteries *(1,3,28)*. Intrathoracic orientation and identification of the target vessel is more challenging than in open procedures. Because of the lack of tactile feedback, it is difficult to evaluate the quality of the target vessel just by visual control. The success rate of TECABG on the arrested heart (intention to treat a patient in closed chest technique without conversion to minithoracotomy) varies between 80% and 95 % depending on factors such as patient selection and experience of the team *(4)*. However, mainly as a result of problems with the identification of the target vessel, inadequate exposition, or cases in which successful realization of endoscopic anastomoses does not seem feasible, many TECABG procedures intraoperatively must be converted to a left side minithoracotomy (MIDCABG). In most of these cases, the target vessel is either confused with neighboring vessels, hidden deep inside the epicardial fatty tissue, bridged by myocardial tissue, or heavily calcified. Our results show that MDCT can identify such morphological traps very often and therefore could improve the success rate of TECABG procedures. First, the selection process of patients is facilitated, thus rendering possible preoperative switching towards alternative surgical techniques. Second, virtual evaluation of the operative site using 3D reformations before surgery allows exact identification of the target vessel, its morphological appearance, and relation to surrounding structures. The surgeon may preoperatively even simulate the surgical approach and the exploration of the vessel. Although our results indicate that invasive coronary angiography more sensitively identified and displayed vascular occlusions, MDCT nevertheless often detected morphological traps that were not visualized with CA. In several patients, MDCT demonstrated that the target vessel was hidden deep inside the epicardial fat or showed an intramural course, and therefore clearly outperformed invasive coronary angiography, which identified these characteristics in fewer patients. The distal bypass touchdown segment often could be predicted correctly only by MDCT, whereas CAG failed to do so. In two patients, only 3D MDCT reformations showed the fatal combination of a prominent superficial diagonal branch and an intramural LCA. In such cases, accidental grafting of the wrong vessel (diagonal branch versus LCA) is a common risk of endoscopic surgery, because spatial orientation is difficult, the field of view restricted, and manual palpation of the vessel not possible (Fig. 6). Moreover, the composition of atherosclerotic plaques often cannot be predicted sufficiently on angiograms *(5)*. Thus, calcified plaques were detected with a markedly lower sensitivity with CAG than on MDCT scans, which always identified these plaques in 100%. If collateral circulation is absent, behind a vascular occlusion on angiograms neither the calcified nor the

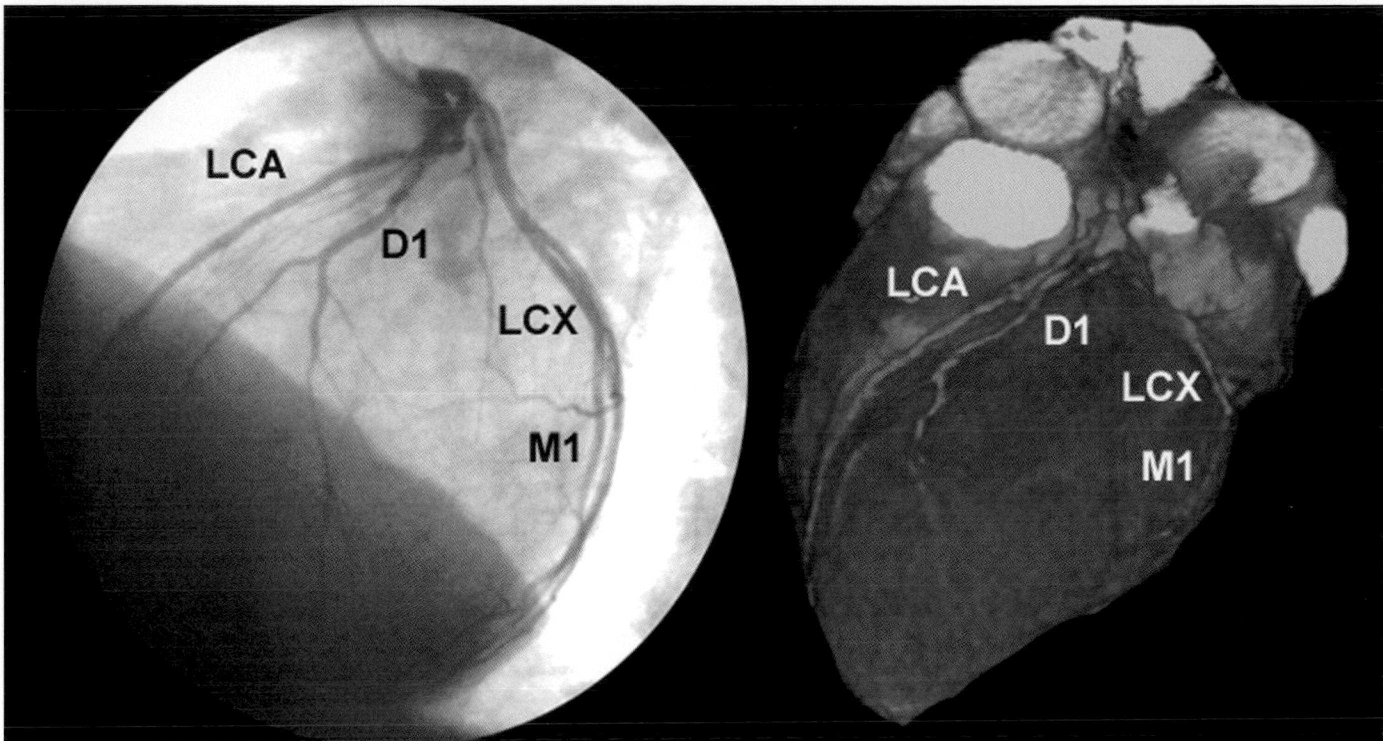

Fig. 6. Comparison between invasive angiography (left), mirror-inverted 15° right anterior oblique projection and multidetector-row CT (MDCT) (right), left anterior oblique, showing how different coronary segments during totally endoscopic coronary artery bypass grafting procedures may easily be confused as a result of the restricted field of view and lack of manual palpation. The patient—the same as shown in Fig. 2—presents a large diagonal branch (D1) running nearly parallel to the left coronary artery (LCA). Both vessels are hidden deep inside the epicardiac fat (compare Fig. 2), and the LCA additionally nestles against the pulmonary trunk. Thus, in cases like this, accidental grafting of the diagonal branch 1 is a common risk. Three-dimensional MDCT reformations provided additional morphological information of the surrounding area, and therefore helped the surgeon to gain a better orientation. D1 designates the first diagonal branch, M1 the first marginal branch, and LCX the left circumflex artery. Reprinted from ref. *35*, with permission from the Radiological Society of North America.

noncalcified plaque will be displayed. MDCT on the contrary will at least detect calcified lesions very precisely *(29–34)*. The results shown above support this assertion. However, such calcifications very often render successful bypass grafting impossible in the region of choice, and thus either prolong operation times or imply intraoperative switching towards alternative surgical procedures.

Four-row MDCT in comparison to 16-row MDCT showed no differences in the detection of calcified plaques. However, the latter provided increased in-plane and temporal resolution, and thus showed less susceptibility to motion artifacts, allowed more coronary artery segments to be visualized, and thus facilitated preoperative allocation of the suited distal bypass touchdown segment. However the data for 16-row scanners are only preliminary and need to be validated through larger studies.

In general MDCT, because of several profound restrictions, must still be regarded solely as a complementary but not alternate technique to invasive angiography. Despite a temporal resolution of up to 105 ms, it remains highly susceptible to motion artifacts—particularly at elevated heart rates—and still offers only poor visualization of coronary artery segments <1 mm.

However, future developments of surgical devices will make preoperative MDCT evaluation of the coronary arteries even more necessary. Thus, new prototypes for TECABG procedures now link transparent flat panels that may be swung over the patient's body with the TECABG main console and slave unit. This combination allows pre- and intraoperative virtual projection of the patient's heart and, if multiple phase image reconstruction has previously been performed, even of the beating heart. With this technique, not only will preoperative planning of port placement be markedly facilitated, but also intraoperative monitoring of the heart's position, the intrathoracic course of the IMA, the localization of the surgical instruments, the position of the target vessel, and the suited bypass touchdown segment.

At the moment, MDCT technique nevertheless is able to provide extended information on the coronary target site, and therefore should be regarded as an ideal additive planning tool for complex minimally invasive procedures such as TECABG or MIDCABG. Combining the advantages of invasive coronary angiography—e.g., high temporal and spatial resolution, blood flow information, assessment of functional parameters and collateral circulation—with the gross morphological superiority of MDCT thus can be of great benefit to the operative outcome.

REFERENCES

1. Falk V, Diegeler A, Walther T, et al. Endoscopic coronary artery bypass grafting on the beating heart using a computer enhanced telemanipulation system. Heart Surg Forum 1999;2:199–205.
2. Falk V, Diegeler A, Walther T, Jacobs S, Raumans J, Mohr FW. Total endoscopic off-pump coronary artery bypass grafting. Heart Surg Forum 2000;3:29–31.
3. Dogan S, Aybek T, Westphal K, Mierdl S, Moritz A, Wimmer-Greinecker G. Computer-enhanced totally endoscopic sequential arterial coronary artery bypass. Ann Thorac Surg 2001;72:610–611.
4. Mohr FW, Falk V, Diegeler A, et al. Computer-enhanced "robotic" cardiac surgery: experience in 148 patients. J Thorac Cardiovasc Surg 2001;121:842–853.
5. Chocron S, Etievent JP, Dussaucy A, et al. Inter-observer reliability in the interpretation of coronary angiograms. Eur J Cardiothorac Surg 1996;10:671–675.
6. Dogan S, Graubitz K, Aybek T, et al. How safe is the port access technique in minimally invasive coronary artery bypass grafting? Ann Thorac Surg 2002;74:1537–1543; discussion 1543.
7. Kirklin JK, Westaby S, Blackstone EH, Kirklin JW, Chenoweth DE, Pacifico AD. Complement and the damaging effects of cardiopulmonary bypass. J Thorac Cardiovasc Surg 1983;86:845–857.
8. Talwalkar NG, Cooley DA. Minimally invasive coronary artery bypass grafting: a review. Cardiol Rev 1998;6:345–349.
9. Duhaylongsod FG. Minimally invasive cardiac surgery defined. Arch Surg 2000;135:296–301.
10. Vassiliades TA, Jr., Rogers EW, Nielsen JL, Lonquist JL. Minimally invasive direct coronary artery bypass grafting: intermediate-term results. Ann Thorac Surg 2000;70:1063–1065.
11. Groh M, Grossi EA. Multivessel coronary bypass grafting with minimal access using cardiopulmonary bypass. Curr Cardiol Rep 1999;1:331–334.
12. Wimmer-Greinecker G, Matheis G, Dogan S, et al. Complications of port-access cardiac surgery. J Card Surg 1999;14:240–245.
13. Glower DD, Komtebedde J, Clements FM, Debruijn NP, Stafford-Smith M, Newman MF. Direct aortic cannulation for port-access mitral or coronary artery bypass grafting. Ann Thorac Surg 1999;68: 1878–1880.
14. Boehm DH, Reichenspurner H, Gulbins H, et al. Early experience with robotic technology for coronary artery surgery. Ann Thorac Surg 1999;68:1542–1546.
15. Kappert U, Schneider J, Cichon R, et al. Wrist-enhanced instrumentation: moving toward totally endoscopic coronary artery bypass grafting. Ann Thorac Surg 2000;70:1105–1108.
16. Loulmet D, Carpentier A, d'Attellis N, et al. Endoscopic coronary artery bypass grafting with the aid of robotic assisted instruments. J Thorac Cardiovasc Surg 1999;118:4–10.
17. Ohnesorge B, Flohr T, Becker C, et al. [Cardiac imaging with rapid, retrospective ECG synchronized multilevel spiral CT]. Radiologe 2000;40:111–117.
18. Ohnesorge B, Flohr T, Becker C, et al. Cardiac imaging by means of electrocardiographically gated multisection spiral CT: initial experience. Radiology 2000;217:564–571.
19. Flohr T, Ohnesorge B. Heart rate adaptive optimization of spatial and temporal resolution for electrocardiogram-gated multislice spiral CT of the heart. J Comput Assist Tomogr 2001;25:907–923.
20. Luisada AA, MacCanon DM. The phases of the cardiac cycle. Am Heart J 1972;83:705–711.
21. Herzog C, Abolmaali N, Balzer JO, et al. Heart-rate-adapted image reconstruction in multidetector-row cardiac CT: influence of physiological and technical prerequisite on image quality. Eur Radiol 2002;12:2670–2678.
22. Fischbach R, Opitz C, Juergens KU, et al. Einfluss des Rekonstruktionsintervalls auf die Qualität der Koronariendarstellung mit Mehrschicht-Spiral CT und retrospektiver EKG-Synchronisation. Fortschr Roentgenstr 2001;173:54.
23. Achenbach S, Ropers D, Holle J, Muschiol G, Daniel WG, Moshage W. In-plane coronary arterial motion velocity: measurement with electron-beam CT. Radiology 2000;216:457–463.
24. Hong C, Becker CR, Huber A, et al. ECG-gated reconstructed multidetector row CT coronary angiography: effect of varying trigger delay on image quality. Radiology 2001;220:712–717.
25. Kopp AF, Ohnesorge B, Flohr T, et al. [Cardiac multidetector-row CT: first clinical results of retrospectively ECG-gated spiral with optimized temporal and spatial resolution]. Rofo Fortschr Geb Rontgenstr Neuen Bildgeb Verfahr 2000;172:429–435.
26. ACC/AHA guidelines for cardiac catheterization and cardiac catheterization laboratories. American College of Cardiology/American Heart Association Ad Hoc Task Force on Cardiac Catheterization. J Am Coll Cardiol 1991;18:1149–1182..
27. Kopp AF, Schroeder S, Baumbach A, et al. Non-invasive characterisation of coronary lesion morphology and composition by multislice CT: first results in comparison with intracoronary ultrasound. Eur Radiol 2001;11:1607–1611.
28. Aybek T, Dogan S, Andressen E, et al. Robotically enhanced totally endoscopic right internal thoracic coronary artery bypass to the right coronary artery. Heart Surg Forum 2000;3:322–324.
29. Gutfinger DE, Leung CY, Hiro T, et al. In vitro atherosclerotic plaque and calcium quantitation by intravascular ultrasound and electron-beam computed tomography. Am Heart J 1996;131:899–906.
30. Becker CR, Kleffel T, Crispin A, et al. Coronary artery calcium measurement: agreement of multirow detector and electron beam CT. AJR Am J Roentgenol 2001;176:1295–1298.
31. Schmermund A, Baumgart D, Gorge G, et al. Coronary artery calcium in acute coronary syndromes: a comparative study of electron-beam computed tomography, coronary angiography, and intracoronary ultrasound in survivors of acute myocardial infarction and unstable angina. Circulation 1997;96:1461–1469.
32. Schroeder S, Kopp AF, Baumbach A, et al. Non-invasive characterisation of coronary lesion morphology by multi-slice computed tomography: a promising new technology for risk stratification of patients with coronary artery disease. Heart 2001;85:576–578.
33. Janowitz WR, Agatston AS, Viamonte M. Comparison of serial quantitative evaluation of calcified coronary artery plaque by ultrafast computed tomography in persons with and without obstructive coronary artery disease. Am J Cardiol 1991;68:1–6.
34. Agatston AS, Janowitz WR, Hildner FJ, Zusmer NR, Viamonte M, Detrano R. Quantification of coronary artery calcium using ultrafast computed tomography. J Am Coll Cardiol 1990;15:827–832.
35. Herzog C, Dogan S, Diebold T, et al. Multi-detector row CT versus coronary angiography: preoperative evaluation before totally endoscopic coronary artery bypass grafting. Radiology 2003;229:200–208.

28 CT Angiography for Assessment of Coronary Bypass Grafts

Marcello De Santis, MD

With the advent of subsecond rotation combined with prospective electrocardiogram (ECG) triggering or retrospective ECG gating, conventional computed tomography (CT) with spiral capability and superior general image quality has challenged electron beam CT (EBCT) in the domain of cardiac imaging. The introduction of multislice CT scanning with the Siemens SOMATOM Volume Zoom with 4 simultaneously scanned slices, half-second rotation, and 250-ms maximum temporal resolution has recently opened new horizons for cardiac CT imaging. ECG-gated multislice spiral CT represents a leap in image quality of CT angiography (CTA) of the coronary arteries. The fast volume coverage allows scanning the heart with 1-mm slice collimation within a single breath-hold (10 cm in 25–30 s) for high-resolution imaging. Three-dimensional reconstruction with approx 1-mm slice width and submillimeter increment provide data of unique quality for visualization of the coronary arteries and of the arterial/venous grafts utilized for surgical revascularization. This chapter will be focused on the clinical background, the previous CT applications in this setting, and the recent results of multidetector-row CT (MDCT) evaluation of coronary artery bypass grafting (CABG).

CORONARY BYPASS GRAFTING—BACKGROUND

Surgical revascularization for atherosclerotic heart disease is one of the milestones in medical history. Relief of angina after revascularization, improvement in exercise tolerance, and the global benefit on survival have attended this approach since the early stages of development (Fig. 1). After many surgical efforts to relieve angina pectoris, including the direct implantation of the internal mammary artery (IMA) into the myocardium (Vineberg procedure), coronary surgery moved into the modern era in the 1950s. The first direct surgical approach to the coronary circulation in a patient was likely performed by Mustard in 1953 using a carotid-to-coronary bypass, but the first clinical use of the IMA to graft a coronary vessel followed an intraoperative misadventure of William Longmire in 1958 after disintegrating a right coronary artery *(1)*. Similarly, the first successful clinical aortocoronary saphenous vein graft (SVG) by DeBakey and Garrett in 1964 salvaged a complicated left anterior descending (LAD) coronary endoarterectomy *(2)*.

In the 1960s, Mason Sones showed the feasibility of selective coronary arteriography and collected a large library of cineangiograms that were studied in depth by Rene Favaloro *(3)*. Sones and Favaloro formed an innovative team that demonstrated the efficacy and safety of SVG interposition and aortocoronary SVGs for single-vessel, left main, and multivessel coronary disease, thus favoring the worldwide application of this approach. Ironically, with demonstration of the dramatic benefits obtainable by saphenous vein grafting came recognition of the ultimately palliative nature of the operation, as a result of the accelerated atherosclerosis that develops within the grafted saphenous vein conduits. During the first year after bypass surgery, up to 15% of venous grafts occlude; between 1 and 6 yr the graft attrition rate is 1% to 2% per year, and between 6 and 10 yr it is 4% per year. By 10 yr after surgery, only 60% of vein grafts are patent and only 50% of patent vein grafts are free of significant stenosis *(4–6)*.

Although the left IMA initially fell from favor as a result of early, ill-founded concerns regarding low flow rates and technical difficulties in implantation, today it is recognized that selection of the left IMA rather than a saphenous vein as the initial conduit is the single most important factor in improved survival, freedom from cardiac events, and long-term graft patency after coronary bypass surgery (85–90% after 10 yr). The favorable effects on mortality and morbidity are observed irrespective of age, gender, or left-ventricular function, and are particularly evident if the left IMA is implanted into a proximally stenosed LAD, in view of the large area of myocardium subtended by this native vessel *(7)* (Fig. 2). The profound and sustained benefits afforded by the IMA grafting have given impetus to both the utilization of other arterial conduits as coronary bypass grafts (right IMA, right gastroepiploic artery, radial artery, inferior epigastric artery, and so on) and the development of minimally invasive coronary artery bypass grafting (MICABG). This innovative technique, first proposed by Benetti and colleagues in 1994, does not involve the use of cardiopulmonary bypass, or of a median sternotomy. Instead, through a small left thoracotomy, the left IMA is harvested with or without the aid of a thoracoscope, the pericardium is opened, and the arterial conduit is grafted to the LAD *(8)*. At present, single-vessel coronary artery disease involving the LAD is the

From: *Contemporary Cardiology: CT of the Heart: Principles and Applications*
Edited by: U. Joseph Schoepf © Humana Press, Inc., Totowa, NJ

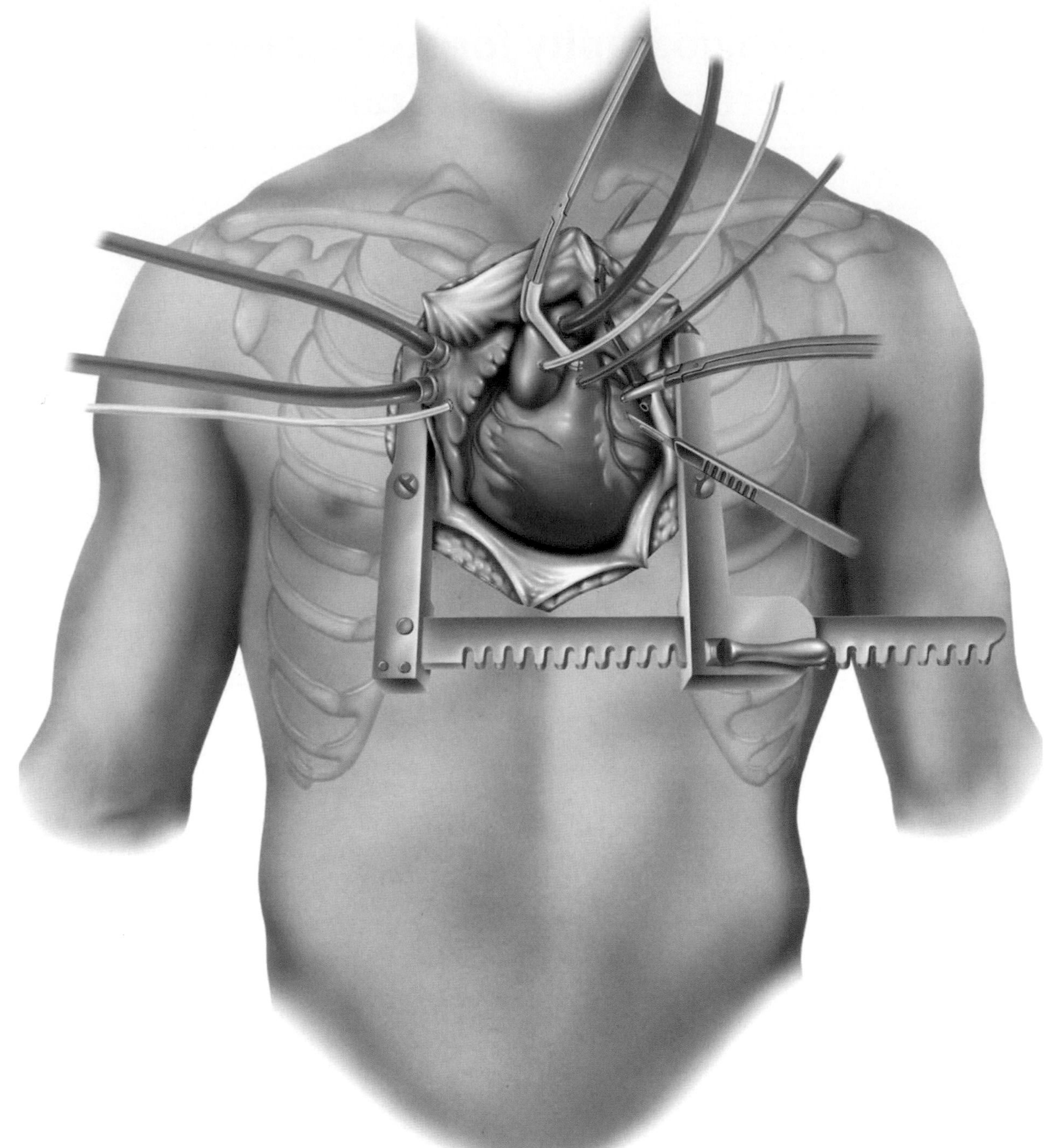

Fig. 1. Schematic drawing of conventional surgical revascularization for coronary artery disease.

primary indication for MICABG. Wider application of the technique, including right IMA or gastroepiploic artery grafting to the right coronary artery, is currently under evaluation.

CORONARY BYPASS GRAFTING—PREVIOUS RESULTS OF CT EVALUATION (CONVENTIONAL SPIRAL CT AND EBCT)

Like any other vascular diagnostic field, coronary bypass grafting was subjected to CT evaluation early after its introduction in clinical practice. In comparison with conventional coronary angiography (CAG), conventional CT scanning with contrast enhancement proved to have the potential to image saphenous vein grafts *(9,10)*, but preliminary promising results on this respect were confined to simple patency assessment (occluded vs not occluded) *(11,12)*. With spiral CT technology, it became possible to scan the entire heart during the arterial phase of contrast enhancement in a single breath-hold, thus significantly reducing both cardiac and respiratory motion artifacts; early spiral CT results, obtained in small populations of CABG patients in comparison with conventional CAG,

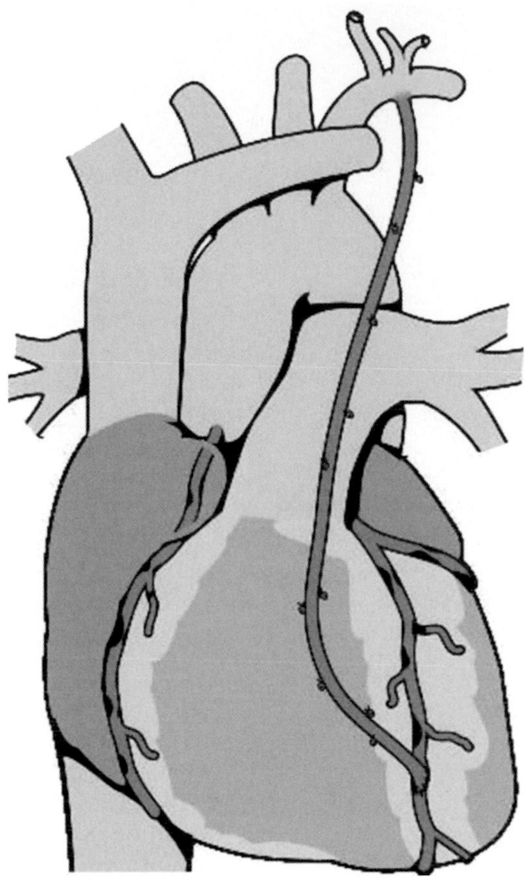

Fig. 2. Schematic visualization of internal mammary artery graft implantation to LAD in the presence of coronary artery disease.

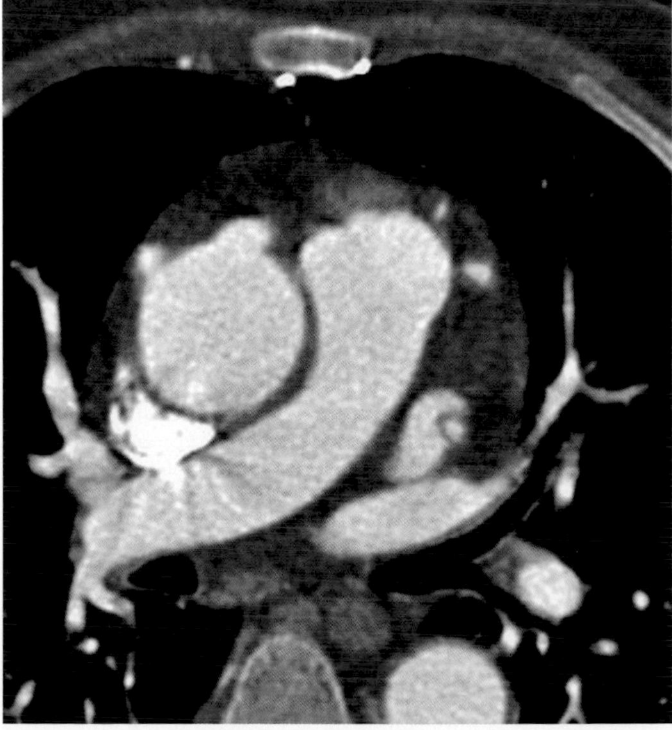

Fig. 3. Source image with clear depiction of the emergence from the ascending aorta of multiple venous grafts.

showed good sensitivity/specificity in terms of venous graft patency, but failed to define both arterial IMA graft and distal anastomosis site patencies *(13)*.

More recent generations of spiral CT single-detector-row scanners with subsecond acquisition (0.75 s) were successfully applied to the contrast-enhanced 3D visualization of venous as well as arterial IMA grafts; in a series of 134 bypass grafts (42 IMA and 92 venous) double-blind evaluated by subsecond spiral CT and conventional CAG, Engelmann et al. found a CT-determined overall sensitivity of 92% for patency with an accuracy of 88% (IMA) and 96% (venous, p = NS) *(14)*. In addition, the newer capabilities of spiral CT imaging allowed the introduction in this setting of a new parameter of CABG patency assessment, i.e., graft flow, which can be qualitatively extracted through the graft length as obtained from multiple 3D reconstruction images at varying Hounsfield unit (HU) thresholds (faster flows correlate with longer graft lengths on most 3D reconstruction thresholds) *(15)*. These refinements in 3D spiral CT angiography of coronary bypass grafting represented a definite step forward in CT vascular imaging and gave rise to the current competition in this respect with EBCT, whose application for CABG patency assessment has scored similar results in two recently reported prospective studies, with overall better evaluation of distal anastomosis sites due to the ECG-triggered EBCT acquisition mode *(16,17)*.

The recent introduction of cardiosynchronization in spiral CT acquisition mode has followed the need to completely suppress cardiac motion when millimeter/submillimeter spatial resolution has to be coupled with high temporal resolution, as recommended in coronary vessel imaging. The crucial importance of this aspect has been recently demonstrated by using an ECG-triggered acquisition approach for spiral CT evaluation of proximal anastomoses in CABG patients *(18)*; despite the suboptimal temporal resolution, optimized timing of scanning as provided by the ECG-triggered mode allowed good visualization of proximal graft anastomoses in all patients, with assessment not only of overall patency (occluded vs not occluded) but also of graft disease, i.e., stenosis detection and grading (Figs. 3,4).

This innovative diagnostic capability, as offered by the cardiosynchronization of CT scanning, explains well the potential of the newer generation of MDCT scanners.

CORONARY BYPASS GRAFTING—PREOPERATIVE APPLICATIONS OF MDCT

The results of several meta-analysis reports on graft failure as well as the spreading application of the minimally invasive approach for CABG surgery have ultimately led to the need for adjunctive preoperative information regarding both the native vessels and the arterial conduits. This information, which can be only partially obtained by using conventional CAG, includes:

1. precise localization of the LAD course (extra- or intramyocardial) and its relationship to adjacent structures
2. emergence, course, size, and branching of the IMAs (and of any other arterial conduit if planned)
3. emergence, course, and size of the left subclavian artery.

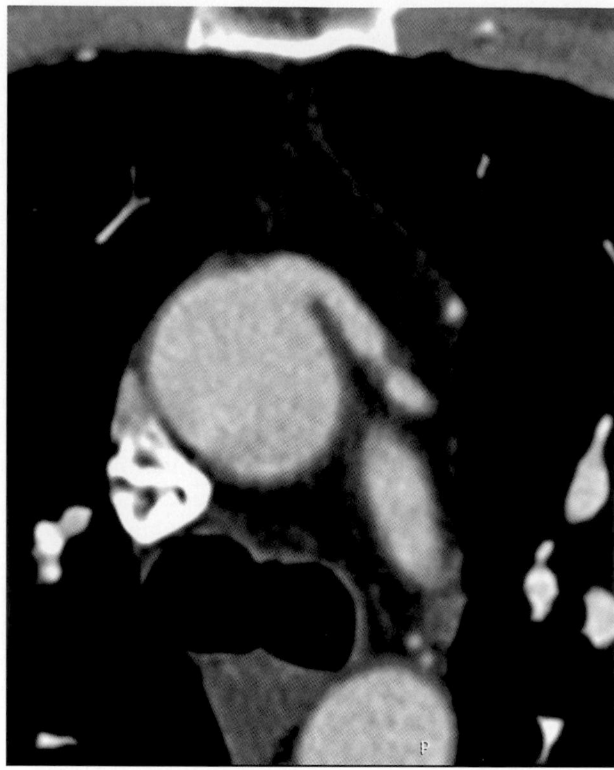

Fig. 4. Source image with visualization of the emergence and proximal portion of a venous graft with a significant stenosis at this level.

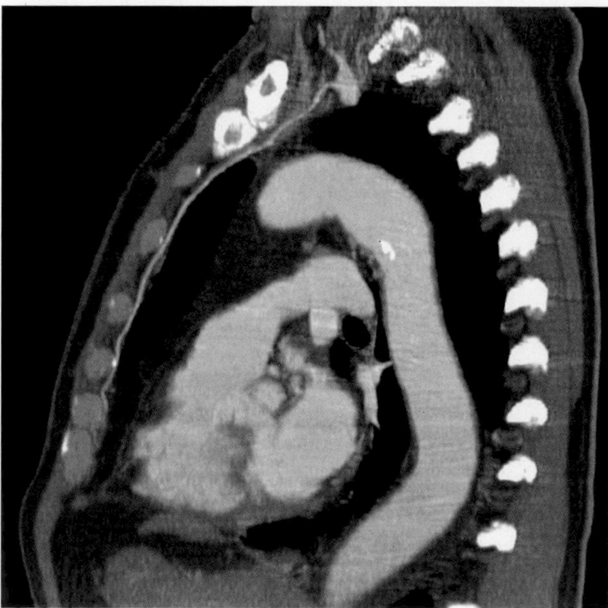

Fig. 5. Sagittal thin maximum intensity projection reconstruction of the entire course of left internal mammary artery.

Intramyocardial LAD course is an absolute contraindication to MICABG, whereas deep, nonpalpable extramyocardial LAD is associated with a more difficult MICABG approach for correct minithoracotomy positioning; in this respect, EBCT with ECG-triggered acquisition has already been applied to visualize LAD anatomy before MICABG surgery with successful results in a small population of patients *(19)*. The application of MDCT technology at higher pitches can be of value in this setting by means of fast contrast-enhanced thoracic examination (3-mm collimation), without prospective triggered or retrospective gated ECG acquisition, and with excellent anatomic depiction of LAD.

The proximal origin of the internal mammary artery, either right or left, is on the concavity of the subclavian artery, just opposite to the thyrocervical trunk, which is the second branch on the convexity of the subclavian artery (the first branch is the vertebral artery). After crossing the subclavian veins, the IMAs line the sternum on both sides for a distance of approx 1–2 cm from the sternal border, and they are accompanied in general by one or two internal mammary veins. After a proximal, medial thymic branch, the IMA anastomoses with the intercostal arteries beyond each rib until it reaches the sixth intercostal space, where it divides into two major branches: the craniocaudal branch enters the sheath of the musculus rectus abdominis and anastomoses with the superior epigastric artery, whereas the major lateral branch follows the cartilaginous arch of the ribs. In a series of 262 consecutive patients undergoing cardiac catheterization prior to CABG, Bauer et al. found surgically significant anomalies, eventually correlated to graft failure, in 79/262 patients (30%) including common origin of another large artery, large side branches, tortuosity, atypical origin/course, hypoplasia, and atherosclerotic lesions, resulting in more difficult IMA preparation in 68/262 patients (26%) and complete modification of surgical strategy in 11/262 patients (4%) *(20)*. These findings, coupled with the above-mentioned LAD anatomic assessment and added to the left subclavian artery evaluation for suspected extensive brachiocephalic atherosclerosis, strongly recommend pre-MICABG fast contrast-enhanced MDCT ungated thoracic examination for optimal surgical planning, as already suggested by our experience in this setting *(21)* (Fig. 5).

Another fundamental preoperative application of MDCT is represented by redo CABG surgery. From an epidemiologic point of view, further revascularization, either reoperative bypass surgery or percutaneous intervention, is required in 4% of patients by 5 yr, 19% of patients by 10 yr, and 31% of patients by 12 yr after initial bypass surgery *(22)*. Despite the increasing numbers of patients undergoing second and third reoperations, repeat revascularization has considerable limitations, taking into account the perioperative morbidity and mortality, which escalate further as the clinical benefits diminish. As compared with initial surgery, reoperation carries a higher mortality rate (3 to 7%), with a high rate of perioperative myocardial infarction (4 to 11.5%). Redo surgery is also associated with less complete relief of angina and with reduction in saphenous vein graft patency as compared with initial bypass surgery *(23,24)*. Extremely meticulous planning of surgical approach is therefore mandatory in this subgroup of redo CABG patients and must be defined taking into account several parameters, both cardiovascular (native CAD, venous-IMA graft patencies, and courses) and thoracic (sternotomy, rib cage, mediastinum, lung

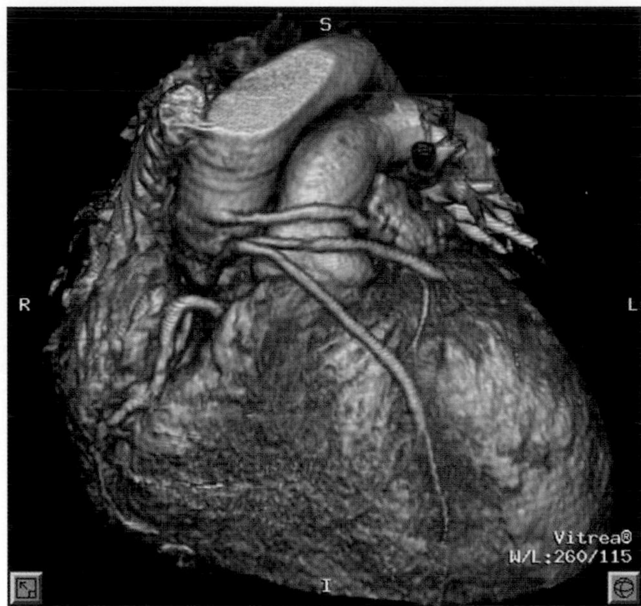

Fig. 6. Volume-rendering 3D reconstruction of multiple venous bypass grafts.

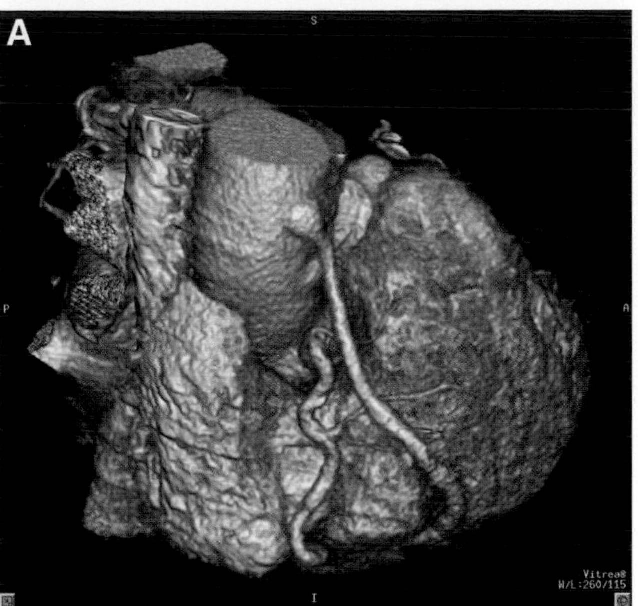

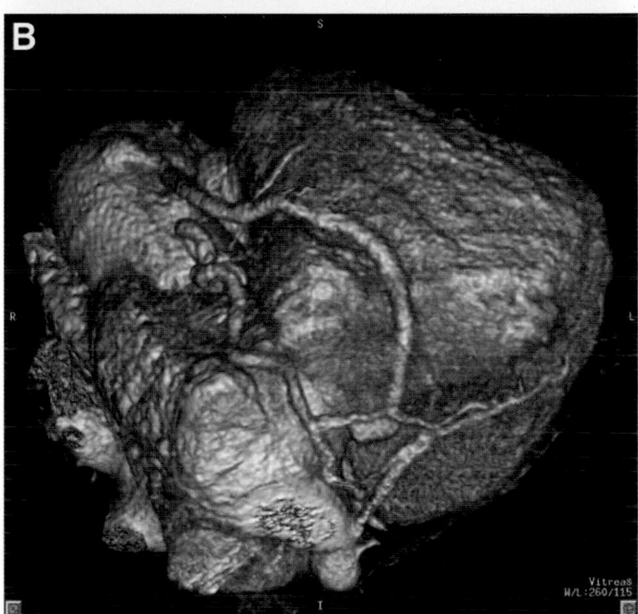

Fig. 7 (A,B). Volume-rendering 3D reconstruction views of a single venous graft to the posterior descending artery in a patient with significant right coronary artery disease.

parenchyma). In this respect, ungated MDCT has already been successfully applied as a preoperative tool in the case of redo CABG surgery *(25)*; 3D visualization of cardiovascular as well as thoracic structures, as offered by the high-resolution MDCT technology, allows user-friendly appreciation of complex post-surgical anatomy and therefore a more confident approach for the surgeon.

CORONARY BYPASS GRAFTING—POSTOPERATIVE APPLICATIONS OF MDCT

To date, few studies have been prospectively addressed to the noninvasive evaluation of coronary bypass grafts by means of ECG-gated MDCT acquisition (Fig. 6). Previous MDCT reports on this respect *(25)* were both restricted to small populations of patients and, much more important, ungated, thus without visualization of distal anastomosis sites. Cardio-synchronization for MDCT evaluation of CABG was first proposed by von Smekal et al. by means of an ECG-triggered approach providing sufficient volume coverage (120- to 140-mm scan range) within a single breath-hold with 0.5-s rotation and 4 × 2.5-mm collimation. However, due to the lack of spatial resolution with 2.5-mm slice width, the distal anastomoses and distal patency of native coronary vessels cannot be evaluated with this approach *(26)*.

Retrospective ECG gating applied to contrast-enhanced MDCT scanning, as already showed in the technical part of this book, is undoubtedly the method of choice for an optimal cardiosynchronization of CTA raw data collection; this approach, coupled with extensive volume coverage and submillimeter spatial resolution, provides unique visualization of arterial-venous grafts almost completely free of cardio-respiratory motion along their entire course at the expense of increased radiation exposure (Fig. 7 A,B). Using 0.5-s rotation, 4 × 1 mm collimation for 1.25-mm slice width, 120 kV, 300 mA, and a spiral pitch between 1.5 and 2.0, a scan range of 120 mm can be covered within a 30- to 35-s breath-hold. Owing to the spiral pitch higher than 1.5, reconstruction is restricted to the single-segment multislice cardiac volume (MSCV) reconstruction algorithm *(27)* with a fixed temporal resolution of 250 ms for heart rates up to approx 74 bpm; this temporal resolution is usually sufficient for motion-free MDCT imaging of coronary bypass grafts and their distal anastomoses, whose motion amplitude is significantly lower than that of native vessels (Figs. 8 and 9). Patient preparation and image postprocessing with 3D reconstruction algorithms are obviously similar to those usually employed for coronary MDCT imaging protocols.

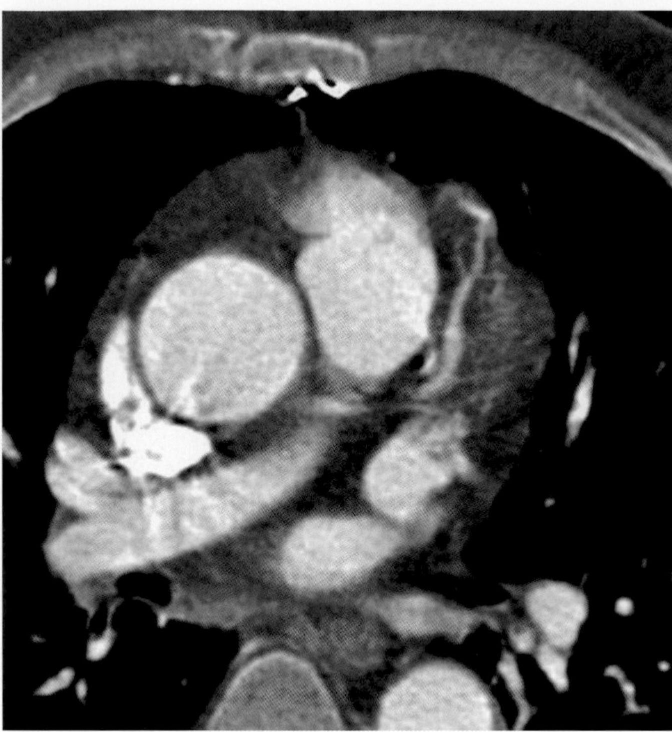

Fig. 8. Source image showing the distal anastomosis site of a left internal mammary artery implantation to left anterior descending artery.

Regarding the preliminary results, Nieman et al. first reported 88% (15/17) of evaluable bypass grafts in a restricted population of four patients, with overall detection of 4/5 graft lesions in comparison to conventional CAG *(28)*. Moreover, a wider population of 65 patients with a total of 182 bypass grafts was prospectively evaluated by Ropers et al., comparing MDCT and conventional CAG results in order to assess overall accuracy in detecting graft occlusion and stenosis *(29)*; higher sensitivity (98%) and specificity (99%) than ever before were obtained by MDCT in terms of bypass graft patency assessment, whereas a satisfactory diagnostic accuracy for the detection of high-grade bypass stenoses (sensitivity 75%, specificity 92%) was achieved when grafts were imaged with sufficient quality (Figs. 10 and 11).

Distal anastomoses visualization represents one of the crucial aspects of bypass grafting MDCT imaging, and its full appreciation depends on the rigorous application of the acquisition technique as well as on the correct utilization of 3D reconstruction algorithms usually available, in order to obtain evidence-based images (Figs. 12–14). In addition, MDCT technology is generally well suited for stenting evaluation and therefore may be successfully applied even in those infrequent cases of graft disease percutaneous treatment (Fig. 15).

The major drawback of such noninvasive approach seems at the moment to be the significant number of unevaluable grafts; as stressed in the study of Ropers et al. *(29)*, only 62% of the patent bypass grafts could be evaluated for the presence or absence of high-grade stenoses. In general, metal and motion artifacts represent the major causes for impaired image quality in this setting, and further improvements of MDCT technology are expected to reduce in the next future the percentage of unevaluable grafts and to optimize visualization and evaluation of distal anastomosis sites.

REFERENCES

1. Shumacker HB. The Evolution of Cardiac Surgery. Indiana University Press, Bloomington, IN: 1992.
2. Garrett HE, Dennis EW, DeBakey ME. Aortocoronary bypass with saphenous vein graft: seven-year follow-up. JAMA 1973;223: 792–794.
3. Favaloro RG. Critical analysis of coronary artery bypass graft surgery: a 30-year journey. J Am Coll Cardiol 1998;31:1B–63B.
4. Campeau L, Enjalbert M, Lesperance J, et al. The relation of risk factors to the development of atherosclerosis in saphenous vein bypass grafts and the progression of disease in the native circulation: a study 10 years after aortocoronary bypass surgery. N Engl J Med 1984;311:1329–1332.
5. Bourassa MG. Fate of venous grafts: the past, the present and the future. J Am Coll Cardiol 1991;5:1081–1083.
6. Fitzgibbon GM, Kafka HP, Leach AJ, et al. Coronary bypass graft fate and patient outcome: angiographic follow-up of 5065 grafts related to survival and reoperation in 1388 patients during 25 years. J Am Coll Cardiol 1996;28:616–626.
7. Loop FD. Internal-thoracic-artery grafts: biologically better coronary arteries. N Engl J Med 1996;334:263–265.
8. Calafiore AM, Angelini GD, Bergsland J, et al. Minimally invasive coronary artery bypass grafting. Ann Thorac Surg 1996;62: 1545–1548.
9. Brundage BH, Lipton MJ, Herfkens RJ, et al. Detection of patent bypass grafts by computed tomography: a preliminary report. Circulation 1980;61:826–831.

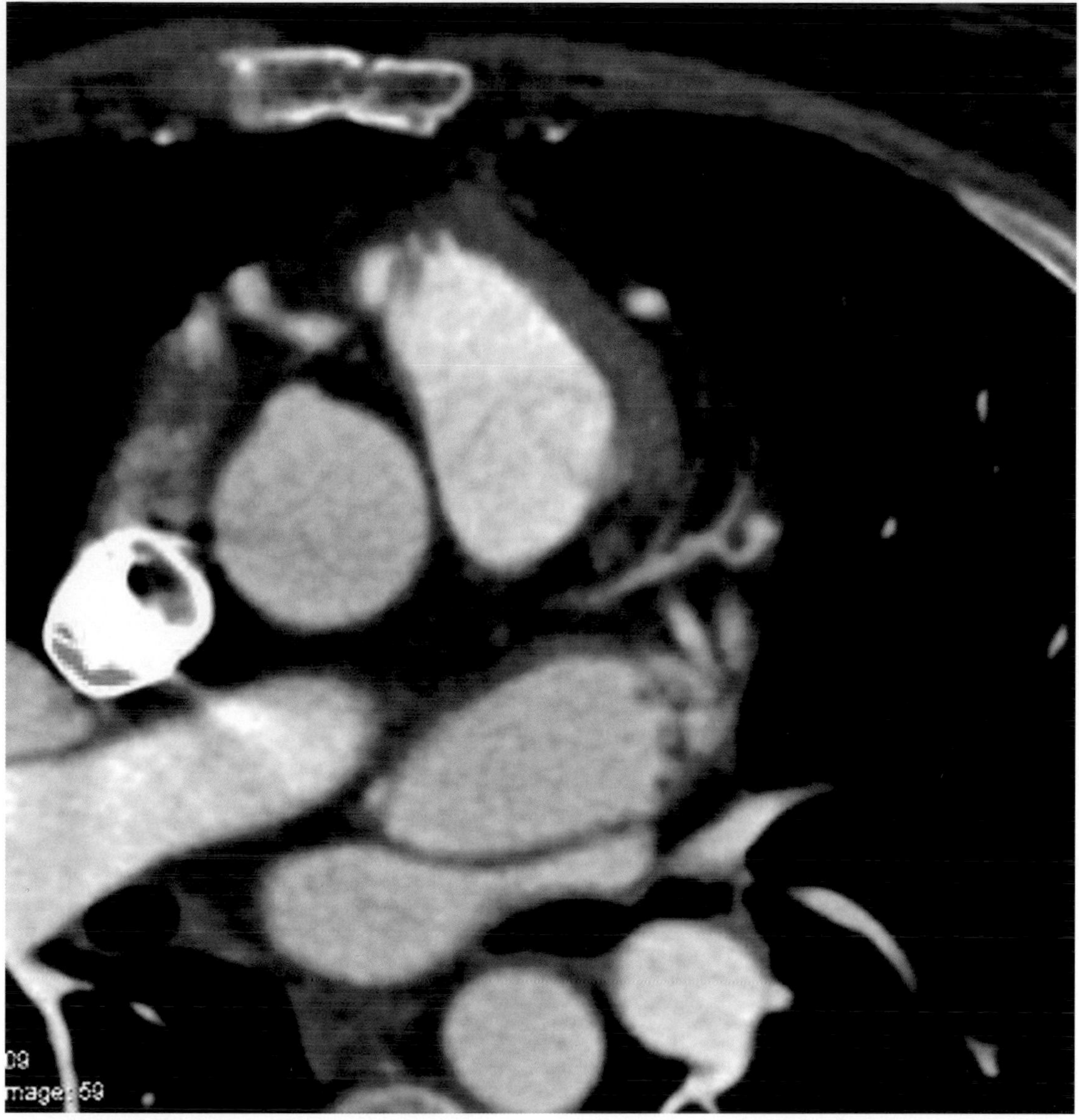

Fig. 9. Source image with evidence of venous graft anastomosis to the second diagonal branch.

10. Ullyot DJ, Turley K, McKay CR, et al. Assessment of saphenous vein graft patency by contrast-enhanced computed tomography. J Thorac Cardiovasc Surg 1982;83:512–518.
11. Godwin JD, Califf RM, Korobkin M, et al. Clinical value of coronary bypass graft evaluation with CT. AJR Am J Roentgenol 1983;140: 649–655.
12. Daniel WG, Dohring W, Stender HS, et al. Value and limitations of computed tomography in assessing aortocoronary bypass graft patency. Circulation 1983;67:983–987.
13. Tello R, Costello P, Ecker CP, et al. Spiral CT evaluation of coronary artery bypass graft patency. J Comput Assist Tomogr 1993;17: 253–259.
14. Engelmann MG, von Smekal A, Knez A, et al. Accuracy of spiral computed tomography for identifying arterial and venous coronary graft patency. Am J Cardiol 1997;80:569–574.
15. Tello R, Hartnell GG, Costello P, et al. Coronary artery bypass graft flow: qualitative evaluation with cine single-detector row CT and comparison with findings at angiography. Radiology 2002;224: 913–918.
16. Ha JW, Cho SY, Shim WH, et al. Noninvasive evaluation of coronary artery bypass graft patencyusing three-dimensional angiography obtained with contrast-enhanced electron beam CT. AJR Am J Roentgenol 1999;172:1055–1059.
17. Lu B, Dai RP, Jing BL, et al. Evaluation of coronary artery bypass graft patency using three-dimensional reconstruction and flow study on electron beam tomography. J Comput Assist Tomogr 2000;24:663–670.
18. von Smekal A, Lachat M, Wildermuth S, et al. Proximal anastomoses of aortocoronary bypasses. Evaluation with ECG-triggered single-slice computerized tomography. Radiologe 2000;40:130–135.
19. Ohtsuka T, Takamoto S, Endoh M, et al. Ultrafast computed tomography for minimally invasive coronary artery bypass grafting. J Thorac Cardiovasc Surg 1998;116:173–174.
20. Bauer EP, Bino MC, von Segesser LK, et al. Internal mammary artery anomalies. Thorac Cardiovasc Surg 1990;38:312–315.
21. De Santis M, Quagliarini F, Leonetti C, et al. MDSCT pre-operative evaluation of internal mammary arteries (IMAs) in patients candidate to minimally invasive coronary artery bypass grafting (MICABG) (abs). ECR, Vienna, Austria: 2003.

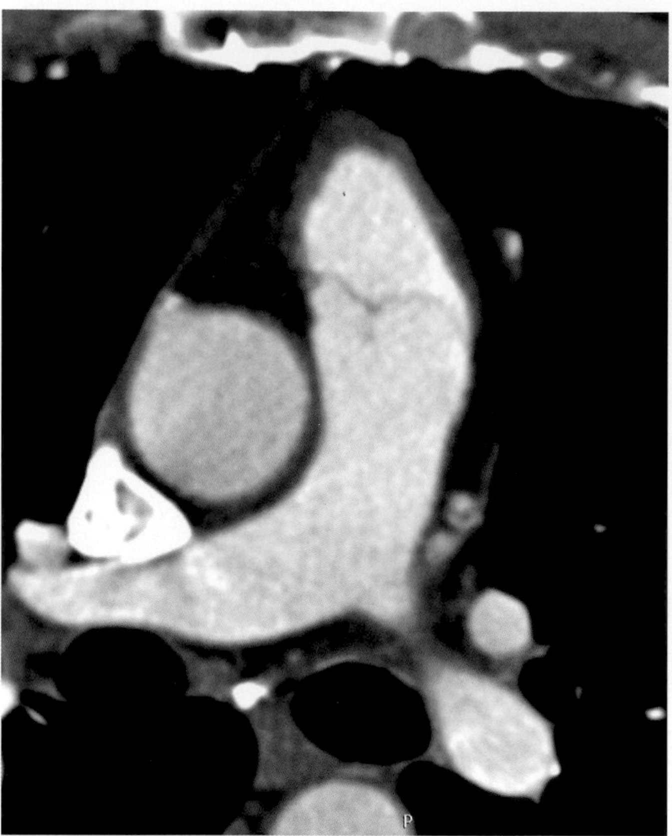

Fig. 10. Axial visualization of a diseased venous graft on the left side of the pulmonary trunk in a patient with internal mammary artery implantation.

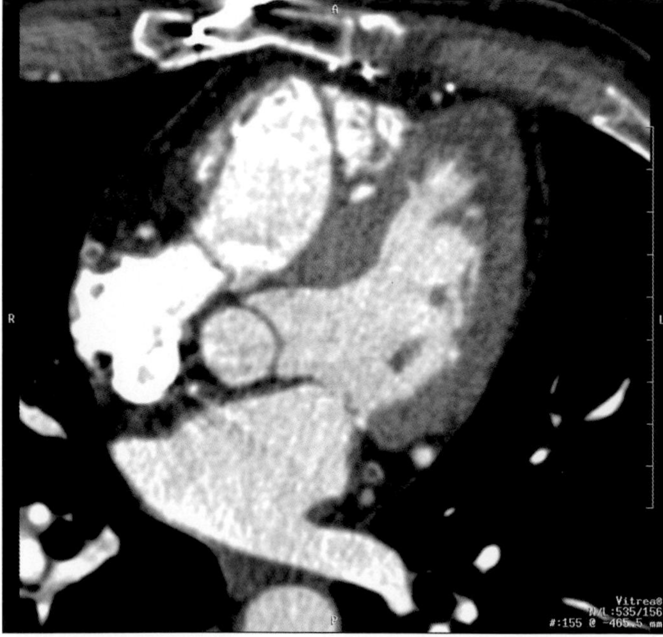

Fig. 11. Axial image showing a completely occluded graft closer to a small patent right coronary artery and an occluded circumflex artery in the presence of patency of the corresponding graft.

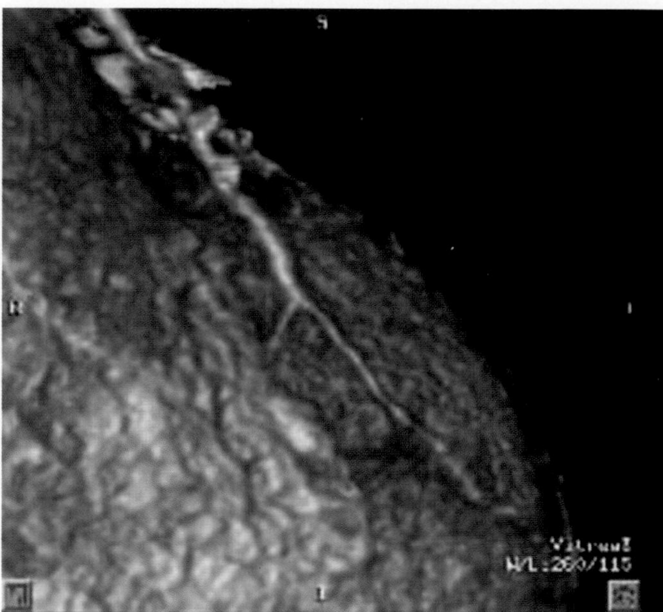

Fig. 12. Volume-rendering 3D reconstruction of a patent distal anastomosis between internal mammary artery graft and left anterior descending artery.

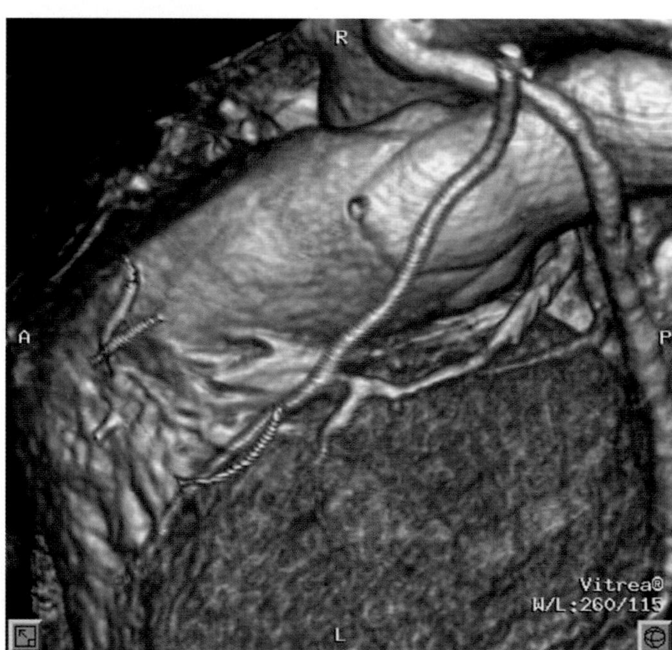

Fig. 13. Volume-rendering 3D reconstruction of a patent internal mammary artery graft implanted to left anterior descending artery.

22. Weintraub WS, Jones EL, Craver JM, et al. Frequency of repeat coronary bypass or coronary angioplasty after coronary artery bypass surgery using saphenous venous grafts. Am J Cardiol 1994;73:103–112.
23. Loop FD, Lytle BW, Cosgrove DM, et al. Reoperation for coronary atherosclerosis: changing practice in 2509 consecutive patients. Ann Surg 1990;212:378–386.

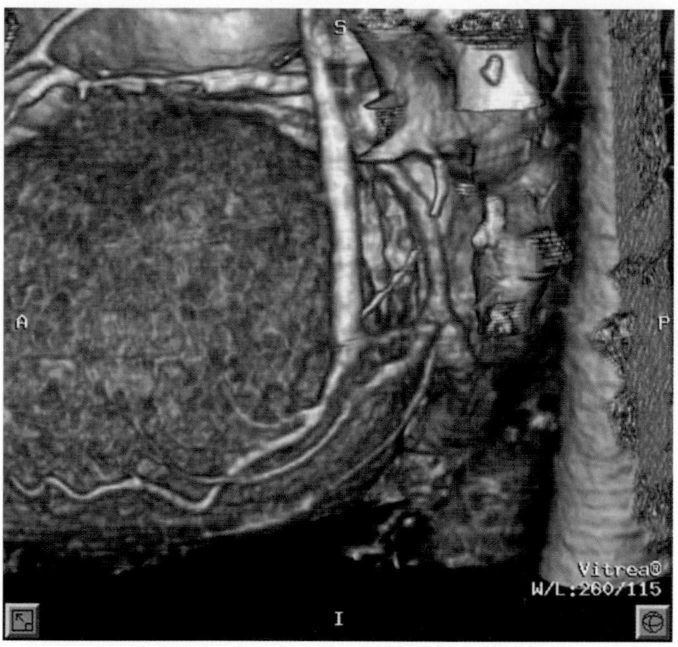

Fig. 14. Volume-rendering 3D reconstruction of a patent distal anastomosis between venous graft and obtuse marginal.

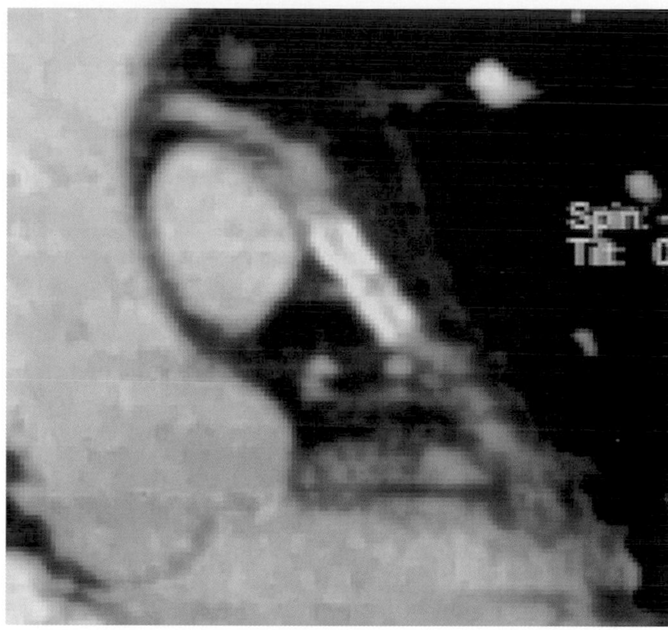

Fig. 15. Multiplanar reformation 3D reconstruction of a patent stent for venous graft disease.

24. Cameron A, Kemp HG Jr, Green GE. Reoperation for coronary artery disease: 10 years of clinical follow-up. Circulation 1988;78 (Suppl I): I/158–I/162.
25. Yamaguchi A, Adachi H, Ino T, et al. Three-dimensional computed tomographic angiography as pre-operative evaluation of a patent internal thoracic artery graft. J Thorac Cardiovasc Surg 2000;120: 811–812.
26. von Smekal A. The potential of cardio-computed tomography. Multislice CT: a practical guide. Proceedings of the 5th International Somatom CT User Conference. Zurich, June 2000.
27. Ohnesorge B, Flohr T, Becker CR, et al. Cardiac imaging by means of electrocardiographically gated multisection spiral CT: initial experience. Radiology 2000;217:564–571.
28. Nieman K, Oudkerk M, Rensing BJ, et al. Coronary angiography with multi-slice computed tomography. Lancet 2001;357 (9256): 599–603.
29. Ropers D, Ulzheimer S, Wenkel E, et al. Investigation of aorto-coronary artery bypass grafts by multislice spiral computed tomography with electrocardiographic-gated image reconstruction. Am J Cardiol 2001;88:792–795.

29 Contrast-Enhanced Electron Beam CT and Multidetector-Row CT in the Evaluation of Coronary Stent Patency

Heiko Pump, MD, Stefan Möhlenkamp, MD, Raimund Erbel, MD, and Rainer Seibel, MD

INTRODUCTION

High-pressure stent implantation is an established technique to maintain luminal integrity following interventional revascularization in native coronary arteries and bypass grafts. Large controlled randomized trials demonstrated superior long-term patency in comparison to percutaneous transluminal coronary angioplasty (PTCA) alone *(8–13)*. The beneficial effects of stent implantation on restenosis can be attributed to larger acute lumen dimensions compared to balloon angioplasty, and the elimination of vessel recoil after intervention *(14,15)*. All currently available stents are made of metal, and they induce significant intimal hyperplasia in some patients. Improvements in antithrombotic and anticoagulation therapy have substantially reduced the rate of in-stent thrombosis *(16–18)*. Brachytherapy and drug-eluting stents have been successfully used in in-stent restenosis *(19–24)*.

Despite these substantial improvements in interventional revascularization, the rate of restenosis remains in the range of >10–20% in routine clinical practice. Considering the still increasing rate in the use of stents, this represents a significant proportion of cases each year. Stent-related restenosis is primarily based on two mechanisms: elastic recoil with luminal narrowing shortly after stent deployment and the induction of intimal cell proliferation caused by the controlled vessel-wall trauma during stent implantation. Optimal strut expansion and stent localization in relation to side branches may have an impact on the long-term outcome.

A noninvasive tool to rule out stent-related stenosis would be of substantial clinical value if only a fraction of recatheterizations could be avoided.

Coronary stents are barely visible with imaging techniques such as high-resolution digital fluoroscopy. In contrast, electron beam computed tomography (EBCT) and multidetector-row computed tomography (MDCT) provide superior spatial resolution that allows visualization of stents both in native coronary arteries and bypass grafts. In our initial investigations we systemically explored the potential of fast-CT imaging to visualize coronary stent morphology *(25,26)* (Fig. 1) and coronary stent patency using contrast-enhanced flow studies *(27–29)*. Technical advances in spatial and temporal resolution in both EBCT and MDCT technology have led to an image quality that may allow broad clinical use of noninvasive contrast-enhanced fast-CT scanning to assess coronary stent morphology and patency.

APPROACHES TO CORONARY STENT IMAGING USING CT

Depending on the aim of the study, it is reasonable to distinguish between morphologic imaging to visualize stent localization (its relation to side branches and stent-related stenosis) on the one hand, and functional imaging (to [semi-] quantitatively evaluate the functional impact of luminal narrowing) on the other. Unattenuated studies have been used in the past to visualize coronary stents, which at the time was hardly possible with any other imaging modality. However, the diagnostic information contained within the resulting images is limited to localize the stent and to distinguish coronary calcification from coronary stents, which in some cases remains difficult even in studies with thin sections. Noninvasive contrast-enhanced coronary CT angiography (CTA) can be used to assess stent patency as per contrast enhancement in the course of the stented artery, where an unenhanced distal coronary artery lumen usually reflects significant in-stent restenosis. Recent improvements in spatial resolution now provide an image quality where visualization of nonocclusive in-stent neointimal hyperplasia seems within reach. Using contrast-enhanced flow studies at rest and after stress, e.g., with infusion of adenosine, may permit noninvasive assessment of coronary flow reserve. These approaches may be used in combination, but the additional diagnostic information must be carefully weighed against additional radiation and use of contrast agent.

ELECTRON BEAM COMPUTED TOMOGRAPHY

In 1994, Eldredge et al. were the first investigators to assess stent patency in native coronary arteries by using EBCT *(30)*.

From: *Contemporary Cardiology: CT of the Heart: Principles and Applications*
Edited by: U. Joseph Schoepf © Humana Press, Inc., Totowa, NJ

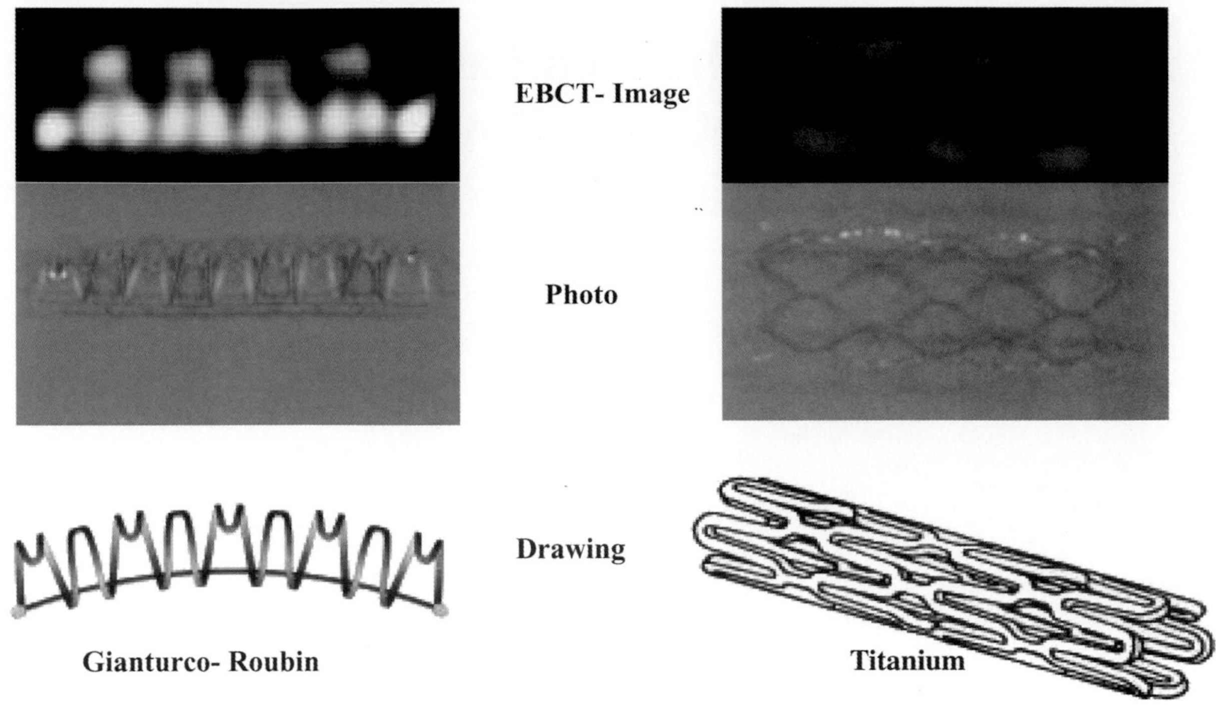

Fig. 1. In vitro study of two stent types after dilatation. Comparison of electron beam CT images, photos, and schematic drawings.

Table 1
Coronary Arterial Stent Patency: Assessment With Electron Beam CT

No. of stented vessels	221
No. of patent vessels at coronary artery (CA) and correctly detected at electron beam CT (EBCT)	189
No. of stent stenosis at CA	23
No. of stent stenosis at CA and correctly detected at EBCT	18
Senstivity for detection of stenoses with EBCT	78%
Specificity for depiction of the absence of stenoses with EBCT	98%
Negative predictive value	97%
Positive predictive value	82%

They performed a contrast-enhanced multisection EBCT and evaluated stent patency with the cineloop and gamma variate-based time density analysis. In 1996 Schmermund et al. reported the assessment of coronary Palmaz–Schatz stents in 22 patients *(27)*. Twenty of 22 patients (91%) could be analyzed by using cineloop evaluation, and in 17 (85%) of these 20 patients, a gamma variate curve was fitted to the segment distal to the stent. In 1998 we reported our findings using various stent types: we found a higher rate of cine loop evaluation (94.8%) and a lower rate of successful distal gamma variate fits (49%) as compared with the study by Schmermund et al. *(28)*. Overall accuracy was 94.3% with a sensitivity of 77%, which is consistent with findings in a larger cohort *(29)* (Table 1). Compared with coronary angiography, EBCT permitted the detection of 18 of 23 high-grade stenoses (sensitivity, 78%) and correctly depicted the absence of high-grade stenoses in 189 of 193 stented vessels (specificity, 98%). The interpretation was false-positive in four vessels (positive predictive value, 82% [18/22 vessels]) and false-negative in five (negative predictive value, 97% [189/194 vessels]). In 1999, we published the results of a prospective study with 44 patients. In correlation with coronary angiography, we found sensitivities of 65% and 84%, respectively, and positive and negative predictive values of 69% and 82%, respectively *(25)*, which is in the same range as other noninvasive tests such as stress ECG.

EBCT SCAN PROTOCOLS

Each examination consists of a single-section volume study and a contrast-enhanced multisection flow study. EBCT in the single-slice mode is performed, beginning at the pulmonary trunk, with 30–45 contiguous 3-mm sections triggered at 80% of the RR interval, and using a 100-ms acquisition time. The localization of the stent and of the calcified plaques is important for the planning of the contrast-enhanced studies. The depiction of each stent and of calcifications with respect to their location is based on typical landmarks, and the analysis is limited to that of major coronary arteries (i.e., proximal, middle, and distal segments) and major side branches (i.e., first diagonal and/or marginal branches). The table position is adjusted so that the stent is positioned between the scanning planes and images can be obtained proximal and distal to the stent. In addition, an incorrect attenuation measurement on the contrast studies caused by calcified plaques can be avoided. Initial circulation time assessment is followed by a multislice flow study, to obtain time-density images from the coronary artery lumen.

This study is performed with a bolus injection of 20 mL of iopromide (370 mg of iodine per milliliter). In the multislice flow study, one bolus injection of 50 mL of iopromide (370 mg of iodine per milliliter) with an injection rate of 7–10 mL/s are performed, which may be followed by a second study during adenosine infusion. In a few cases, the scan volume may not encompass the entire length of the stented segment, especially in patients with multiple stents, so that dual injections may be required to image proximal and distal segments. The multislice flow study protocol consists of 8-mm slices, eight levels,10 times per level, electrocardiogram triggered at 80% of the RR interval on every second heartbeat, and a 50-ms acquisition time.

In the second step, the multisection flow study results are analyzed and the images obtained at each level are combined in a cineloop for qualitative assessment based on the examiner's visual inspection of the images. In the third step, integrated scanner software or off-line assessment can be used for densitometric evaluation in a time-attenuation analysis of the contrast-enhanced studies using a gamma variate, which can be fitted to the data. The slope of the curve in comparison to that in the aorta may be used for semi-quantitative estimation of epicardial blood flow.

SUGGESTED EBCT CRITERIA FOR PATENCY, STENOSIS, AND OCCLUSION

Initially, coronary stent patency was assessed only under resting conditions. The degree of opacification of the segment distal to the stent was used to distinguish occluded from patent vessels. The coronary stent was defined to be patent if distal vessel opacification was similar to that in control vessels of similar size in the cineloop. An automated fit of a gamma variate was used as an additional observer-independent tool to define stent patency, because in most cases a gamma variate can be fitted only if the time-density curve shows a typical flow profile (Fig. 2A,B). Further, in a nonobstructed coronary artery, the delay in opacification after aortic root enhancement is usually brief, which can be used as an additional criterion for stent patency.

The criteria of absence of hyperattenuation distal to the stent in the cineloop or hyperattenuation proximal to the stent but weak contrast enhancement distally and no fitted gamma variate curve raise the suspicion of luminal narrowing or vessel occlusion (Fig. 3).

In most cases, cineloop evaluation is sufficient to confirm stent patency. A comparison with the other coronary arteries usually leads to the correct diagnosis. The time-attenuation analysis and gamma variate curve application are important additional elements in confirming the obstruction in cases in which there was weak contrast enhancement distal to the stent. Prolonged circulation time with insufficient contrast enhancement, arrhythmia, inadequate breath-holding, and calcifications in distal segments are frequent reasons for insufficient image quality.

MULTIDETECTOR-ROW CT

The development of mechanical MDCT systems with increased scan speed and the introduction of retrospective gating were very important steps in the noninvasive visualization of the heart and the coronary vessels *(31)*. The multirow CT technology, with 1-mm or even submillimeter section thickness and dedicated ECG-gated image reconstruction algorithms provide an improved spatial resolution compared with EBCT. The minor temporal resolution of MDCT compared with EBCT remains a drawback today, and in some cases it is necessary to treat patients with oral or intravenous metoprolol prior to imaging to achieve a heart rate less than 60 beats per minute (bpm). The increased gantry rotation speed (420 ms) of the second-generation MDCT may have the potential to expand the range of heart rates.

In contrast to the prospective ECG-gated EBCT scan protocol, the MDCT examination is performed as a spiral scan combined with simultaneously digitized ECG. To our knowledge, the performance of multisection flow studies with densitometric measurements and cineloop evaluations are not considered as standard tools in the evaluation of the coronary arteries, and in most cases, software options are not routinely available commercially.

4-ROW MDCT

Initially, a 4 × 2.5-mm collimation with simultaneous ECG recording is used to obtain retrospectively reconstructed 3-mm sections of the whole heart to localize the coronary stents and to determine coronary calcifications.

After determination of the scanning delay with a bolus injection of 15 mL contrast agent, a contrast-enhanced 4-row MDCT (130–150 cc contrast agent, flow rate 4 cc/s) is performed by using a 4 × 1-mm collimation and a 500 ms rotation time. The axial images are reconstructed retrospectively in 1-mm slice thickness with a 50% slice overlap. Usually, maximum intensity projection (MIP) reconstructions, 3D reconstructions in volume-rendering technique (VRT), and the axial source images are used for the evaluation of stent patency.

16-ROW CT

A 1.5-mm collimation with simultaneous ECG recording and a 420-ms rotation time is used to obtain retrospectively reconstructed 3-mm sections of the whole heart for stent localization and determination of coronary calcium (Fig. 4).

The 0.75-mm collimation with a 420-ms rotation time is used for the contrast-enhanced study. The optimal scan delay is determined by direct visualization and measurement of the hyperattenuation in the vessel lumen during the contrast-agent injection by placing a region of interest in the ascending aorta. A total of 130–150 cc contrast agent with a flow rate of 5 cc/s is injected. Cross-sectional images are reconstructed with a slice thickness of 0.75 mm in 0.5-mm intervals. On the basis of the cross-sectional images, sliding thin-slab MIP, and 3D reconstructions—VRT—the coronary arteries are evaluated.

SUGGESTED MDCT CRITERIA FOR PATENCY, STENOSIS, AND OCCLUSION

The coronary stent is considered to be patent if the examiner visualizes the hyperattenuated vessel proximal and distal to the stented target vessel on the axial slices and the generated 2- and 3D reconstructions compared with the other coronaries (Figs. 5A–C). Weak contrast enhancement distal to the stent or in the stent lumen are signs of hemodynamically relevant

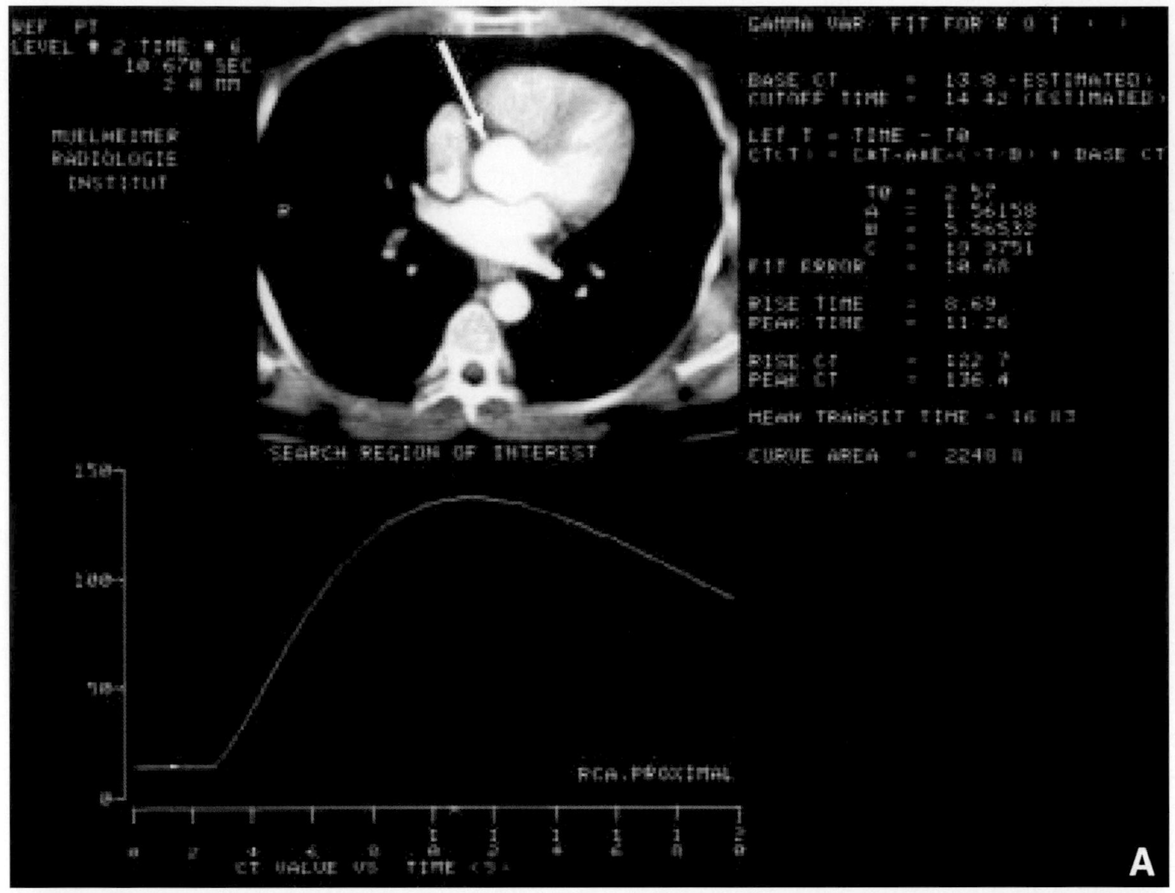
REF PT
LEVEL # 2 TIME # 6
10.670 SEC
2.0 MM
MUELHEIMER
RADIOLOGIE
INSTITUT
GAMMA VAR. FIT FOR R.O.I.
BASE CT = 13.8 (ESTIMATED)
CUTOFF TIME = 14.42 (ESTIMATED)
LET T = TIME - T0
T0 = 2.57
A = 1.56158
B = 5.56532
C = 10.9751
FIT ERROR = 10.68
RISE TIME = 8.69
PEAK TIME = 11.26
RISE CT = 122.7
PEAK CT = 136.4
MEAN TRANSIT TIME = 16.83
CURVE AREA = 2248.8
SEARCH REGION OF INTEREST
RCA.PROXIMAL
CT VALUE VS TIME (S)
A

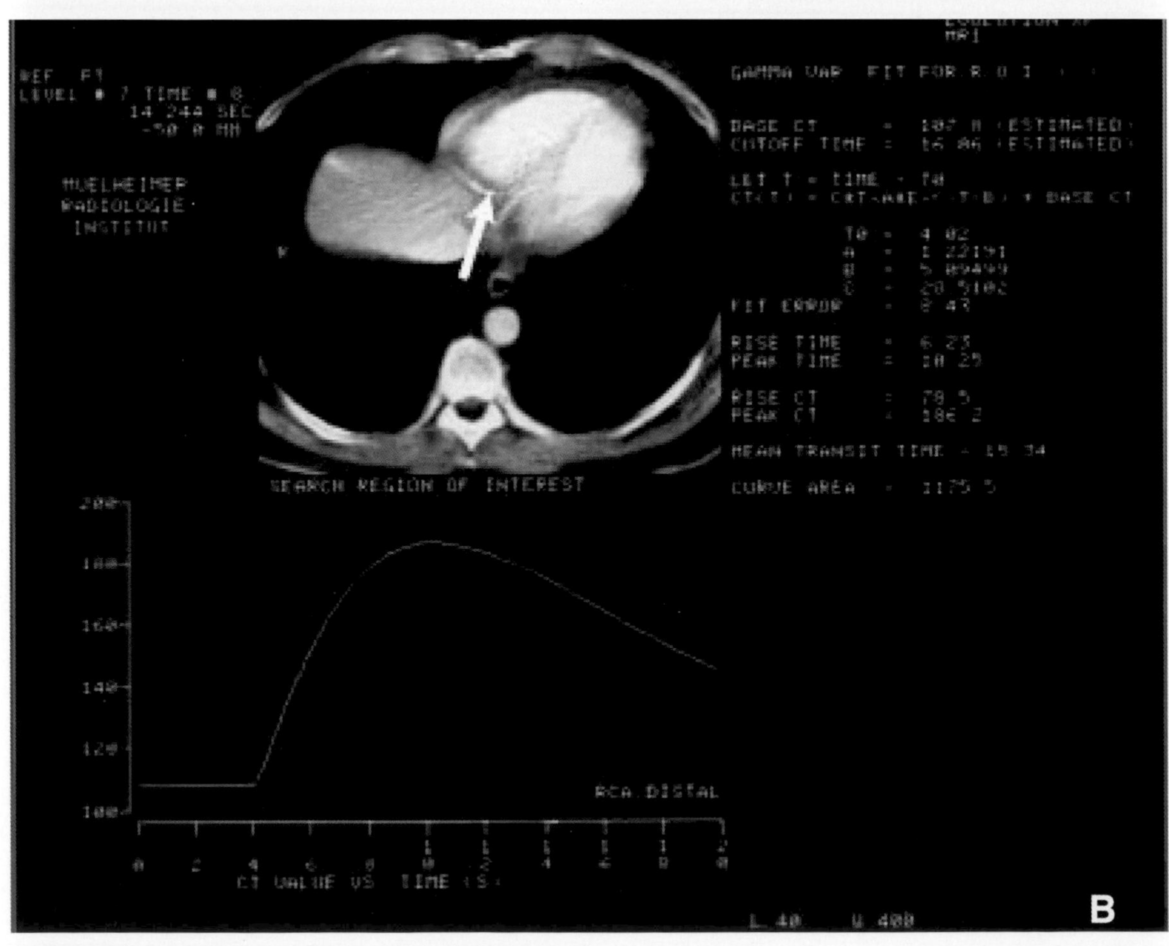
REF PT
LEVEL # 7 TIME # 8
14.244 SEC
-50.0 MM
MUELHEIMER
RADIOLOGIE
INSTITUT
GAMMA VAR. FIT FOR R.O.I.
BASE CT = 107.8 (ESTIMATED)
CUTOFF TIME = 16.86 (ESTIMATED)
LET T = TIME - T0
T0 = 4.02
A = 1.22191
B = 5.89499
C = 20.5102
FIT ERROR = 8.43
RISE TIME = 6.23
PEAK TIME = 10.25
RISE CT = 78.5
PEAK CT = 186.2
MEAN TRANSIT TIME = 15.34
CURVE AREA = 1175.5
SEARCH REGION OF INTEREST
RCA DISTAL
CT VALUE VS TIME (S)
L 40 W 400
B

Fig. 2. **(A)** *(opposite page)* Time attenuation measurement obtained proximal to a patent stent in the right coronary artery with electron beam CT. The gamma variate curve demonstrates a typical arterial curve. The arrow indicates the deposition of the region of interest. **(B)** Time attenuation measurement obtained distal to the patent stent in the same patient with gamma variate curve. The arrow indicates the depostition of the region of interest in the distal vessel region of the right coronary artery.

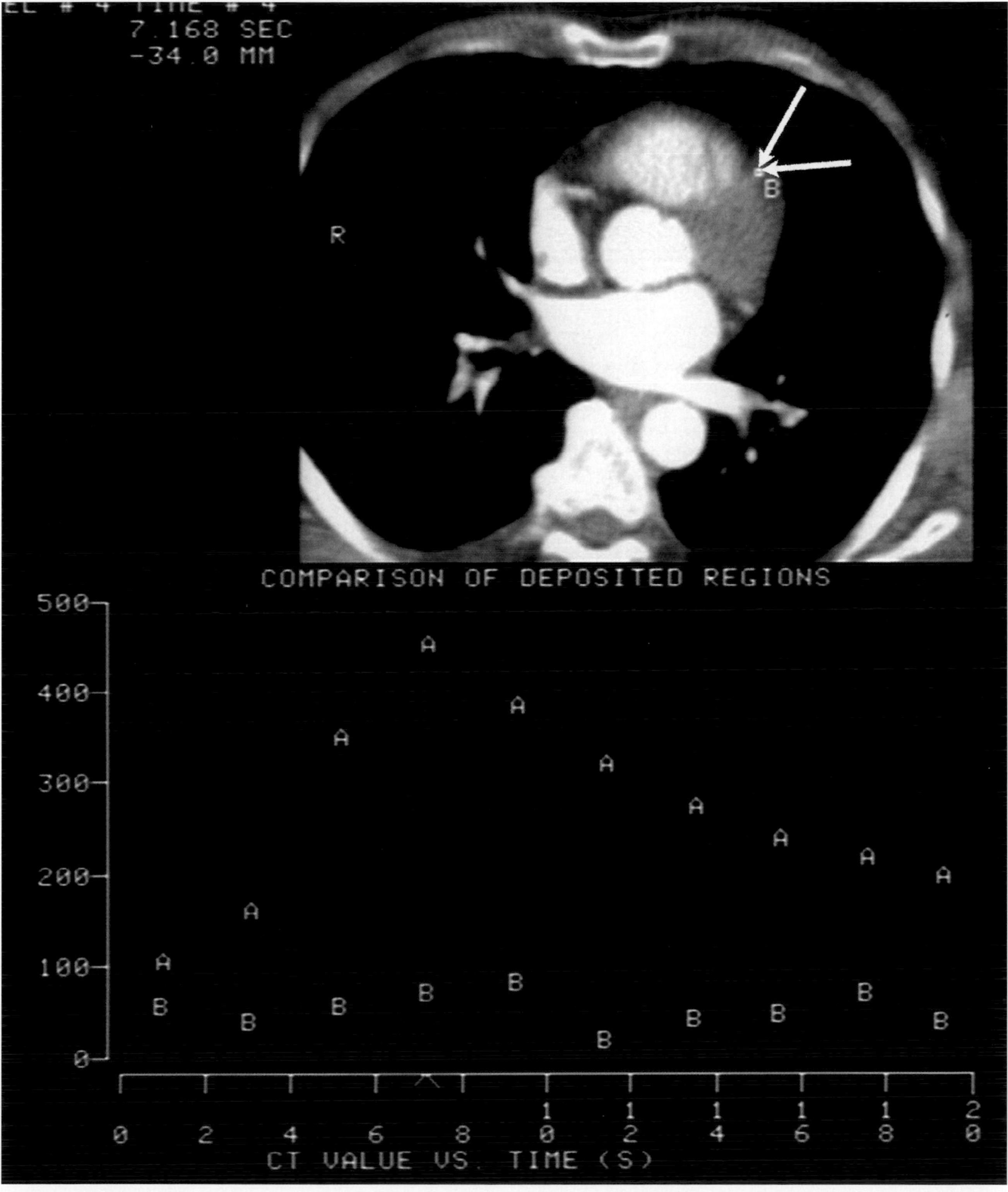

Fig. 3. Transverse electron beam CT scan shows a high-grade left anterior descending arterial stenosis distal to the stent. The region of interest (B) is placed in a hypoattenuating distal vessel region (arrows). The unconnected dots below the 100-HU mark (B) indicate the ROI placed in the hypoattenuating distal vessel region. A, gamma variate curve of the ascending aorta.

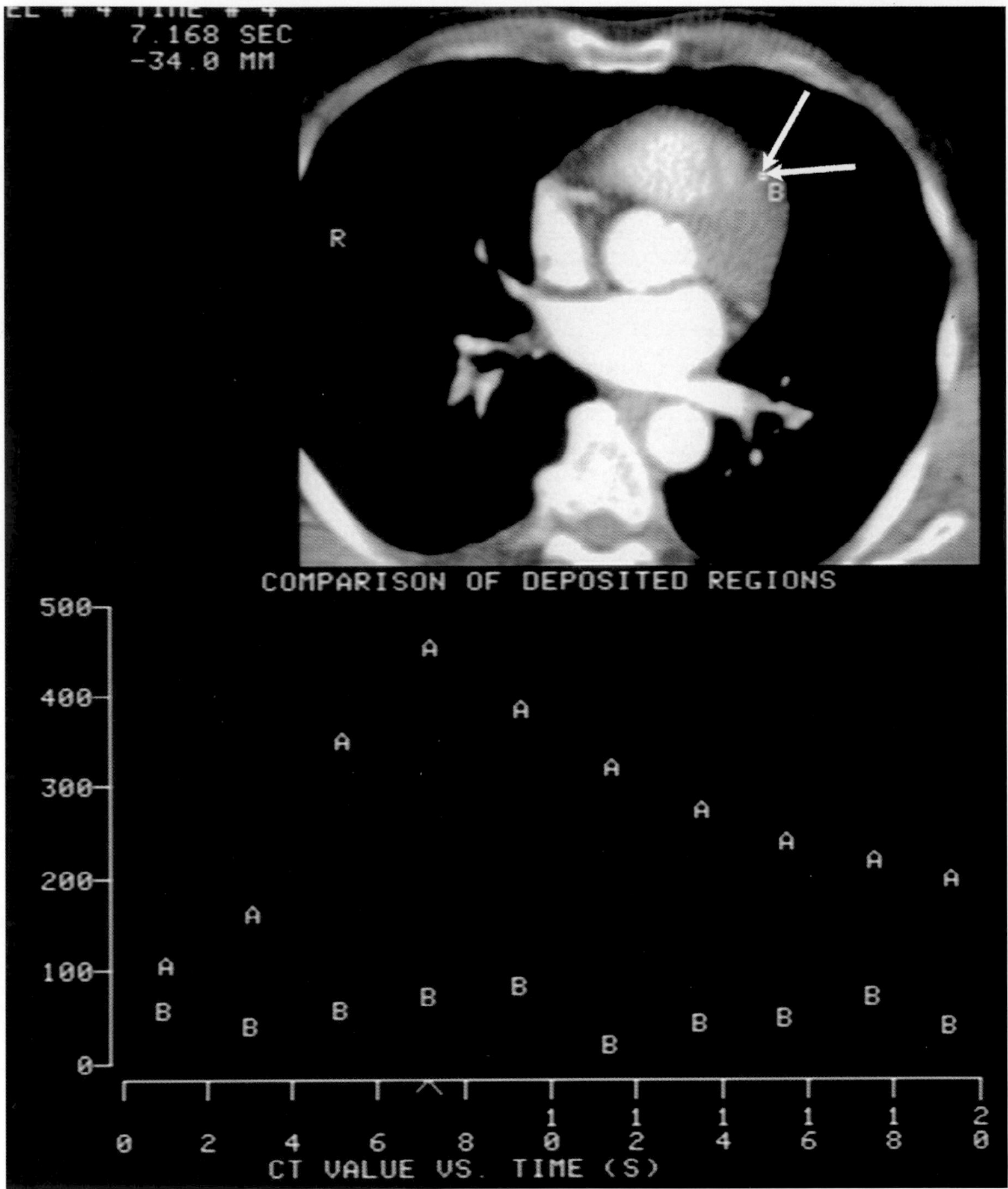

Fig. 4. Transverse CT scan (16-row CT) of stents placed in the left anterior descending artery and the first diagonal branch.

stenosis or occlusion (Figs. 6A,B). The visualization of in-stent stenosis remains a problem caused by high-contrast artifacts of the stainless steel stent struts, which make an exact differentiation between struts noncalcified plaques, and calcified plaques impossible. The newest development of dedicated reconstruction algorithms and improved in-plane resolution might reduce these artifacts *(32)*, and it may be possible to differentiate between stent struts and neoproliferation.

SUMMARY

Currently, exact quantification of stenosis is possible only with coronary angiography. The time-attenuation analysis allows only the differentiation between a patent stent, high-grade stenosis, and stent occlusion, but no exact quantification of the coronary arterial flow.

Overlapping contrast-enhanced single-section EBCT examination is widely used in the noninvasive visualization of the

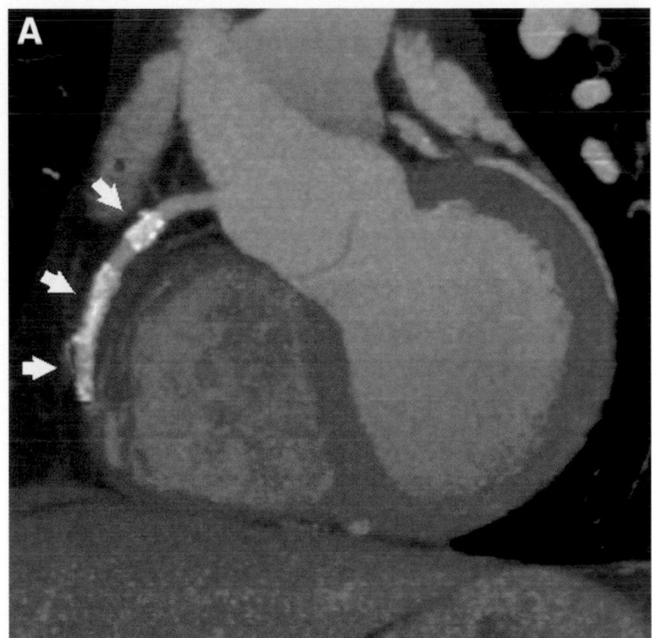

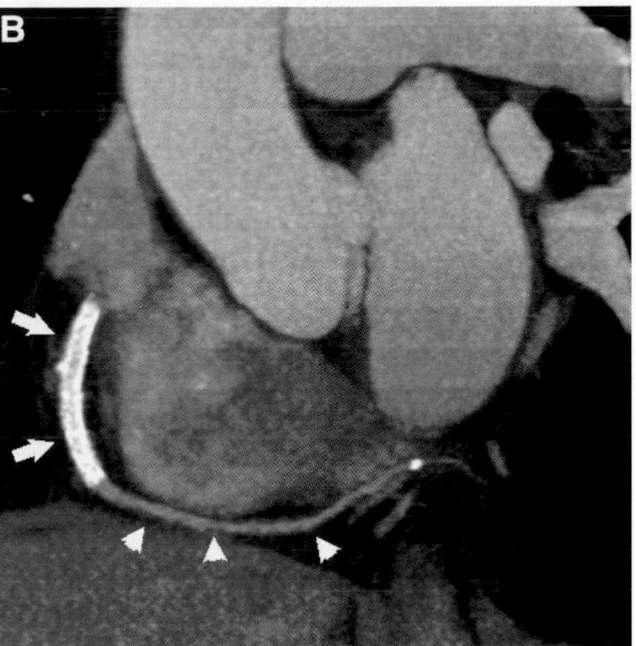

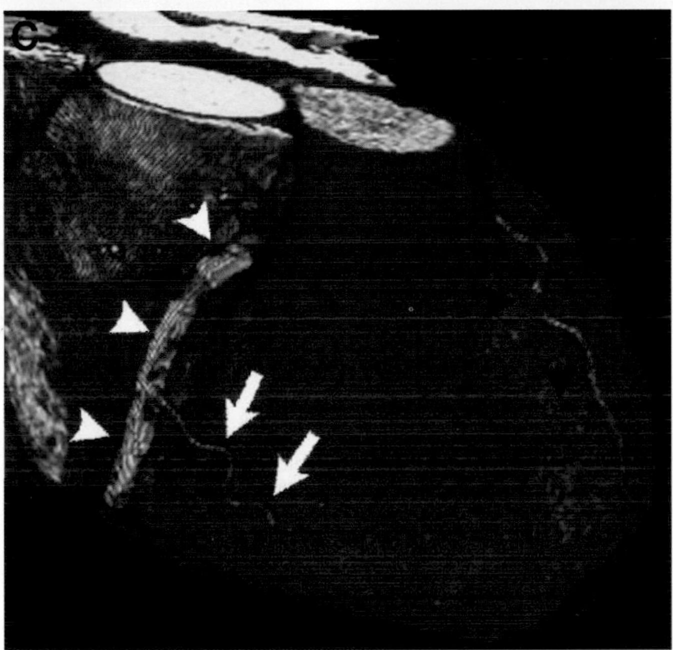

Fig. 5. (**A**) Maximum intensity projection of a 16-row CT dataset. Visualization of the proximal and middle segment of the right coronary artery with patent stents (arrows). (**B**) Maximum intensity projection of the same patient. Visualization of the middle and distal segments of the right coronary artery with patent stents (arrows) and a patent distal vessel segment (arrowheads). (**C**) Volume-rendering technique of the same patient. The white arrowheads show the stents in the proximal and middle vessel region of the right coronary artery. Visualization of a side branch (arrows) and of the left anterior descending (black arrowheads).

coronary system, and several studies have demonstrated the high sensitivity and specificity in the detection of high-grade stenosis in native coronary arteries *(33,34)*, but the detection of in-stent stenosis with EBCT remains an unsolved problem.

MDCT technology, especially the acquisition of a 3D data set with isotropic voxels, scan protocols developed for stent imaging, and postprocessing modalities may in future lead to a better visualization of the stent lumen.

The major drawback of MDCT is the significant increase of the effective radiation dose. Hunold et al. measured doses in the range from 6.7 to 10.9 mSv for male patients and 8.1 to 13.0 mSv for female patients in contrast-enhanced MDCT, and 1.5 and 2.0 mSv for male and female patients in electron beam CTA, respectively *(35)*. These data are consistent with reports from others. The development of new scan techniques might lead to a significant decrease of the radiation dose.

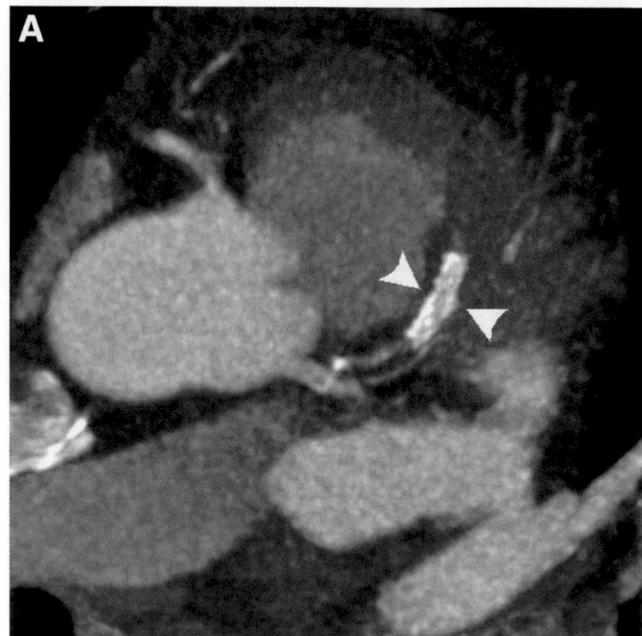

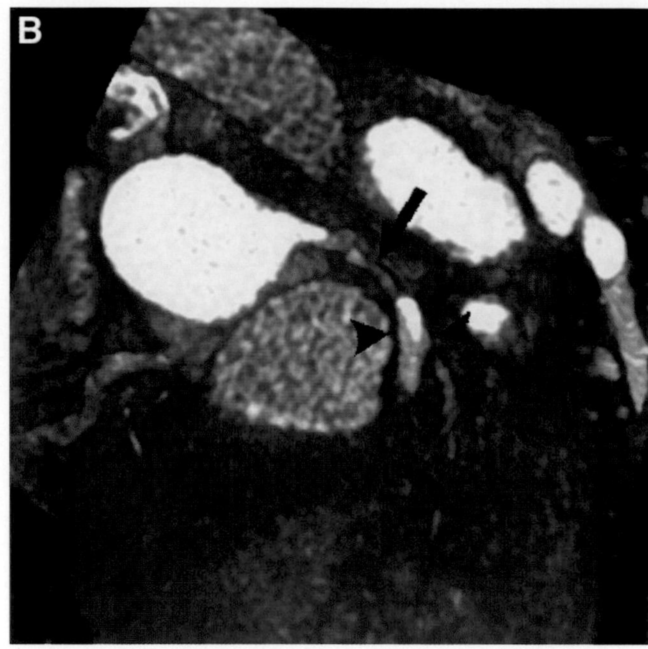

Fig. 6. (**A**) Maximum intensity projection of a stent occlusion in the left anterior descending artery. Weak contrast enhancement proximal to the stent. There is no attenuation in the vessel region distally of the stent. Arrowheads indicate the stent. (**B**) Volume-rendering technique of the same patient. The arrow indicates the vessel region proximal of the stent, the arrowheads indicate the stent.

Noninvasive imaging of coronary artery stents, stent patency, and in-stent restenosis is a clinically attractive application of fast computed tomography. Currently, spatial resolution, especially in submillimeter distances from the stainless steel struts, is not always sufficient to quantitate in-stent stenosis with an accuracy high enough for clinical purposes. However, improvements in scanner technology are in sight that might overcome this problem. Further, functional imaging at the coronary artery or myocardial level *(36)* using indicator dilution principles and additional infusion of adenosine may further enhance diagnostic accuracy of noninvasive assessment of coronary stent patency.

REFERENCES

1. Sigwart U, Puel J, Mirkovitch V, Joffre F, Kappenberger L. Intravascular stents to prevent occlusion and restenosis after transluminal angioplasty. N Engl J Med 1987;316:701–706.
2. Haude M, Erbel R, Straub U, Dietz U, Schatz R, Meyer J. Results on intracoronary stents for management of coronary dissection after balloon angioplasty. Am J Cardiol 1991;67:691–969.
3. Roubin GS, Cannon AD, Agrawal SK, et al. Intracoronary stenting for acute and threatened closure complicating percutaneous transluminal coronary angioplasty. Circulation 1992;85:916–927.
4. De Feyter PJ, De Scheerder I, van den Brand M, Laarman GJ, Suryarpranata H, Serrruys PW. Emergency stenting for refractory acute coronary artery occlusion during coronary angioplasty. Am J Cardiol 1990;66:1147–1150.
5. Herman HC, Buchbinder M, Cleman MW, et al. Emergent use of balloon-expandable coronary artery stenting for failed percutaneous transluminal coronary angioplasty. Circulation 1992;86:812–819.
6. Fischman DL, Leon MB, Baim DS, et al. A randomized comparison of coronary-stent placement and balloon angioplasty in patients with coronary artery disease: Stent Restenosis Study Investigators. N Engl J Med 1994;331:496–501.
7. Serruys PW, de Jaegere P, Kiemeneji I, et al. A comparison of balloon-expandable stent implantation with balloon angioplasty in patients with coronary artery disease: Benestent Study Group. N Engl J Med 1994;331:489–495.
8. Serruys PW, Emanuelsson H, van der Giessen W, et al. Heparin-coated Palmaz-Schatz stents in human coronary arteries: early outcome of the Benestent-II pilot study. Circulation 1996;93: 412–422.
9. Erbel R, Haude M, Höpp HW, et al. Coronary-artery stenting compared with balloon angioplasty for restenosis after initial balloon angioplasty: Restenosis Stent (REST) Study Group. N Engl J Med 1998;339:1672–1678.
10. Antoniucci D, Valenti R, Santoro GM, et al. Restenosis after coronary stenting in current clinical practice. Am Heart J 1998;135: 510–518.
11. DiMario C, Reimers B, Almagor Y, et al. Procedural and follow-up results with a new balloon expandable stent in unselected lesions. Heart 1998;79:234–241.
12. De Gregorio J, Kobayashi Y, Albiero R, et al. Coronary artery stenting in the elderly: short-term outcome and long-term angiographic and clinical follow-up. J Am Coll Cardiol 1998;32: 577–583.
13. Bittl JA. Advances in coronary angioplasty. N Engl J Med 1996;335:1290–1302.
14. Kuntz RA, Gibson CM, Nobuyoshi M. Generalized model of restenosis after conventional balloon angioplasty, stenting and diretional atherectomy.J Am Coll Cardiol 1993;21:15–25.
15. Kuntz RA, Safian RD, Carozza JP Jr., et al. The importance of acute luminal diameter in determining restenosis after coronary artherectomy or stenting. Circulation 1992;86:1827–1835.
16. Pan M, Suarez de Lezo J, Velasco F, et al. Reduction of thrombotic and hemorrhagic complications after stent implantation. Am Heart J 1996;132(6):1119–1126.
17. Spinler S, Cheng J. Antithrombotic therapy after intracoronary stenting. Pharmacotherapy 1997;17(1):74–90.
18. Leon MB, Baim DS, Popma JJ, Gordon PC, et al. A clinical trial comparing three antithrombotic-drug regimens after coronary-

artery stenting. Stent Anticoagulation Restenosis Study Investigators. N Engl J Med 1998;339(23):1665–1671.

19. Teirstein PS, Massullo V, Jani S, et al. Catheter-based radiotherapy to inhibit restenosis after coronary stenting. N Engl J Med 1997;336: 1697–1703.
20. Leon MB, Teirstein PS, Moses JW, et al. Localized intracoronary gamma-radiation therapy to inhibit the recurrence of restenosis after stenting. N Engl J Med 2001;344:250–256.
21. Serruys PW, Emanuelsson H, van der Giessen W, et al. Heparin-coated Palmaz-Schatz stents in human coronary arteries. Early outcome of the Benestent-II Pilot Study. Circulation 1996;93(3): 412–422.
22. Morice MC, Serruys PW, Sousa JE, et al. A randomized comparison of a sirolimus-eluting stent with a standard stent for coronary revascularization. N Engl J Med 2002;346(23):1773–1780.
23. Fattori R, Piva T. Drug-eluting stents in vascular intervention. Lancet 2003 (18);361(9353):247–249.
24. Verin V, Popowski Y, de Bruyne B, et al. Endoluminal beta-radiation therapy for the prevention of coronary restenosis after balloon angioplasty. The Dose-Finding Study Group. N Engl J Med 2001; 344:243–249.
25. Möhlenkamp S, Pump H, Baumgart D, et al. Minimally invasive evaluation of coronary stents with electron beam computed tomography: in vivo and in vitro experience. Cath Cardiovasc Interv 1999;48(1):39–47.
26. Möhlenkamp S, Schmermund A, Pump H, et al. Characterization of balloon expandable coronary stent morphology using electron beam computed tomography. Materialwiss Werkst 1999;30:793–800.
27. Schmermund A, Haude M, Baumgart D, et al. Non-invasive assessment of coronary Palmaz-Schatz stents by contrast enhanced electron beam computed tomography. Eur Heart J 1996;17:1546–1553.
28. Pump H, Möhlenkamp, C. Sehnert, et al. Electron beam CT in the noninvasive assessment of coronary stent patency. Acad Radiol 1998;5:858–862.
29. Pump H, Möhlenkamp S, Sehnert, et al. Coronary arterial stent patency: assessment with electron-beam CT. Radiology 2000;214: 447–452.
30. Elredge WJ, Santolan EC, Taylor MA, et al. Noninvasive assessment of intracoronary stent patency using ultrafast computed tomography (abstract). Am J Card Imaging 1994;8 (Suppl):12.
31. Achenbach S, Ulzheimer S, Baum U. Noninvasive coronary angiography by retrospectively ECG-gated multislice spiral CT. Circulation 2000;102:2823.
32. Flohr T, Bruder H, Stierstorfer, et al. New technical developments in multislice CT, part 2: sub-millimeter 16-slice scanning and increased gantry rotation speed for cardiac imaging. Fortschr Röntgenstr 2002; 174:1022–1027.
33. Moshage EL, Achenbach S, Seese B, et al. Coronary artery stenoses: three-dimensional imaging with electrocardiographically triggered contrast agent-enhanced, electron-beam CT. Radiology 1995;196: 707–714.
34. Achenbach S, Moshage W, Ropers D, et al. Value of electron beam computed tomography for the noninvasive detection of high-grade coronary artery stenoses and occlusions. N Engl J Med 1998;339: 1964–1971.
35. Hunold P, Vogt FM, Schmermund A, et al. Radiation exposure during cardiac CT: effective doses at multi-detector row CT and electron-beam CT. Radiology 2003;226:145–152.
36. Möhlenkamp S, Behrenbeck TR, Lerman A, et al. Coronary microvascular functional reserve: quantification of long-term changes with electron-beam CT preliminary results in a porcine model. Radiology 2001;221(1):229–236.

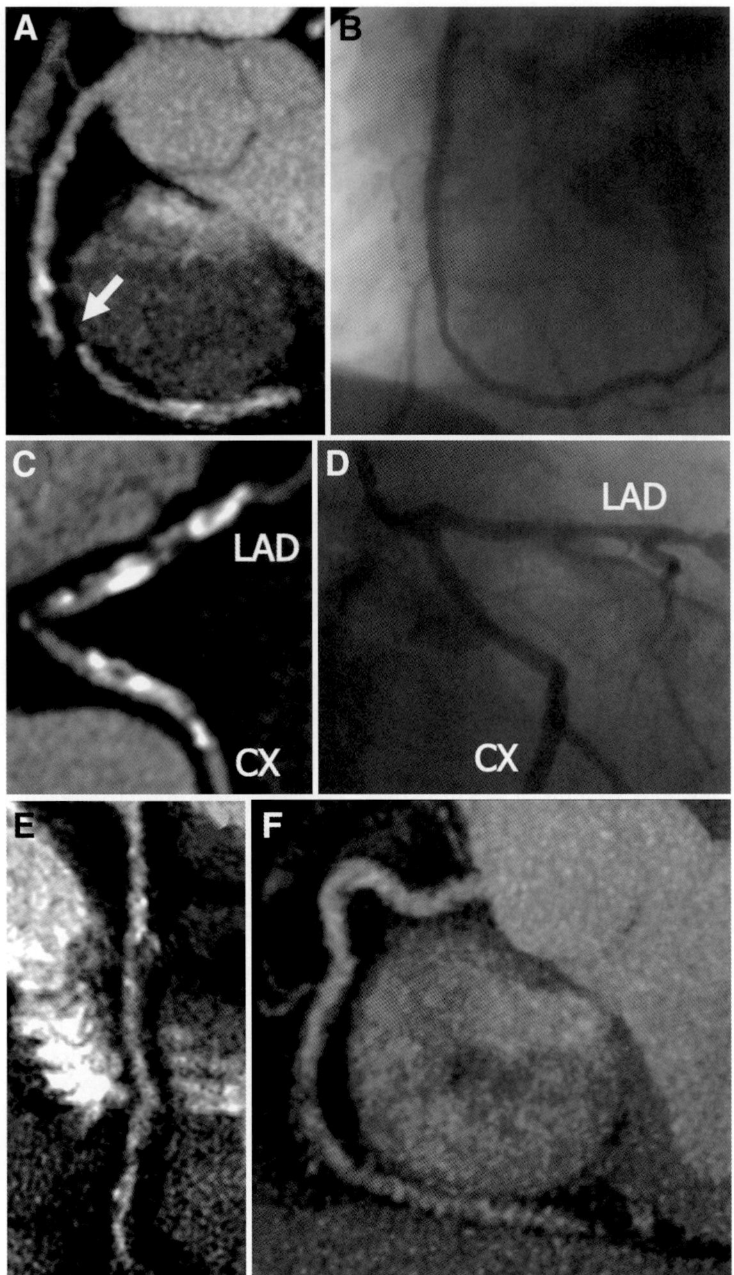

Fig. 2. Image artifacts. The accuracy of Multislice CT can be affected by a number of artifacts. Consecutive slabs are reconstructed during different cardiac phases in the occurrence of irregular heartbeats, which results in stair-step artifacts or in complete discontinuity of the artery (arrow), as in this case **(A,B)**. The presence of extensive calcification of the left anterior descending (LAD) and circumflex coronary artery (CX) limits the assessability as a result of partial-volume artifacts and beam hardening **(C,D)**. At faster heart rates, image-degrading motion artifacts occur **(E)**. Particularly in overweight patients, the attenuation by the surrounding tissue, such as the liver, can decrease the signal-to-noise ratio. In this case, the distal right coronary artery, which runs at the same level as the liver, is poorly assessable **(F)**.

The RCA, which has a large motion radius and short motion-sparse period during the diastole, is a branch that is most affected by motion artifacts caused by residual cardiac motion during the image reconstruction interval. Visualization of the LCx also suffers from motion artifacts. Occasionally it can be difficult to distinguish the small LCx from the adjacent contrast-enhanced cardiac vein. The fact that proximal vessels are better visualized than more distal branches is only partially related to diameter size. Both the middle segment of the RCA as well as the LCx have a larger motion radius compared to the proximal segments. The more distal branches and side branches are most difficult to visualize. In a study that compared the assessability of the different coronary segments with a minimal diameter of 2.0 mm, the proximal RCA was evaluable in 88%, compared to 61% of the middle and 60% of the distal segments. Assessment of the proximal LAD was possible in 89%, com-

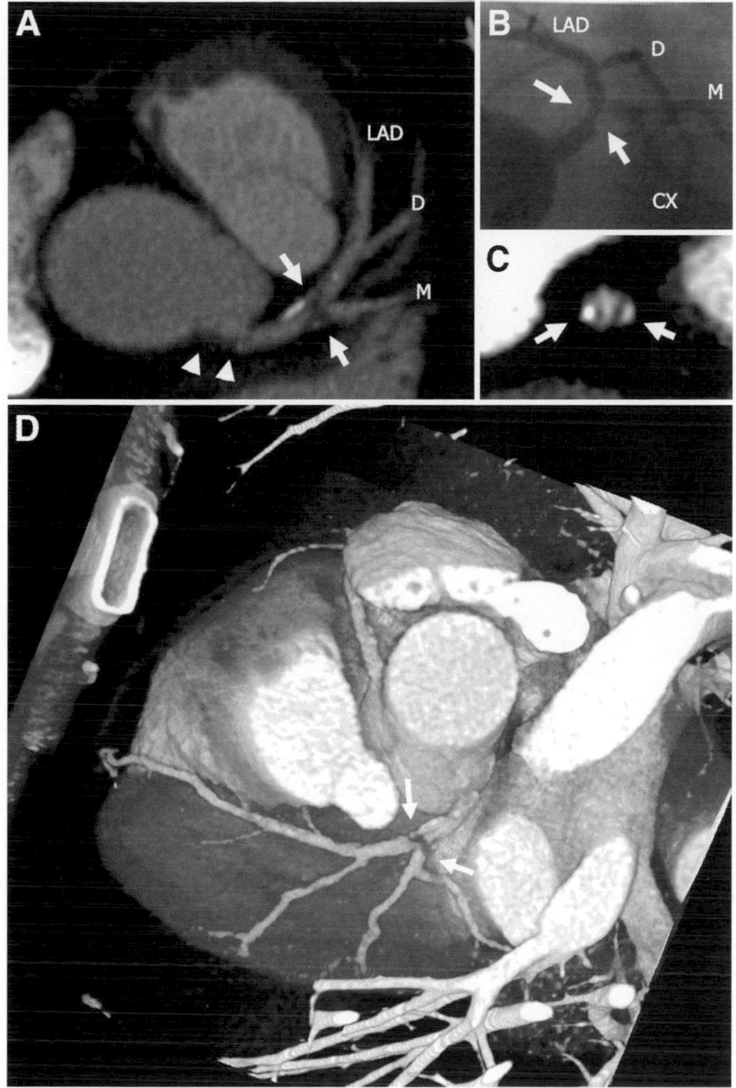

Fig. 3. Lesions in the left main bifurcation. A significant lesion (arrow), consisting of two partially calcified plaques, is situated at the distal part of the left main coronary artery, obstructing both the left anterior descending (LAD) as well as the left circumflex branch (CX) (**A** and **D**). The cross-section of the vessel confirms the distinct configuration of the lesions (**C**). Additionally, more non-calcified plaque material (arrowhead) can be observed in the proximal part of the left main artery (arrowheads) (**A**). Diagnonal (D) and marginal (M) branch.

pared to 77% of the middle and 75% of the distal segments. In this study, the proximal and the middle segments of the LCx were equally difficult to evaluate—57% and 56%, respectively*(19)*.

DETECTION OF CORONARY OBSTRUCTION

When considering only the coronary arteries or segments that were imaged with sufficient image quality, the sensitivity of 4-slice MSCT to detect significant coronary obstruction, defined as ≥50% lumen diameter reduction, ranges between 75% and 95%, and the specificity between 76% and 99% *(10–16)*. As can be expected, the sensitivity and specificity are inversely correlated, as well as the number of excluded segments and the diagnostic performance in the assessable segments. The positive and negative predictive value ranged between 56% and 99%, and 93% and 99%, respectively. Compared to >50% lesions, Achenbach et al. found a higher diagnostic performance for the detection of lesions with a lumen diameter reduction of at least 70% *(11)*. The results show that exclusion of disease in a normal vessel is less challenging than the classification of a diseased vessel as significantly stenosed or not, particularly in the presence of extensive calcification. The apparent size of the calcium deposits causes overestimation of the total plaque size, which results in false-positive assessments. According to some investigators, MSCT coronary angiography may be most valuable as a tool to exclude significant lesions in patients with a relatively low pretest likelihood for the presence of stenoses, and not for the staging of patients with very high likelihood and expectedly advanced coronary artery degeneration. Figs. 3–8 are examples of MSCT imaging of coronary obstruction with corresponding conventional X-ray angiograms.

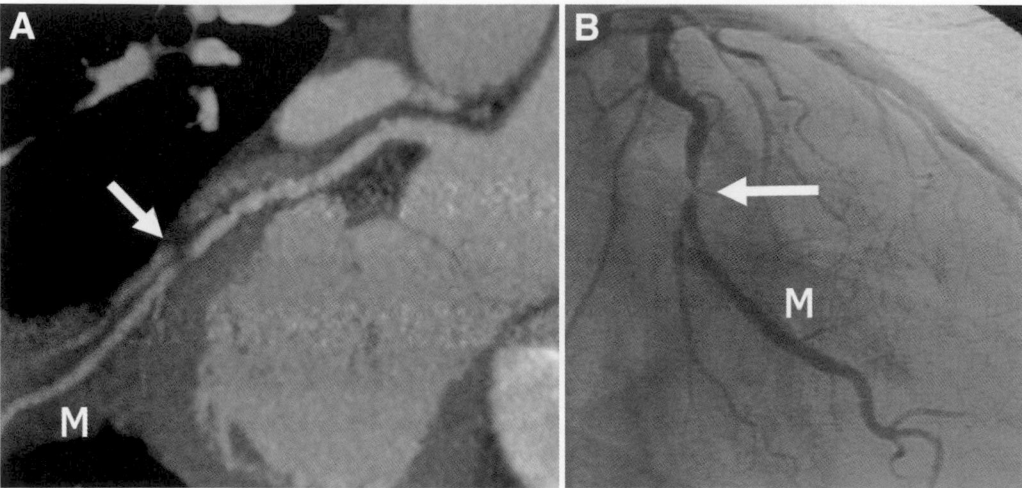

Fig. 4. Significant lesion in the left circumflex coronary artery. A significant lesion (arrow) was found in the mid-segment of the left circumflex branch, just proximal of the bifurcation of a major marginal branch (M), both by multislice CT (**A**) and conventional angiography (**B**).

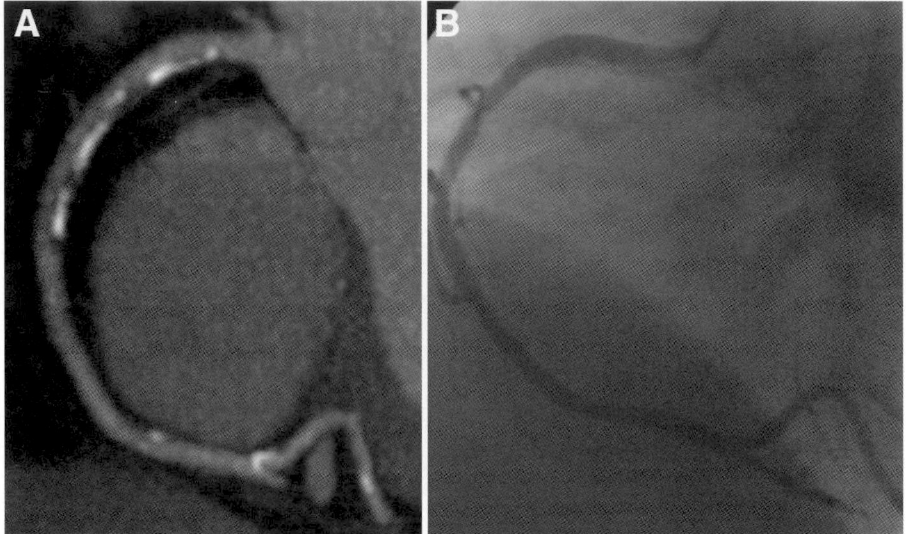

Fig. 5. Diffuse coronary artery disease. This right coronary artery shows extensive atherosclerotic degeneration, with calcified and noncalcified plaque material along the entire length of the proximal inner curve, and separate lesions more distally (**A**). Although the MSCT shows no severe stenosis, the absence of significant lesions was more straightforward on the conventional angiogram.

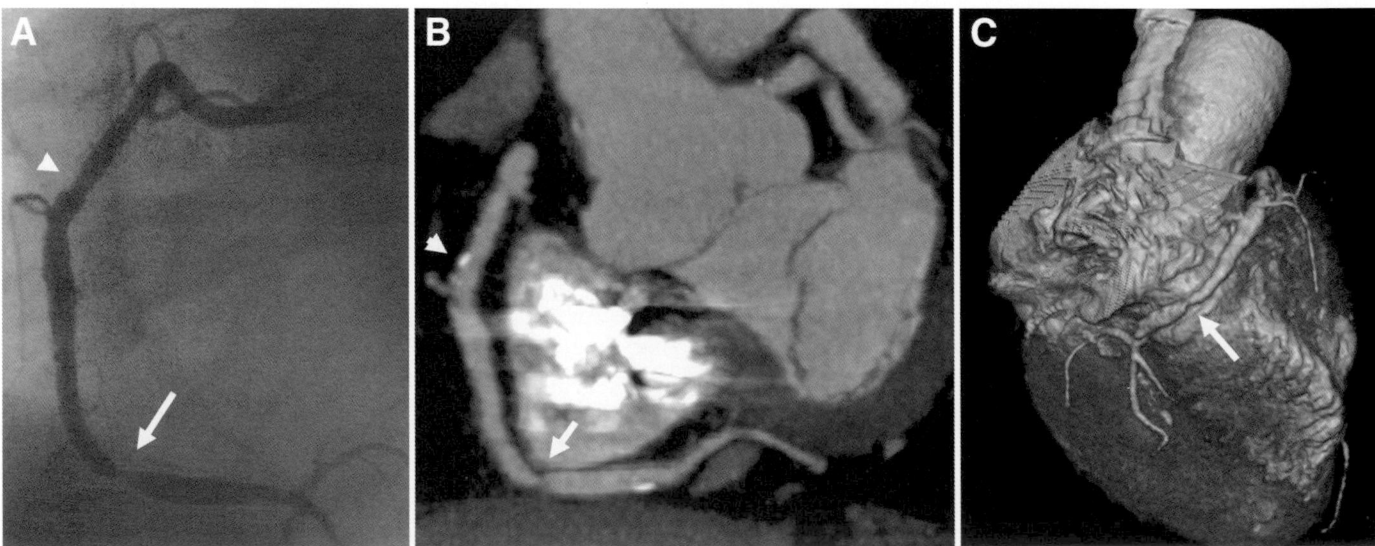

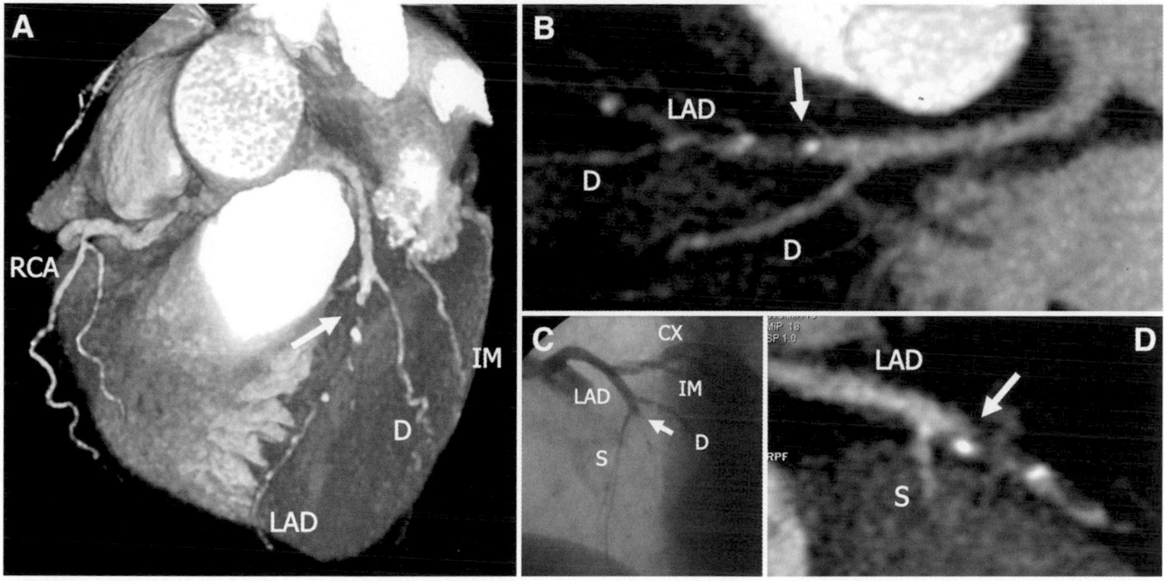

Fig. 6. Occlusion of the left anterior descending coronary artery. Three-dimensional reconstruction (**A**) and curved multiplanar reconstruction (**B**) of a CT coronary angiogram, showing an occluded (arrow) left anterior descending coronary artery (LAD) (**B**), which was confirmed by conventional coronary angiography (**C**). A sagittal cross-section shows in detail the different plaque components, both calcified and noncalcified, as well as some residual contrast enhancement within the obstructed segment (**D**). Right coronary artery (RCA), diagonal (D), intermediate (IM), and circumflex branch (CX).

In a study comparing the diagnostic accuracy of MSCT in relation to the proximity of the coronary segment, a sensitivity and specificity of 92% and 96% were found in the largest proximal segments (RCA1, LM, LAD6), 85% and 90% for the middle segments (RCA2, LAD7, LCx11), 71% and 94% for the distal segments (RCA3, LAD8, LCx13), and 50% and 89% for the side branches *(19)*. In the study by Kopp et al., the sensitivity to detect stenotic lesions significantly increased, to 97/99%, by selectively assessing the proximal and middle coronary segments *(14)*.

The segments and vessels that were excluded from analysis because of inadequate image quality contained a substantial number of undetected lesions. If these lesions in nonevaluable vessels are included in the analysis as false-negative interpretations, the sensitivity is much lower in most studies, between 49% and 93% *(10–16)*.

16-SLICE MSCT CORONARY ANGIOGRAPHY

To date two studies have been published comparing MSCT and conventional coronary angiography using 16-slice MSCT *(17,18)*. The advantages offered by this new technique are a faster rotation time of 0.42 s, an extended number of narrower detector rows (0.75 mm), and shorter total scan time of approx 20 s. For the ECG-gated protocol, the 12 central detector rows were applied. To optimize the image quality, consistent heart rate control was incorporated into both protocols. In the study by Nieman et al., patients with a prescan heart rate over 65 beats

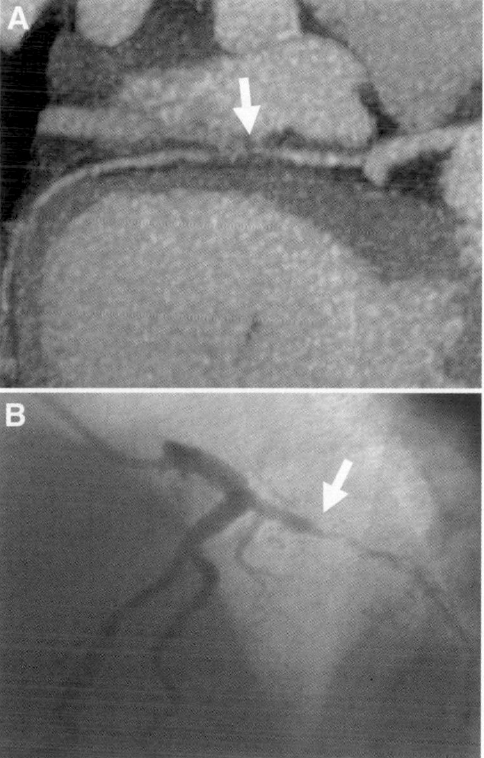

Fig. 7. Occlusion of the left circumflex coronary artery. Curved maximum intensity projection of a predominantly noncalcified occlusion (arrow) of the left circumflex branch (**A**), confirmed by conventional coronary angiography (**B**). The distal segment is filled collaterally by the left anterior descending coronary artery.

Fig. 8. *(oppositer page, bottom left)* Stenosis of the distal right coronary artery. Using thin-slab maximum intensity projection (**B**) and volume rendering (**C**), a stenotic lesion (arrow) is demonstrated in the distal right coronary artery. Also minor wall irregularities, caused by small calcified lesions (arrowheads), can be observed, and were confirmed by conventional angiography (**A**).

Table 2
Patient-Based Diagnostic Performance of Multislice CT (MSCT) Coronary Angiography

	4-slice MSCT (19) Segment-based (N = 53)		*16-slice MSCT (17) Vessel-based (N = 58)*	
	Accuracy	Predictive value	Accuracy	Predictive value
No lesions	9/14 (64%)	9/19 (47%)	7/7 (100%)	7/8 (88%)
Single lesion/vessel	9/23 (39%)	9/15 (60%)	12/16 (75%)	12/20 (60%)
Multiple lesions/vessel	11/16 (69%)	11/19 (58%)	26/35 (74%)	26/30 (87%)
Overall	29/53 (55%)	29/53 (55%)	45/58 (78%)	45/58 (78%)

per minute (bpm) were given an oral dose of 100 mg metoprolol 1 h prior to the examination, decreasing the average heart rate to 57 bpm. Ropers et al. used 50 mg of atenolol to decrease the heart rates of all patients with >60 bpm, down to an average heart rate of 62 bpm. Only 7% and 12% of the coronary branches contained sections with a poor image quality. Compared to the other branches, the RCA was still most vulnerable to image quality degradation. Nieman et al., irrespectively of the image quality, evaluated all branches with a minimal lumenal diameter of 2.0 mm, and found a sensitivity and specificity of 95% and 86% to detect significantly stenosed branches. The positive and negative predictive value were 80% and 97% *(17)*. All four missed lesions were located in the LCx and marginal branches, no lesions were missed in the LM, LAD, or RCA. The 20 overestimations included 7 lesions with a subsignificant (40–49%) diameter reduction, according to quantitative coronary angiography. Including only the evaluable (88%) vessels (minimal diameter 1.5 mm), Ropers et al. found a sensitivity and specificity of 92% and 93% to detect significant stenoses. Without exclusion of nonevaluable lesions, the sensitivity was 73% *(18)*.

PATIENT-BASED ASSESSMENT

Understanding that different methods of data analysis and presentation were used is important to compare the results of the previously mentioned studies. For instance, by using an evaluation based on the individual coronary segments, the relative and absolute number of nondiseased segments is much larger, compared to the number of nondiseased branches in case of a main branch–based analysis. One of the consequences is that for the segment-based studies, the specificity is often better compared to the those of the branch-based studies. Perhaps a more comparable indicator of the clinical applicability of MSCT coronary angiography is the diagnostic accuracy based on the individual patients. Using 4-slice MSCT, Giesler et al. showed that in 39 out of 100 patients (39%), all vessels could be evaluated *(15)*. In the study by Knez et al., the accuracy to detect no, single, double, or triple vessel disease was 74% (32/43 patients) after exclusion of the nonassessable segments *(12)*. Nieman et al. reported a 56% (45/78 patients) accuracy to distinguish no, single, or multivessel disease, without the exclusion of nonassessable segments *(16)*. A high heart rate affects also the diagnostic accuracy per patient in a negative way *(16)*. By 16-slice MSCT, Nieman et al. reported a patient-based accuracy to distinguish no, single, or multivessel disease of 78% (Table 2) *(17)*. In this study, the number of diseased vessels was overestimated in a number of patients, but none with significant coronary stenoses were falsely evaluated as normal, without exclusion of nonassessable segments. Ropers et al. correctly assessed 85% as having one or more lesions *(18)*.

CONSIDERATIONS AND LIMITATIONS

TEMPORAL RESOLUTION AND THE HEART RATE

Coronary Motion

The coronary arteries are in constant motion, and therefore an infinitely short acquisition or reconstruction time is required to acquire completely motionless images. Angiography studies have shown that during diastole a brief moment of near-immobility occurs *(20)*. The moment and duration of this window of imaging opportunity varies per person and per vessel, but always shortens at higher heart rates. Generally, the RCA moves at a wider radius and has a shorter motion-sparse period compared to the left coronary artery. The RCA is therefore most vulnerable to motion artifacts caused by cardiac motion (Fig. 2).

Temporal Resolution

The temporal resolution of 4-slice MSCT scanners is 250 ms at low heart rates. At a heart rate of 50 bpm the duration of the heart cycle measures 1200 ms, of which 21% is required for the reconstruction of a set of axial slices. At a heart rate of 80 bpm the ratio is 33%, and at 120 bpm the ratio is 50%, thereby increasing the occurrence of motion artifacts. Considering the fact that the shortening of the diastolic phase at higher heart rates is more substantial than the shortening of the systolic phase, the negative effect of a fast heart rate on the image quality is even more profound. At higher heart rates, multi-segment reconstruction algorithms can improve the effective temporal resolution by combining data from consecutive heart cycles. However, this reduction is highly dependent on the actual heart rate, and does not always result in an improvement of image quality. Using a bi-segmental reconstruction algorithm at a rotation time of 500 ms, a heart rate of 68 bpm results in an effective temporal resolution of 125 ms, while at 80 bpm the noncomplementary configuration of the X-ray source and detector array allows no reduction at all, maintaining a 250-ms effective temporal resolution. Up to approx 75 bpm, the relative temporal resolution, the ratio of the image reconstruction interval to the RR interval, is less than 30%. The use of more than two segments for reconstruction of a set of slices, which potentially reduces the duration of the image reconstruction interval per cycle to less than 100 ms, requires a very slow table advance, resulting in an increased radiation exposure to the patient.

Motion Artifacts

Motion artifacts are probably the most important limitation of MSCT coronary angiography, and lead to substantial numbers of nonassessable investigations. The high number of nonassessable vessels reduces the clinical applicability of the technique. Two studies evaluated the diagnostic accuracy of MSCT in relation to the heart rate of the patient. Giesler et al. divided 100 patients into four groups and showed that in patients with a heart rate below 60 bpm, motion artifacts occurred in only 8% of the coronary arteries, compared to 18% at a heart rate between 61 and 70 bpm, 41% at a heart rate between 71 and 80 bpm, and 22% at a heart rate of more than 80 bpm. The respective percentage of nonassessable vessels (22%, 23%, 50%, and 24%) resulted in a degrading overall sensitivity to detect >70% coronary diameter narrowing—67%, 55%, 35%, and 22%, for the respective heart-rate groups *(15)*. In a study by Nieman et al., 78 patients were equally divided into 3 groups according to the average heart rate during MSCT coronary angiography. In the low-heart-rate group (56±4 bpm), intermediate-heart-rate group (67±3 bpm), and high-heart-rate group (82±9 bpm), the number of assessable segments were 78%, 73%, and 54%, resulting in an overall sensitivity to detect >50% lumenal stenosis of 82%, 61%, and 32%, respectively. The accuracy of MSCT to classify patients as having no, single, or multivessel disease, without exclusion of nonassessable segments, was 73%, 54%, and 42%, for each respective group *(16)*. Based on these and other experiences, many centers have introduced the administration of antichronotropic medication, such as β-blockers, particularly in patients with higher heart rates, to reduce the occurrence of motion artifacts and improve the accuracy of MSCT coronary angiography.

State-of-the-art scanners now have a rotation time below 500 ms, and combined with sufficient heart-rate control, the reliability of MSCT has substantially improved (Table 1). It needs to be established up to what heart rate these faster scanners can acquire motion-sparse images, but it seems unlikely that a rotation time of 400 ms or more provides sufficient image quality in the majority of patients with a heart rate over 80 bpm, when the coronary arteries are concerned.

RESPIRATION AND THE SCAN TIME

Respiratory motion is suppressed during scanning by maintaining an inspiratory breath-hold. Using 4-slice scanners the relatively long scan time of 35–45 s that is required to scan the entire heart at a narrow collimation can be too long in a substantial number of patients. In addition to respiratory motion artifacts, the long breath-hold increases the patient's heart rate, resulting in an increased occurrence of cardiac motion artifacts. The new generation MSCT scanners are equipped with up to 16 slices and have a faster rotation, which results in a total scan time below 20 s. A breath-hold of 20 s can be performed by most patients, and does not result in a significant acceleration of the heart rate.

ARRHYTHMIA

Inappropriate ECG-synchronization results in interslice discontinuity (Fig. 2). Contrary to prospectively ECG-triggered modalities, such as EBCT and most MRI sequences, ECG-gated spiral CT image reconstruction allows for retrospective editing of the ECG. This can be useful to correct for inappropriate interpretation of the ECG by the reconstruction algorithm, and provides an opportunity to manually insert R-wave indicators in case of ECG noise. Editing of the ECG will not suffice in patients with continuous arrhythmia. For instance, during atrial fibrillation, the end-diastolic volume constantly varies because of the alternating filling time. Thereby, the heart will be displaced and have a different shape and position at each consecutive heart cycle and acquisition. Apart from cardiac motion artifacts, this results in severe and noncorrectable interslice discontinuity and noninterpretable results. On the other hand, nonsinus rhythm, delayed conduction, or otherwise unusual configuration of the ECG is no contra-indication for MSCT, as long as the RR interval variation is within an acceptable range.

HIGHLY ATTENUATING MATERIAL

STENTS AND SURGICAL MATERIAL

Material with strong X-ray attenuating characteristics, such as metal and calcium, cause beam hardening and partial volume artifacts. Because stents are positioned within the coronary, adjacent to the lumen, assessment of the lumen diameter is impaired. In patients who underwent bypass grafting, sternal wires and vascular clips can cause streak artifacts that hamper proper assessment of the bypass grafts as well as coronary arteries. Both patient groups will be discussed in more detail in following chapters. Occasionally, pacemaker wires in the right heart can cause identical artifacts, obscuring the RCA. In case of biventricular pacing systems, with wires positioned in the cardiac veins, assessment of the left circumflex and the left anterior descending coronary arteries is severely hampered.

Calcifications

Calcium deposits also cause a strong attenuation of the X-ray and are the most frequent cause of high-density artifacts, such as partial-volume and beam-hardening artifacts. Partial-volume artifacts are directly but not solely related to the size of the voxel, or three-dimensional image elements. The direct result is that calcified plaque material appears larger than it actually is, thereby increasing the apparent severity of the lumen narrowing and complicating accurate assessment (Fig. 2). By experience, most reviewers will take the overestimation into account when assessing the lumen diameter of a calcified lesion. Nevertheless, an accurate semi-quantitative assessment of coronary arteries with extensive coronary calcification remains less reliable, and patients with suspected or known advanced coronary artery disease are therefore not the most suitable candidates for CT coronary angiography.

All studies comparing MSCT and conventional coronary angiography report that extensive calcification of the coronary arteries prevented assessment of a substantial number of segments and resulted in a number of false-positive or false-negative interpretations of significant stenoses *(10–19)*. In order to avoid contrast-enhanced CT angiography in these individuals, some proposed to perform a low-dose nonenhanced scan in all patients prior to angiography, to determine the amount of calcium in the coronary arteries and exclude unsuitable candidates.

Table 3
Diagnostic Performance of Electron Beam CT to Detect Coronary Stenosis, Using Conventional Coronary Angiography As the Standard of Reference

		A	*N*	*Assess.*	*D*	*Prev*	*Excl.*	*Se*	*Sp*	*PPV*	*NPV*	*Se*[a]
Nakanishi *(3)*	3.0	–	37	Vessel	50%	0.8	—	74%	94%	68%	93%	74%
Reddy *(4)*	3.0	–	23	Vessel	50%	1.3	10%	88%	78%	65%	94%	77%
Schmermund *(5)*	3.0	+	28	Segment	50%	1.1	28%	82%	88%	57%	96%	70%
Rensing *(6)*	1.5	+	37	Segment	50%	1.1	81%	77%	94%	73%	95%	63%
Achenbach *(7)*	3.0	–	125	Vessel	70%	0.8	25%	92%	94%	78%	98%	70%
Budoff *(8)*	3.0	–	52	Vessel	50%	≥1.1	11%	78%	91%	78%	91%	NR
Achenbach *(9)*	3.0	–	36	Vessel	75%	≥1.0	20%	92%	94%	85%	92%	NR

A, use of atropine; Assess., method of assessment; D, diameter reduction considered significantly stenosed; Prev, number of stenotic vessel per patient; Excl., percentage of excluded segments/branches. Sensitivity (Se), specificity (Sp), positive (PPV) and negative predictive value (NPV) regarding the assessable segments/branches; NR, not reported.
[a]Sensitivity including missed lesions in nonassessable segments/branches.

EBCT AND MR CORONARY ANGIOGRAPHY

ELECTRON-BEAM COMPUTED TOMOGRAPHY

EBCT Coronary Angiography

In 1997 the first studies comparing EBCT with conventional angiography were published. All but one study were performed using an 1.0-mm overlapping 3.0-mm slice thickness *(3–5, 7–9)*. In one study, a nonoverlapping 1.5-mm detector collimation was applied *(6)*. The nonmechanical EBCT is a sequential CT scanner. Prospectively triggered by the patient's electrocardiogram (ECG), the scanner acquires a single slice, after which the table advances to the next slice position. The acquisition is performed during the diastolic phase, and the exact timing of the electron generation is based on the preceding heart cycles. Because of the lack of mechanically rotating elements, the slice acquisition time is very short: 100 ms. The one-slice sequential scan design requires a long scan time and breath-hold to cover the entire heart. To increase the scan coverage, atropine can be injected to increase the heart rate, and consequently the number of slices that can be acquired within a certain breath-hold time *(6)*.

Comparative Studies Against Conventional Angiography

Table 3 lists the results from the comparative publications between contrast-enhanced EBCT and conventional coronary angiography for the purpose of the detection of significant coronary artery obstruction. The study populations ranged from 23 to 125 patients. The use of atropine to increase the number of acquisitions per breath-hold was reported in two studies *(6,7)*. At low heart rates, breath-hold durations of >50 s were reported. In one study no segments were excluded *(3)*; in the others, between 10% and 28% of the segments and vessels were excluded due to impaired image quality. Similar to MSCT, noninterpretability was caused by motion artifacts and extensive calcification. Considering the assessable segments and vessels, the sensitivity to detect significant lumenal narrowing ranged from 74% to 92%. The specificity ranged from 63% to 94%. The positive and negative predictive value ranged from 57% to 85% and 91% to 98%, respectively. If lesions in nonassessable vessels were included as false-negative results, the overall sensitivity decreased to 63% and 77%, although these figures were reported in only five studies. Contrary to the MSCT studies, many of the EBCT studies were limited to the proximal and middle coronary segments *(6,7)*.

Future Developments

A recently introduced generation of EBCT scanners acquires two slices simultaneously, and is capable of scanning several times during one heart cycle, which increases the radiation exposure, but allows for retrospective selection of the data set at the optimal phase. The slice acquisition time has been decreased to 50 ms, which will further improve the image quality with regard to motion artifacts. Whether the use of thinner slices and faster scan times has a negative effect on the contrast-to-noise ratio is currently unknown. Future studies will need to determine the incremental diagnostic value of this new EBCT technology.

MAGNETIC RESONANCE IMAGING

As a result of the lack of X-radiation and use of less harmful and optional contrast media, MRI is an attractive modality for noninvasive imaging, including coronary angiography. Various scanning techniques and data-acquisition sequences have been explored and compared to conventional coronary angiography. The first experiences in 1993 were very promising, reporting a sensitivity and sensitivity to detect significant coronary stenosis of 90% and 92% in 39 patients *(1)*. Currently, respiratory-gated volumetric acquisitions of the entire heart are acquired, or smaller targeted volumes are acquired during a single breath-hold. Intravenous injection of contrast media is possible but is not mandatory to image the coronary artery lumen. Many comparative studies using different 2- and 3D techniques have been published, with widely varying results *(2)*. Between 4% and 48% of the vessels and segments needed to be excluded because of insufficient image quality. The sensitivity and specificity to detect significant coronary obstruction ranged from 38% to 93% and 54% to 97%, respectively *(2)*. A recent multicenter trial using a respiratory-gated free-breathing scan protocol and a study population of 109 patients was published by Kim et al. in 2001 *(21)*. The investigators reported a sensitivity of 93% and specificity of 42% to detect significant lesions in the assessable (84%) proximal and middle coronary segments. The overall sensitivity, including lesions in nonassessable segments, was not reported.

Despite its benign nature, MR coronary angiography is complicated by a relatively low 3D image resolution of rarely less than 1 mm^3, long scanning time, and inconsistent image quality. Compared to CT, the acquisition of the coronary MR is time-consuming and requires dedicated scanners and image sequences as well as experienced operators.

DISCUSSION

MSCT is currently the most accurate noninvasive angiographic modality for the detection of coronary stenosis. Despite the use of radiation and contrast media, MSCT coronary angiography is a relatively safe and simple procedure. All data can be acquired within 20 s, often providing predictable image quality, depending on the heart rate and the coronary calcium status of the patient. The contrast-to-noise ratio is high and the 3D resolution of the current generation scanners is less than 0.3 mm^3. This high spatial resolution allows imaging of small branches, often neglected in the MR and EBCT studies.

CLINICAL IMPLEMENTATION OF MSCT CORONARY ANGIOGRAPHY

However, within the foreseeable future, MSCT coronary angiography will not replace coronary angiography as the reference coronary imaging tool. Conventional angiography is performed without severe complications in the vast majority of patients. Conventional angiography consistently provides high-quality data, with an excellent spatial resolution that allows quantitative assessment of the severity of the stenotic lesion. Apart from motion artifacts, image noise, or calcium-related artifacts, with a slice thickness between 0.5 and 1.0 mm, MSCT can not be expected to provide comparable quantitative assessments. Conventional angiography can also be complemented by functional flow assessment and advanced plaque-imaging techniques. Finally, conventional angiography can immediately be followed by a percutaneous interventional procedure to treat the obstructive problem.

In patients with a modest heart rate, MSCT could, however, provide a useful and reliable alternative to diagnostic catheter-based angiography for the initial detection and localization of coronary stenoses. Additionally, because of its noninvasive nature, MSCT coronary angiography can be introduced into the diagnostic work-up of patients with anginal complaints at an earlier stage, when catheter-based angiography is not yet indicated. Potential applications are the exclusion of an acute coronary obstruction in patients with atypical chest pain at the emergency ward, coronary artery stenosis in patients who need major (noncardiac) surgery, or obstructive disease in patients with inconclusive stress test. MSCT may also be valuable when repeated angiographic follow-up is indicated, or after percutaneous coronary intervention or coronary artery bypass surgery (Table 4).

Table 4
Potential Applications of CT Coronary Angiography

Early detection of stenoses in nonsymptomatics
Exclusion of coronary disease:
high-risk patients
prior to major (noncardiac) surgery
Detection and/or exclusion of stenoses:
Atypical (unstable) chest pain
Nonconclusive stress tests
Substitution for diagnostic X-ray coronary angiography
Prior to percutaneous coronary intervention
High risk patients: aortic disease
Adjuvant to coronary angiography:
Plaque characterization
Complicated coronary intubation
Follow-up:
Percutaneous coronary intervention
Bypass surgery

ADDITIONAL VALUE OF MSCT CORONARY ANGIOGRAPHY

Besides being a noninvasive alternative to conventional coronary angiography, MSCT provides additional and possibly valuable information with respect to the coronary artery wall that is not provided by standard X-ray coronary angiography (Figs. 1, 3, and 5). Nonstenotic atherosclerotic material is visualized well, and the value of plaque characterization by MSCT is currently being investigated and will be discussed in the following chapters *(22)*. Furthermore, MSCT presents a 3D depiction of the coronary arteries, which can be useful when a coronary anomaly is suspected *(23)*. Diseased vessels can easily be related to an infarcted or perfusion-depleted myocardial segment. Besides the coronary arteries, the MSCT scan includes high-quality volumetric information on the entire heart and lower lungs, resulting in (accidental) early detection of abnormalities, including pericardial disease, intra-cardiac thrombi, morphologic valvular disease (calcifications, thickening), lung tumors, and so on. Finally, the raw MSCT data can be used for reconstruction of different cardiac phases, to evaluate the ventricular performance: ventricular cavity volumes, ejection fraction, and regional myocardial wall thickening *(24)*.

FURTHER IMPROVEMENT

To further improve the quality and quantitative potential of MSCT coronary angiography, fundamental characteristics such as the spatial and temporal resolution need to be further optimized. Evaluation of three-dimensional MSCT angiograms may become more efficient and better reproducible with dedicated post-processing tools. More sophisticated tools that combine an accurate, reproducible assessment with presentable overviews are currently being developed, and will improve the clinical implementation of MSCT coronary angiography as a noninvasive tool to localize obstructive coronary artery disease.

REFERENCES

1. Manning WJ, Li W, Edelman RR, et al. A preliminary report comparing magnetic resonance coronary angiography with conventional angiography. N Engl J Med 1993;328–832.
2. Fayad ZA, Fuster V, Nikolaou K, et al. Computed tomography and magnetic resonance imaging for noninvasive coronary angiography and plaque imaging. Current and potential future concepts. Circulation 2002;106:2026–2034.
3. Nakanishi T, Ito K, Imazu M, et al. Evaluation of coronary artery stenoses using electron-beam CT and multiplanar reformation. J Comput Assist Tomogr 1997;21:121–127.

4. Reddy G, Chernoff DM, Adams JR, et al. Coronary artery stenoses: assessment with contrast-enhanced electron-beam CT and axial reconstructions. Radiology 1998;208:167–172.
5. Schmermund A, Rensing BJ, Sheedy PF, et al. Intravenous electron-beam computed tomographic coronary angiography for segmental analysis of coronary artery stenoses. J Am Coll Cardiol 1998;31: 1547–1554.
6. Rensing BJ, Bongaerts A, van Geuns RJ, et al. Intravenous coronary angiography by electron beam computed tomography: a clinical evaluation. Circulation 1998;98:2509–2512.
7. Achenbach S, Moshage W, Ropers D, et al. Value of electron-beam computed tomography for the noninvasive detection of high-grade coronary artery stenoses and occlusions. N Engl J Med 1998;339: 1964–1971.
8. Budoff MJ, Oudiz RJ, Zalace CP, et al. Intravenous three-dimensional coronary angiography using contrast-enhanced electron beam computed tomography. Am J Cardiol 1999;83:840–845.
9. Achenbach S, Ropers D, Regenfus M, et al. Contrast enhanced electron beam computed tomography to analyse the coronary arteries in patients after acute myocardial infarction. Heart 2000;84:489–493.
10. Nieman K, Oudkerk M, Rensing BJ, et al. Coronary angiography with multi-slice computed tomography. Lancet 2001;357:599–603.
11. Achenbach S, Giesler T, Ropers D, et al. Detection of coronary artery stenoses by contrast-enhanced, retrospectively electrocardiographically-gated, multislice spiral computed tomography. Circulation 2001;103:2535–2538.
12. Knez A, Becker CR, Leber A, et al. Usefulness of multislice spiral computed tomography angiography for determination of coronary artery stenoses. Am J Cardiol 2001;88:1191–1194.
13. Vogl TJ, Abolmaali ND, Diebold T, et al. Techniques for the detection of coronary atherosclerosis: multi-detector row CT coronary angiography. Radiology 2002;223:212–220.
14. Kopp AF, Schröder S, Küttner A, et al. Non-invasive coronary angiography with high resolution multidetector-row computed tomography: results in 102 patients. Eur Heart J 2002;23:1714–1725.
15. Giesler T, Baum U, Ropers D, et al. Noninvasive visualization of coronary arteries using contrast-enhanced multidetector CT: influence of heart rate on image quality and stenosis detection. AR Am J Roentgenol 2002;179:911–916.
16. Nieman K, Rensing BJ, van Geuns RJ, et al. Non-invasive coronary angiography with multislice spiral computed tomography: impact of heart rate. Heart 2002;88:470–474.
17. Nieman K, Cademartiri F, Lemos PA, et al. Reliable noninvasive coronary angiography with fast submillimeter multislice spiral computed tomography. Circulation 2002;106:2051–2054.
18. Ropers D, Baum U, Pohle K, et al. Detection of coronary artery stenoses with thin-slice multi-detector row spiral computed tomography and multiplanar reconstruction. Circulation 2003;107(5): 664–666.
19. Nieman K, Rensing BJ, van Geuns RJM, et al. Usefulness of multislice computed tomography for detecting obstructive coronary artery disease. Am J Cardiol 2002;89:913–918.
20. Wang Y, Watts R, Mitchell I, et al. Coronary MR angiography: selection of acquisition window of minimal cardiac motion with electrocardiography-triggered navigator cardiac motion prescanning—initial results. Radiology 2001;218:580–585.
21. Kim WY, Daniel PG, Stuber M, et al. Coronary magnetic resonance angiography for the detection of coronary stenoses. N Engl J Med 2001;345:1863–1869.
22. Schroeder S, Kopp AF, Baumbach A, et al. Noninvasive detection and evaluation of atherosclerotic coronary plaques with multislice computed tomography. J Am Coll Cardiol 2001;37:1430–1435.
23. Ropers D, Gehling G, Pohle K, et al. Anomalous course of the left main or left anterior descending coronary artery originating from the right sinus of Valsalva. Identification of four common variations by electron beam tomography. Circulation 2002;105:e42–e43.
24. Dirksen MS, Bax JJ, de Roos A, et al. Usefulness of dynamic multislice computed tomography and left ventricular function in unstable angina pectoris and comparison with echocardiography. Am J Cardiol 2002;90:1157–1160.

31 Complementary Use of Coronary Calcium Scoring and CT Angiography

Alexander W. Leber, MD

INTRODUCTION

Electron-beam computed tomography (EBCT) and multislice CT (MSCT) are used for the detection and quantification of coronary calcium, which is a good indicator of coronary atherosclerosis and total plaque burden *(1–6)*. It is suggested that the coronary calcium score can be used to predict future coronary events in asymptomatic patients *(3–7)*. However, acute coronary events are initiated by rupture or superficial erosion of vulnerable coronary plaques, and these plaques are not necessarily calcified *(8–11)*. Therefore, for purposes of risk stratification, the assessment of noncalcified plaques seems to be necessary as well. Besides estimation of plaque burden and risk stratification, evidence from several studies suggests that the CT-derived calcium score can be helpful in identifying coronary artery disease (CAD) in symptomatic patients *(12,13)*. In most studies, coronary calcium score cut-off points have been presented, revealing high sensitivities and specificities to diagnose or to exclude coronary stenoses *(12,13)*. On an individual basis, however, the estimation of luminal obstruction based on a calcium score cut-off point remains difficult. Therefore the consensus of most studies is that the use of age- and gender-related percentiles is preferable *(12–14)*. Patients with scores in the highest percentile have a high likelihood for a relevant stenosis, and in the lower percentiles, stenoses can be excluded. According to these findings, scores in the intermediate percentiles have no diagnostic value *(14)*. Furthermore, recent studies have reported that, especially in young patients and in patients with unstable coronary artery disease, coronary stenoses may be present in the absence of any coronary calcium *(14,15)*. Both EBCT and MSCT offer the opportunity to visualize coronary arteries directly after the administration of contrast agent *(16–18)*. It has been demonstrated that noncalcified plaques and coronary stenoses can be detected by CT angiography (CTA) *(16–20)*. Therefore, the complementary use of calcium scoring and CTA provides incremental information with regards to stenosis detection, determination of plaque burden, and plaque morphology. However, it has to be kept in mind that noninvasive angiography, in contrast to calcium scoring, is more demanding, requiring the administration of contrast agent and additional radiation exposure.

From: *Contemporary Cardiology: CT of the Heart: Principles and Applications*
Edited by: U. Joseph Schoepf © Humana Press, Inc., Totowa, NJ

CALCIUM SCORING COMBINED WITH CTA TO DETERMINE PLAQUE BURDEN AND PLAQUE MORPHOLOGY

Despite advances in our understanding of the pathogenesis of atherosclerosis, coronary heart disease is still the leading cause of death in Western societies. Approx 50% of all myocardial infarctions occur in patients with no prior symptoms. It is well established that the risk for plaque rupture is predicted by plaque burden and plaque composition. Reliable and accurate assessment of the composition of coronary atherosclerosis is currently achieved mainly by invasive methods like intracoronary ultrasound or angioscopy *(21)*. Since these are invasive procedures, they are not suitable for preventive investigations in asymptomatic patients. EBCT and MSCT enable an accurate identification and quantification of calcified coronary plaques noninvasively *(1–4)*. The extent of coronary calcium roughly reflects total plaque burden, and it is suggested that the coronary calcium score is a powerful predictor of future coronary events *(4–13)*. However, myocardial infarction is initiated by rupture or superficial erosion of vulnerable coronary plaques, and these plaques are not necessarily calcified, as calcium is considered to be a frequent feature of stable lesions. Furthermore, calcified plaques reflect only the peak of the entire atherosclerotic burden, and the ratio of calcified to noncalcified plaques is highly variable among individuals *(7–11)*. In animal studies and in a study using intravascular ultrasound, it has been demonstrated that an increase of plaque density in noncalcified plaques is part of a stabilization processes under drug therapies (i.e., statin therapy) *(22,23)*. For a more precise determination of plaque burden and to monitor the course of coronary atherosclerosis, it is therefore necessary to determine also noncalcified plaques. Recently it has been demonstrated that besides the detection of calcified plaques, after the administration of contrast agent, MSCT also allows the identification of noncalcified plaques with high accuracy (Fig. 1). Furthermore, noncalcified plaques can be further differentiated on the basis of their CT density *(19,20)*. In a first clinical study, coronary calcium scores in patients with myocardial infarction were significantly lower than in stable CAD, whereas the number of

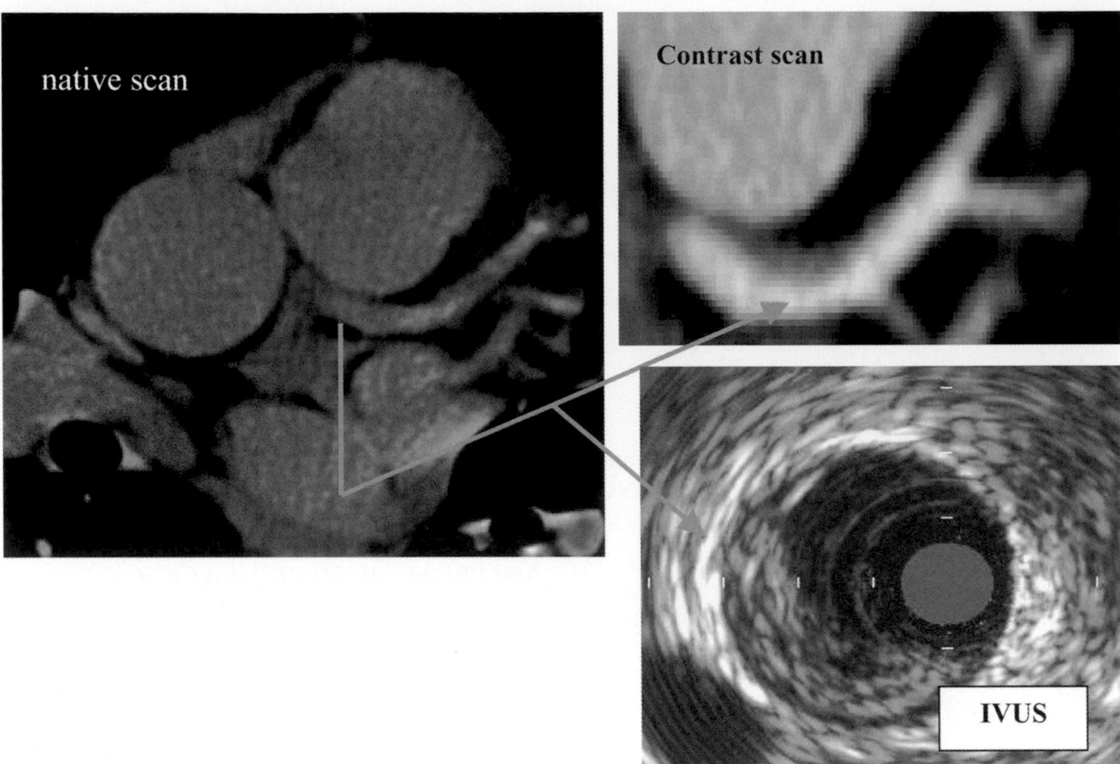

Fig. 1. Detection of noncalcified plaques by multislice CT in relation to intravascular ultrasound (IVUS).

noncalcified plaques was higher, resulting in a similar plaque burden among both groups. This study demonstrated that by determining only calcified lesions, total plaque burden was significantly underestimated in patients with myocardial infarction *(15)*. In another study, Schroeder and colleagues found that in a set of 68 asymptomatic patients with a distinctive risk profile, 53% of patients revealed calcified and noncalcified lesions, and 12.5% of patients revealed only noncalcified lesions *(24)*. These initial results indicate that the possibility to identify and quantify noncalcified plaques may improve future attempts to detect and monitor coronary atherosclerosis in its preclinical stage. However the prognostic impact of noncalcified plaques is unknown so far, and it has to be determined in future large-scale studies. Therefore, contrast-enhanced scans for atherosclerosis screening should be performed only in the setting of research trials. To date there is no evidence to implement coronary plaque imaging by MSCT in the clinical practice.

CALCIUM SCORING AND CTA TO EVALUATE PATIENTS WITH SUSPECTED CORONARY STENOSES

Evidence from several studies suggests that CT-derived calcium scores can be helpful in identifying CAD in patients with chest pain. However, the estimation of luminal obstruction based on the calcium score remains difficult *(1–7)*. In most studies, calcium score cut-off points have been presented, revealing high sensitivities and specificities to diagnose or to exclude coronary stenoses. However, on an individual basis the estimation of luminal obstruction based on a calcium score cut-off point remains difficult. Therefore, the consensus of most studies is that the use of age- and gender-related percentiles (score ranges) is preferable. A review of the literature reveals that on average patients with scores in the highest percentile (>75th percentile) have a high likelihood (>75% of cases) for a relevant stenosis, and in the lower percentiles (< 25th) stenoses can be excluded in more than 85% of cases. According to these findings, scores in the intermediate percentiles (25th–75th) reveal an accuracy that is statistically not different from chance. By using intravenous contrast-enhanced EBCT angiography and MSCT angiography, which allows the visualization of coronary stenoses in the proximal and mid portions of the coronary arteries, calcium scoring can effectively be supported *(14)*. EBCT angiography has been evaluated by a number of investigators *(18,25–30)*. In most studies, high sensitivities (range 93–78%) and high specificities (range 98–88%) for the detection of significant coronary stenoses have been reported after excluding 20–30% of coronary segments because of nondiagnostic image quality. Similar results have been found for 4-slice CT *(18,17)*. With the development of 16-slice CT technology, noninvasive coronary angiography has become clinically more robust and more accurate, allowing the assessment of almost all coronary segments with diagnostic image quality *(16,31)*. However, heavily calcified coronary plaques, which

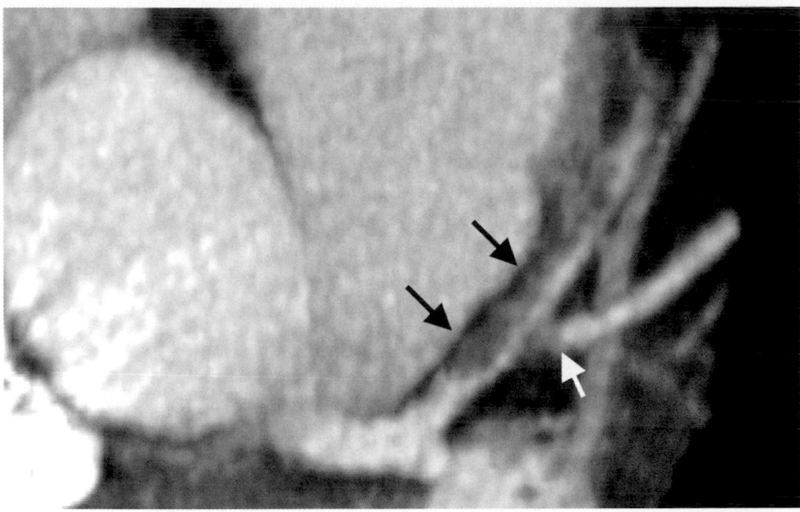

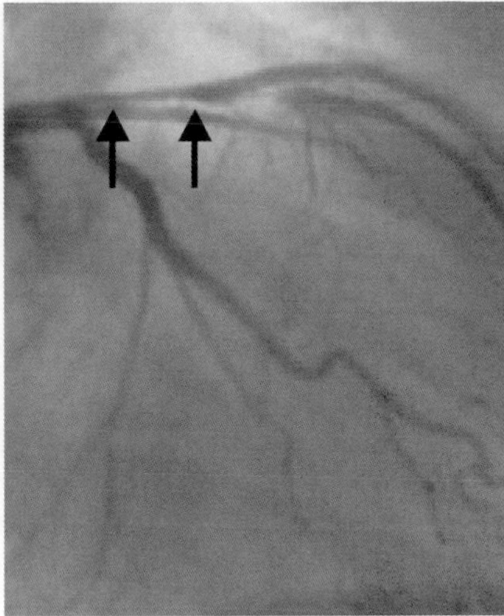

Fig. 2. High-grade stenosis of the left anterior descending artery and the first diagonal branch in a patient with no coronary calcium.

on the one hand can obscure coronary stenoses and on the other hand may cause hardening artifacts that can resemble stenoses, are still a major limitation impairing diagnostic accuracy of all CT technologies. Especially this limitation might be overcome by a combined approach of calcium scoring and CTA.

CALCIUM SCORING AND CTA IN PATIENTS WITH HIGH CALCIUM SCORES

There is only one study evaluating the complementary use of EBCT calcium scoring and EBCT angiography to diagnose significant coronary stenoses *(14)*. In this study it was demonstrated that in the case of high coronary calcium scores the diagnostic accuracy of EBCT angiography is severely affected. Of 31 patients with scores >310, EBCT angiography revealed diagnostic image quality in 27 patients. Accuracy for detecting coronary stenoses was 77% and was statistically not different from calcium scoring alone. While on the one hand extensive calcifications hinder the evaluation of CT angiograms, on the other hand they indicate advanced atherosclerosis with a high probability for the presence of at least one high-grade stenosis. Therefore, it is reasonable to avoid contrast-enhanced scans in patients with severe calcium scores.

CTA IN PATIENTS WITH INTERMEDIATE BORDERLINE CALCIUM SCORES

As already mentioned, intermediate calcium scores are very difficult to handle, and in the clinical setting in the individual patient they have no diagnostic value. In a first study comparing calcium scoring and EBCT angiography, intermediate calcium scores (sensitivity <85% and specificity <80%) were found in 33% of patients. In a review of the literature, equivocal calcium scores occur in up to 50% of patients *(1–7)*. In these patients, CTA is of particular benefit. In a recent study, EBCT angiography guided the correct diagnosis in 80% of patients with equivocal calcium scores (Fig. 2). By transferring this observation to recent 16-slice CT studies, it is likely that this technology with improved spatial and temporal resolution will provide a significant improvement of diagnostic accuracy.

CT ANGIOGRAPHY IN PATIENTS WITH NO CORONARY CALCIUM OR LOW CALCIUM SCORES

The results of the available studies indicate that exclusion of any coronary calcium provides an extremely high negative predictive value ranging from 90 to 99% to rule out coronary stenoses. Almost the same values are obtained for calcium scores below the 25th percentile. However, there is evidence that especially in young patients, in smokers, and in patients with acute chest pain, the diagnosis of a significant luminal obstruction is not a rare finding *(32)*. In a set of patients with atypical chest pain, 4 of 31 patients revealed a significant stenosis despite a low or zero calcium score *(14)*. In 3 of these 4 patients, EBCT angiography identified a high-grade stenosis. In another study, 2 of 21 patients with myocardial infarction had no coronary calcium, but CTA by 4-slice CT identified the culprit stenoses (Fig. 3) *(15)*. Therefore, an additional CTA will add incremental diagnostic safety in symptomatic patients who are younger than 40 yr, who are smokers, and who probably report from a more unstable course of chest pain.

POSSIBLE FUTURE CLINICAL ALGORITHM FOR THE COMPLEMENTARY USE OF CALCIUM: SCORING AND CTA

Owing to the lack of prospective studies in large patient cohorts, to date there exists neither a clinical recommendation nor a clinical guideline to routinely perform coronary calcium scoring or CTA in general practice. The algorithm and related flowchart represented by Fig. 4 provides a better understanding of the utility of the combined CT modalities for future diagnostic strategies.

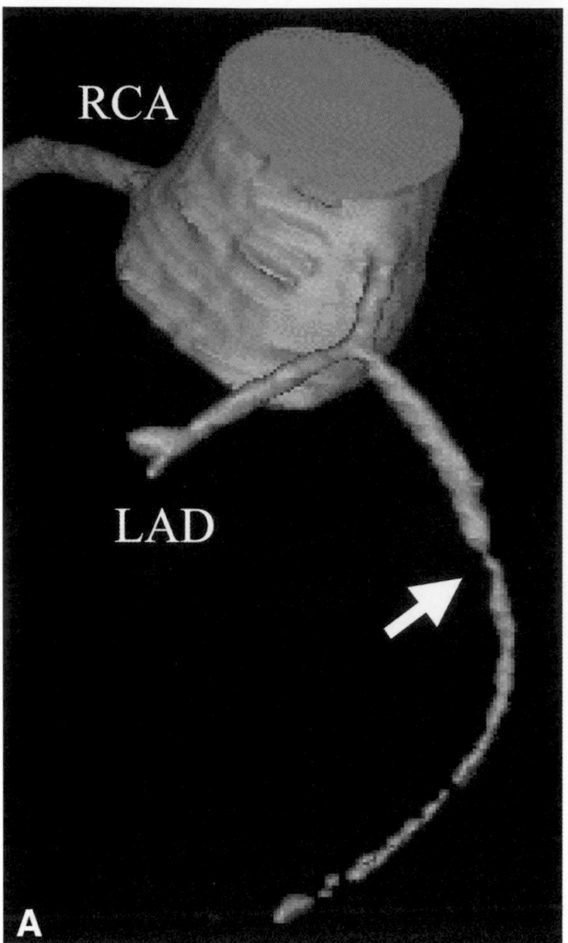

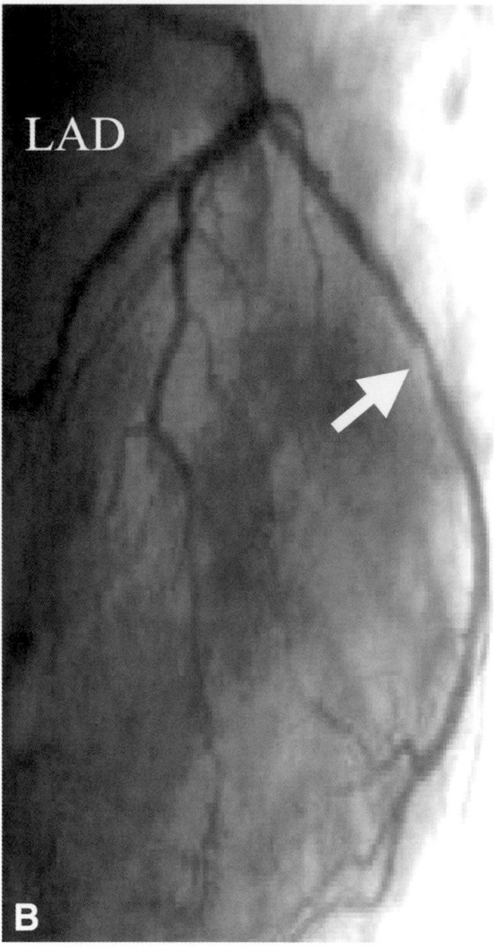

Fig. 3. Proximal 65% stenosis of the left anterior descending artery (arrows) in a patient with a borderline calcium score (176). **(A)** selective coronary angiography. **(B)** Electron beam CT (EBCT) angiography, volume-rendering technique. **(C)** EBCT angiography, shaded surface rendering technique. Figure taken from Leber et al. *(14)*.

REFERENCES

1. Wexler L, Brundage B, Crouse J, et al. Coronary artery calcification: pathophysiology, epidemiology, imaging methods, and clinical implications. A statement for health professionals from the American Heart Association Writing Group. Circulation 1996;94: 1175–1192.
2. Knez A, Becker C, Becker A, et al. Determination of coronary calcium with multi-slice spiral computed tomography: a comparative study with electron-beam CT. Int J Cardiovasc Imaging 2002;18: 295–303.
3. Wayhs R, Zelinger A, Raggi P. High coronary artery calcium scores pose an extremely elevated risk for hard events. J Am Coll Cardiol 2002;39:225–230.
4. Wong ND, Budoff MJ, Pio J, Detrano RC. Coronary calcium and cardiovascular event risk: evaluation by age- and sex-specific quartiles. Am Heart J 2002;143:456–459.
5. Detrano RC, Doherty TM, Davies MJ, Stary HC. Predicting coronary events with coronary calcium: pathophysiologic and clinical problems. Curr Probl Cardiol 2000;25:374–402.
6. Pohle K, Ropers D, Maffert R, et al. Coronary calcifications in young patients with first, unheralded myocardial infarction: a risk factor matched analysis by electron beam tomography. Heart 2003;89: 625–628.
7. O'Malley PG, Taylor AJ, Jackson JL, Doherty TM, Detrano RC. Prognostic value of coronary electron-beam computed tomography for coronary heart disease events in asymptomatic populations. Am J Cardiol 2000;85:945–948.
8. Virmani R, Kolodgie F, Burke A, et al. Lessons from sudden coronary death: a comprehensive morphological classification scheme for atherosclerotic lesions. Arterioscler Thromb Vasc Biol 2000;20(5):1262–1275.
9. Kragel A, Reddy S, Wittes J, et al. Morphometric analysis of the composition of atherosclerotic plaques in the four major epicardial coronary arteries in acute myocardial infarction and in sudden coronary death. Circulation 1989;80(6):1747–1756.
10. Virmani R, Burke A, Farb A. Coronary risk factors and plaque morphology in men with coronary disease who died suddenly. Eur Heart J 1998;19:678–680.
11. Virmani R, Burke AP, Kolodgie FD, et al. Prognostic value of coronary calcification and angiographic stenoses in patients undergoing coronary angiography. J Am Coll Cardiol 1996;27:285–290.
12. Guerci AD, Spadaro LA, Popma JJ, et al. Relationship of coronary calcium score by EBCT to arteriographic findings in asymptomatic and symptomatic adults. Am J Cardiol 1997;79:128–133.
13. Haberl R, Becker A, Leber A, et al. Correlation of coronary calcification and angiographically documented stenoses in patients with suspected coronary artery disease: results of 1,764 patients. J Am Coll Cardiol 2001;37(2):451–457.
14. Leber A, Knez A, Mukherjee R, et al. Usefulness of calcium scoring using electron beam computed tomography and noninvasive coronary angiography in patients with suspected coronary artery disease. Am J Cardiol 2001;88(3):219–223.
15. Leber AW, Knez A, White CW, et al. Composition of coronary atherosclerotic plaques in patients with acute myocardial infarction

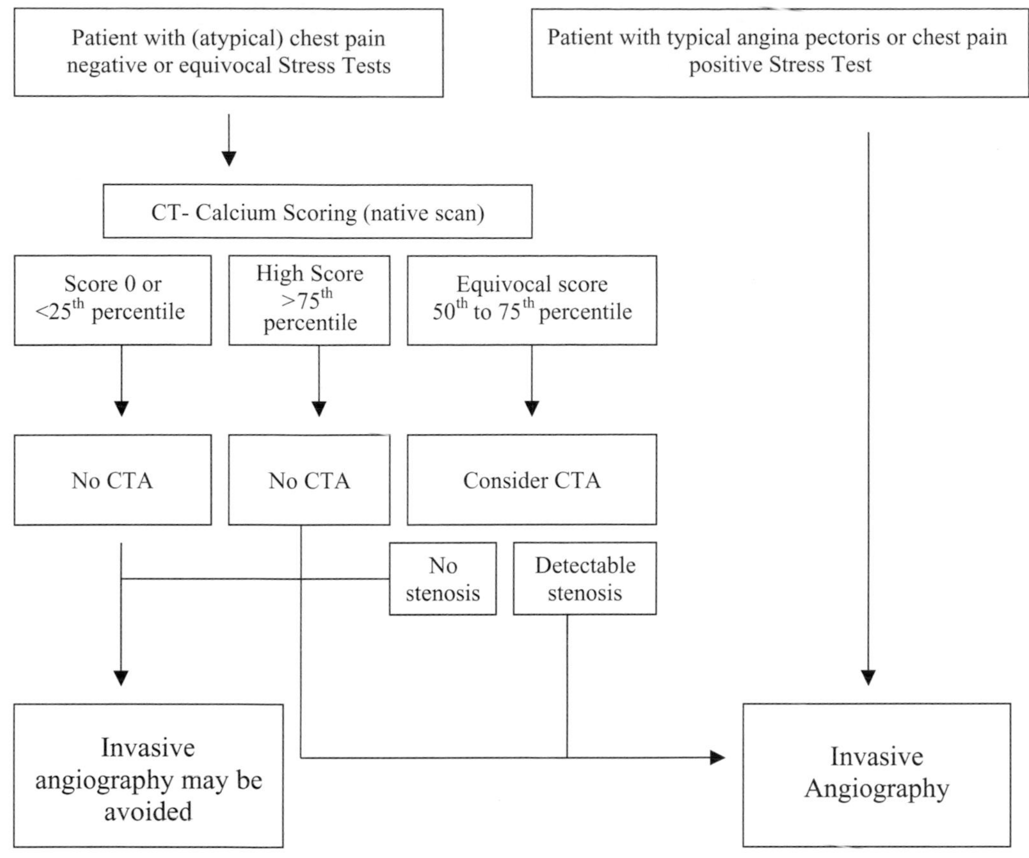

Fig. 4. Proposed algorithm for the complementary use of calcium scoring and CT coronary angiography.

and stable angina pectoris determined by contrast-enhanced multislice computed tomography. Am J Cardiol 2003;91:714–718.

16. Nieman K, Cademartiri F, Lemos PA, Raaijmakers R, Pattynama PM, de Feyter PJ. Reliable noninvasive coronary angiography with fast submillimeter multislice spiral computed tomography. Circulation 2002;106:2051–2054.
17. Achenbach S, Ulzheimer S, Baum U, et al. Noninvasive coronary angiography by retrospectiveely gated multislice spiral CT. Circulation 2000;102:2823–2828.
18. Leber AW, Knez A, Becker C, et al. Non-invasive intravenous coronary angiography using electron beam tomography and multislice computed tomography. Heart 2003;89:633–639.
19. Schroeder S, Kopp AF, Baumbach A, et al. Noninvasive detection and evaluation of atherosclerotic coronary plaques with multislice computed tomography. J Am Coll Cardiol 2001;37:1430–435.
20. Leber AW, Knez A, Becker A, et al. Accuracy of multi detector spiral CT in identifying and differentiating the composition of coronary atherosclerotic plaques. A comparative study with intracoronary ultrasound. J Am Coll Cardiol 2004;43:1241–1247.
21. Waxman S. Characterization of the unstable lesion by angiography, angioscopy, and intravascular ultrasound. Cardiol Clin 1999;17: 295–305.
22. Schartl M, Boksch W, Koschyk D, et al. Use of intravascular ultrasound to compare effects of different strategies of lipid-lowering therapy on plaque volume and composition in patients with coronary artery disease. Circulation 2001;104(4):387–389.
23. Gomberg-Maitland, Fuster V, Fayad Z, et al. Statins and plaque stability. J Cardiovasc Risk 2003;10(3):161–167.
24. Schroeder S, Kopp A, Kuettner A, et al. Prevalence of noncalcified plaques in asymptomatic patients with a high atherosclerotic risk profile. Z Kardiol 2002;Suppl.
25. Moshage WE, Achenbach S, Seese B, Bachmann K, Kirchgeorg M. Coronary artery stenoses: three-dimensional imaging with electrocardiographically triggered, contrast agent-enhanced, electron-beam CT. Radiology 1995;196:707–714.
26. Chernoff DM, Ritchie CJ, Higgins CB. Evaluation of electron beam CT coronary angiography in healthy subjects. AJR Am J Roentgenol 1997;169:93–99.
27. Reddy GP, Chernoff DM, Adams JR, Higgins CB. Coronary artery stenoses: assessment with contrast-enhanced electron-beam CT and axial reconstructions. Radiology 1998;208:167–172.
28. Schmermund A, Rensing BJ, Sheedy PF, Bell MR, Rumberger JA. Intravenous electron-beam CT coronary angiography for segmental analysis of coronary artery stenoses. J Am Coll Cardiol 1998;31(7): 1547–1554.
29. Achenbach S, Moshage W, Ropers D, Nossen J, Daniel WG. Value of electron beam computed tomography for the noninvasive detection of high-grade coronary-artery stenoses and occlusions. N Engl J Med 1998;339:1964–1971.
30. Rensing BJ, Bongaerts A, van Geuns RJ, van Ooijen P, M Oudkerk, PJ de Feyter. Intravenous coronary angiography by electron beam computed tomography: a clinical evaluation. Circulation 1998;98(23):2509-2512.
31. Ropers D, Baum U, Pohle K, et al. Detection of coronary artery stenoses with thin-slice multi-detector row spiral computed tomography and multiplanar reconstruction. Circulation 2003;107: 664–666.
32. Schmermund A, Baumgart D, Adamzik M, et al. Comparison of electron-beam computed tomography and intracoronary ultrasound in detecting calcified and noncalcified plaques in patients with acute coronary syndromes and no or minimal to moderate angiographic coronary artery disease. Am J Cardiol 1998;81:141–146.

32 CT vs Magnetic Resonance for Imaging of the Coronary Arteries

ARMIN HUBER, MD

Coronary arteries are small tortuous vessels with physiological motion by respiratory motion and cardiac contraction. The noninvasive imaging of normal and diseased coronary arteries by magnetic resonance (MR) angiography has undergone numerous technical improvements since its introduction in 1993. Early coronary MR techniques used a combination of segmental acquisition of the k-space data and breath-holding. More recent techniques allow use of both electrocardiogram (ECG) triggering and respiratory gating, eliminating the need for patient breath-holding. Thus the acquisition time can be longer than a single breath-hold, and spatial resolution can be increased substantially. Three generations of MR coronary angiography techniques have been described and can be used with or without contrast agents.

Potential clinical applications of MR imaging (MRI) of the coronary arteries include coronary lesion detection, delineation of congenital coronary artery anomalies, characterization of previously known coronary lesions with imaging of the vessel wall, coronary anatomy after transplantation, and quantification of coronary flow reserve by velocity encoding MR of the coronaries at rest and under adenosine stress.

Electron beam computed tomography (EBCT) has been the method of choice to image coronary arteries by computed tomography (CT), as the temporal resolution of 100 ms was much higher than that of helical CT. Unenhanced EBCT of the coronary arteries is useful to detect and quantify coronary calcifications. Variable studies have been reported about contrast-enhanced CT angiography (CTA) of the coronary arteries with EBCT (Fig. 1). One of the major limitations is the slice thickness of 3 mm or the limited volume that can be imaged during a breath-hold when the slice thickness is reduced. Another limitation is limited signal-to-noise ratio (SNR) that can be achieved with EBCT.

Since introduction of multislice CT with retrospective ECG gating, contrast-enhanced data sets of the coronary arteries can be acquired with high spatial resolution, thin slice thickness, and high SNR. The drawback of lower temporal resolution compared to electron beam CTA is compensated by retrospectively chosen optimal temporal window for data reconstruction during the RR cycle and therefore reduction of motion artifacts. In order to achieve longer rest time of the coronary arteries during diastole, β-blockers are used to reduce heart rate. Multislice CT allows for reliable detection and quantification of coronary calcifications in unenhanced data sets acquired with low-dose ECG triggering or in contrast-enhanced CTA data sets acquired with ECG gating. As coronary CTA is possible with higher image quality compared to EBCT, calcium screening is possible with comparable diagnostic accuracy *(1,2)*, and multislice CTs are widely available and useful for many other indications than cardiac imaging, multislice CT replaced EBCT in the majority of centers.

MR angiography (MRA) is possible with high diagnostic accuracy comparable to that of digital subtraction angiography in many vascular territories, such as renal arteries, carotid arteries, and the peripheral vascular tree *(3,4)*. The technique that shows the highest diagnostic accuracy and short acquisition times is contrast-enhanced 3D MRA with T1-weighted 3D gradient echo sequences. For coronary MRA, it is still not clear which MRA technique will be the technique of choice in future.

Pioneering work with first-generation coronary MRA started 1993. The MRA technique was a 2D gradient-echo technique, which means that one slice is acquired during a single breath-hold with ECG triggering and segmented k-space acquisition. The initial enthusiasm of the first very positive and promising preclinical reports could not be reproduced by other investigators, who found more negative results. Initial clinical testing of the first-generation coronary MRA technique was reported by Manning et al. *(5)*. They examined 39 patients and determined the diagnostic accuracy of MRA compared to conventional coronary angiography for detection of stenosis and occlusions. In this first study, coronary MR had a sensitivity of 90% and a specificity of 92% for correctly identifying individual vessels with 50% or greater angiographic stenosis. The corresponding positive and negative predictive values were 0.85 and 0.95. The overall sensitivity and specificity for correctly classifying individual patients as having or not having serious coronary disease were 97% and 70%. Subsequent attempts of imaging the coronary arteries by MRA by other investigators to reproduce these results have not been successful. Duerinckx et al. found that a sensitivity of 90% for lesion detecting by using first-generation coronary MRA was optimistic and could not be reproduced in a double-blinded pro-

From: *Contemporary Cardiology: CT of the Heart: Principles and Applications*
Edited by: U. Joseph Schoepf © Humana Press, Inc., Totowa, NJ

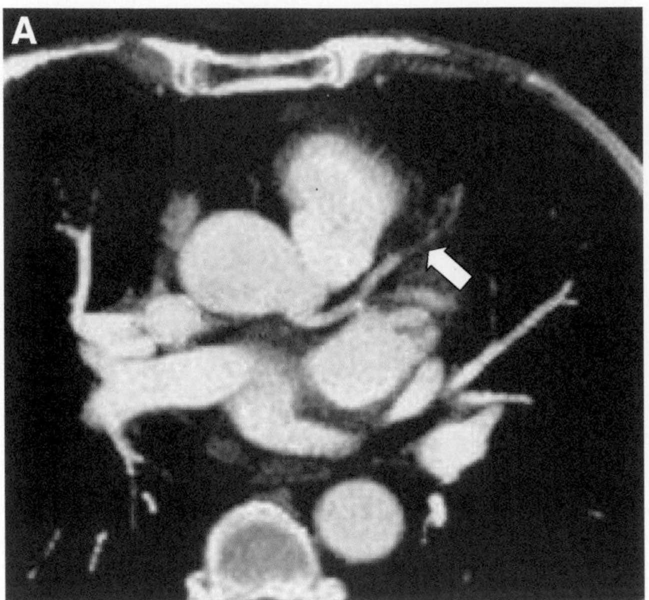

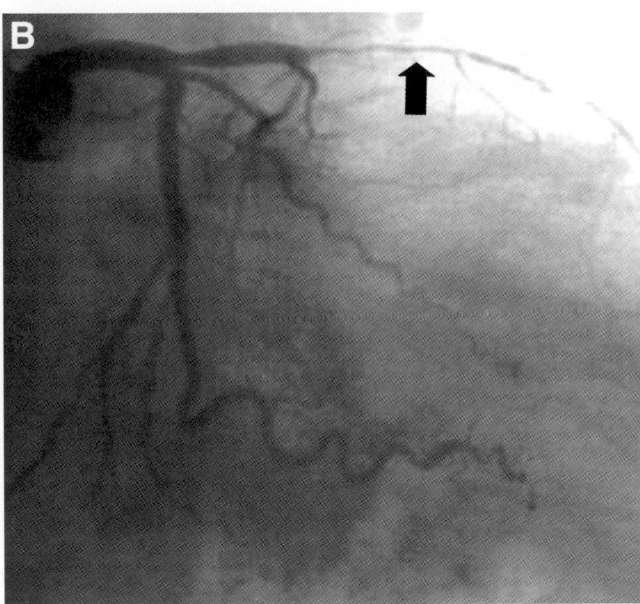

Fig. 1. (A) Thin-slice maximum intensity projection reconstruction of electron beam CT angiography data set shows high-grade stenoses of the left anterior descending artery (arrow). **(B)** Right anterior oblique projection of conventional coronary angiography shows high-grade stenoses of the left anterior descending artery (arrow).

spective study *(6)*. In some of the patients, very promising data sets with spectacular image quality could be acquired; however, first-generation coronary MRA was not consistent enough to reproduce the results first reported by Manning et al. Post et al. found a sensitivity for detection of significant coronary artery lesions of 36% in an initial study and results of 33% to 75% in an follow-up study *(7)*. An important practical problem of the first-generation 2D coronary MRA is the potential of overreading or underreading coronary artery lesions. As only one slice can be acquired during a single breath-hold, the course of tortuous coronary arteries is not strictly in plane. Thus more slices than one have to be acquired during different breath-holds to assess a longer part of one vessel, and partial-volume effects can decrease diagnostic accuracy as well as different respiratory positions.

To overcome the problems of single–slice, single-breath-hold acquisitions, the second-generation techniques introduce respiratory gating. With the combination of respiratory gating and ECG triggering, a continuous high-resolution data set of the entire heart can be acquired with a 3D technique. The respiratory gating can be performed with bellows, respiratory belts, and with noninvasive navigator pulses positioned on the dome of the right diaphragm (Fig. 2). Most studies used noninvasive navigator pulses. The advantages of these techniques are the ability to image the coronaries despite their tortuous course continuously in a high-resolution data set (Figs. 3,4). The spatial resolution can be increased, as the scan time for one data set is not restricted to the length of a single breath-hold. A disadvantage is that the entire examination time can be very long because of the double trigger/gating technique (respiratory and ECG). Another disadvantage is that usual extravascular contrast agents are not suitable to increase SNR because the acquisition time is too long compared to the first pass time of the contrast agent. Moreover, the navigator techniques usually are based on a time-of-flight MRA technique, which means the degree of stenosis is overestimated by flow voids and the SNR is limited. Recent techniques allow the combination of 3D TrueFISP and 3D Flash techniques (Figs. 5,6) with respiratory navigator gating. For respiratory gating, different techniques can be used. First, retrospective respiratory gating with continuous data acquisition and retrospective selection of suitable data at the same diaphragm position; second, prospective respiratory gating with acquisition of data only at the correct diaphragm position; and third, slice correction algorithms with correction of data position dependent on the diaphragm position, with a correction factor of 0.3 to 0.6. For second-generation techniques with 3D acquisition and respiratory gating, various values for diagnostic accuracy were found. Müller et al. found a sensitivity of 87% and a specificity of 97%. Huber et al. found a sensitivity of 73% and a specificity of 50% *(8)*, and Nikolaou et al. found a sensitivity and specificity of and 71%/72% and 53%/60% for navigator echo MRA with and without the use of a slice interpolation technique *(9)*. One of the major problems is that excellent image quality can be achieved in some of the patients, but image quality is variable and cannot be reproduced reliably at a high standard. Therefore, diagnostic accuracy decreases in larger patient populations. In contrast to the already reported studies, Lethimonnier used a navigator technique with prospective instead of retrospective respiratory gating *(10)*. This technique reduces the acquisition time, but diagnostic accuracy could not be improved compared to the studies with retrospective respiratory gating.

Kim et al. examined 109 patients scheduled for X-ray coronary angiography with free-breathing coronary MRA *(11)*.

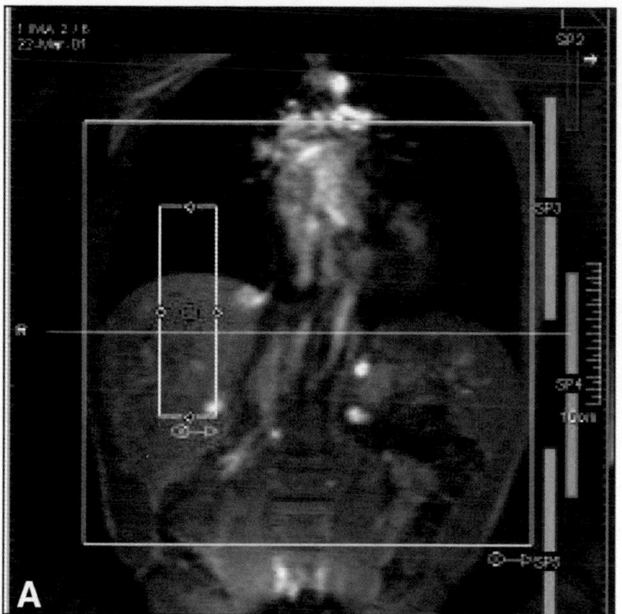

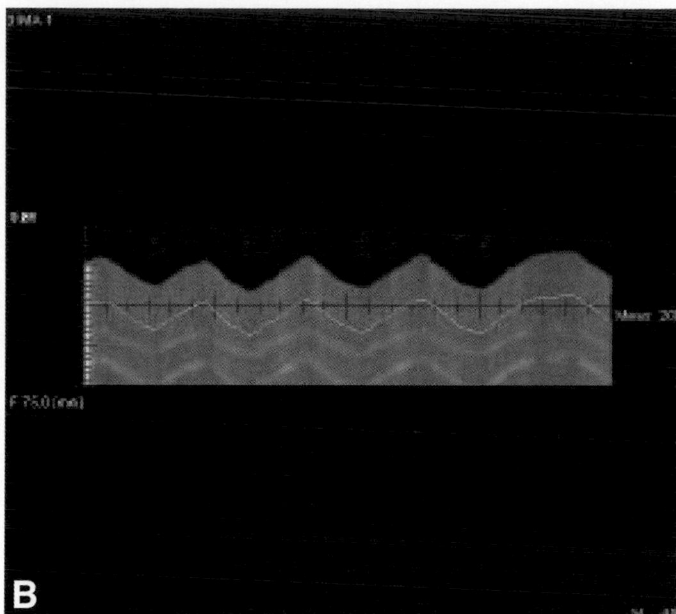

Fig 2. (**A**) Slab of navigator pulse positioned on the dome of the right diaphragm. (**B**) Noninvasive prospective detection of the position of the diaphragm during respiratory cycle.

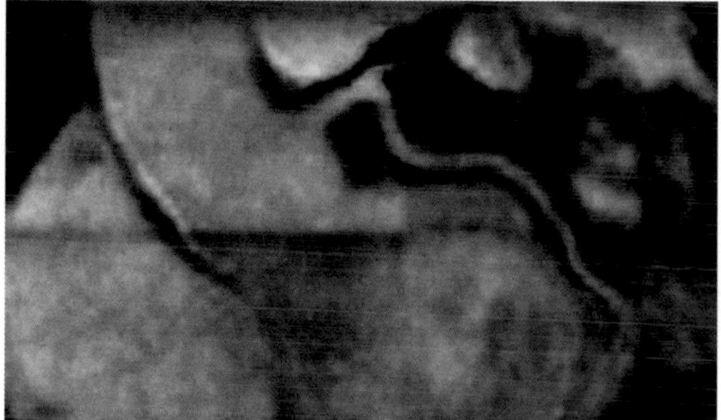

Fig. 3. Circumflex artery: multiplanar reformation reconstruction of high-resolution magnetic resonance (MR) coronary angiography data set acquired with retrospectively gated navigator echo MR angiography technique. Modified from ref. *8*.

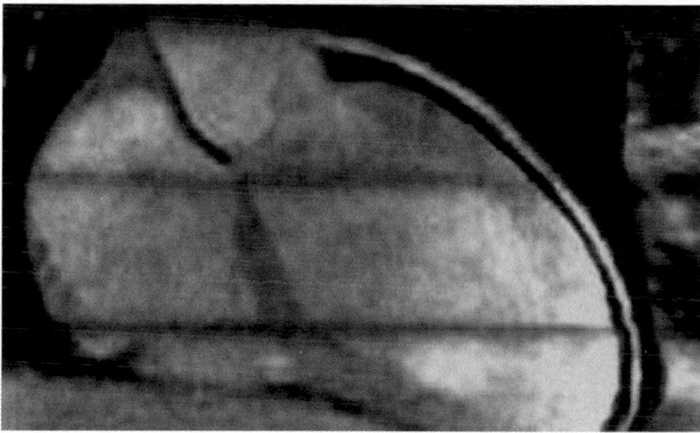

Fig. 4. Left anterior descending artery: multiplanar reformation reconstruction of high-resolution magnetic resonance (MR) coronary angiography data set acquired with retrospectively gated navigator echo MR angiography technique. Modified from ref. *8*.

They found that 84% of the proximal and middle segments of coronary arteries were interpretable on MRA; 83% of clinically significant lesions (more than 50% reduction in diameter on X-ray angiography) were identified. However, the sensitivity, specificity, and accuracy for patients with disease of the left main coronary artery or three-vessel disease were 100%, 85%, and 87%. The negative predictive values for any coronary artery disease and for left main artery or three-vessel disease were 81% and 100%.

The third-generation techniques allow acquisition of a whole 3D slab during a single breath-hold with the use of strong gradient systems and fast T1- or T2-weighted gradient echo pulse sequence techniques, either 3D Flash or 3D TrueFISP.

Kessler et al. used a single transverse 3D slab that covers only the proximal coronary artery tree *(12)*. The pulse-sequence technique is similar to a contrast-enhanced T1w 3D gradient-echo technique, which is used for many other vascular territories with high image quality and high diagnostic accuracy. However, with the combination of ECG triggering and the reduction of scan time to a single breath-hold, spatial resolution is limited and the acquisition time in the RR cycle is relatively long (250 ms). Compared to multislice CT, the acquisition window during the RR cycle is similar; however, the prospective ECG-triggering technique leads to a lower image quality concerning cardiac motion artifacts than the retrospectively ECG-gated technique, which is used for CTA in multislice CTA of the coronary arteries. Wielopolski et al. introduced the volume coronary artery targeted scan (VCAT) technique *(13)*. This technique uses seven to nine small 3D slabs to cover the entire coronary artery tree. With the use of

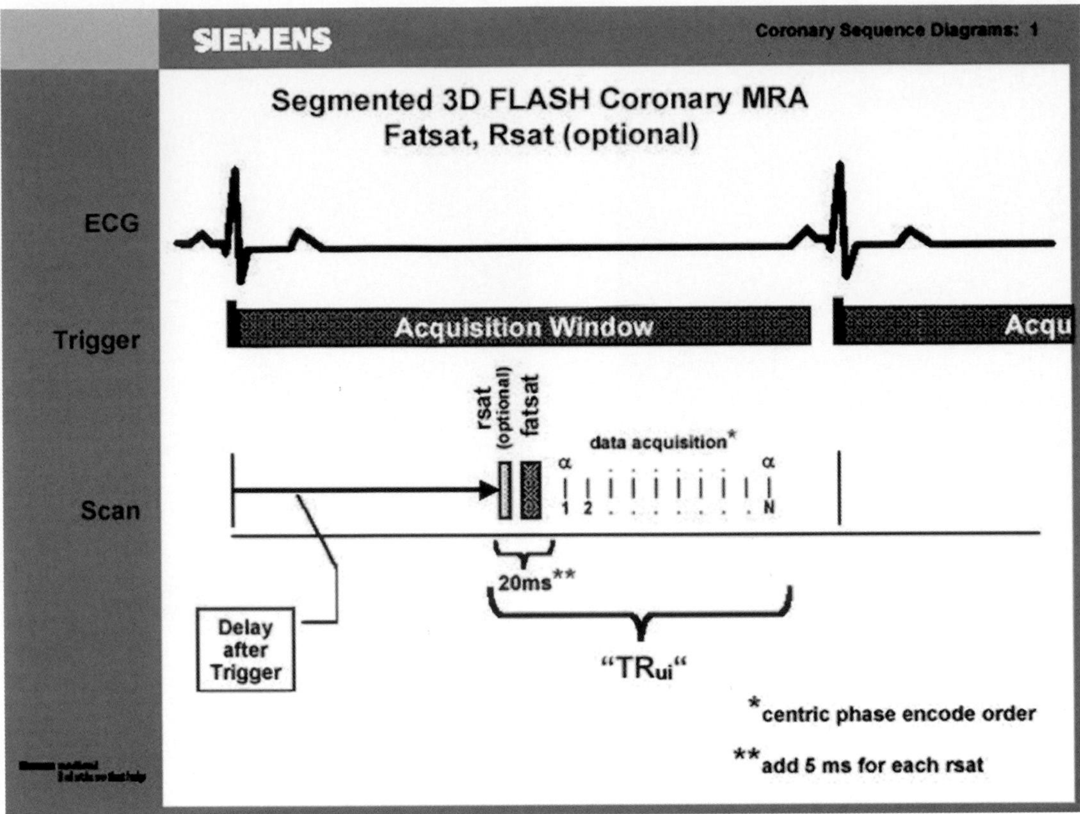

Fig. 5. Drawing shows segmented data acquisition during RR interval with prospective respiratory gating and prospective electrocardiogram gating with 3D Flash technique.

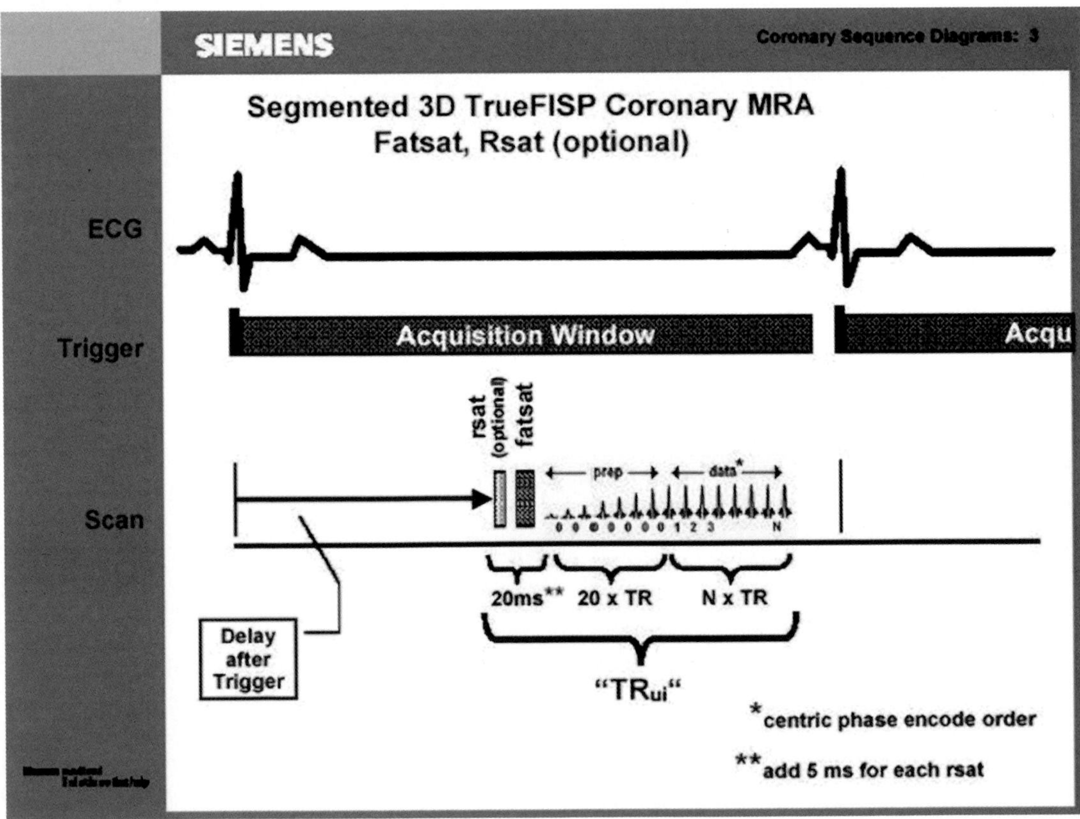

Fig. 6. Drawing shows segmented data acquisition during RR interval with prospective respiratory gating and prospective electrocardiogram gating with 3D TrueFISP technique.

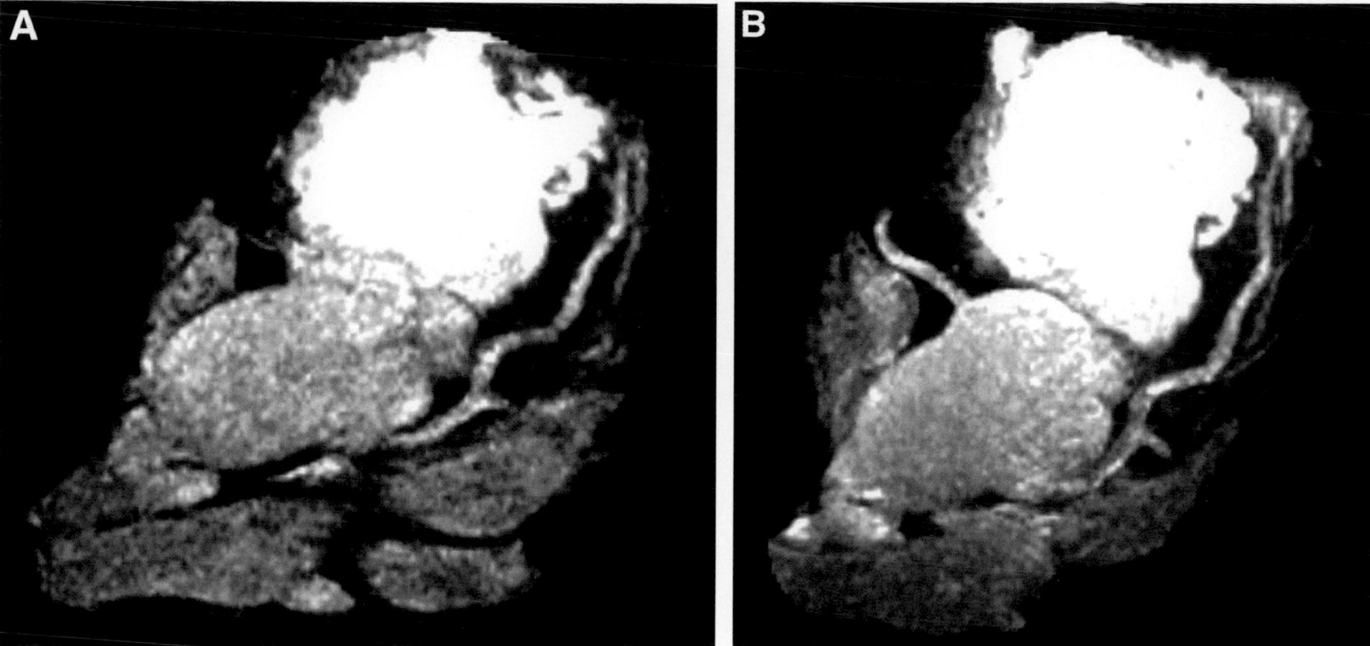

Fig. 7. **(A)** Magnetic resonance (MR) coronary angiography. 3D TrueFISP breath-hold technique has a lower spatial resolution but a shorter scan time than the respiratory triggered technique. **(B)** MR coronary angiography. 3D TrueFISP respiratory triggered technique has a higher spatial resolution but a longer scan time than the respiratory triggered technique.

small 3D slabs instead of a single proximal 3D slab, spatial resolution can be improved significantly. The disadvantage of this technique is that a usual extravascular contrast agent cannot be used for seven or nine injections. Usually, at least a single dose of Gd-DTPA (0.1 mmol/L) is necessary to perform contrast-enhanced MRA successfully. Thus, the number of contrast-material injections is restricted to three, which is not enough for seven or nine 3D slabs. Therefore, the VCAT techniques can be used unenhanced with limited signal-to-noise ratio or with the use of an intravascular contrast agent. The T2 weighted 3D TrueFISP pulse sequence is another method to image the coronary without contrast material, either with a breath-hold approach or with a respiratory triggered technique (Fig. 7). The advantage of this technique is that fluid and blood has an intrinsic high contrast in TrueFISP sequences without the use of contrast material.

The heart can be imaged with the use of two different CT modalities: one employs nonmechanical movement of the X-ray source (i.e., EBCT) and the other involves the motion of the X-ray source and table, combined with multiple detectors to acquire the data in spiral or helical fashion (i.e., multidetector-row CT [MDCT]). In order to freeze cardiac motion, a cardiac-dedicated CT system was developed in 1982 on the basis of a nonmechanical movement of the X-ray source and fixed detector arrays. The EBCT uses a single, curved anode with four tungsten targets underneath the patient, and a focused electron beam that is rapidly swept across these targets to produce an X-ray fan beam detected by two detector rows above the patient.

Mechanical MDCT systems were introduced in 1998, and allow for scanning with one X-ray tube and 4 detector rows in a single gantry rotating twice per second around the patient. Continuous gantry rotation and table movement causes the projection data to be obtained along a spiral or helical path. A new generation of MDCT permits working with 16 detector rows in a single gantry rotation and therefore improves spatial resolution and reduces scan time of the entire heart by 50%. With helical CT, it was not possible to image the coronary arteries with high spatial resolution and reduction of cardiac motion by ECG triggering. The introduction of helical CT with multirow detectors (4 rows) allows for a coverage of the entire heart during a single breath-hold (40 s) with high spatial resolution and thinner slice thickness (1.25 mm) than is possible with EBCT (3 mm). However, the acquisition window during the RR cycle is limited by a rotation time of 500 ms. This is five times longer than with EBCT. The first step to reduce the acquisition window is to use a 180-degree sector for image reconstruction instead of a 360-degree sector. That means the acquisition window is reduced to 250 ms. The second step to improve image quality is to choose the right delay time in the RR cycle retrospectively after the scan to reconstruct the images at the time of minimal motion during the RR interval. Hong et al. showed that the rest time of each coronary artery is different in each individual and is variable in different individuals *(14)*. Furthermore, the length of the rest time is dependent on the patient's heart rate. That means high image quality can be achieved in patients with low heart rates (under 65 beats per min [bpm]). Therefore, the third step to cope with the problem of the long acquisition window is to decrease the patient's heart rate with a β-blocker. If it is not possible to decrease the patient's heart rate, a segmented algorithm can be used to acquire the data for one 180-degree sector reconstruction over two RR intervals. However, this method can cause additional motion artifacts.

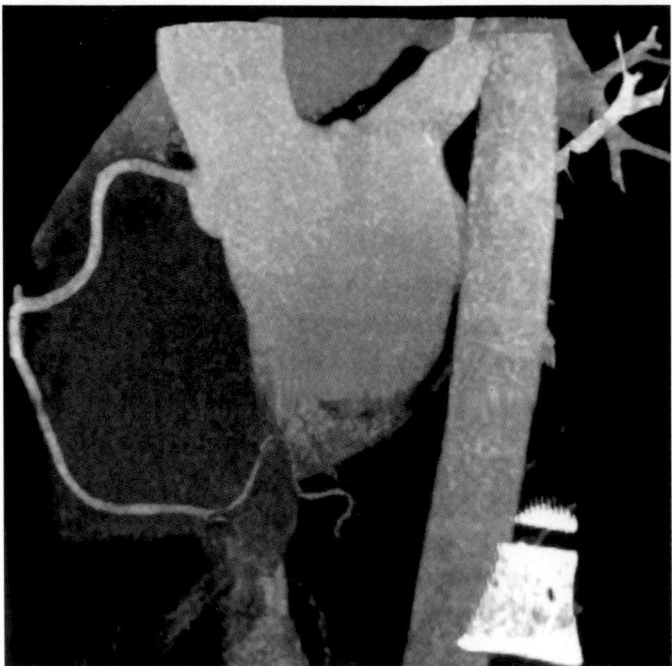

Fig. 8. Maximum intensity projection reconstruction of a multislice CT angiography (16 row) data set shows normal anatomy of right coronary artery.

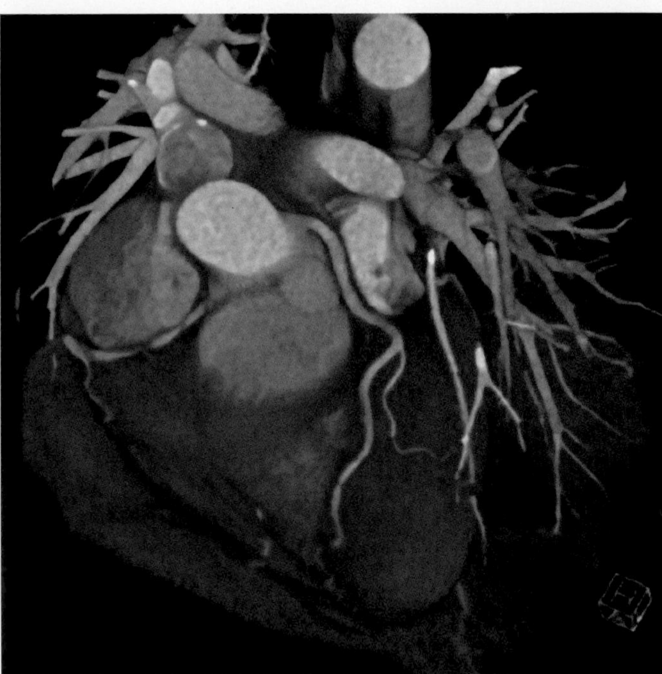

Fig. 9. 3D reconstruction of a multislice CT angiography (16 row) data set shows normal anatomy of left anterior descending artery and a diagonal branch.

Compared to EBCT, multislice CT has a higher spatial resolution, especially a smaller slice thickness and a higher SNR and contrast-to-noise ratio (CNR), as it is possible to apply a higher radiation dose. In spite of the fact that the acquisition window of multislice CTA of coronary arteries is much longer than with coronary MRA or EBCT, cardiac motion artifacts can be suppressed sufficiently in the majority of patients with retrospective ECG gating, where patient's heart rate can be reduced under 65 bpm (Figs. 8,9).

CTA using EBCT was performed in various studies with similar imaging parameters. In all studies, a single-slice mode was used with a high in-plane matrix (512 × 512); the temporal resolution was 100 ms in all studies (Table 1). The percentage of depicted vessels with adequate image quality ranged from 72% to 90%—i.e., in all studies a certain number of vessel segments with reduced image quality had to be excluded from further evaluation *(15–20)*.

Nieman et al. found a sensitivity and specificity for a comparison of multislice CTA (4 slices) with conventional coronary angiography of 82% and 93% and positive and negative predictive value of 66% and 97% in detection of stenosis (=50%) *(21)*. Knez et al. found a sensitivity and specificity of 83% and 78% for the detection of stenosis (=50%) and 67% for the detection of occlusions, a specificity of 98% and a negative predictive value of 96% *(22)*. Achenbach et al. excluded 32% of the examined vessels and found a sensitivity and specificity of 85% and 76% *(23)*. Becker et al. found a sensitivity, specificity, and negative predictive value for the detection of stenoses (>50%) with multislice CTA of 81%, 90%, and 97%, respectively *(24)*. However, the agreement for determining the degree of stenoses with multislice CT was only moderate ($\kappa = 0.58$). Vogel et al. analyzed different CT reformation techniques in assessing the coronary arteries examined with multislice CT, including 3D reformations, virtual endoscopic reformations, multiplanar reformations, and transverse source images *(25)*. The highest diagnostic accuracy was found at transverse scanning.

In comparison to conventional coronary angiography, several studies show that the sensitivity of multislice CTA in detection of coronary artery stenosis cannot replace invasive angiography. However, the high negative predictive value in all studies suggests use of the method in patients with a low pretest probability for having coronary artery disease, who would be scheduled for coronary angiography to exclude coronary heart disease. One limitation in detecting coronary artery stenosis is the difficulty of correctly determining the degree of narrowing of the luminal diameter. Another limitation is the high density of coronary artery wall calcifications. In regions of strongly calcified vessels, the assessment of coronary artery stenosis is very difficult. Compared to CT of the coronaries, coronary MRA has the advantage that calcified plaques show low signal intensity and do not decrease diagnostic accuracy for the assessment of coronary artery stenosis. The advantage of multislice CTA is that calcified plaques can be identified and quantified in the same data set that is acquired after contrast-material application for CTA *(26)*.

Table 1 shows sensitivity and specificity of different noninvasive coronary angiography methods in comparison to conventional coronary angiography, and the number of excluded patients or vessel segments from the evaluation because of low image quality. The results show that none of the three methods—MRA, contrast-enhanced EBCT, or contrast-enhanced MDCT—can replace conventional invasive coronary

Table 1
Sensitivity and Specificity of Coronary CT and Magnetic Resonance (MR) Angiography Studies As Compared With Conventional Angiography (Stenosis =50%)

Techniques	*No. of patients*	*No. of patients, vessels, or segments excluded (%)*	*Sensitivity %*	*Specificity %*
CT angiography with electron-beam CT				
Nakanishi et al. 1997 *(16)*	37	4 patients (11%)	74	94
Achenbach et al. 2000 *(17)*	36	29 vessels (20%)	92	94
Schmermund et al. 1998 *(18)*	28	93 segments (28%)	82	88
Reddy et al. 1998 *(19)*	23	7 vessels (10%)	88	63
Buddoff et al. 1999 *(20)*	52	23 vessels (11%)	78	91
Achenbach et al. 1998 *(21)*	125	124 vessels (25%)	92	94
CT angiography with multidetector CT				
Niemann et al. 2002 *(22)*	53	55 segments (30%)	82	93
Knez et al. 2001 *(23)*	44	29 segments (6%)	78	98
Achenbach et al. 2001 *(24)*	64	82 vessels (32%)	85	76
Becker et al. 2002 *(25)*	28	81	90	
Vogl et al. 2002 *(26)*	64	38 segments (19%)	75	99
MR angiography, first generation, 2D breath-hold				
Manning et al. 1993 *(5)*	39	9 vessels (6%)	90	92
Post et al. 1997 *(7)*	35	15 vessels (11%)	63	89
MR angiography second generation, 3D retrospective respiratory gating				
Post et al. 1996 *(38)*	20	3 vessels (4%)	38	95
Mueller et al. 1997 *(39)*	35	35 segments (14%)	83	94
Sandstede et al. 1999 *(40)*	30	7 patients (23%)	81	89
Huber et al. 1999 *(9)*	20	45 segments (31%)	79	54
Sardanelli et al. 2000 *(41)*	42	39 segments (14%)	82	89
Gonschior et al. 2001 *(42)*	20	45 segments (31%)	79	54
Nikolaou et al. 2001 *(10)*	40	75 segments (27%)	72	60
3D prospective respiratory gating				
Lethimonnier 1999 *(11)*	20	3 patients (15%)	65	93
Kim et al. 2001 *(12)*	109	123 segments (16%)	93	42
MR angiography third generation, 3D breath-hold				
Van Geuns et al. 2000, unenhanced *(43)*	38	85 segments (31%)	68	97
Regenfus et al. 2000, contrast-enhanced *(44)*	50	82 segments (23%)	86	91

angiography. However, multislice CTA is a promising method in excluding coronary artery disease in patients with a low pretest probability of having coronary artery disease, as all studies show a high negative predictive value and a high specificity. The study performed by Kim et al. shows that coronary MRA has the potential role to detect or exclude three-vessel disease or stenoses of the left main coronary artery *(11)*.

Moreover, contrast-enhanced multislice CTA can detect not only calcified plaques but also noncalcified plaques *(27,28)* and indicate atherosclerosis in an early stage. That means multislice CTA, as a result of its high CNR, can demonstrate not only the reduction of luminal diameter by noncalcified plaques but also noncalcified plaques in regions where no significant stenosis is located . Owing to their risk for plaque rupture, first attempts were made to classify noncalcified plaques by their density using multislice CTA.

Fuster and Fayad showed that the coronary artery wall can be imaged with MRI with T1, T2, and PD weighted TSE pulse sequences, which allow imaging of atherosclerotic plaques with different contrast depending on the pulse sequence *(29,30)*. High-resolution MR has emerged as the potential leading noninvasive in vivo imaging modality for atherosclerotic plaque characterization. MR differentiates plaque components on the basis of biophysical and biochemical parameters such as chemical composition and concentration, water content, physical state, molecular motion, or diffusion. MR provides imaging without ionizing radiation and can be repeated over time. In vivo MR plaque imaging and characterization have been performed utilizing a multicontrast approach with high-resolution black blood spin echo– and fast spin echo–based MR sequences. The signal from the blood flow is rendered black through preparatory pulses (e.g., radio-frequency spatial saturation or inversion recovery pulses) to better image the adjacent vessel wall. High-resolution black-blood MR of both normal and atherosclerotic human coronary arteries was performed for direct assessment of coronary wall thickness and the visualization of focal atherosclerotic plaque in the wall. The difference in maximum wall thickness between the normal subjects and patients (>40% stenosis) was statistically significant. The coronary MR plaque imaging study by Fayad et al. was performed during breath-holding to minimize respiratory motion, with a spatial resolution of $0.46 \times 0.46 \times 2.0$ mm^3. To alleviate the need for the patient to hold his or her breath, Botnar et al. *(31)* have combined the black-blood fast spin echo (FSE) method and a real-time navigator for respiratory gating and real-time slice position correction, and achieved a near isotropic spatial resolution ($0.7 \times 0.7 \times 1$ mm^3). This method provided a quick way to image a long segment of the coronary artery wall, and may be useful for rapid coronary plaque burden measurement. Future studies need to address the possibilities.

As shown in animal experimental studies, MR is a powerful tool to serially and noninvasively investigate the progression and regression of atherosclerotic lesions in vivo *(32,33)*. In asymptomatic, untreated, hypercholesterolemic patients with carotid and aortic atherosclerosis, Corti et al. *(34)* showed that MR can be used to measure the efficacy of lipid-lowering therapy with statin. Atherosclerotic plaques were assessed with MR at different times after lipid-lowering therapy. Significant regression of atherosclerotic lesions was observed, despite the early and expected hypolipidemic effect of the statins. Changes in the vessel wall were observed for 12 mo. As with previous experimental studies, there was a decrease in the vessel wall area and no alteration in the lumen area after 12 mo *(35,36)*. Recently, a case-controlled study demonstrated substantially reduced carotid plaque lipid content without change in overall lesion area in patients treated for 10 y with an aggressive lipid-lowering regime compared with untreated control *(37)*.

Comparing multislice CTA and MRI of the vessel wall, CTA is the imaging method that allows to examine the coronary arteries lumen, and detect calcified plaques and noncalcified plaques during a single breath-hold *(26–28)*. However MRI has the potential to classify the plaques that are already identified with different pulse sequence and different contrast at a defined region. In contrast to multislice CTA, the scan time is much longer with MRI. Therefore, for a screening approach, multislice CTA is superior to MRI in detection of vessel wall plaques.

Coronary artery stents are a major problem for noninvasive imaging methods. EBCT, multislice CT, and MRI show artifacts at the regions where stents are implanted. Therefore, in-stent re-stenosis cannot be assessed directly, as the stent lumen is not visible without artifacts. One method to identify in-stent re-stenosis is velocity encoding MRI of the coronary arteries. Nagel et al. performed a study comparing intracoronary flow wire examinations at rest and under adenosine stress, and determined the coronary flow reserve both with MRI and with invasive measurements *(44)*. They found very promising results, which allow identification of in-stent re-stenosis noninvasively and determine their hemodynamical relevance.

REFERENCES

1. Becker CR, Kleffel T, Crispin A, et al. Coronary artery calcium measurement: agreement of multirow detector und electron beam CT. AJR Am J Roentgenol 2002;176:1295–1298.
2. Knez A, Becker C, Becker A, et al. Determination of coronary calcium with multi-slice spiral computed tomography: a comparative study with electron-beam CT. Int J Cardiovasc Imaging 2002;18:295–303.
3. Huber A, Scheidler J, Wintersperger B, et al. Moving-table MR angiography of the peripheral runoff vessels: comparison of body coil and dedicated phased array coil systems. AJR Am J Roentgenol 2003;180:1365–1373.
4. Schoenberg SO, Essig M, Bock M, et al. Comprehensive MR evaluation of renovascular disease in five breathholds. J Magn Reson Imaging 1999;10:347–356.
5. Manning WJ, Li W, Edelman RR. A preliminary report comparing magnetic resonance coronary angiography with conventional angiography. N Engl J Med 1994;328:828–832.
6. Duerinckx AJ, Urman MK. Two-dimensional coronary MR angiography: analysis of initial clinical results. Radiology 1994;193(3): 731–738.
7. Post JC; van Rossum AC, Hofman MBM, et al. Clinical utility of two-dimensional magnetic resonance angiography in detecting coronary artery disease. Eur Heart J 1997;18:426–433.
8. Huber A, Nikolaou K, Gonschior P, et al. Navigator echo-based respiratory gating for three-dimensional MR coronary angiography: results from healthy volunteers and patients with proximal coronary artery stenoses. AJR Am J Roentgenol 1999;173:95–101.
9. Nikolaou K, Huber A, Knez A, et al. Navigator echo-based respiratory gating for 3D-MR coronary angiography: reduction of scan time using a slice-interpolation technique. J Comput Assist Tomogr 2001;25:378–387.
10. Lethimonnier F, Furber A, Morel O, et al. Three-dimensional coronary artery MR imaging using prospective real-time respiratory navigator and linear phase shift processing: comparison with conventional coronary angiography. Magn Reson Imaging 1999;17: 1111–1120.
11. Kim YW, Danias PG, Stuber M, et al. Coronary magnetic resonance angiography for the detection of coronary stenoses. Circulation 2001;247:1863–1869.
12. Kessler W, Laub G, Achenbach S, Ropers D, Moshage W, Daniel WG. Coronary arteries: MR angiography with fast contrast-enhanced three-dimensional breath-hold imaging—initial experience. Radiology 1999;210:566–572.
13. Wielopolski PA, van Geuns RJ, de Feyter PJ, Oudkerk M. Breath-hold coronary MR angiography with volume-targeted imaging. Radiology 1998;209:209–219.
14. Hong C, Becker CR, Huber A, et al. ECG-gated, retrospectively reconstructed multidetector-row CT coronary angiography: effect of varying trigger delay on image quality. Radiology 2001;220: 712–717.
15. Nakanishi T, Ito K, Imazu M, et al. Evaluation of coronary artery stenoses using electron-beam CT and multiplanar reformations. J Comput Assist Tomogr 1997;21:121–127.
16. Achenbach S, Ropers D, Regenfus M, et al. Contrast enhanced electron beam computed tomography to analyse the coronary arteries in patients after acute myocardial infarction. Heart 2000;84:489–493.
17. Schmermund A, Rensing BJ, Sheedy PF, Bell MR, Rumberger JA. Intravenous electron-beam computed tomographic coronary angiography for segmental analysis of coronary artery stenoses. J Am Coll Cardiol 1998;31(7):1547-1554.
18. Reddy GP, Chernoff DM, Adams JR, et al. Coronary artery stenoses: assessment with contrast-enhanced electron-beam CT and axial reconstructions. Radiology 1998;208:167–172.
19. Budoff MJ, Oudiz RF, Zalace CP, et al. Intravenous three-dimensional coronary angiography using contrast enhanced electron beam computed tomography. Am J Cardiol 1999;83:840–854.
20. Achenbach S, Moshage W, Ropers D, et al. Value of electron-beam computed tomography for the noninvasive detection of high-grade

coronary-artery stenoses and occlusions. N Engl J Med 1998;339: 1964–1971.

21. Niemann K, Rensing BJ, van Geuns RJ, et al. Usefulness of multislice computed tomography for detecting obstructive coronary artery disease. Am J Cardiol 2002;89:913–918.
22. Knez A, Becker CR, Leber A, et al. Usefulness of multislice spiral computed tomography angiography for determination of coronary artery stenoses. Am J Cardiol 2001;88:1191–1194.
23. Achenbach S, Giesler T, Ropers D, et al. Detection of coronary artery stenoses by contrast-enhanced, retrospectively electrocardiographically-gated, multislice spiral computed tomography. Circulation 2001;103:2535–2538.
24. Becker CR, Knez A, Leber A, et al. Detection of coronary artery stenoses with multislice helical CT angiography. J Comput Assist Tomogr 2002;26(5):750–755.
25. Vogl TJ, Abolmaali ND; Dibold T, et al. Techniques for the detection of coronary atherosclerosis: multi-detector row CT coronary angiography. Radiology 2002;223:212–220.
26. Hong C, Becker CR, Schoepf UJ, et al. Coronary artery calcium: absolute quantification in nonenhanced and contrast-enhanced multi-detector row CT studies. Radiology 2002;223:474–480.
27. Becker CR, Knez A, Leber A, Treede H, Haberl R, Reiser MF. [Angiography with multi-slice spiral CT. Detecting plaque, before it causes symptoms.] MMW Fortschr Med 2001;143(16): 30–32.
28. Leber AW, Knez A, White CW, et al. composition of coronary atherosclerotic plaques in patients with acute myocardial infarction and stable angina pectoris determined by contrast-enhanced multislice computed tomography. Am J Cardiol 2003;91:714–718.
29. Fayad ZA, Nahar T, Fallon JT, et al. In vivo MR evaluation of atherosclerotic plaques in the human thoracic aorta: a comparison with TEE. Circulation 2000;101:2503–2509.
30. Fayad ZA, Fuster V, Fallon JT, et al. Noninvasive in vivo human coronary artery lumen and wall imaging using black-blood magnetic resonance imaging. Circulation 2002;102:506–510.
31. Botnar RM, Kim WY, Bornert P, et al. 3D coronary vessel wall imaging utilizing a local inversion technique with spiral image acquisition. Magn Reson Med 2001;46:848–854.
32. McConnel MV; Aikawa M, Maier SE, et al. MRI of rabbit atherosclerosis in response to dietary cholesterol lowering. Arterioscler Thromb Vasc Biol 1999;19:1956–1959.
33. Helft G, Worthley SG, Fuster V, et al. Progression and regression of atherosclerotic lesions monitoring with serial noninvasive magnetic resonance imaging. Circulation 2002;105:993–998.
34. Corti R, Fayad ZY; Fuster V, et al. Effects of lipid-lowering by simvastation on human atherosclerotic lesions: a longitudinal study by high-resolution, noninvasive magnetic resonance imaging. Circulation 2001;104:249–252.
35. Zhao XQ, Yuan C, Hatsukami TS, et al. Effects of prolonged intensive lipid-lowering therapy on the characteristics of carotid atherosclerotic plaques in vivo by MRI: a case-controlled study. Arterioscler Thromb Vasc Biol 2001;21(10):1623-1629.
36. Manning WJ, Li W, Edelman RR. A preliminary report comparing magnetic resonance coronary angiography with conventional angiography. N Engl J Med 1993;328:828–832.
37. Post JC; van Rossum AC; Hofman MBM, et al. Three-dimensional respiratory-gated MR angiography of coronary arteries: comparison with conventional coronary angiography. AJR Am J Roentgenol 1996;166:1399–1404.
38. Mueller MF, Fleisch M, Kroeker R, et al. Proximal coronary artery stenosis: three-dimensional MRI with fat saturation and navigator echo. J Magn Reson Imaging 1997;7:644–651.
39. Sanstede JJ, Pabst T, Beer M, et al. Three-dimensional MR coronary angiography using the navigator technique compared with conventional coronary angiography. AJR Am J Roentgenol 1999;172:135–139.
40. Sardanelli F, Molinari G, Zandrino F, et al. Three-dimensional, navigator-echo MR coronary angiography in detecting stenoses of the major epicardial vessels, with conventional coronary angiography as the standard of reference. Radiology 2000;214:808–814.
41. Gonschior P, Pragst I, Valassis G, et al. High-resolution MR angiography: results in diseased arteries. J Invasive Cardiol 2001; 13:151–157.
42. van Geuns RJ, Wielopolski PA, de Bruin HG, et al. MR coronary angiography with breath-hold targeted volumes: preliminary clinical results. Radiology 2000;217:270–277.
43. Regenfus M, Ropers D, Achenbach S, et al. Noninvasive detection of coronary artery stenosis using contrast-enhanced three-dimensional breath-hold magnetic resonance coronary angiography. J Am Coll Cardiol 2000;36:44–50.
44. Nagel E, Thouet T, Klein C, et al. Noninvasive determination of coronary blood flow velocity with cardiovascular magnetic resonance in patients after stent deployment. Circulation 2003;107:1738–1743.

Contrast-Enhanced CT of the Heart: *Principles of Atherosclerosis and Vessel Wall Imaging*

VI

33 Pathology and Pathophysiology of Coronary Atherosclerotic Plaques

RENU VIRMANI, MD, ALLEN P. BURKE, MD, FRANK D. KOLODGIE, PhD, ANDREW FARB, MD, ALOKE V. FINN, MD, AND HERMAN GOLD, MD

INTRODUCTION

The death rate from coronary artery disease has declined in the past few decades through greater understanding of risk factors of coronary heart disease as well as through better treatment, including the creation of coronary care units. However, because of the lack of an animal model of unstable plaque, our understanding of atherosclerotic plaque morphology comes only from static histology of lesion morphology in patients dying of acute coronary syndromes *(1)*. Although transgenic models of atherosclerosis have markedly enhanced our understanding of certain aspects of plaque progression and regression, they have failed thus far to explain the relationship of the coagulation parameters and plaque morphology that precipitate coronary thrombosis *(1)*. Until we are able to create a better model or study plaque morphology prospectively and determine the mechanisms and the anatomic markers of progression, we will make progress very slowly. This review is based on examination of human coronary artery pathology in patients dying a sudden coronary death, in order to ascertain the pathologic lesion morphologies that are linked to plaque progression and thrombosis, which will be necessary for us to be able to recognized by invasive or noninvasive means the prospective lesions that are likely to produce symptoms.

CLASSIFICATION OF ATHEROSCLEROSIS

Our understanding of atherosclerosis has been enhanced by the development of the various classifications that have come from the insights of scientists like Virchow, who was a pioneer in pathology. Systematic studies of lesion development, described by the giants of atherosclerosis including Robert Wissler, Herbert Stary (Table 1), Henry McGill, and Michael Davies in the last century, have made enormous contributions to the better understanding of early lesions, the influence of risk factors on plaque progression, and the role of plaque rupture in the occurrence of luminal thrombosis.

The cellular participants of atherosclerosis include smooth muscle cells, endothelial cells, macrophages, T- and B-lymphocytes, red cells, platelets, neutrophils, and basophils. The noncellular components include lipid, proteoglycans, collagen, elastic fibers, calcium, iron (hemosiderin), and blood components, including fibrin and factor VIII. These various components help to form the various lesions that are recognized as part of the atherosclerotic process. These include adaptive intimal thickening (AIT), intimal xanthomas, pathologic intimal thickening (PIT), fibroatheroma, thin-cap fibroatheroma, plaque rupture, plaque erosion, calcified nodule, fibrocalcific plaque, healed plaque rupture, and fibrous plaque (either from healed plaque erosion or propagated thrombus). The best-known of the classifications is the American Heart Association report by Stary et al. *(2,3)*. The various lesions of atherosclerosis will be described and the plaque morphologies that lead to coronary thrombosis along with the precursor lesion of plaque rupture, also known as thin-cap fibroatheroma or vulnerable plaque.

ADAPTIVE INTIMAL THICKENING (AIT)

AIT occurs in most arteries once flow is established in utero or soon after birth, consisting primarily of smooth muscle cells, which are strongly α-actin positive and surrounded by a proteoglycan-rich matrix (Fig. 1A). Macrophages are rarely detected. These lesions are most prominent at branch points and are considered by many to be precursor lesions of atherosclerosis. Kim et al. have shown in hypercholesterolemic swine that atherosclerotic lesions arise almost exclusively from intimal cell masses. Similarly, we have observed that lesions of pathologic intimal thickening with lipid pools arise at sites of branch points where adaptive intimal thickening is prominent, and therefore are most likely the precursor lesions of atherosclerosis.

INTIMAL XANTHOMAS (FATTY STREAK)

We have used the microscopic term intimal xanthoma for fatty streak, the corresponding designation for the lesion as grossly seen in the aorta. We believe intimal xanthoma is not a lesion of atherosclerosis, as it eventually regresses in humans. The Pathobiologic Determinants of Atherosclerosis in Youth (PDAY) study showed that fatty streaks are prominent in the third decade in the thoracic aorta, but regress later in life. The site of advanced lesions is generally the abdominal aorta, where fatty streaks are relatively uncommon. Fatty streaks are rich in macrophages (hence the term *xanthoma*) but lack necrotic cores or lipid pools (Fig. 1B).

From: *Contemporary Cardiology: CT of the Heart: Principles and Applications*
Edited by: U. Joseph Schoepf © Humana Press, Inc., Totowa, NJ

Table 1
Atherosclerotic Plaque Classifications

		Virmani et al.	
		Initial	*Progression*
Early plaques	Type I: Microscopic detection of lipid droplets in intima and small groups of macrophage foam cells	Intimal thickening	None
	Type II: Fatty streaks visible on gross inspection, layers of foam cells, occasional lymphocytes and mast cells	Intimal xanthoma	None
	Type III (intermediate): Extracellular lipid pools among layers of smooth muscle cells	Pathologic intimal thickening	Thrombosis (erosion)
Intermediate plaque	Type IV: Well-defined lipid core; may develop surface disruption (fissure)	Fibrous cap atheroma	Thrombosis (Erosion)[a]
Late lesions	Type Va: New fibrous tissue overlying lipid core (multilayered fibroatheroma)[b]	Thin cap fibroatheroma	Thrombus (rupture)
		Healed plaque rupture, erosion	Repeated rupture or erosion with or without total occlusion
	Type Vb: Calcification[c]	Fibrocalcific plaque (with or without necrotic core)	
	Type Vc: Fibrotic lesion with minimal lipid (could be result of organized thrombi)		
Miscellaneous/ complicated features	Type VIa: Surface disruption	Calcified nodule	Thrombus (usually nonocclusive)
	Type VIb: Intraplaque hemorrhage		
	Type VIc: Thrombosis		

[a] May further progress with healing (healed erosion).
[b] May overlap with healed plaque ruptures.
[c] Occasionally referred to as type VII lesion. Modified from ref. *26*.

PATHOLOGIC INTIMAL THICKENING (PIT)

PIT lesion is also rich in smooth muscle cells in a proteoglycan matrix (Fig. 2A). However, the area close to the media shows loss of smooth muscle cells and an accumulation of fat as a lipid pool, which stains positive with oil red O. A significant number of smooth muscle cells close to the media show accumulation of intracellular fat and may appear foamy, best appreciated by transmission electron microscopy. The smooth muscle cells may appear as ghosts with surrounding thickened basement membrane, which stains strongly Periodic Acid Schiff (PAS) positive *(3a)*. The surrounding matrix also stains positive for oil red O and often shows the presence of monohydrate cholesterol, which may appear as cholesterol crystals (lipid pools). There may be macrophage infiltration in the superficial regions of the plaque, but these macrophages are not in proximity to the lipid pools. It is believed that smooth muscle cells are undergoing apoptosis, degeneration, and calcification *(22)*. We believe that pathologic intimal thickening is the precursor lesion of the fibroatheroma.

FIBROUS CAP ATHEROMA

Fibrous cap atheromas are lesions with a necrotic core and a thick fibrous cap (Fig. 2B). The necrotic core is rich in acellular debris and varies in size. The fibrous cap covers the necrotic core completely, is rich in smooth muscle cells within a collagen/proteoglycan matrix, and may contain macrophages and lymphocytes. The thickness of the fibrous cap varies; a thin cap is believed to impart instability, and therefore warrants a separate designation of thin cap fibroatheroma.

We believe that the necrotic core originates from foam cell infiltration of the lipid pool and eventual breakdown of the foamy cell, which occurs as a result of apoptosis or necrosis. How the necrotic core enlarges and becomes rich in free cholesterol is poorly understood. Hemorrhage into a plaque, either through the breakdown of the vasa vasorum or possibly through plaque fissuring, may play an important role. It is possible that the vasa vasorum become leaky, allowing fibrinogen to leak into the plaque if pressure within them rises, as they have a poorly developed basement membrane and often lack pericytes and smooth muscle cells. In support of this concept is the frequent finding of fibrin, by immunohistochemical methods, within the necrotic core.

THIN FIBROUS CAP ATHEROMA

The original description of Stary et al. did not mention the thin fibrous cap atheroma (TCFA) as a precursor lesion of plaque rupture. Partly based on their morphologic resemblance to acute ruptures, we believe that they are the precursor lesions. The TCFA is defined as a lesion with a necrotic core and an overlying fibrous cap that is <65 μm and infiltrated by macrophages (>25 per high power magnification [0.03-mm diameter field]) *(4)* (Fig. 3). The thickness criterion of TCFA was

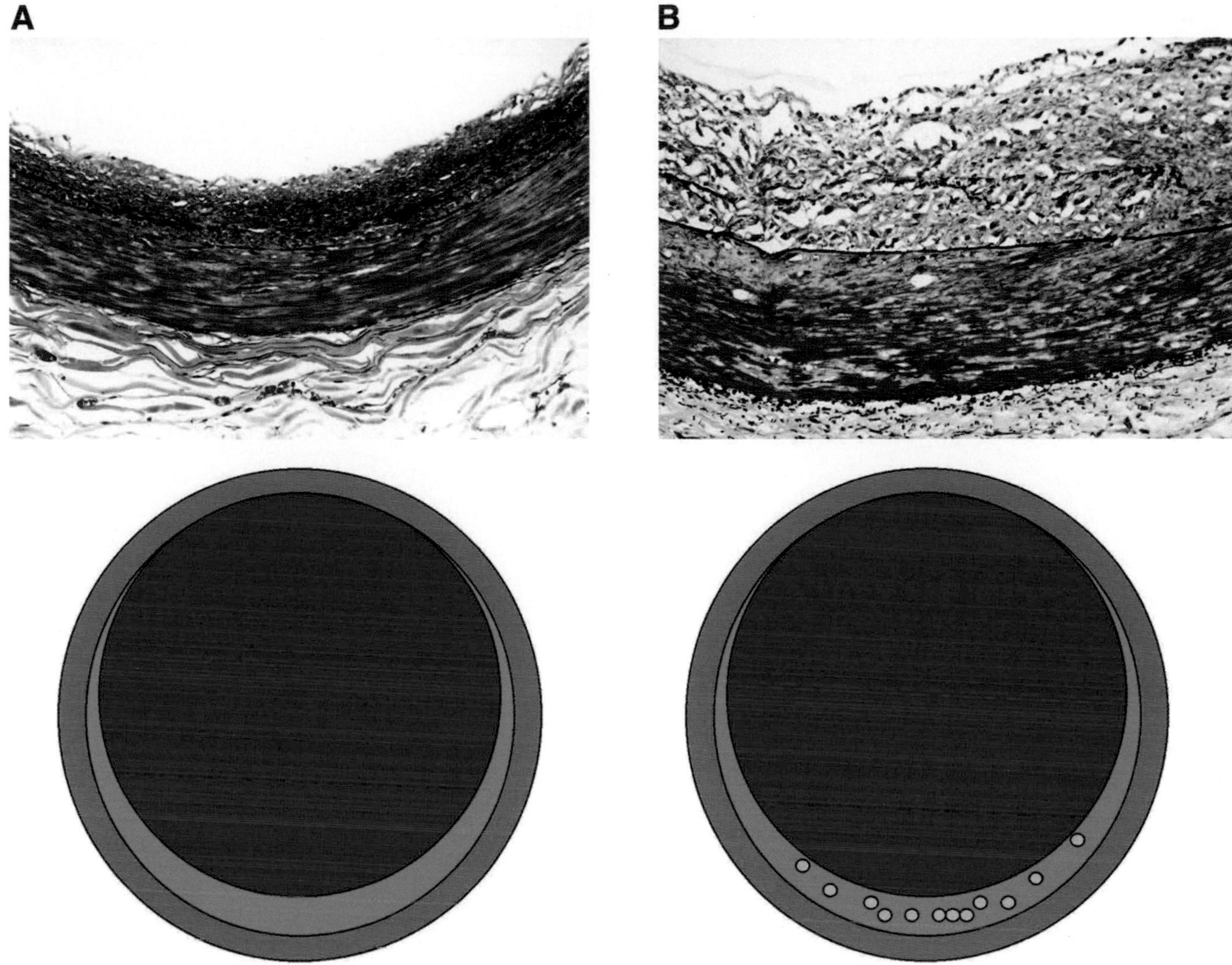

Fig. 1. Adaptive intimal thickening (**A**) and intimal xanthoma (**B**). Lesions uniformly present in all populations, although intimal xanthomas are more prevalent with exposure to a Western diet. Intimal xanthomas are commonly produced in animal models; however, they usually do not develop into progressive atherosclerotic lesions. Both lesions occur soon after birth; the intimal xanthoma (otherwise known as a fatty streak) is known to regress. Intimal thickening consists mainly of smooth muscle cells in a proteoglycan-rich matrix, while intimal xanthomas primarily contain macrophage-derived foam cells, T lymphocytes, and varying degrees of smooth muscle cells. Reproduced from ref. *1*, with permission.

chosen because 95% of fibrous caps adjacent to acute plaque rupture measured <65 μm, with a mean cap thickness of 23 ± 19 μm. We have also compared other morphologic characteristics between plaque rupture and TCFA. The necrotic core is smaller than that seen in rupture (Table 2). In addition, the percent area occupied by the necrotic core is greater in rupture than TCFA, although we were unable to determine any significant differences in length (Table 2).The cross-sectional luminal narrowing of TCFA is less than that of acute rupture; nearly 80% of TCFAs had luminal narrowing <75% in contrast to rupture (Fig. 4).

LESIONS WITH THROMBI

From studies carried out in patients dying sudden coronary death, we have observed three main causes of luminal thrombi: plaque rupture (the precursor of which is presumably the TCFA), erosion, and calcified nodule (Fig. 5). The most frequent cause of thrombosis being plaque rupture (over 60%), plaque erosion is the second most frequent (about 35%), whereas calcified nodule is a rare cause of thrombosis (<5%). These three types of thrombosis occur, respectively, in the setting of a TCFA, fibroatheroma or pathologic intimal thickening, and a calcified plaque with or without a necrotic core (Fig. 1).

PLAQUE RUPTURE

Plaque rupture is defined as a disruption, discontinuous fibrous cap, underlying necrotic core, and superimposed luminal thrombus. Ruptured plaques that result in occlusive luminal thrombi almost invariably have a large necrotic core, which occupies =25% of the plaque area in 80% of cases. Plaque rupture is the major underlying mechanism of luminal throm-

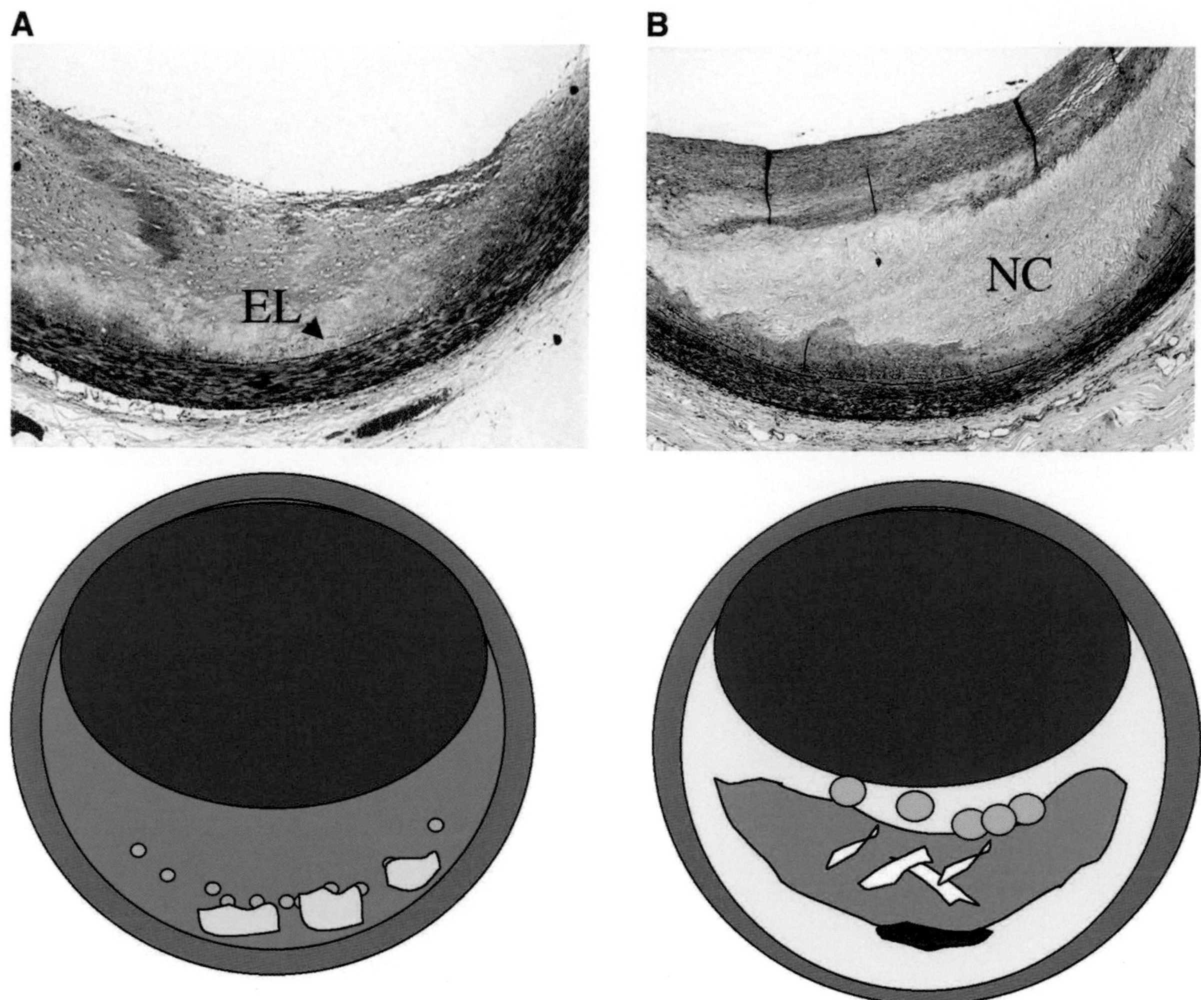

Fig. 2. Pathological intimal thickening (**A**) vs atheroma (**B**). Pathological intimal thickening is a poorly defined entity sometimes referred to in the literature as an "intermediate lesion." True necrosis is not apparent, and there is no evidence of cellular debris; some lipid may be present deep in the lesion near the elastic lamina (EL), but it is dispersed. The fibrous cap overlying the areas of lipid is rich in smooth muscle cells and proteoglycans. Some scattered macrophages and lymphocytes may also be present, but are usually sparse. The more definitive lesion or fibrous cap atheroma classically shows a "true" necrotic core (NC), containing cholesterol esters, free cholesterol, phospholipids, and triglycerides. The fibrous cap consists of smooth muscle cells in a proteoglycan-collagenous matrix, with a variable number of macrophages and lymphocytes. The media underneath the plaque is often thin. Reproduced from ref. *1*, with permission.

Table 2
Approximate Sizes of Necrotic Core in Fibroatheroma, Thin Cap Atheroma, and Acute Rupture

	Plaque type		
Dimension	*Fibroatheroma*	*Thin cap atheroma*	*Acute plaque rupture*
Length, mm, mean/range	6 mm (range 1–18 mm)	8 mm (range 2–17 mm)	9 mm (range 2.5 ± 22)
Cross sectional area, mm^2	1.2 ± 2.2	1.7 ± 1.1	4.1 ± 5.5
% cross sectional area	15 ± 20%	23 ± 17%	34 ± 17%

Reproduced from ref. *27* with permission.

bosis in sudden death (60%), acute myocardial infarction (75%), and unstable angina (70%), and is rarely present in stable angina *(5–7)*. The mechanism of rupture is poorly understood; however, it is generally believed that macrophages infiltrate the cap and release matrix metalloproteinases, which are responsible for the breakdown of the collagens *(8,9)*. There is also evidence that macrophage myeloperoxidase may be responsible for the disruption of the fibrous cap by producing

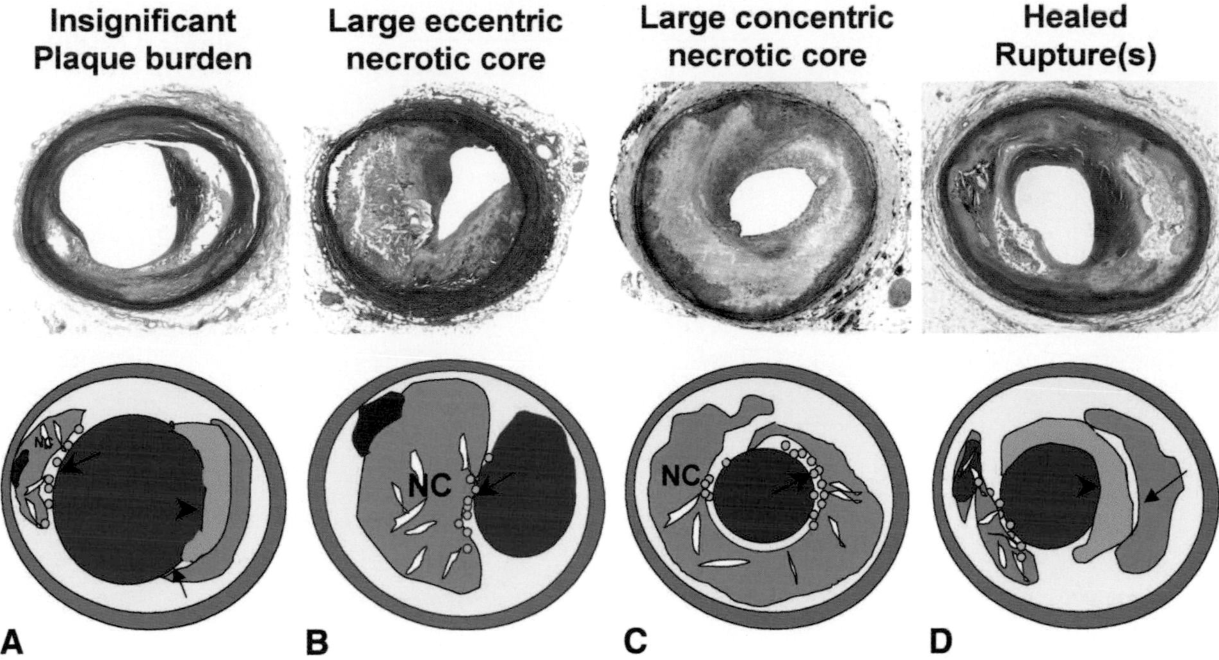

Fig. 3. Morphologic variants of the thin-cap atheroma. Thin caps may emerge in fibroatheromas with insignificant plaque burden and insignificant luminal narrowing, in fibroatheromas with large cores that are eccentric or eccentric, and frequently in plaques with evidence of prior rupture. **(A)** In this plaque with insignificant plaque burden, there is an area of proteoglycan-rich smooth muscle cells (arrowheads) suggestive of a prior rupture, and multiple areas of thin caps (arrows). **(B)** The necrotic core (NC) is large, with an area of thinned cap (arrow). **(C)** The necrotic core (NC) is concentric with an extensive area of cap thinning (arrow). **(D)** There may be a healed rupture (arrows) with a proteoglycan-rich smooth muscle cell reparative layer (arrowhead).

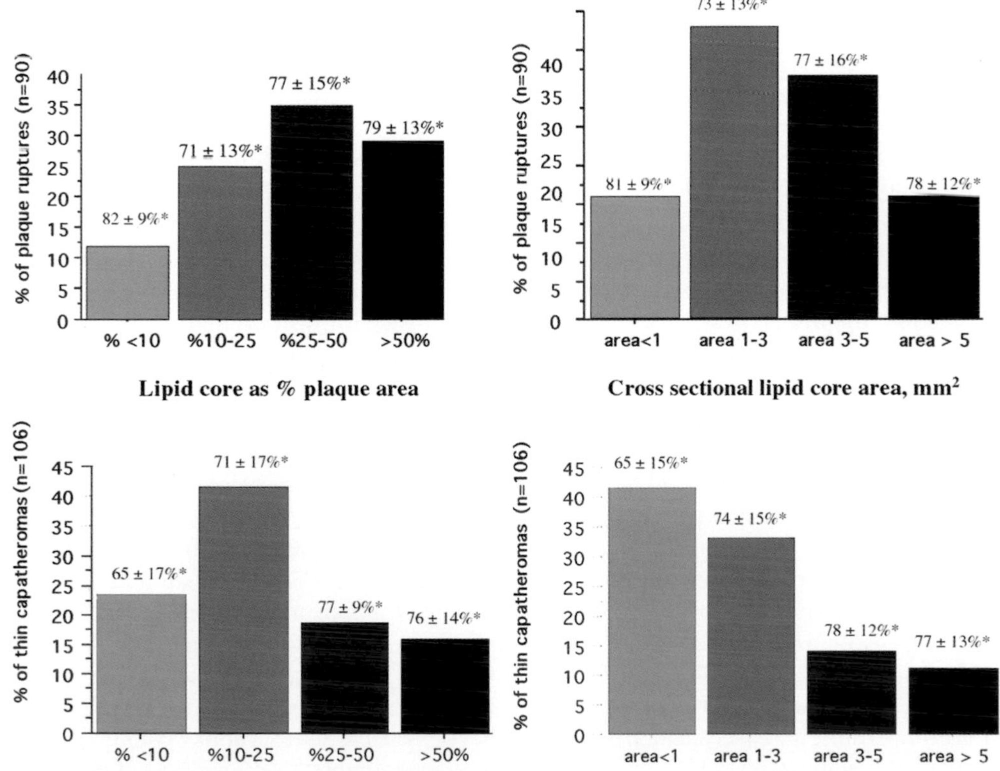

Fig. 4. The distribution frequency of plaque ruptures **(A,B)** and thin-cap atheromas **(C,D)** by size of lipid core or lipid core as a percent of plaque area (*x* axis). The majority of plaque ruptures occur when lipid core area forms 25–50% of plaque area, or 1–3 mm^2 lipid core area. In the case of thin-cap atheromas, the degree of cross-sectional area luminal narrowing and area of necrotic core is shifted to the left (lesser or smaller) as compared to plaque ruptures. Reproduced from ref. *27*, with permission.

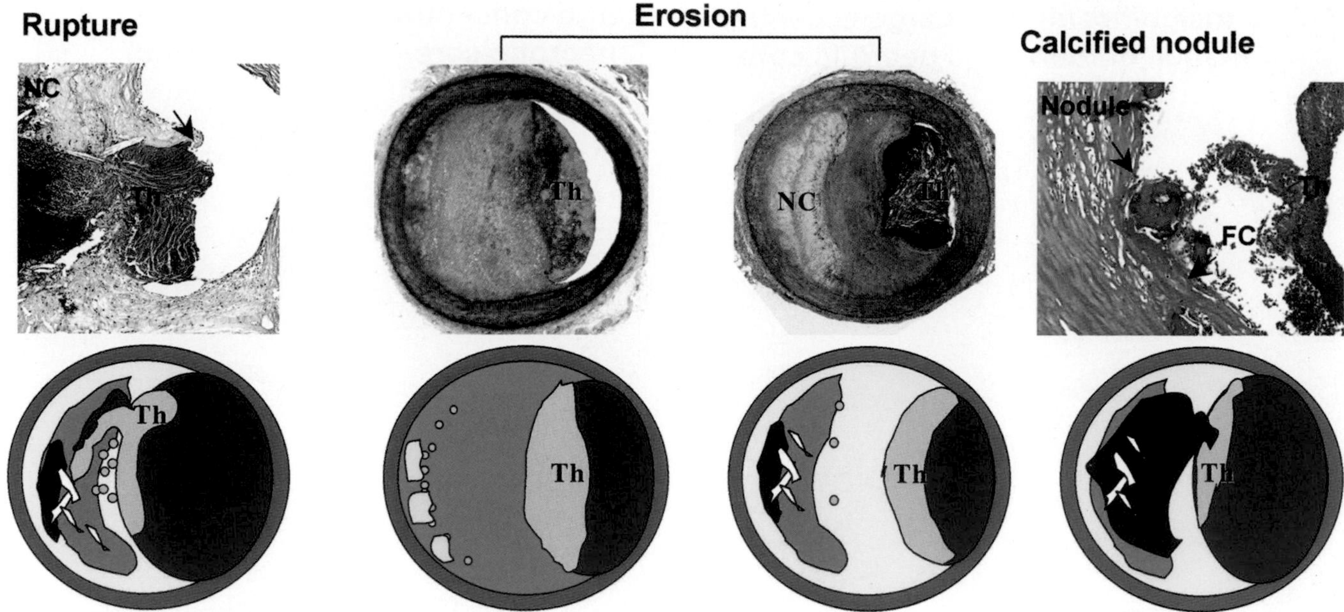

Fig. 5. Lesions with thrombi. Ruptured plaques are thin fibrous-cap atheromas with luminal thrombi (Th). These lesions usually have an extensive necrotic core containing large numbers of cholesterol crystals, and a thin fibrous cap (<65 μm) infiltrated by foamy macrophages and a paucity of T-lymphocytes. The fibrous cap is thinnest at the site of rupture and consists of a few collagen bundles and rare smooth muscle cells. The luminal thrombus is in communication with the lipid-rich necrotic core. Erosions occur over lesions rich in smooth muscle cells and proteoglycans. Luminal thrombi overly areas lacking surface endothelium. The deep intima of the eroded plaque often shows extracellular lipid pools, but necrotic cores are uncommon; when present, the necrotic core does not communicate with the luminal thrombus. Inflammatory infiltrate is usually absent, but if present, it is sparse and consists of macrophages and lymphocytes. Calcified nodules are plaques with luminal thrombi showing calcific nodules protruding into the lumen through a disrupted thin fibrous cap (FC). There is absence of endothelium at the site of the thrombus, and inflammatory cells (macrophages, T-lymphocytes) are absent. Reproduced from ref. *1*, with permission.

the pro-oxidant species, hypochlorous acid. We have shown that up to 15% of macrophages within ruptured fibrous caps are rich in myeloperoxidase. We have observed that the numbers of plaque hemorrhages in the coronary arteries of patients dying suddenly with acute plaque rupture are greater than in patients with severe coronary disease dying with other forms of thrombosis or without coronary thrombosis. These data suggest that hemorrhage, due to plaque fissure or rupture of vasa vasorum, may be precursors to plaque rupture. Davies has shown that 11% of hearts have plaque fissure with intra-intimal thrombus, 2% have intimal thrombus as the only mechanism of sudden death, while rupture with thrombosis was identified in 74%, and only 5% had no acute coronary lesion *(10)*. We have observed vasa vasorum to be more prominent in patients dying suddenly during exercise with plaque rupture, compared to patients dying at rest. Also, hemorrhage into a plaque was more frequent in patients dying during exercise than in patients dying at rest *(11)*. The rupture site has been reported to be the shoulder region in a majority of cases. However, we observed the most frequent site to be the central region of the cap (42%), followed by shoulder (36%) and circumferential (4%). In 18% of ruptures, it was not possible to determine the exact location because of extensive destruction of the rupture site *(11)*.

PLAQUE EROSION

Plaque erosion is defined as an acute thrombus in direct contact with intimal plaque rich in smooth muscle cells within a proteoglycan matrix, and an absence of endothelium *(1,6)*. There are relatively few macrophages and lymphocytes adjacent to the thrombus in the majority of plaque erosions. Plaque erosion accounts for 20% of all sudden coronary deaths and 35% of coronary thrombi in patients dying suddenly with coronary thrombosis *(1,6)*. The mean age of patients dying with plaque erosion is less than that of patients dying with acute rupture, and there is less severe narrowing at sites of thrombosis in plaque erosion. Plaque erosion accounts for over 80% of thrombi occurring in women less than 50 yr of age. The lesions tend to be eccentric and are infrequently calcified *(6)*. Plaque erosions tend to embolize more frequently than plaque rupture (74%, vs 40%, respectively) *(6)*. The risk factors for erosion are poorly understood; similar to acute rupture, there is an increased risk among smokers, but there appears to be a lesser association with dyslipidemia, as compared to plaque rupture. The underlying plaque in erosions is generally pathologic intimal thickening or fibrous cap atheroma. The most frequent location for both erosion and rupture is the proximal left anterior descending coronary artery (nearly two-thirds of patients) followed by the right coronary artery and the left circumflex. However, patients dying with plaque erosion frequently do not have extensive disease, unlike patients dying with stable plaque or plaque rupture. Over one-half of deaths are seen in patients with single-vessel disease, and one-quarter with double-vessel disease. The etiology of plaque erosion is poorly understood; however, it is believed that coronary vasospasm may be involved.

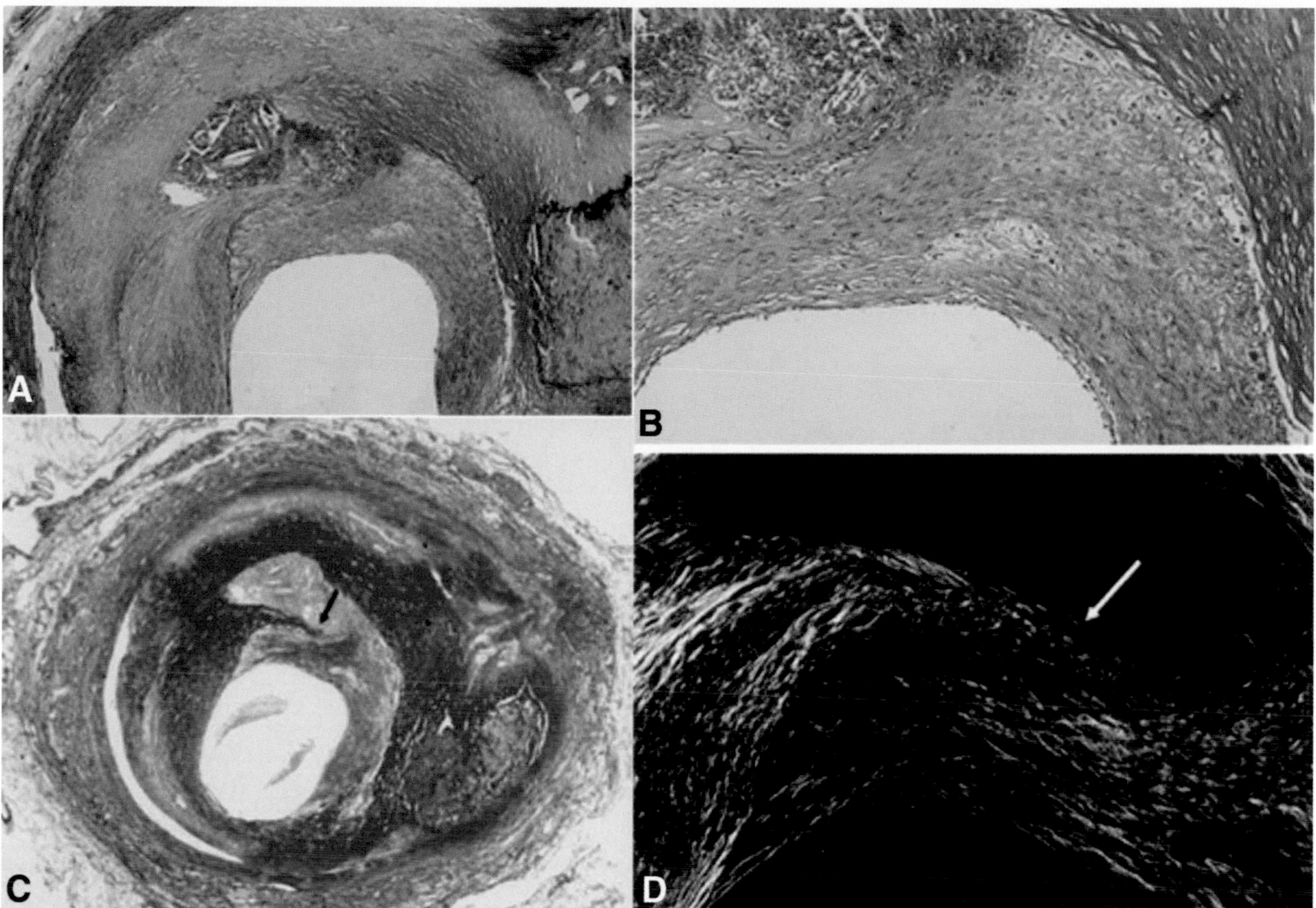

Fig. 6. Healed plaque rupture. **(A)** demonstrates areas of intraintimal lipid-rich core with hemorrhage and cholesterol clefts. **(B)** shows a higher magnification of the looser smooth muscle cell formation within a collagenous proteoglycan–rich neointima showing a clear demarcation with the more fibrous regions of the old plaque to the right. **(C)** and **(D)** demonstrate the layers of collagen by Sirius red staining. **(C)**, note the area of dense dark red collagen surrounding the lipid hemorrhagic cores seen in corresponding view in panel **A**. **(D)** demonstrates an image taken with polarized light. The dense collagen (Type 1) which forms the fibrous cap is lighter reddish-yellow and is disrupted (arrow), with the newer greenish Type III collagen on the right and above the rupture site. (**A** and **B**, Movat pentachrome). Reproduced from ref. *28*, with permission.

CALCIFIED NODULE

The least frequent lesion that results in coronary luminal thrombus is the calcified nodule, a plaque that contains calcified plates at the site of luminal disruption. There may or may not be necrotic core within the plaque, but the characteristic features are the breakage of calcified plates, often with a fibrotic reaction, interspersed fibrin, a disrupted surface, and an overlying thrombus. Occasionally, bone formation with osteoblasts and osteoclasts is present *(1)*. The lesion is located in the mid-right coronary artery in 50% of cases, generally in a heavily calcified segment. It is more common in older male individuals than women. We have observed these lesions in the carotid arteries as well as the coronaries, and speculate that their development may be related to the repeated episodes of plaque hemorrhage.

HEALED PLAQUE RUPTURES

Not all plaque ruptures result in symptoms; therefore, there should be morphologic hallmarks that could be recognized within plaques that are representative of a previous site of thrombus. Healed ruptures in the coronary vascular bed are readily detected microscopically by the identification of the breaks in the fibrous cap, which is rich in type I collagen, and an overlying repaired lesion, which is richer in type III collagen. The healed lesion can be more easily recognized by Movat stain (healed site identified by the brilliant blue-green color of the proteoglycan-rich matrix) and confirmed by picrosirius red staining and polarized microscopy. When viewed under polarized light, this stain highlights the breaks in the fibrous cap, which is rich in collagen type I, as yellow-red birefringence with an underlying necrotic core (Fig. 6). The plaque overlying the fibrous cap consists of smooth muscle cells in a proteoglycan matrix, which is rich in type III collagen and has green birefringence under polarized light (sirius red stained) *(11)*.

We and others believe that healing of a disrupted plaque is the main stimulus for plaque progression and is a major factor in causing chronic high-grade coronary stenosis once a late atherosclerotic necrotic core with a thin fibrous cap has formed *(12)*. This mechanism would explain the phasic rather than

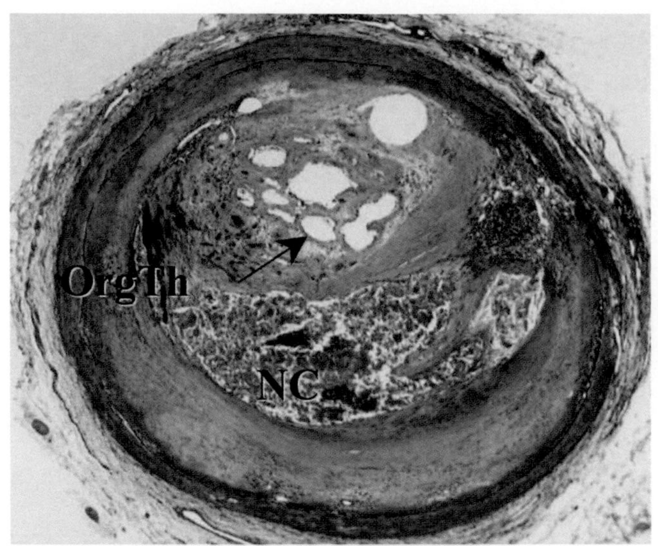

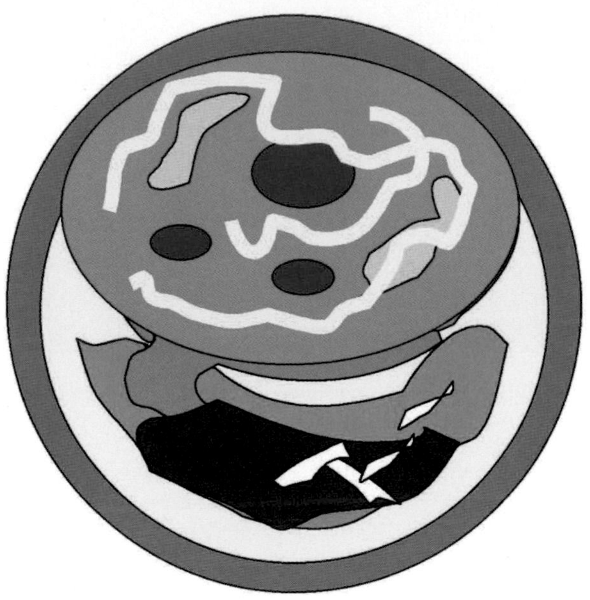

Fig. 7. Total occlusion. Plaques with total occlusion from prior thrombi contain mostly smooth muscle cells in a collagen-proteoglycan-rich matrix with capillaries and inflammatory cell infiltrate. This section shows a necrotic core (NC), although this is not always present, and the lumen is filled with an organized thrombus (orgTh) with multiple capillary channels.

linear progression of coronary disease observed in angiograms carried out annually in patients with chronic ischemic heart disease *(12)*. However, these are speculations that need to be proven when we can prospectively recognize the sites of vulnerability and follow up the lesional morphologies with advanced imaging techniques. We have also shown that these lesions are the most heavily calcified as compared to acute rupture or thin-cap fibroatheroma, suggesting that healing of a ruptured plaque also results in greater extent of calcification *(13)*.

TOTAL OCCLUSIONS (*see* FIG. 7)

Among patients dying sudden coronary death without prior symptoms, total occlusion is a frequent finding at autopsy. The frequency is as high as 40% when there are no other sites with acute plaque rupture. Healed myocardial infarcts are seen in 90% of patients with a total occlusion *(1)*. The lumen is composed of dense collagen and/or proteoglycans with interspersed capillaries, arterioles, smooth muscle cells, and macrophages. In the case of total occlusions secondary to thrombi, the proximal and distal ends organize initially, followed by the middle segment, which may demonstrate entrapped red cells and fibrin without cellular ingrowth for long periods. Sites of total occlusion are often associated with negative remodeling of the vessel, probably related to collagen replacement of the thrombus with eventual crosslinking, resulting in artery shrinkage. There is often little calcification within total occlusions, probably because the plaque has formed via organized thrombus, as opposed to successive ruptures of necrotic cores with preserved blood flow.

FIBROUS AND FIBROCALCIFIC PLAQUES

A subset of coronary artery plaques have little evidence of lipid pool or necrotic core formation, and are designated as fibrous or fibrocalcific plaques, depending on the presence of calcification. The mechanism of plaque enlargement of such plaques is unknown, but may be in some cases related to propagated thrombus or healed plaque erosions (Fig. 8). These lesions are rich in type I collagen, but type III collagen and proteoglycans may also be present. The calcium deposition may be related to calcified apoptotic smooth muscle cells in the absence of a significant influx of macrophages and other inflammatory cells. The term *fibrous plaque* has not been typically used in formal classifications of coronary artery atherosclerosis, partly because it is a general category that may represent an etiologically diverse set of lesions.

PLAQUE HEMORRHAGE

As mentioned above, the interrelationship between intraplaque hemorrhage, fibrin, necrotic core, and vasa vasorum has not been fully explained. Most vasa vasorum originate from the parent artery and ramify plexogenically in the adventitia *(14)*. There is a clear relationship between numbers of vasa vasorum (Fig. 9) and blood flow through them, and mass of coronary plaque *(15)*. In addition, increased vasa vasorum are associated with atherosclerotic plaque expansion *(14)*, and plaque regression is paralleled by a decrease in blood flow through the vasa vasorum *(16)*. Further evidence for a dynamic relationship between vasa vasorum and the atherosclerotic process are the fact that they respond to vasoconstrictor stimuli, and that their density is associated with exertional plaque rupture *(11)*.

The mechanisms by which vasa vasorum contribute to plaque growth are poorly understood. Plaque iron content is a surrogate marker of preceding hemorrhage, and correlates with plaque neovascularization *(14)*. The frequency of iron deposition in the coronary plaques is higher in patients with acute coronary syndrome than in those dying of noncardiac causes *(17)*. Since plaque hemorrhage is a frequent phenomenon, especially in advanced plaques, it is not surprising that some of the free cholesterol may have its origin from the red cell membrane *(18)*. The increase in iron content correlated with

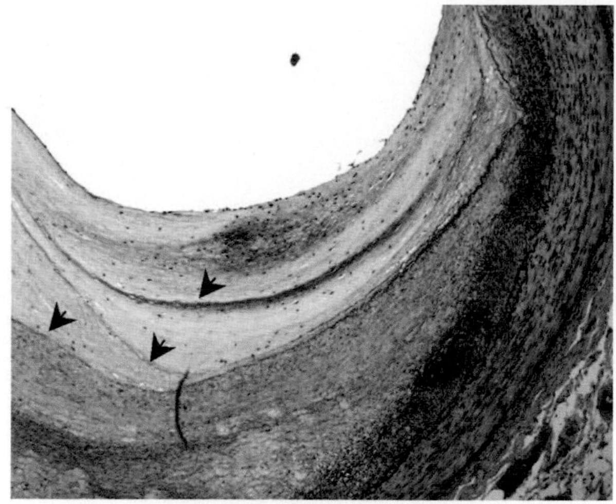

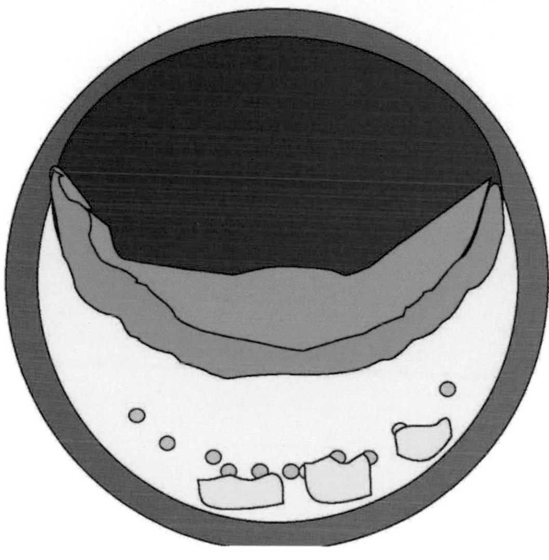

Fig. 8. Healed erosion shows deep multilayering of collagen separated by elastin layers (arrowheads) and a paucity of smooth muscle cells. The superficial plaque is rich in smooth muscle cells, collagen, and proteoglycans.

intraplaque hemorrhage as identified by glycophorin A staining, a red-cell specific anion-exchange protein. In a recent study of pulmonary artery atherosclerotic plaques by Arbustini et al., glycophorin A positive erythrocyte membranes were shown to be a major component of the necrotic core in patients with chronic thromboembolic pulmonary hypertension *(19)*.

Rupture of vasa vasorum is not the sole etiology of intraplaque hemorrhage. As Constantinides originally suggested, plaque hemorrhage may occur from cracks or fissures originating from the lumen *(20)*. Intraplaque hemorrhage, whether from vasa vasorum or the lumen, may be critical to the lesion progression, as it may provide a significant source of nonmetabolic cholesterol *(21)*.

CORONARY CALCIFICATION

In early coronary atherosclerotic plaques, coronary calcification is identified using sensitive histochemical stains, such as the von Kossa stain. When such tests are applied to fatty streaks, there is little if any calcium present. However, pathologic intimal thickening and fibrous plaques have a high propensity for microscopic calcification, especially when there is evidence of smooth muscle cell apoptosis. The biology of intimal calcification within atherosclerotic regions is complex, and involves smooth muscle cell matrix vesicles (related to apoptotic bodies), bone-associated proteins, lipids, and inflammation in the formation of extracellular intimal calcifications *(22)*. Almost all necrotic cores with apoptotic smooth muscle cells contain calcification (at least 90%), and those cores with predominantly macrophage infiltrates are less likely to initially calcify. The nature of the calcifications differs by cell type, in that fibrous cores contain finely granular calcifications, occasionally coalescing into masses, whereas macrophage "necrotic" cores often contain larger crystalline deposits. Calcification of fibrous plaques in which there is smooth muscle cell death cores progresses to plate-like sheets of calcification and often pipestem-like arteries. However, calcification of necrotic, inflamed, macrophage-rich cores tends to be more irregular, resulting in a radiographic appearance of irregular calcification. Ultrastructural study of coronary plaques will demonstrate calcifications in close contact with dying smooth muscle cells, macrophages, and surrounding cholesterol clefts (Fig. 10). In less than 5% of plaques, actual ossification may occur, with osteoblasts, osteoclasts, and even marrow formation (Fig. 11).

Calcification does not in itself appear to play a role in the thrombotic process, except under the unusual circumstances of nodular calcification. Successive ruptures or fissures of the fibrous cap result in layering of the plaque, and the deeper layers close to the internal elastic lamina typically demonstrate more severe calcification than the surface layers.

We have performed quantitative analysis of calcified matrix in intermediate and later plaque stages, including fibroatheromas, acute and healed plaque ruptures, total occlusions, and plaque erosion. In contrast to rupture, plaque erosion does not expose the contents of the necrotic core to the lumen. Eroded plaques, perhaps partly as a function of their pathogenesis, do not typically occur in calcified arteries, and demonstrate far less calcified matrix than acute or healed ruptures. The degree of calcification by plaque type is illustrated in Fig. 12.

The relationship between coronary plaque calcification and plaque instability has been debated. Biomechanical studies have calculated stress at different regions of the plaque. Mathematical models using large-strain finite element analysis have shown that increased lipids are associated with areas of weakness of the fibrous cap, but not calcification *(23)*. Although calcification is a good marker for plaque burden, absolute calcium scores do not indicate plaques that are unstable or prone to result in clinical events. It has been stated that calcification is a "disease marker" as opposed to a "process marker," unlike markers of inflammation*(24)*. These findings are corroborated by autopsy studies that demonstrate a good correlation between plaque size and morphometric analysis of calcification, but no correlation between residual lumen and calcification (Table 3). Few studies have correlated the radiologic pattern of calcification with plaque instability *(25)*, but there is some suggestion that speckled or fragmented calcification patterns as determined radiologically are most likely associated with unstable plaque

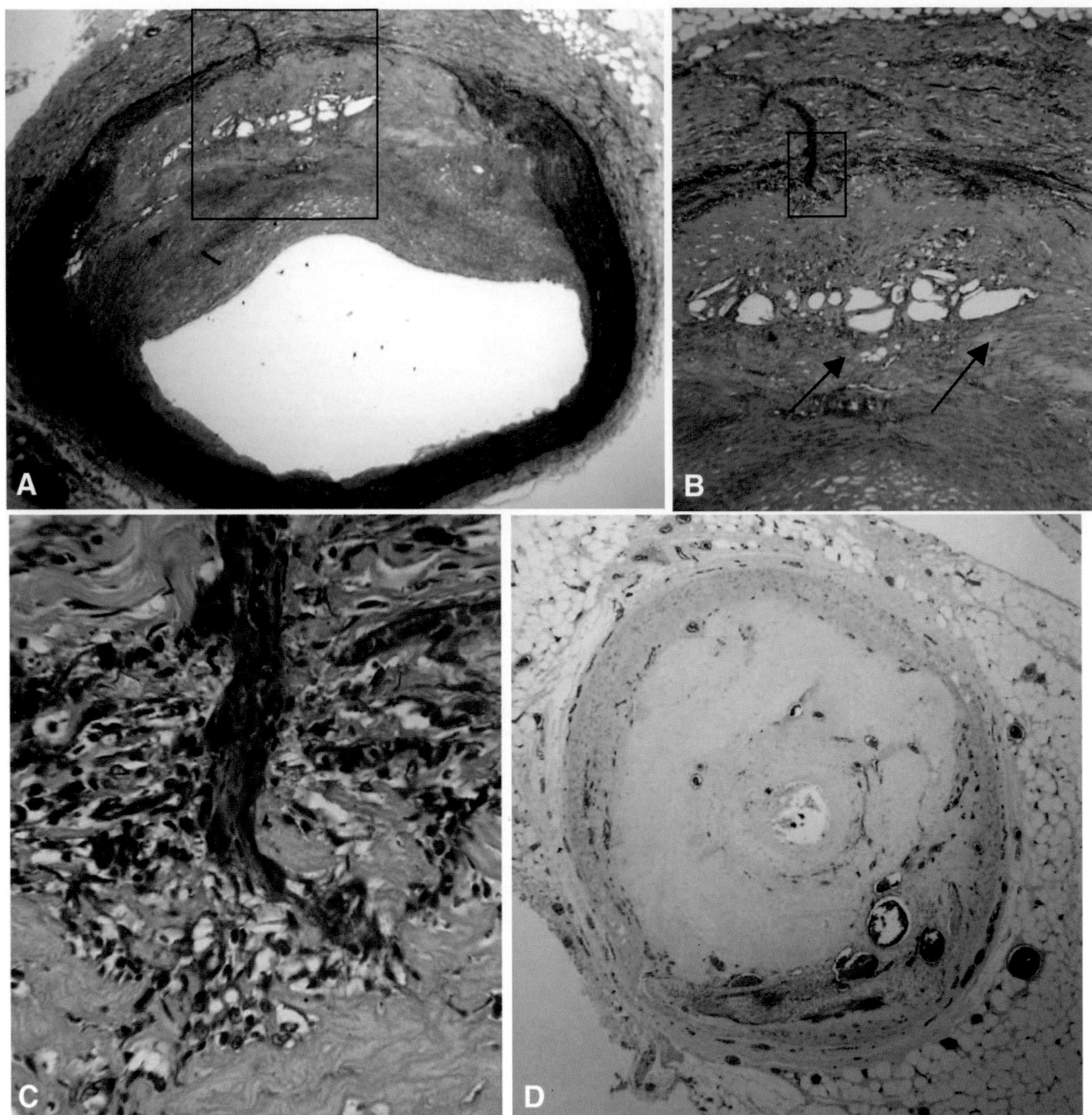

Fig. 9. Vasa vasorum within plaque. (**A**) At low magnification, there is thinning of the media with dilated spaces within the plaque. (**B**) A higher magnification of the boxed area in (**A**) shows dilated channels to be blood vessels (arrows). (**C**) A higher magnification of the boxed area in *B* shows a muscular artery feeder vessel traversing the media. (**D**) A different segment of near-total occlusion stained with *Ulex europaeus* lectin highlighting neovessels brown within the adventitia and intima.

types (Fig. 13). It remains to be determined whether imaging of calcification morphology (instead of simply burden) will be beneficial in assessing patient risk for coronary events.

REFERENCES

1. Virmani R, Kolodgie FD, Burke AP, Farb A, Schwartz SM. Lessons from sudden coronary death: a comprehensive morphological classification scheme for atherosclerotic lesions. Arterioscler Thromb Vasc Biol 2000;20:1262–275.
2. Stary HC, Chandler AB, Glagov S, et al. A definition of initial, fatty streak, and intermediate lesions of atherosclerosis. A report from the Committee on Vascular Lesions of the Council on Arteriosclerosis, American Heart Association. Circulation 1994;89:2462–2478.
3. Stary HC, Chandler AB, Dinsmore RE, et al. A definition of advanced types of atherosclerotic lesions and a histological classi-

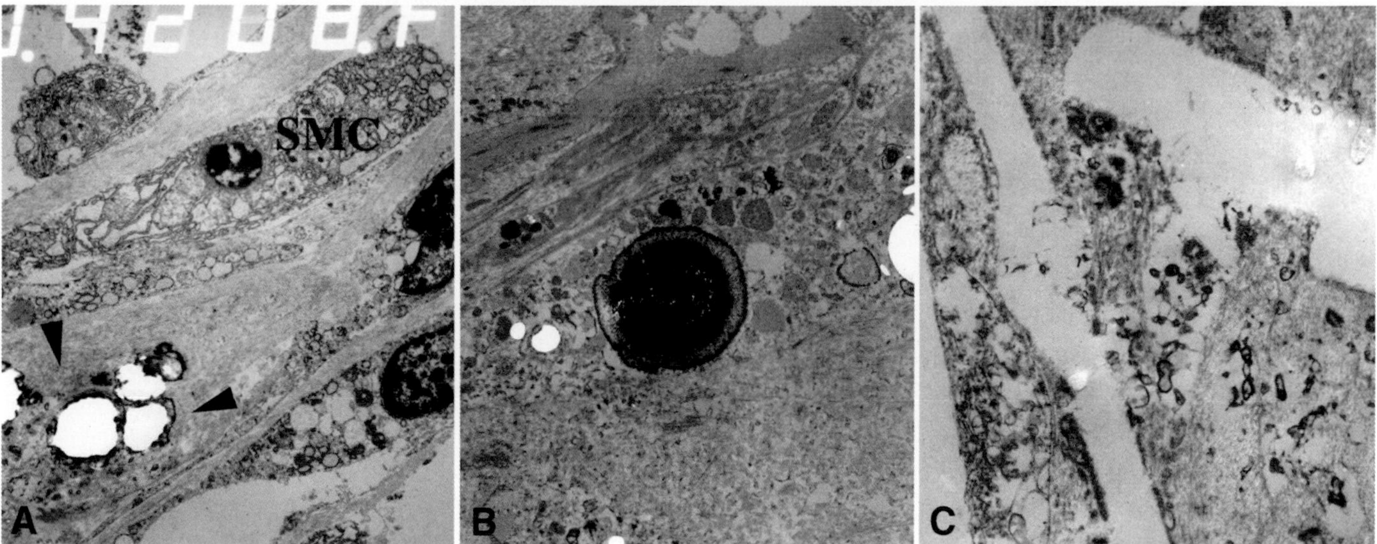

Fig. 10. Ultrastructural images of coronary atherosclerotic plaques show extracellular calcifications adjacent to an apoptotic smooth muscle cell (SMC) (**A**), spherical calcification associated with degenerating smooth muscle cell organelles (**B**), and small calcifications surrounding cholesterol clefts in area of macrophage degeneration (**C**).

fication of atherosclerosis. A report from the Committee on Vascular Lesions of the Council on Arteriosclerosis, American Heart Association. Circulation 1995;92:1355–1374.

3a. Kockx MM, De Meyer GRY, Muhring J, Jacob W, Bult H, Herman AG. Apoptosis and related proteins in different stages of human atherosclerotic plaques. Circulation 1998;97:2307–2315.

4. Burke AP, Farb A, Malcom GT, Liang YH, Smialek J, Virmani R. Coronary risk factors and plaque morphology in men with coronary disease who died suddenly. N Engl J Med 1997;336:1276–1282.

5. Arbustini E, Dal Bello B, Morbini P, et al. Plaque erosion is a major substrate for coronary thrombosis in acute myocardial infarction. Heart 1999;82:269–272.

6. Farb A, Burke AP, Tang AL, et al. Coronary plaque erosion without rupture into a lipid core. A frequent cause of coronary thrombosis in sudden coronary death. Circulation 1996;93:1354–363.

7. Roberts WC, Kragel AH, Gertz SD, Roberts CS, Kalan JM. The heart in fatal unstable angina pectoris. Am J Cardiol 1991;68: 22B–27B.

8. Libby P. Molecular bases of the acute coronary syndromes. Circulation 1995;91:2844–2850.

9. Libby P, Sukhova G, Lee RT, Galis ZS. Cytokines regulate vascular functions related to stability of the atherosclerotic plaque. J Cardiovasc Pharmacol 1995;25 Suppl 2:S9–12.

10. Davies MJ, Thomas A. Thrombosis and acute coronary-artery lesions in sudden cardiac ischemic death. N Engl J Med 1984;310:1137–1140.

11. Burke AP, Farb A, Malcom GT, Liang Y, Smialek JE, Virmani R. Plaque rupture and sudden death related to exertion in men with coronary artery disease. JAMA 1999;281:921–926.

12. Mann J, Davies MJ. Mechanisms of progression in native coronary artery disease: role of healed plaque disruption. Heart 1999;82: 265–268.

13. Burke AP, Weber DK, Kolodgie FD, Farb A, Taylor AJ, Virmani R. Pathophysiology of calcium deposition in coronary arteries. Herz 2001;26:239–244.

14. Kumamoto M, Nakashima Y, Sueishi K. Intimal neovascularization in human coronary atherosclerosis: its origin and pathophysiological significance. Hum Pathol 1995;26:450–456.

15. Heistad DD, Armstrong ML. Blood flow through vasa vasorum of coronary arteries in atherosclerotic monkeys. Arteriosclerosis 1986;6:326–331.

16. Williams JK, Armstrong ML, Heistad DD. Vasa vasorum in atherosclerotic coronary arteries: responses to vasoactive stimuli and regression of atherosclerosis. Circ Res 1988;62:515–523.

17. Virmani R, Roberts WC. Extravasated erythrocytes, iron, and fibrin in atherosclerotic plaques of coronary arteries in fatal coronary heart disease and their relation to luminal thrombus: frequency and significance in 57 necropsy patients and in 2958 five mm segments of 224 major epicardial coronary arteries. Am Heart J 1983; 105:788–797.

18. Alberts B, Bray D, Lewis J, Raff M, Roberts K, Watson JD (eds). Molecular Biology of the Cell. Garland, Inc., New York: 1983;260.

19. Arbustini E, Morbini P, D'Armini AM, et al. Plaque composition in plexogenic and thromboembolic pulmonary hypertension: the critical role of thrombotic material in pultaceous core formation. Heart 2002;88:177–182.

20. Constantinides P. Plaque fissures in human coronary thrombosis J Atheroscler Res 1966;6:1–17.

21. Pasterkamp G, Virmani R. The erythrocyte: a new player in atheromatous core formation. Heart 2002;88:115–116.

22. Proudfoot D, Shanahan CM. Biology of calcification in vascular cells: intima versus media. Herz 2001;26(4):245–251.

23. Huang H, Virmani R, Younis H, Burke AP, Kamm RD, Lee RT. The impact of calcification on the biomechanical stability of atherosclerotic plaques. Circulation 2001;103:1051–1056.

24. Hunt ME, O'Malley PG, Vernalis MN, Feuerstein IM, Taylor AJ. C-reactive protein is not associated with the presence or extent of calcified subclinical atherosclerosis. Am Heart J 2001;141: 206–210.

25. Burke AP, Taylor A, Farb A, Malcom GT, Virmani R. Coronary calcification: insights from sudden coronary death victims. Z Kardiol 2000;89:49–53.

26. Virmani R, Burke AP, Kolodgie FD, Farb A. Vulnerable plaque: the pathology of unstable coronary lesions. J Intervent Cardiol 2002;15:439–446.

27. (No authors listed.) Can atherosclerosis imaging techniques improve the detection of patients at risk for ischemic heart disease? Proceedings of the 34th Bethesda Conference. Bethesda, MD, USA. October 7, 2002. J Am Coll Cardiol. 2003;41(11):1856–1917.

28. Burke AP, Kolodgie FD, Farb A, et al. Healed plaque ruptures and sudden coronary death : evidence that subclinical rupture has a role in plaque progression. Circulation 2001;103(4):934–940.

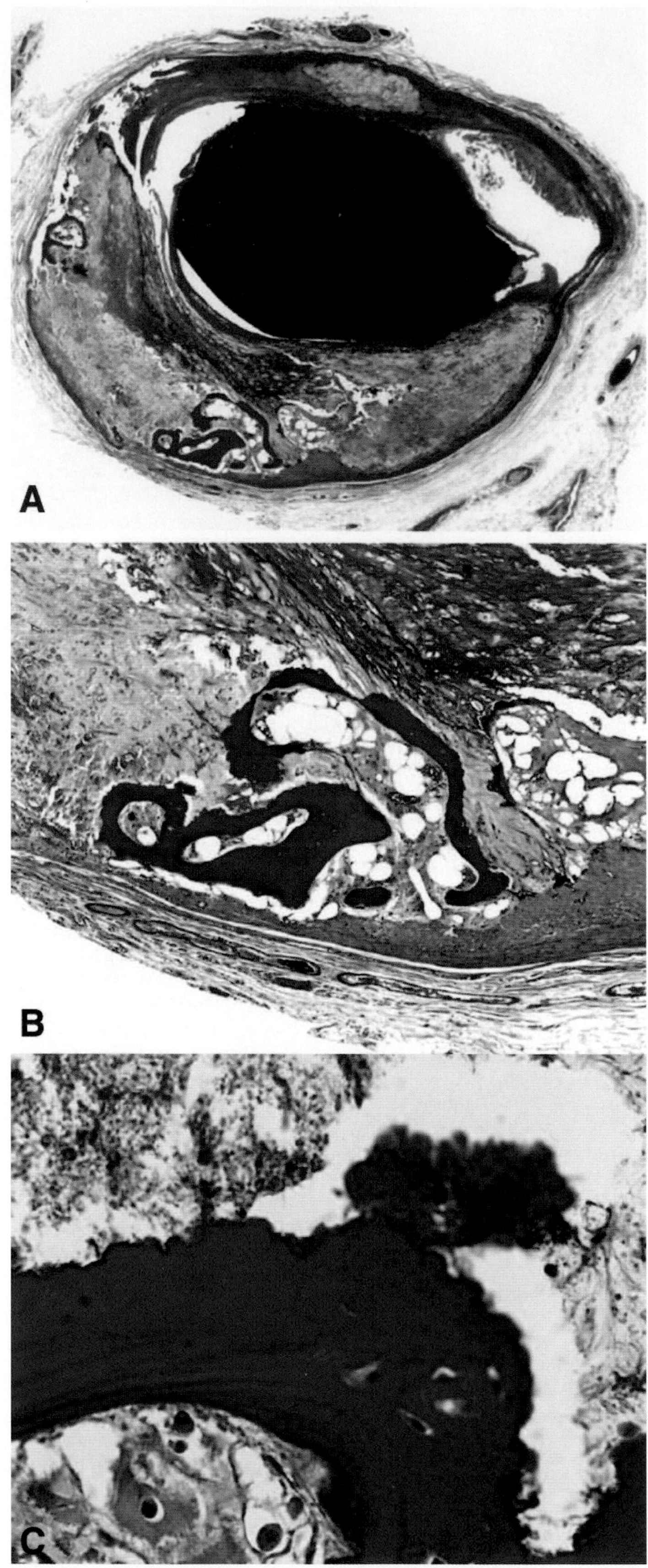

Fig. 11. Ossification in coronary plaque. (**A**) demonstrates a low-magnification image of a coronary artery section (proximal left anterior descending artery) in the left anterior descending coronary artery of an obese elderly woman with hypertensive atherosclerotic heart disease. (**A**) is a low magnification of the cross-section of the artery; contrast material (black) was injected into the artery postmortem. (**B**) demonstrates the bony trabeculae and (**C**) a higher magnification of lacunae containing osteoblasts.

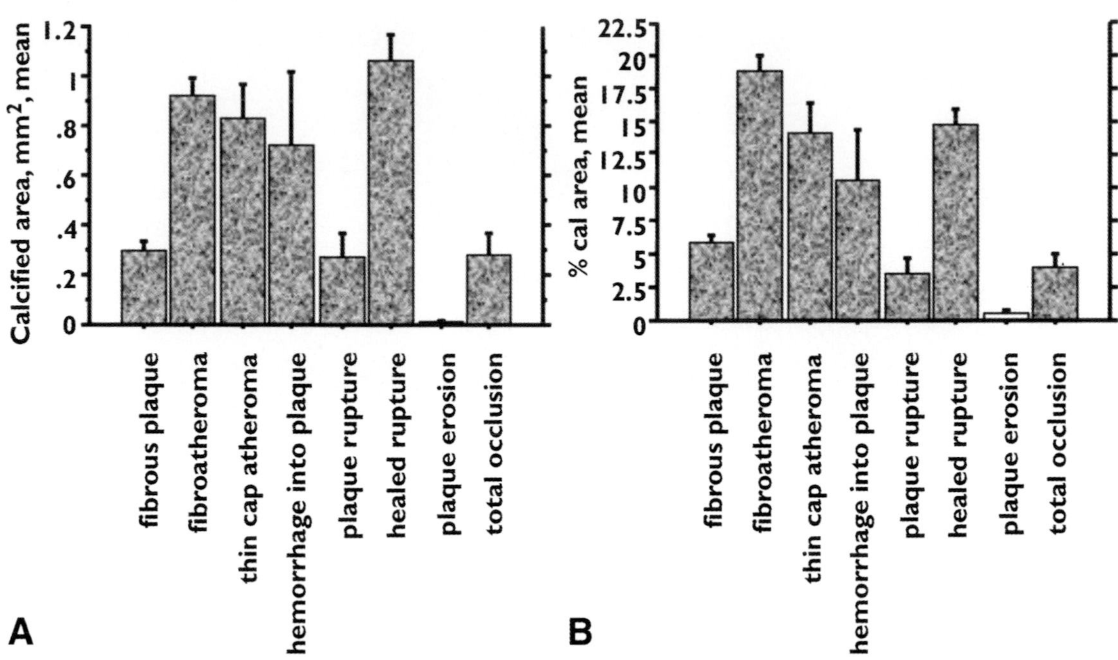

Fig. 12. Amount of calcification by plaque morphology. Morphometric measurements were made of calcified matrix in several hundred coronary lesions classified by plaque type. (**A**) Healed ruptures demonstrated the greatest mean area of calcification; plaque erosions demonstrate almost no calcification. (**B**) When expressed as a percentage of the plaque area, total occlusion and plaque ruptures have relatively little calcium, and plaque erosions the least. Fibroatheroma and healed ruptures demonstrate the greatest amount of calcified matrix. Reproduced from ref. *13*, with permission.

Table 3
Relationship Between Calcification and % Luminal Narrowing and Residual Lumen, by Arterial Section

Artery	*Calcified area vs % luminal narrowing (simple regression)*						*Calcified area vs residual lumen area (simple regression)*	
	Men			*Women*			*Men and women (combined)*	
	r^a	*p*	*DF*	r^a	*p*	*DF*	r^b	*p*
LM	.20	.20	30	.15	.59	14	.14	.58
PLAD	.56	<.0001	122	.15	.27	53	.07	.53
MLAD	.45	<.0001	91	.50	<.0001	66	.10	.29
DLAD	.64	.0003	27	.31	.11	24	.18	28
LD	.59	.001	26	.75	.0004	17	.13	.71
PLC	.30	.01	78	.25	.07	51	.11	.32
MLC	.02	.90	35	.31	.29	13	.21	.40
LOM	.60	.0001	34	.72	0.01	11	.13	.30
PRC	.12	.15	143	.09	.54	54	.09	.38
MRC	.29	.001	127	.63	<.0001	68	.09	.37
DRC	.32	.0004	116	.36	.06	27	.17	.29

[a]T values are all positive (positive correlation).

[b]T values are negative (plad, mrc, drc, ld) or positive (lm, lom, mlad, plc, mlc, prc).

Abbreviations: LM, left main; PLAD, proximal left anterior descending; MLAD, mid left anterior descend-ing; DLAD, distal left anterior descending; LD, left diagonal; PLC, proximal left circumflex; MLC, mid left circumflex; LOM, left obtuse marginal; PRC, proximal right coronary; MRC, mid right coronary; DRC, distal right coronary; df, degrees of freedom.

Segments are bolded showing *r* values > 0.4 and a significant correlation $p < 0.05$. Reproduced from ref. *13*, with permission.

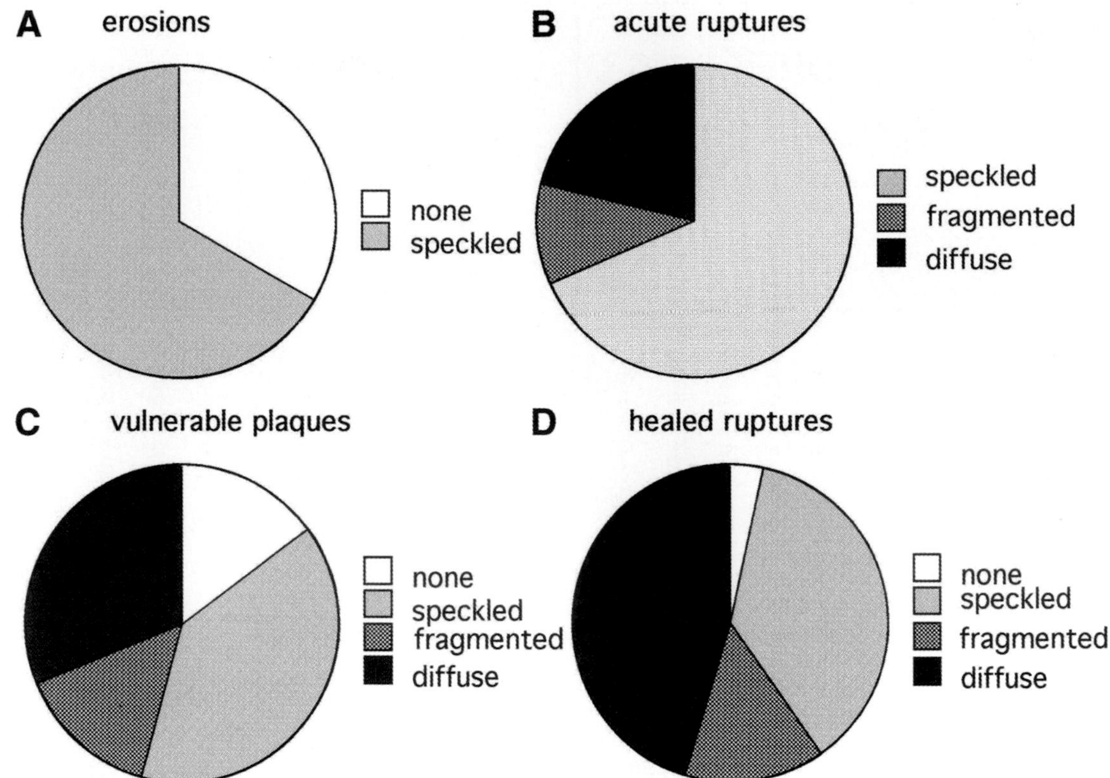

Fig. 13. Relationship between plaque morphology and radiographic calcification. Plaque erosions (**A**) were exclusively present in areas with stippled or no calcification. Plaque ruptures (**B**) were most frequently seen in areas of speckled calcification, but were also present in blocked or diffuse calcification. Curiously, there were no ruptures in segments devoid of any calcification. Thin-capped atheromas were most frequently present in areas of speckled calcification (**C**), but were also seen in heavily calcified or uncalcified areas, suggesting that calcification pattern is not helpful in diagnosing these lesions. Healed ruptures are almost always seen in areas of calcification, and most frequently in diffusely calcified areas (**D**). Reproduced from ref. *13*, with permission.

34 Pathogenesis of the Vulnerable Atherosclerotic Plaque

Masanori Aikawa, MD, PhD

INTRODUCTION

Vascular inflammation plays a major role in the development of chronic coronary atherosclerosis and the onset of acute coronary syndromes, including myocardial infarction, a leading cause of death in the United States *(1)*. Macrophage accumulation and the consequent expression of proteolytic and thrombogenic molecules critically contribute to the formation of "vulnerable" plaque prone to disruption and thrombus formation, leading to fatal obstruction of the coronary arteries. A number of clinical investigations suggest hypercholesterolemia as one of the major coronary risk factors. Preclinical studies demonstrate that hypercholesterolemia promotes accumulation of oxidatively modified low-density lipoprotein (oxLDL) in the arterial wall, inducing endothelial cell (EC) activation and, in turn, invasion of inflammatory cells such as macrophages (Fig. 1) *(1–3)*. Recent advances in vascular medicine provide evidence that lipid-lowering therapy prevents acute coronary complications in patients, most likely by functionally improving inflammation of atheroma *(1,4)*. This chapter will discuss the biology of vascular inflammation and acute coronary complications, as well as evidence of mechanisms by which lipid lowering stabilizes the vulnerable plaque.

FEATURES TYPICAL OF THE VULNERABLE PLAQUE PRONE TO ACUTE MYOCARDIAL INFARCTION (*see* FIG. 2)

Our classical view suggested that myocardial infarction usually occurs in a critically stenosed coronary artery, detectable by angiography. However, pathologic and angiographic studies in the 1980s determined that fissure or rupture of the thin fibrous cap in coronary atheroma containing preserved lumen often triggers acute fatal thrombosis *(5–7)*. Several factors contribute to the physical instability and thrombogenicity of the atherosclerotic plaque (Fig. 1). Atheroma with a higher risk for disruption and thrombosis often contain a prominent accumulation of macrophages, key players in any inflammatory diseases *(8–10)*. Lesional macrophages in such vulnerable plaques express high levels of various proteinases, including members of the matrix metalloproteinase (MMP) family *(11,12)*. Among them, interstitial collagenases (MMP-1/collagenase-1, MMP-8/collagenase-2, and MMP-13/collagenase-3) found in human atheroma can cleave interstitial collagen macromolecules (Fig. 3) *(13–15)*.

Macrophage-derived collagenases of the MMP family may cause formation of a collagen-poor, thin fibrous cap overlying macrophage- and lipid-rich plaques, another feature typical of the vulnerable plaque. Collagen, which tolerates much greater tensile stress than elastin, usually determines the stability and durability of a wide variety of tissues *(16)*. Using computer modeling, Loree et al. demonstrated the inverse relationship between cap thickness and peak circumferential stress in the plaque *(17,18)*. Burk et al. from Virmani's group reported that thin fibrous caps measure approx 60–70 µm thick, and measurement near the site of rupture can be as little as 25 µm *(19)*. Therefore, the collagen-poor, thin fibrous cap caused by collagenolytic activity is likely responsible for instability and consequent physical disruption of atherosclerotic plaques.

Macrophages in atheroma also overexpress tissue factor, a strong initiator of the blood coagulation cascade, and plasminogen activator inhibitor 1 (PAI-1), which inhibits fibrinolysis *(20,21)*. The fibrous cap usually separates thrombogenic macrophages from various coagulation factors in circulating blood. However, physical disruption of the cap causes direct contact between blood containing coagulation factors and macrophage-derived tissue factor, possibly accelerating thrombus formation. Simultaneously, anti-fibrinolytic PAI-1 stabilizes the clot, which may favor massive, obstructive thrombosis in the coronary arteries.

OXIDATIVE STRESS AND EC ACTIVATION MEDIATE FORMATION OF THE VULNERABLE PLAQUE

Clinical and epidemiologic studies suggest that elevated plasma levels of low-density lipoprotein (LDL) increase the risk of acute coronary syndromes, including acute myocardial infarction, unstable angina, and cardiac sudden death *(22–24)*. Beginning early in the 20th century, a number of preclinical investigations using animal models demonstrated that hypercholesterolemia induces experimental atheroma formation *(25–28)*. In vitro studies, however, long suggested that native

From: *Contemporary Cardiology: CT of the Heart: Principles and Applications*
Edited by: U. Joseph Schoepf © Humana Press, Inc., Totowa, NJ

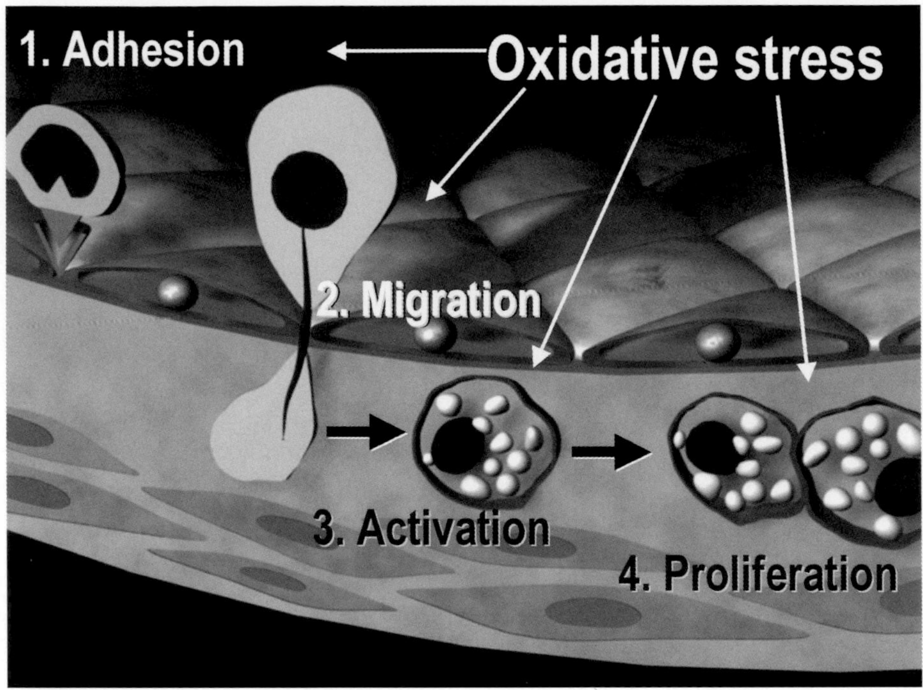

Fig. 1. Monocyte recruitment and macrophage accumulation in atheroma. Oxidative stress induces endothelial cell activation and enhances expression of adhesion molecules such as vascular cell adhesion molecule-1, which binds monocytes in the circulating blood (1). Monocytes then migrate into the intima in response to chemokines including monocyte chemoattractant protein-1 (MCP-1) (2). Oxidative stress induces MCP-1 expression. Monocytes differentiate into macrophages in the intima (3). Several molecules such as macrophage-colony stimulating factor induce macrophage differentiation and activation. Activated macrophages express a number of molecules related to atherogenesis, plaque instability and thrombogenicity. Macrophage proliferation likely plays an important role in formation of the atherosclerotic plaques rich in this cell type (4). Oxidative stress also induces macrophage activation and proliferation. Adapted from ref. *3*, with permission.

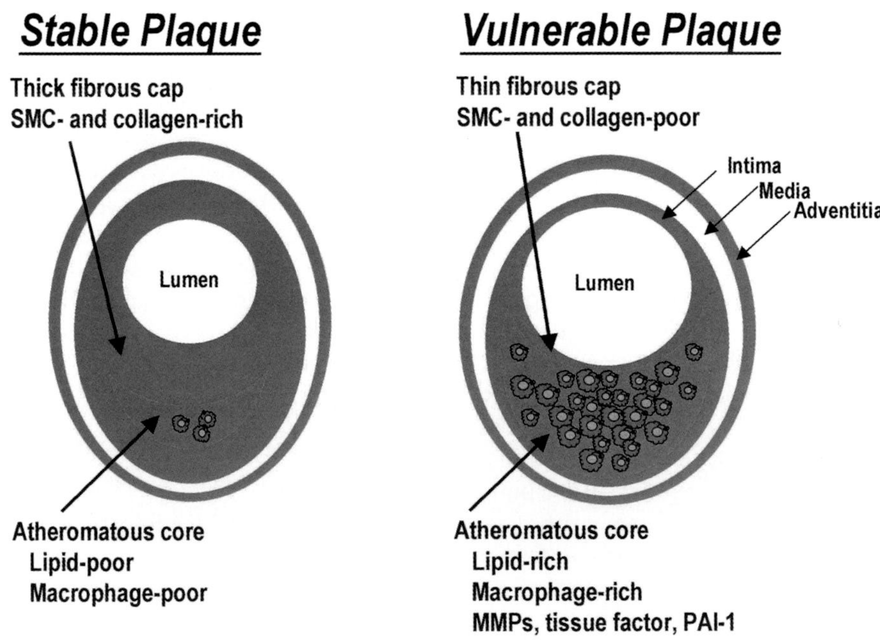

Fig. 2. Diagram demonstrating pathological and biological features typical of the "vulnerable" atherosclerotic plaque. The so-called vulnerable plaque usually contains prominent macrophage accumulation and lipid pool in its atheromatous core, underlying a thin, collagen-poor fibrous cap. Macrophages produce matrix metalloproteinases (MMPs) including collagenases, which may weaken the fibrous cap and promote physical disruption. Tissue factor and plasminogen activator inhibitor 1 (PAI-1) produced by macrophages may accelerate formation of massive thrombus and inhibit fibrinolysis at the sites of rupture, and likely contribute to fetal obstruction of the coronary artery. Smooth muscle cells (SMCs) in the fibrous cap tend to undergo apoptosis and are likely responsible for collagen loss. Intimal SMCs also express MMPs and tissue factor. Activated endothelial cells promote monocyte recruitment and macrophage accumulation in atheroma.

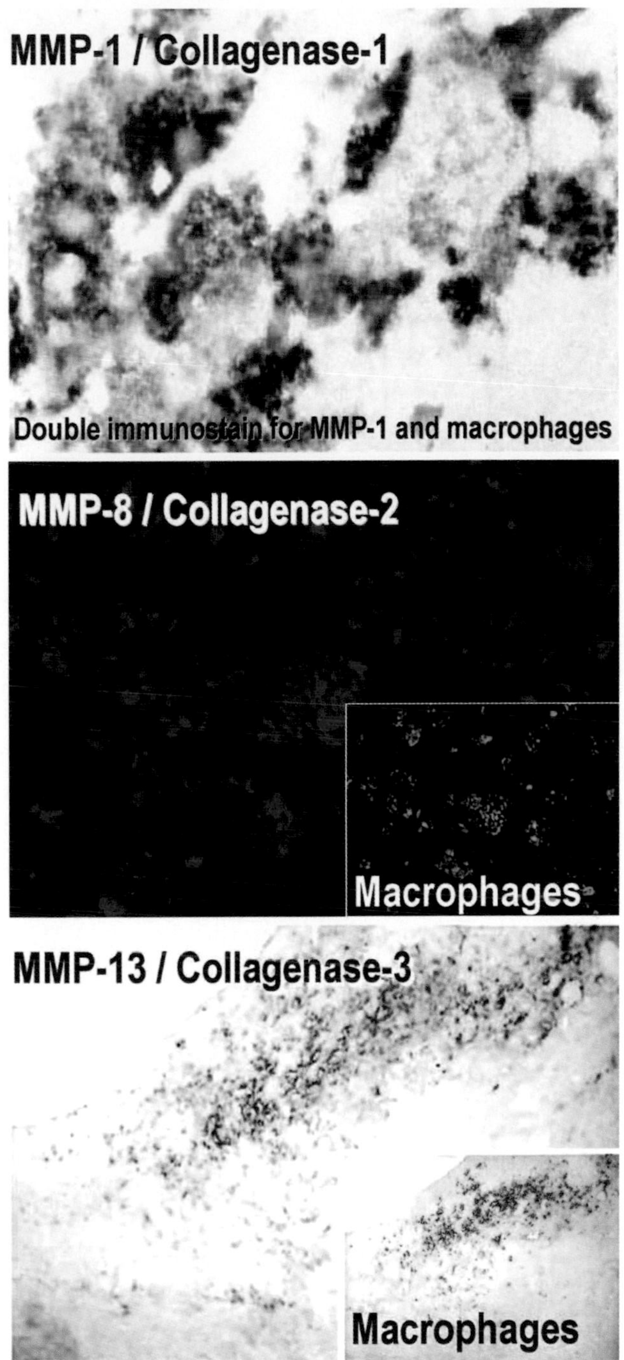

Fig. 3. Macrophage expression of collagenases of the MMP family in human atheroma. Immunohistochemistry detected MMP-1/collagenase-1, MMP-8/collagenase-2, and MMP-13/collagenase-3 in atheroma of the human carotid artery. Both collagenases colocalize with macrophages detected by CD68 antibody. Adapted from refs. *13–15*, with permission.

LDL itself does not induce features associated with atheroma (e.g., transformation of monocyte/macrophages into lipid-laden foam cells). In the late 1980s, the "oxidation hypothesis" finally linked LDL with atherogenesis by introducing evidence that oxLDL is proinflammatory *(29)*. Since then, vascular biology has provided much evidence that hypercholesterolemia induces oxidative stress, leading to vascular inflammation and atherosclerosis *(30)*.

The excess LDL that accumulates in the artery wall as a result of hypercholesterolemia can be oxidatively modified *(31,32)*. Human and experimental atheroma both contain oxLDL *(33–35)*. Atherosclerotic lesions intrinsically produce excess reactive oxygen species (ROS) such as superoxide anion (O_2^-), promoting further oxidative modification of LDL *(32)*. OxLDL instigates an inflammatory response on arterial ECs. In vitro studies suggest that oxLDL and its derivatives increase

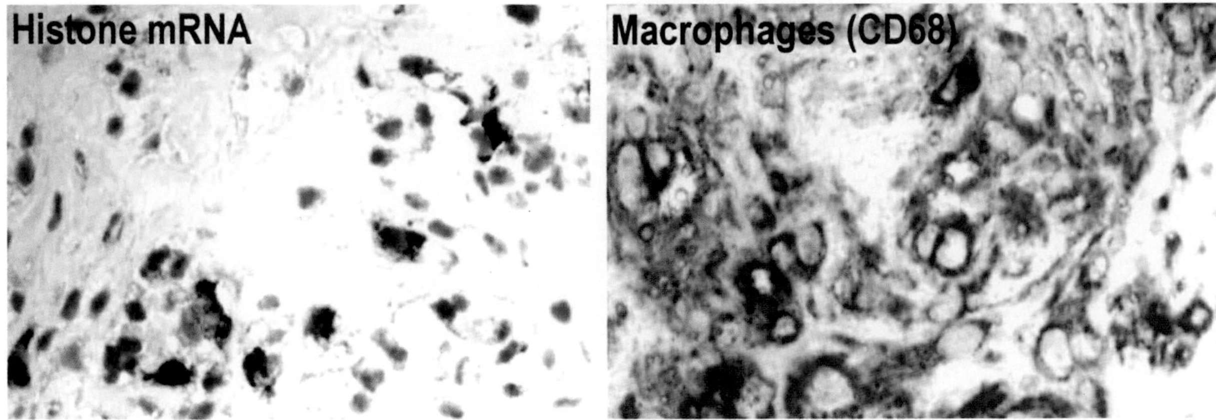

Fig. 4. Macrophage growth in human atheroma. *In situ* hybridization detected histone mRNA expression, a sensitive marker for DNA replication, in the intima of a human carotid artery. mRNA signals colocalized with macrophages detected by immunohistochemistry for CD68 on a serial section. Scale bar: 50 μm. Original magnification: ×400. Adapted from ref. *45*, with permission.

expression of cell-adhesion molecules, including vascular cell-adhesion molecule 1 (VCAM-1) and chemokines such as monocyte chemoattractant protein 1 (MCP-1), both of which critically contribute to leukocyte recruitment into the intima (Fig. 1) *(36–38)*. Preclinical studies employing genetically altered mice demonstrate in vivo evidence supporting the role of VCAM-1 and MCP-1 in the formation of macrophage-rich atheroma *(39–41)*. In rabbits, high-cholesterol diet induces EC expression of VCAM-1 *(35,42)*.

Macrophage proliferation may play an important role in the development of vascular inflammation (Fig. 4) *(43–45)*. OxLDL induces macrophage proliferation in vitro *(46)* and also activates nuclear factor-κB (NF-κB), a key transcription factor that regulates a wide variety of atherosclerosis-associated genes *(47)*. Furthermore, the discovery of macrophage scavenger receptors that selectively take up oxLDL and induce foam-cell formation improved our understanding of the role hypercholesterolemia plays in vascular inflammation and atherogenesis *(48)*.

Nitric oxide (NO) exerts antiatherogenic actions by inhibiting monocyte adhesion to ECs or suppressing expression of VCAM-1 and MCP-1 by EC *(49–52)*. Apparently normal ECs constitutively express endothelial NO synthase (eNOS), which produces NO from L-arginine. However, eNOS expression decreases in human atherosclerotic arteries *(53)*. Oxidative stress decreases eNOS expression by cultured ECs as well as bioavailability of NO *(54)*.

Superficial erosion of the plaque due to EC detachment may also contribute to the onset of acute coronary syndromes *(55)*. Rajavashisth et al. reported that oxLDL induces EC expression of membrane type 1–matrix metalloproteinase (MT1-MMP), an activator of MMP-2 *(56)*. MMP-2 cleaves type IV collagen, a major component of the basement membrane underlying the endothelium, thus suggesting that EC activation by oxidative stress may cause plaque erosion.

Additionally, activated ECs may affect the fibrinolytic balance in atheroma. Relatively normal ECs express the tissue-type plasminogen activator (t-PA), a fibrinolytic molecule. On the other hand, activated ECs increase the production of endogenous inhibitors of plasminogen activators (i.e., PAI-1) *(57)*. Such fibrinolytic imbalance may stabilize clots and favor fatal, occlusive thrombus formation.

PLAQUE STABILIZATION: MECHANISMS BY WHICH LIPID LOWERING BY HMG-COA REDUCTASE INHIBITORS PREVENTS ACUTE CORONARY SYNDROMES

Since the 1990s, clinical studies have established that lipid-lowering therapy by HMG-CoA reductase inhibitors (statins) prevents the onset of acute coronary events despite no or modest reduction in angiographic stenoses *(3,58,59)*. This discrepancy raised the concept that lipid lowering may modify the vulnerable plaque in a functional manner ("stabilization") rather than simply shrinking the lesion ("regression") *(60,61)*. A number of animal studies previously focused on regression of atheroma by lipid lowering *(62,63)*; however, more recent preclinical studies, including our own, improved mechanistic understanding of the clinical benefits of lipid lowering and furnished the "plaque stabilization" hypothesis *(1,4)*. Clinical and preclinical studies also suggest that statins have various direct or pleiotopic effects independent of lipid lowering *(1,64)*.

Our studies on plaque stabilization have employed mainly rabbit models of atherosclerosis *(28)*. Beginning early in the 20th century, accumulating knowledge has suggested that atherosclerotic lesions of hypercholesterolemic rabbits mimic chronic coronary atherosclerosis in humans *(25,26,28)*. We found that rabbit aortic atherosclerosis created by both mechanical injury and high-cholesterol diet contained a number of features associated with vulnerable plaques in humans: prominent macrophage accumulation, a thin and collagen-poor fibrous cap, and expression of MMP and tissue factor *(65,66)*. Potent inflammatory mediators CD154 (or CD40 ligand) and CD40, which induce MMP and tissue factor expression, also occur in rabbit atheroma *(66)*. To address the effects of lipid lowering itself without direct vascular effects of statins, we examined the way these features change in hypercholesterolemic rabbits during lipid lowering by diet alone (Table 1)

Table 1
Effects of Lipid Lowering on Atheroma of Hypercholesterolemic Rabbits

	Diet	*Statins*
Macrophage accumulation	Decreased	Decreased
Macrophage proliferation	ND	Decreased
Macrophage apoptosis	ND	No change
MMP expression/activity	Decreased	Decreased
Collagen content	Increased	Increased[a]
Tissue factor expression/activity	Decreased	Decreased
PAI-1 expression	ND	Decreased
CD154 (CD40L) expression	Decreased	Decreased
PDGF-β expression	Decreased	ND
SMC maturity	Increased	ND
SM1 and SM2, a marker for mature SMCs	Increased	ND
SMemb, a nonmuscle or embryonic myosin	Decreased	ND
ROS production (O_2^-)	Decreased	ND
LDL accumulation	Decreased	Decreased
oxLDL accumulation	Decreased	Decreased
Plasma autoantibody for oxLDL	Decreased	ND
VCAM-1	Decreased	ND
MCP-1	Decreased	ND
eNOS	Increased	ND
Microvessels	Decreased	ND

ND, not determined; MMP, matrix metalloproteinase; PAI-1, plasminogen activator inhibitor 1; PDGF-β, platelet-derived growth factor beta; SMC, smooth muscle cells; ROS, reactive oxygen species; oxLDL, oxidatively modified low-density lipoprotein; VCAM-1, vascular cell-adhesion molecule 1; MCP-1, monocyte chemoattractant protein 1; eNOS, endothelial NO synthase.

[a]No change with fluvastatin.

(1,4,35,65–67). Dietary cholesterol lowering in rabbit atheroma reduced macrophage accumulation expressing MMPs including MMP-1/collagenase-1 and, in parallel, increased interstitial collagen content, a key determinant of plaque stability (Fig. 5) *(65)*. A rabbit study by Kockx et al. and a clinical study by Crisby et al. reported a similar finding of increased collagen content in atherosclerotic plaques by lipid lowering *(68,69)*. These studies suggest that lipid lowering prevents acute coronary syndromes in part by increasing the mechanical strength of atheroma.

Lipid lowering also reduced expression and activity of tissue factor, suggesting decreased thrombogenic potential, another major contributor to acute coronary events *(66)*. Additionally, inflammatory mediators CD154 and CD40 decreased substantially during cholesterol lowering *(66)*. More recently, we reported that lipid lowering by statin treatment also reduces expression of MMPs, tissue factor, and their inducer CD154 in hypercholesterolemic rabbits (Fig. 6) *(45,70)*.

Smooth muscle cells (SMCs) in the fibrous cap of rabbit atheroma exhibited immature phenotype compared to those in apparently normal media found in human atheroma *(67,71)*. However, dietary lipid lowering promoted accumulation of SMCs of more mature phenotype in the fibrous cap, expressing fewer MMPs and less tissue factor than those found in baseline lesions *(66,67)*.

We furthermore tested the hypothesis that cholesterol lowering reduces oxidative stress and EC activation in atheroma (Table 1) *(35)*. Atherosclerotic aortas of cholesterol-fed rabbits produced high levels of ROS, including superoxide anion (O_2^-). Baseline lesions in hypercholesterolemic rabbits contained a prominent accumulation of oxLDL underlying activated ECs that expressed VCAM-1 (Fig. 7A, top panels). In contrast, few if any ECs in atheroma expressed eNOS, in agreement with a previous study on human atheroma *(53)*. However, lipid lowering by diet alone reduced ROS production to levels similar to those found in normal aortas. Dietary lipid lowering reduced oxLDL accumulation and VCAM-1 expression concomitantly (Fig. 7A bottom panels, and 7B) *(35)*. In contrast, lipid lowering by diet increased eNOS expression substantially. ECs, SMCs, and macrophages in human atheroma express MCP-1, a potent chemokine that induces monocyte recruitment into the arterial wall *(72)*. In aortic atheroma of cholesterol-fed rabbits, ECs as well as SMCs and macrophages contained immunoreactive MCP-1 *(35)*. However, this chemokine was almost undetectable after cholesterol lowering. After lipid lowering, aortic ECs also exhibited a more normal ultrastructure compared with those of the atherosclerotic intima, which had features typical of activated ECs (Fig. 8). Taken together, these pre-clinical and clinical results suggest that cholesterol lowering reduces oxidative stress and ameliorates EC dysfunction, favoring stabilization of the vulnerable plaque.

CLINICAL SIGNIFICANCE OF PLEIOTROPIC EFFECTS OF STATINS

Accumulating preclinical evidence using animal models or in vitro systems demonstrates that statins possess effects other than reduction of cholesterol synthesis, including anti-inflammatory effects on vascular cells *(1,64)*. We reported that cerivastatin inhibited M-CSF-induced macrophage growth in vitro with clinically achievable concentrations *(45)*. This treatment

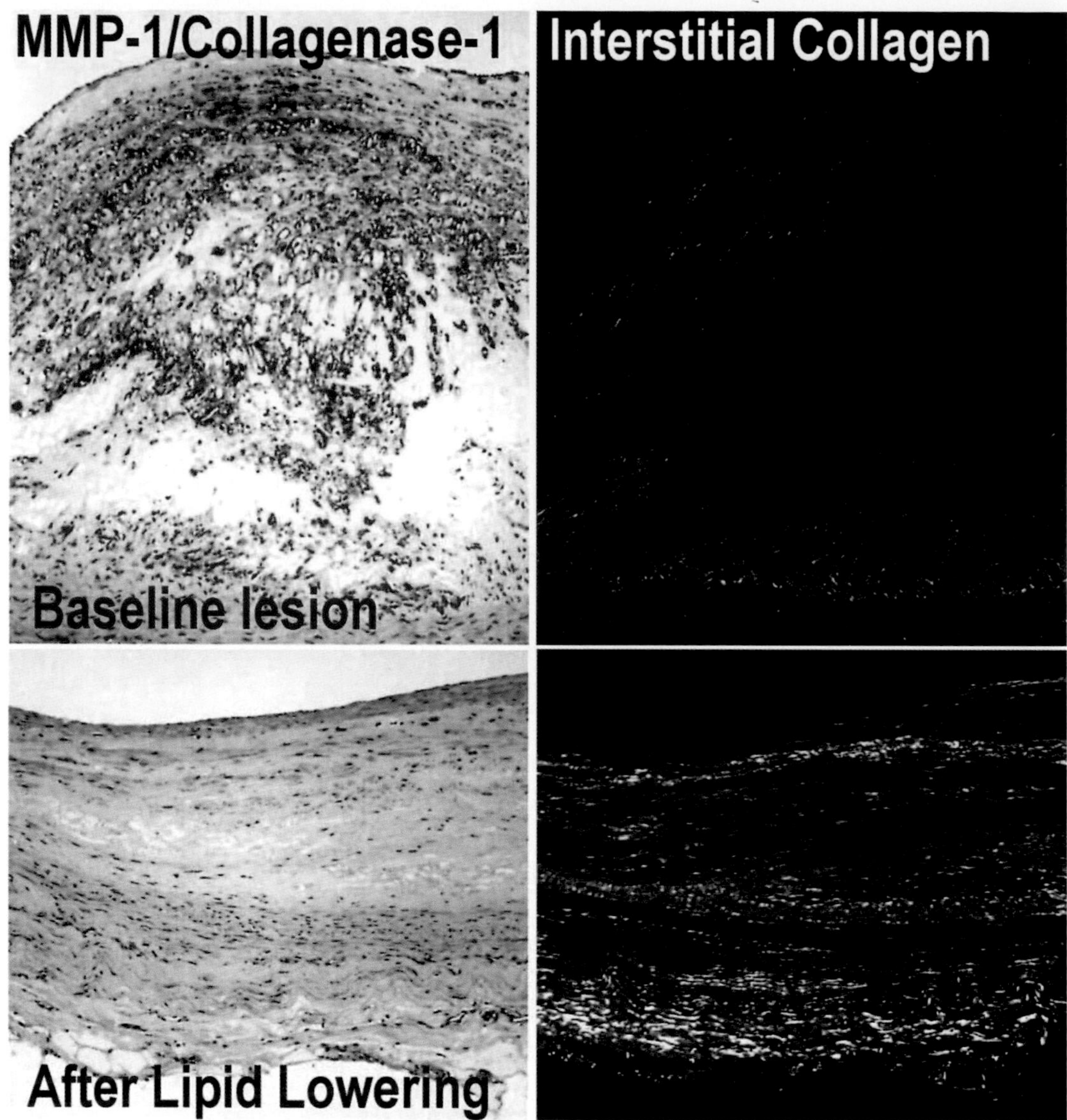

Fig. 5. Lipid lowering by diet alone reduces MMP-1/collagenase-1 expression and increases interstitial collagen content in rabbit atheroma. Top panels: The rabbit aortic lesion after 4 mo on a high-cholesterol diet (baseline lesion) contained high level of MMP-1/collagenase-1 expression, a potent collagenolytic enzyme. Picrosirius red staining with polarization barely detected accumulation of interstitial collagen on a serial section of this collagenase-rich plaque. Bottom panels: 16 mo of dietary lipid lowering decreased MMP-1/collagenase-1 expression and, in parallel, increased collagen content, a key determinant of plaque stability. Original magnification: ×10. From ref. *65*, with permission.

also reduced macrophage activation as examined by decreased MMP-9 activity and tissue factor expression *(45)*. Previous studies employing fluvastatin and simvastatin demonstrated similar findings regarding macrophage proliferation and activation in vitro *(73–75)*. These cholesterol-independent, antimacrophage effects should favor stabilization of the vulnerable plaque. Thus far, however, no unambiguous clinical evidence suggests that such pleiotropic effects substantially increase the benefits of statin treatment in patients.

Like other classes of drugs, statins have variable lipophilic properties. Unlike hydrophilic compounds, lipophilic compounds are generally cell permeant, and their effects on peripheral tissues or cultured cells are usually more direct. For instance, lipophilic statins suppress proliferation or induce apoptosis of cultured SMCs more effectively than do hydrophilic statins *(70,76,77)*. Clinical trials for all statins, however, have shown benefits somewhat similar to the prevention of acute coronary syndromes. Insufficient cell permeability of hydrohilic pravastatin is not reflected by significant risk reduction in clinical trials. Moreover, both lipophilic and hydrophilic statins possess anti-inflammatory effects independent of LDL reduction in patients, as determined by plasma levels of hsCRP *(78,79)*. Thus, the mechanisms by which all statins with different lipophilic properties produce cholesterol-independent, anti-inflammatory effects remain obscure. Concentrations of statins used in in vitro investigations often exceed those achievable in

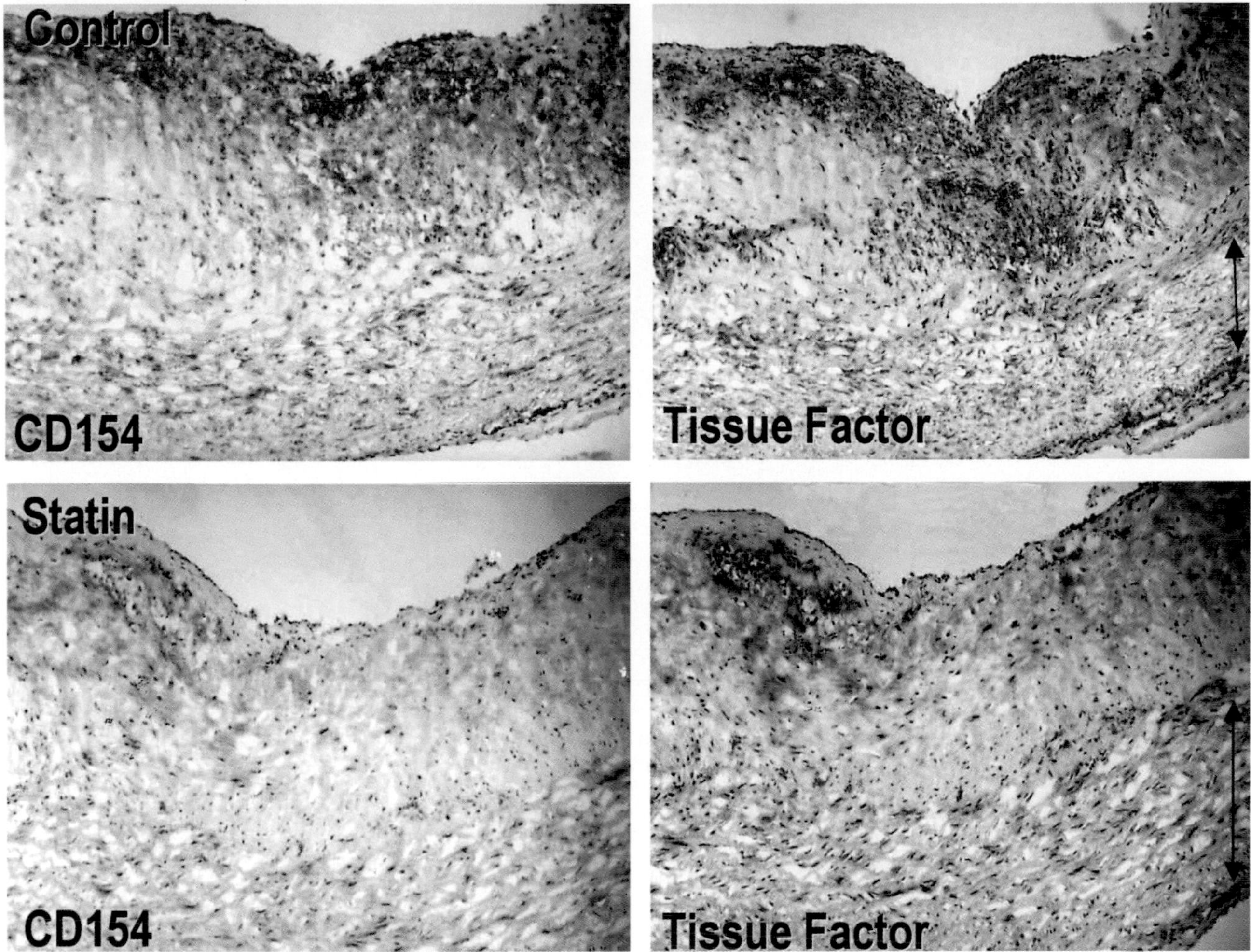

Fig. 6. Lipid lowering by statin treatment reduces expression of CD154 and tissue factor in atheroma of hypercholesterolemic rabbits. The aortic intima of 34-mo-old Watanabe heritable hyperlipidemic rabbits, a model of endogenous hypercholesterolemia, exhibited expression of tissue factor, a strong activator of blood coagulation, and its inducer CD154 (or CD40 ligand). With cerivastatin treatment for 32 mo, expression of both CD40L and TF decreased substantially. The arrow indicates the tunica media. Scale bar: 200 μm. From ref. *45*, with permission.

patients, further stirring controversy about the clinical importance of their pleiotropic effects. On the other hand, animal studies including our own clearly suggest that lipid lowering by diet alone improves a number of features associated with vascular inflammation and activation. Clinical statin trials also demonstrate that aggressive cholesterol lowering produces a greater reduction of inflammatory burden than does more moderate therapy. These preclinical and clinical data suggest the importance of lowering lipids by diet therapy, lifestyle changes, and, if necessary, statins.

FUTURE PERSPECTIVES

In the last two decades, advances in clinical and basic cardiovascular medicine forged several missing links between coronary risks and the onset of acute thrombotic complications. In particular, discoveries regarding the role of oxidative stress in vascular inflammation substantially improved our mechanistic understanding of the pathogenesis of coronary thrombosis. Based on clinical and our own preclinical evidence, this chapter has also underscored the importance of lipid management in the prevention of acute coronary syndromes. New targets for antiinflammatory therapies beyond lipid lowering may include inhibition of the renin-angiotensin-aldosterone system and activation of peroxisome proliferator-activated receptors (PPARs) *(4,80–83)*. Interestingly, inhibitors for these pathways, like statins, have seemingly pleiotropic effects on vascular inflammation as well. In addition to screening conventional coronary risk factors (e.g., LDL levels), sensitive but inexpensive biomarkers for new risk factors (e.g., hsCRP) may identify currently unattended high-risk patients. Moreover, novel imaging modalities will probably detect not only luminal stenoses but also more "qualitative" features, including the biological processes typical of the vulnerable plaque *(84)*. These new approaches should provide more effective and individualized strategies for the prevention of acute thrombotic complications of atherosclerosis.

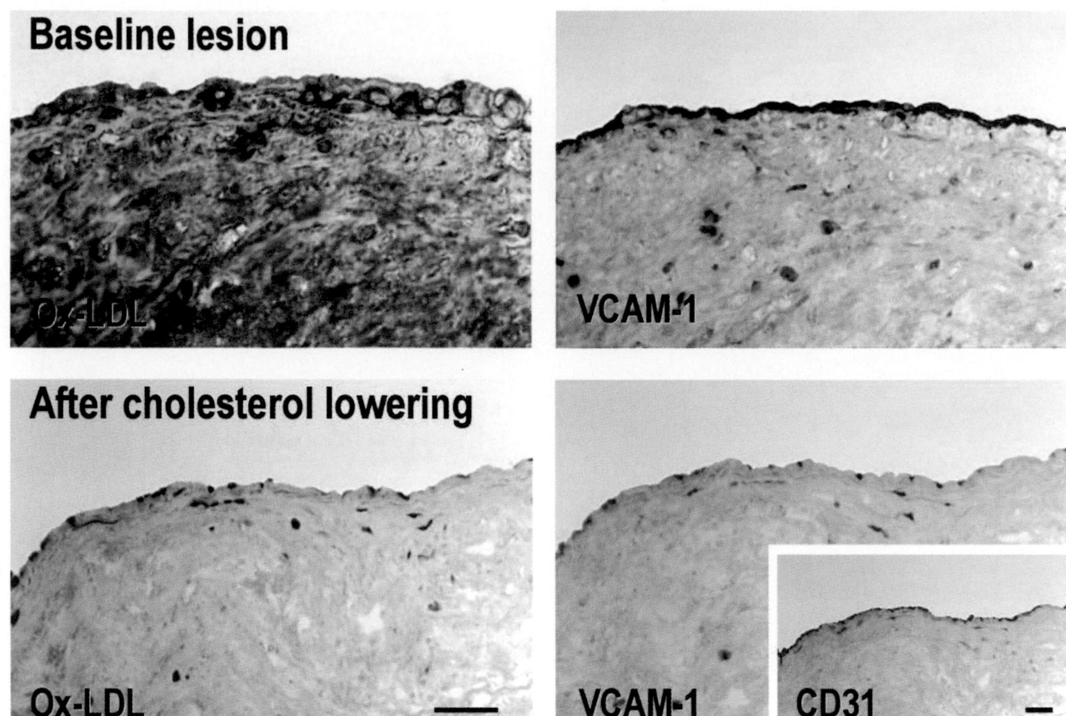

Fig. 7. Dietary lipid lowering reduces oxidatively modified low-density lipoprotein (oxLDL) accumulation and vascular cell-adhesion molecule 1 (VCAM-1) expression in rabbit atheroma. Top panels: OxLDL epitopes (MDA-lysine) accumulated in the aortic intima beneath activated endothelial cells (ECs) expressing VCAM-1 in hypercholesterolemic rabbits which consumed the atherogenic diet for 4 mo (baseline). Bottom panels: OxLDL epitopes (MDA-lysine) and VCAM-1 expression by ECs were almost undetectable in the intima of rabbit aorta after 16 mo of lipid lowering, while CD31, an EC marker, indicated an intact monolayer. The atheroma from control animals that continued the atherogenic diet for 16 mo sustained oxLDL and VCAM-1. Scale bar: 50 μm. Original magnification ×400. From ref. *35*, with permission.

ACKNOWLEDGMENT

The author acknowledges a number of colleagues and collaborators for their tremendous contributions to the study concepts and experiments that this chapter mentioned. This work was supported in part by grants from the National Institutes of Health, National Heart, Lung, and Blood Institute (PO1 HL48743 and Merit Award to Dr. Peter Libby, SCOR P50HL56985 to Drs. Libby and Aikawa, and R01HL66086 to Dr. Aikawa), and Japan Heart Foundation (to Dr. Aikawa). We also acknowledge Karen E. Williams for her excellent editorial assistance.

REFERENCES

1. Aikawa M, Libby P. The vulnerable atherosclerotic plaque; pathogenesis and therapeutic approachhh. Cardiovasc Pathol 2004;13(3): 125–138.
2. Munro JM, Cotran RS. The pathogenesis of atherosclerosis: atherogenesis and inflammation. Lab Invest 1988;58:249–261.
3. Libby P, Aikawa M. Evolution and stabilization of vulnerable atherosclerotic plaques. Jpn Circ J 2001;65:473–479.
4. Libby P, Aikawa M. Stabilization of atherosclerotic plaques: new mechanisms and clinical targets. Nature Medicine 2002;8:1257–1262.
5. Davies MJ, Thomas AC. Plaque fissuring—the cause of acute myocardial infarction, sudden ischaemic death, and crescendo angina. Br Heart J 1985;53:363–373.
6. Hackett D, Davies G, Maseri A. Pre-existing coronary stenoses in patients with first myocardial infarction are not necessarily severe. Eur Heart J 1988;9:1317–1323.
7. Ambrose JA, Tannenbaum MA, Alexopoulos D, et al. Angiographic progression of coronary artery disease and the development of myocardial infarction. J Am Coll Cardiol 1988;12:56–62.
8. Davies MJ, Richardson PD, Woolf N, Katz DR, Mann J. Risk of thrombosis in human atherosclerotic plaques: role of extracellular lipid, macrophage, and smooth muscle cell content. Br Heart J 1993;69:377–381.
9. van der Wal AC, Becker AE, van der Loos CM, Das PK. Site of intimal rupture or erosion of thrombosed coronary atherosclerotic plaques is characterized by an inflammatory process irrespective of the dominant plaque morphology. Circulation 1994;89:36–44.
10. Moreno PR, Falk E, Palacios IF, Newell JB, Fuster V, Fallon JT. Macrophage infiltration in acute coronary syndromes. Implications for plaque rupture. Circulation 1994;90:775–778.
11. Nagase H, Woessner JF Jr. Matrix metalloproteinases. J Biol Chem 1999;274:21491–21494.
12. Brinckerhoff CE, Matrisian LM. Matrix metalloproteinases: a tail of a frog that became a prince. Nat Rev Mol Cell Biol 2002;3: 207–214.
13. Galis ZS, Sukhova GK, Lark MW, Libby P. Increased expression of matrix metalloproteinases and matrix degrading activity in vulnerable regions of human atherosclerotic plaques. J Clin Invest 1994; 94:2493–2503.
14. Sukhova G, Schoenbeck U, Rabkin E, et al. Evidence of increased collagenolysis by interstitial collagenases-1 and -3 in vulnerable human atheromatous plaques. Circulation 1999;99:2503–2509.
15. Herman MP, Sukhova GK, Libby P, et al. Expression of neutrophil collagenase (matrix metalloproteinase-8) in human atheroma: a novel collagenolytic pathway suggested by transcriptional profiling. Circulation 2001;104:1899–1904.
16. Lee RT, Libby P. The unstable atheroma. Arterioscler Thromb Vasc Biol 1997;17:1859–1867.

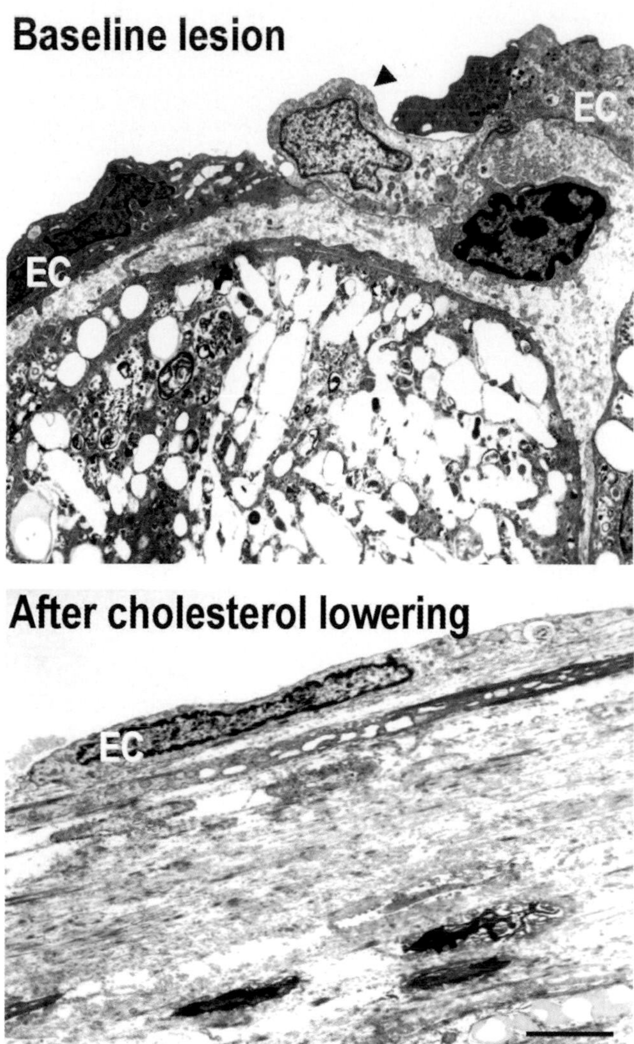

Fig. 8. Ultrastructure of activated endothelial cells (ECs) in rabbit atheroma and its normalization by lipid lowering. Top panel: ECs in aortic atheroma of cholesterol-fed rabbits showed a cuboidal or rounded structure, typical of an "activated" phenotype. Monocytic cell (indicated by the arrowhead) appears to be entering the intima through the gap between ECs. The circular cells containing abundant lipid particles in subendothelial space of the aorta of the baseline lesion are probably macrophage-derived foam cells. Bottom panel: The aortic ECs of the treated animals had a more squamous morphology. The size, density, and amount of cytoplasmic organelles of ECs of the atheroma of the treated animals are substantially smaller than those in the hypercholesterolemic animals. Accumulation of organized collagen fibrils was more prominent in the intima of the treated animals than in atheroma of the high-cholesterol-fed rabbits. Original magnification: ×3000. From ref. *35*, with permission.

17. Loree HM, Kamm RD, Stringfellow RG, Lee RT. Effects of fibrous cap thickness on peak circumferential stress in model atherosclerotic vessels. Circ Res 1992;71:850–858.
18. Loree HM, Tobias BJ, Gibson LJ, Kamm RD, Small DM, Lee RT. Mechanical properties of model atherosclerotic lesion lipid pools. Arterioscler Thromb 1994;14:230–234.
19. Burke AP, Farb A, Malcom GT, Liang YH, Smialek J, Virmani R. Coronary risk factors and plaque morphology in men with coronary disease who died suddenly. N Engl J Med 1997;336:1276–1282.
20. Wilcox JN, Smith KM, Schwartz SM, Gordon D. Localization of tissue factor in the normal vessel wall and in the atherosclerotic plaque. Proc Natl Acad Sci USA 1989;86:2839–2843.
21. Lupu F, Bergonzelli GE, Heim DA, et al. Localization and production of plasminogen activator inhibitor-1 in human healthy and atherosclerotic arteries. Arterioscler Thromb 1993;13:1090–1100.
22. Stamler J, Shekelle R. Dietary cholesterol and human coronary heart disease. The epidemiologic evidence. Arch Pathol Lab Med 1988; 112:1032–1040.
23. Libby P, Aikawa M, Schonbeck U. Cholesterol and atherosclerosis. Biochim Biophys Acta 2000;1529:299–309.
24. LaRosa JC, Hunninghake D, Bush D, et al. The cholesterol facts. A summary of the evidence relating dietary fats, serum cholesterol, and coronary heart disease. A joint statement by the American Heart Association and the National Heart, Lung, and Blood Institute. The Task Force on Cholesterol Issues, American Heart Association. Circulation 1990;81:1721–1733.
25. Anitschkow N, Chalatow S. On experimental cholesterin steatosis and its significance in the origin of some pathological processes (1913). Reprinted in Arteriosclerosis 1983;3:178–182.
26. Vesselinovitch D. Animal models and the study of atherosclerosis. Arch Pathol Lab Med 1988;112:1011–1017.

27. Armstrong ML, Heistad DD. Animal models of atherosclerosis. Atherosclerosis 1990;85:15–23.
28. Aikawa M, Fukumoto Y, Rabkin E, Libby P. Rabbit models of atherosclerosis. In: Simon DI, Rogers C (eds), Vascular Disease and Injury: Preclinical Research. Humana Press, Totowa, NJ: 2000; 175–191.
29. Steinberg D, Parthasarathy S, Carew TE, Khoo JC, Witztum JL. Beyond cholesterol. Modifications of low-density lipoprotein that increase its atherogenicity. N Engl J Med 1989;320:915–924.
30. Libby P. Inflammation in atherosclerosis. Nature 2002;420:868–874.
31. Steinberg D, Parthasarathy S, Carew TE, Khoo JC, Witztum JL. Beyond cholesterol. Modifications of low-density lipoprotein that increase its atherogenicity. N Engl J Med 1989;320:915–924.
32. Berliner JA, Navab M, Fogelman AM, et al. Atherosclerosis: basic mechanisms. Oxidation, inflammation, and genetics. Circulation 1995;91:2488–2496.
33. Haberland ME, Fong D, Cheng L. Malondialdehyde-altered protein occurs in atheroma of Watanabe heritable hyperlipidemic rabbits. Science 1988;241:215–218.
34. Yla-Herttuala S, Palinski W, Rosenfeld ME, et al. Evidence for the presence of oxidatively modified low density lipoprotein in atherosclerotic lesions of rabbit and man. J Clin Invest 1989;84:1086–1095.
35. Aikawa M, Sugiyama S, Hill C, et al. Lipid lowering reduces oxidative stress and endothelial cell activation in rabbit atheroma. Circulation 2002;106:1390–1396.
36. Kume N, Cybulsky MI, Gimbrone MA Jr. Lysophosphatidylcholine, a component of atherogenic lipoproteins, induces mononuclear leukocyte adhesion molecules in cultured human and rabbit arterial endothelial cells. J Clin Invest 1992;90:1138–1144.
37. Khan BV, Parthasarathy SS, Alexander RW, Medford RM. Modified low density lipoprotein and its constituents augment cytokine-activated vascular cell adhesion molecule-1 gene expression in human vascular endothelial cells. J Clin Invest 1995;95:1262–1270.
38. Cushing SD, Berliner JA, Valente AJ, et al. Minimally modified low density lipoprotein induces monocyte chemotactic protein 1 in human endothelial cells and smooth muscle cells. Proc Natl Acad Sci USA 1990;87:5134–5138.
39. Cybulsky MI, Iiyama K, Li H, et al. A major role for VCAM-1, but not ICAM-1, in early atherosclerosis. J Clin Invest 2001;107: 1255–1262.
40. Gu L, Okada Y, Clinton SK, et al. Absence of monocyte chemoattractant protein-1 reduces atherosclerosis in low density lipoprotein receptor-deficient mice. Mol Cell 1998;2:275–281.
41. Boring L, Gosling J, Cleary M, Charo IF. Decreased lesion formation in CCR2–/– mice reveals a role for chemokines in the initiation of atherosclerosis. Nature 1998;394:894–897.
42. Li H, Cybulsky MI, Gimbrone MA Jr., Libby P. An atherogenic diet rapidly induces VCAM-1, a cytokine-regulatable mononuclear leukocyte adhesion molecule, in rabbit aortic endothelium. Arterioscler Thromb 1993;13:197–204.
43. Rosenfeld ME, Ross R. Macrophage and smooth muscle cell proliferation in atherosclerotic lesions of WHHL and comparably hypercholesterolemic fat-fed rabbits. Arteriosclerosis 1990;10:680–687.
44. Gordon D, Reidy MA, Benditt EP, Schwartz SM. Cell proliferation in human coronary arteries. Proc Natl Acad Sci USA 1990;87: 4600–4604.
45. Aikawa M, Rabkin E, Sugiyama S, et al. An HMG-CoA reductase inhibitor, cerivastatin, suppresses growth of macrophages expressing matrix metalloproteinases and tissue factor in vivo and in vivo. Circulation 2001;103:276–283.
46. Sakai M, Kobori S, Miyazaki A, Horiuchi S. Macrophage proliferation in atherosclerosis. Curr Opin Lipidol 2000;11:503–509.
47. Collins T, Cybulsky MI. NF-kappaB: pivotal mediator or innocent bystander in atherogenesis? J Clin Invest 2001;107:255–264.
48. Kodama T, Freeman M, Rohrer L, Zabrecky J, Matsudaira P, Krieger M. Type I macrophage scavenger receptor contains alpha-helical and collagen-like coiled coils. Nature 1990;343:531–535.
49. Tsao PS, McEvoy LM, Drexler H, Butcher EC, Cooke JP. Enhanced endothelial adhesiveness in hypercholesterolemia is attenuated by L-arginine. Circulation 1994;89:2176–2182.
50. De Caterina R, Libby P, Peng HB, et al. Nitric oxide decreases cytokine-induced endothelial activation. Nitric oxide selectively reduces endothelial expression of adhesion molecules and proinflammatory cytokines. J Clin Invest 1995;96:60–68.
51. Khan BV, Harrison DG, Olbrych MT, Alexander RW, Medford RM. Nitric oxide regulates vascular cell adhesion molecule 1 gene expres-sion and redox-sensitive transcriptional events in human vascular endothelial cells. Proc Natl Acad Sci USA 1996;93: 9114–9119.
52. Tsao PS, Wang B, Buitrago R, Shyy JY, Cooke JP. Nitric oxide regulates monocyte chemotactic protein-1. Circulation 1997;96: 934–940.
53. Oemar BS, Tschudi MR, Godoy N, Brovkovich V, Malinski T, Luscher TF. Reduced endothelial nitric oxide synthase expression and production in human atherosclerosis. Circulation 1998;97: 2494–2498.
54. Liao JK, Shin WS, Lee WY, Clark SL. Oxidized low-density lipoprotein decreases the expression of endothelial nitric oxide synthase. J Biol Chem 1995;270:319–324.
55. Farb A, Burke AP, Tang AL, et al. Coronary plaque erosion without rupture into a lipid core. A frequent cause of coronary thrombosis in sudden coronary death. Circulation 1996;93:1354–1363.
56. Rajavashisth TB, Liao JK, Galis ZS, et al. Inflammatory cytokines and oxidized low density lipoproteins increase endothelial cell expression of membrane type 1-matrix metalloproteinase. J Biol Chem 1999;274:11924–11929.
57. Schneiderman J, Sawdey MS, Keeton MR, et al. Increased type 1 plasminogen activator inhibitor gene expression in atherosclerotic human arteries. Proc Natl Acad Sci USA 1992;89:6998–7002.
58. Gotto AM, Farmer JA. Lipid-lowering trials. In: Braunwald E, Zipes DP, Libby P (eds), Heart Disease: A Text Book of Cardiovascular Medicine. W.B. Saunders, Philadelphia: 2001;126–146.
59. Libby P, Aikawa M. Mechanisms of plaque stabilization with statins. Am J Cardiol 2003;91:4B–8B.
60. Brown BG, Zhao XQ, Sacco DE, Albers JJ. Lipid lowering and plaque regression. New insights into prevention of plaque disruption and clinical events in coronary disease. Circulation 1993;87: 1781–1791.
61. Libby P. Molecular bases of the acute coronary syndromes. Circulation 1995;91:2844–2850.
62. Small DM. George Lyman Duff memorial lecture. Progression and regression of atherosclerotic lesions. Insights from lipid physical biochemistry. Arteriosclerosis 1988;8:103–129.
63. Wissler RW, Vesselinovitch D. Can atherosclerotic plaques regress? Anatomic and biochemical evidence from nonhuman animal models. Am J Cardiol 1990;65:33F–40F.
64. Liao JK. Isoprenoids as mediators of the biological effects of statins. J Clin Invest 2002;110:285–288.
65. Aikawa M, Rabkin E, Okada Y, et al. Lipid lowering by diet reduces matrix metalloproteinase activity and increases collagen content of rabbit atheroma: a potential mechanism of lesion stabilization. Circulation 1998;97:2433–2444.
66. Aikawa M, Voglic SJ, Sugiyama et al. Dietary lipid lowering reduces tissue factor expression in rabbit atheroma. Circulation 1999;100: 1215–1222.
67. Aikawa M, Rabkin E, Voglic SJ, et al. Lipid lowering promotes accumulation of mature smooth muscle cells expressing smooth muscle myosin heavy chain isoforms in rabbit atheroma. Circ Res 1998;83:1015–1026.
68. Kockx MM, De Meyer GR, Buyssens N, Knaapen MW, Bult H, Herman AG. Cell composition, replication, and apoptosis in atherosclerotic plaques after 6 months of cholesterol withdrawal. Circ Res 1998;83:378–387.
69. Crisby M, Nordin-Fredriksson G, Shah PK, Yano J, Zhu J, Nilsson J. Pravastatin treatment increases collagen content and decreases lipid content, inflammation, metalloproteinases, and cell death in human carotid plaques: implications for plaque stabilization. Circulation 2001;103:926–933.
70. Fukumoto Y, Libby P, Rabkin E, et al. Statins alter smooth muscle cell accumulation and collagen content in established atheroma of

Watanabe heritable hyperlipidemic rabbits. Circulation 2001;103: 993–999.

71. Aikawa M, Sivam PN, Kuro-o M, et al. Human smooth muscle myosin heavy chain isoforms as molecular markers for vascular development and atherosclerosis. Circ Res 1993;73:1000–1012.
72. Rollins BJ. Chemokines. Blood 1997;90:909–928.
73. Sakai M, Kobori S, Matsumura T, et al. HMG-CoA reductase inhibitors suppress macrophage growth induced by oxidized low density lipoprotein. Atherosclerosis 1997;133:51–59.
74. Colli S, Eligini S, Lalli M, Camera M, Paoletti R, Tremoli E. Vastatins inhibit tissue factor in cultured human macrophages. A novel mechanism of protection against atherothrombosis. Arterioscler Thromb Vasc Biol 1997;17:265–272.
75. Bellosta S, Via D, Canavesi M, et al. HMG-CoA reductase inhibitors reduce MMP-9 secretion by macrophages. Arterioscler Thromb Vasc Biol 1998;18:1671–1678.
76. Guijarro C, Blanco-Colio LM, Ortego M, et al. 3-Hydroxy-3-methylglutaryl coenzyme a reductase and isoprenylation inhibitors induce apoptosis of vascular smooth muscle cells in culture. Circ Res 1998;83:490–500.
77. Negre-Aminou P, van Vliet AK, van Erck M, van Thiel GC, van Leeuwen RE, Cohen LH. Inhibition of proliferation of human smooth muscle cells by various HMG-CoA reductase inhibitors; comparison with other human cell types. Biochim Biophys Acta 1997;1345:259–268.
78. Ridker PM, Rifai N, Pfeffer MA, et al. Inflammation, pravastatin, and the risk of coronary events after myocardial infarction in patients with average cholesterol levels. Cholesterol and Recurrent Events (CARE) Investigators. Circulation 1998;98:839–844.
79. Ridker PM, Rifai N, Lowenthal SP. Rapid reduction in C-reactive protein with cerivastatin among 785 patients with primary hypercholesterolemia. Circulation 2001;103:1191–1193.
80. Weiss D, Sorescu D, Taylor WR. Angiotensin II and atherosclerosis. Am J Cardiol 2001;87:25C–32C.
81. Bocan TM, Krause BR, Rosebury WS, et al. The ACAT inhibitor avasimibe reduces macrophages and matrix metalloproteinase expression in atherosclerotic lesions of hypercholesterolemic rabbits. Arterioscler Thromb Vasc Biol 2000;20:70–79.
82. Perrey S, Legendre C, Matsuura A, et al. Preferential pharmacological inhibition of macrophage ACAT increases plaque formation in mouse and rabbit models of atherogenesis. Atherosclerosis 2001; 155:359–370.
83. Ziouzenkova O, Perrey S, Marx N, Bacqueville D, Plutzky J. Peroxisome proliferator-activated receptors. Curr Atheroscler Rep 2002;4:59–64.
84. Fayad ZA, Fuster V. Clinical imaging of the high-risk or vulnerable atherosclerotic plaque. Circ Res 2001;89:305–316.

35 Multidetector-Row CT Imaging of Clinical and Preclinical Coronary Atherosclerosis

Christoph R. Becker, MD

PREREQUISITE FOR THE ASSESSMENT OF CORONARY ATHEROSCLEROSIS

Complete assessment of coronary atherosclerosis with multidetector-row computed tomography (MDCT) requires motion-free, contrast-enhanced images with the highest spatial resolution available. Because of the rather long exposure time with MDCT (approx 200 ms), patient preparation with β-blocker may be necessary. Optimal results will be achieved if the heart rate of the patient is below 60 beats per minute (bpm). The spatial resolution is given by the detector element size. The current reasonably achievable near isotropic spatial resolution is approx 0.4 mm^3.

A timely, accurate, and homogenous vascular lumen enhancement is essential for full diagnostic capability of coronary MDCT angiography studies and to assess coronary atherosclerosis. Higher contrast enhancement is superior to identify small vessels in MDCT. However, coronary atherosclerosis is commonly associated with calcifications that may interfere with dense contrast material and hinder the assessment of the residual lumen. In a randomized control group study, we investigated different contrast agent densities as well as peripheral venous injection rates to determine the optimal contrast protocol for the assessment of coronary atherosclerosis. We found that a contrast medium flow rate of 1 g/s iodine resulted in an enhancement of approx 250–300 Hounsfield units (HU), which allows for delineation of intermediate (91 ± 21 HU) as well as highly dense plaques (419 ± 194 HU) *(1)*.

The final vessel enhancement will also depend on physiological parameters such as cardiac output and central blood volume. The cardiac output and central blood volume (correlates with body weight) is inversely related with the final enhancement *(2)*. It needs to be considered that in patients with heart rates above 60 bpm, β-blockers are now frequently applied to achieve good image quality *(3,4)*. The consequent lower cardiac output may lead to a higher final enhancement in these patients. Because MDCT imaging of the coronary arteries is performed during the first pass of the contrast medium, the central blood volume plays a minor role for the final enhancement.

From: *Contemporary Cardiology: CT of the Heart: Principles and Applications*
Edited by: U. Joseph Schoepf © Humana Press, Inc., Totowa, NJ

ASSESSMENT OF CORONARY ATHEROSCLEROSIS

The morphology of calcifications may already give a first hint for the presence or absence of significant stenoses in the coronary arteries. From electron beam CT (EBCT) studies, Kajinami et al. reported that the positive predictive value for significant stenosis (=75%) was 0.04 and 0.17 in none, 0.18 and 0.59 in spotty (Fig. 1), 0.32 and 0.87 in long, 0.40 and 0.84 in wide, and 0.56 and 0.96 in diffuse (Fig. 2) coronary calcifications, respectively *(5)*.

Besides displaying the coronary artery lumen, MDCT as a cross-sectional modality is able to display the coronary artery wall. Coronary calcifications can easily be assessed even without contrast media, and represent an advanced stage of atherosclerosis. However, as different stages of coronary atherosclerosis may be present simultaneously, calcifications may also be associated with lesions of more early stages of the disease. The entire extent of coronary atherosclerosis will be underestimated by assessing coronary calcifications alone *(6)*. Calcified as well as noncalcified lesions can be completely assessed by contrast-enhanced MDCT of the coronary arteries.

In our initial experience, it seems that different histological stages of atherosclerosis will present with different morphological pattern in MDCT. Because of the limited spatial resolution, it cannot be expected to assess a thinned fibrous cap (65 µm) that is approx 10 times beyond the current resolution of MDCT (750 µm). In addition, contrast uptake as an indicator of inflammatory processes is unlikely to be detected by MDCT. In extremely large atheromas, a lipid core may be visible with negative density values corresponding to fat. More commonly, atheromas may present as well-defined and homogenous humps in the coronary artery wall, without calcifications (Fig. 3). The density of these plaques may vary between 40 and 60 HU, and may reflect the ratio between lipid and fibrous tissue. These kinds of plaques are most often found in asymptomatic patients. Plaque with densities above 80 HU may be considered to contain predominantly fibrous tissue. Fibrous plaques may also frequently be associated with calcifications (Fig. 4), indicating an advanced stage of atherosclerotic disease as well as coronary artery disease, and may therefore be found in patients with chronic and stable angina.

Other types of plaques (Table 1) present with low densities (20 HU) and inhomogeneous structure with irregular defined

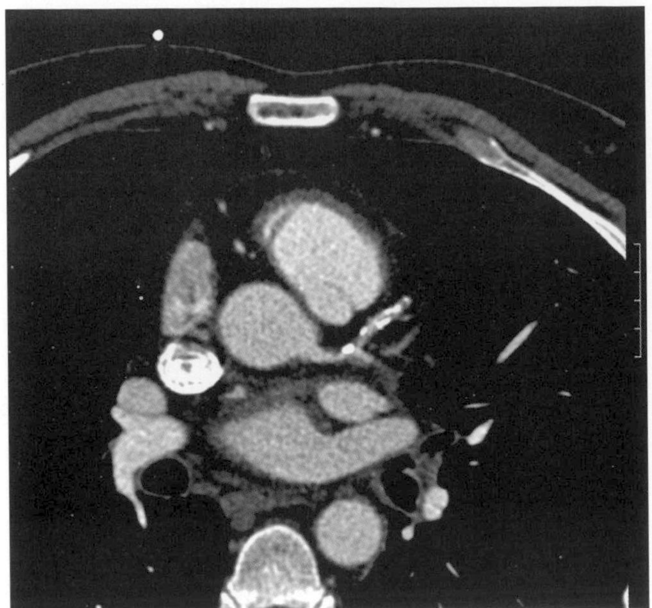

Fig. 1. The positive predictive value of spotty coronary calcifications (calcified nodules) for predicting coronary artery stenosis is between 18% and 59%.

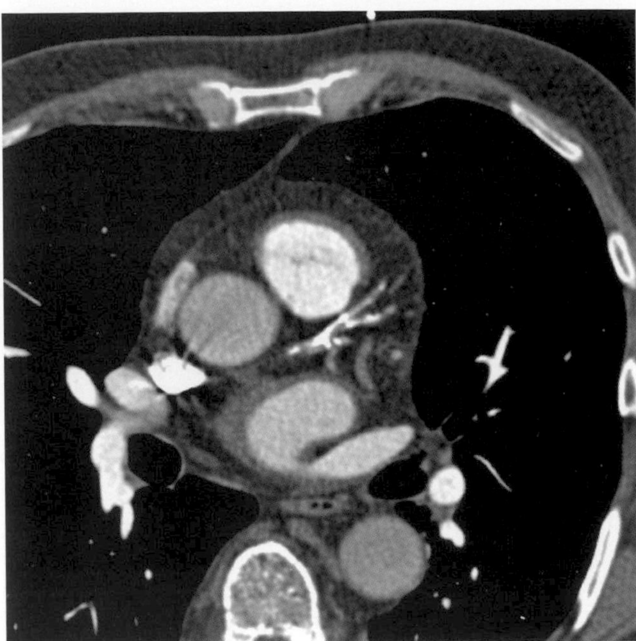

Fig. 2. The positive predictive value of diffuse coronary calcifications is between 56% and 96%.

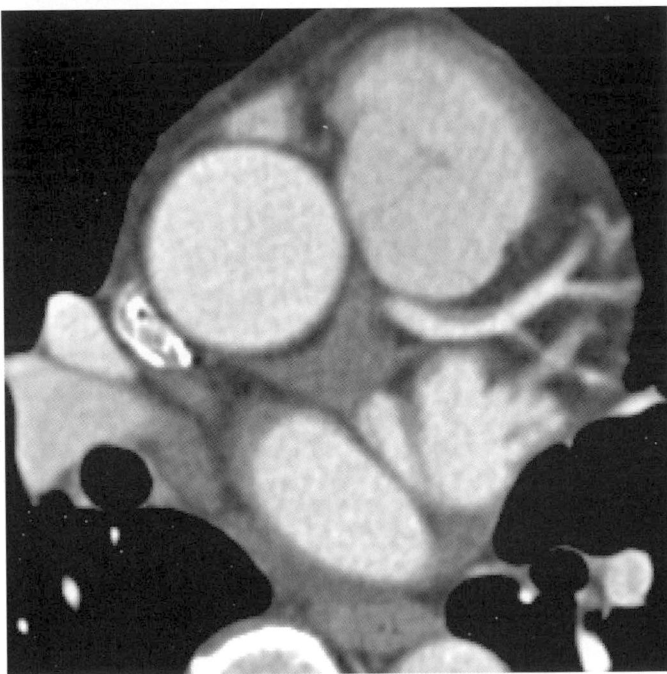

Fig. 3. Homogenous and well-defined lesion with approx 40-HU density in asymptomatic patients most likely corresponds to atheromas.

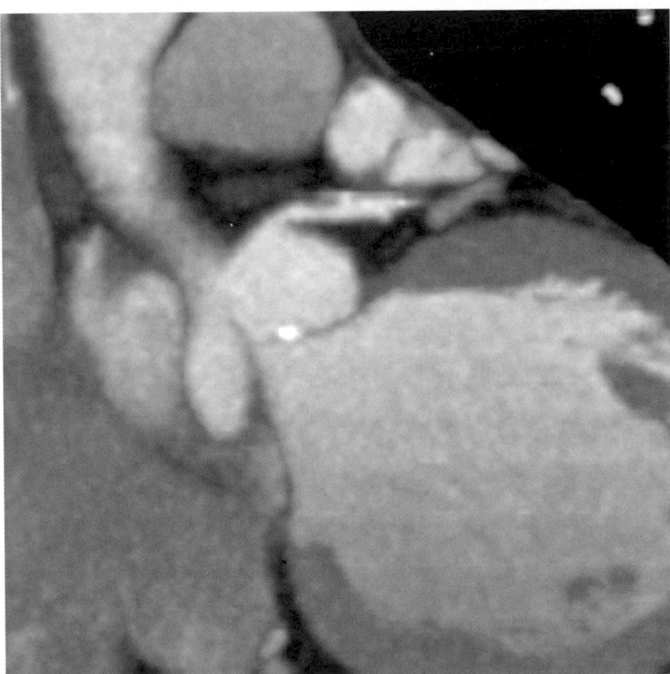

Fig. 4. Homogenous plaques with approx 100-HU density and calcifications correspond most likely to fibro-calcified plaques and may be found in patients with chronic stable angina.

borders (Fig. 5). We have frequently observed these kinds of lesions in patients with acute and unstable angina. We currently believe that these plaques may correspond to intra-coronary thrombi. In some cases, the entire coronary artery may be filled with low-density material with a bright rim surrounding it, indicating a complete thrombus occlusion. Acute thrombus occlusion may lead to enlargement of the coronary artery vessel, whereas in chronic vessel occlusion, organizing fibrous tissue may lead to shrinkage and increased density of the vessel.

As mentioned above, spotty, calcified lesions may commonly be associated with minor wall changes in conventional coronary angiography *(5)*. However, it is known that such calcified nodules may also be the source of unheralded plaque rupture and consequent thrombosis, and may lead to sudden

Table 1
Coronary Artery Plaque Entities and Morphological Appearance in Multidetector-Row CT

Plaque entity	*AHA type*	*Calcification*	*Density*	*Shape*	*Remodelling*	*Symptoms*
Atheroma	IV	No	approx 40 HU	Smooth	Positive	No
Fibroatheroma	Va	No	approx 60 HU	Smooth	Positive/negative	No
Fibrotic lesion	Vc	No	approx 100 HU	Smooth	Positive/negative	No
Fibrocalcified plaque	Vb	Yes	approx 100 HU or absent	Smooth	Negative	Chronic stable angina
Thrombus	VI	No	approx 20 HU	Irregular	High-grade stenosis or occlusion	Acute unstable angina

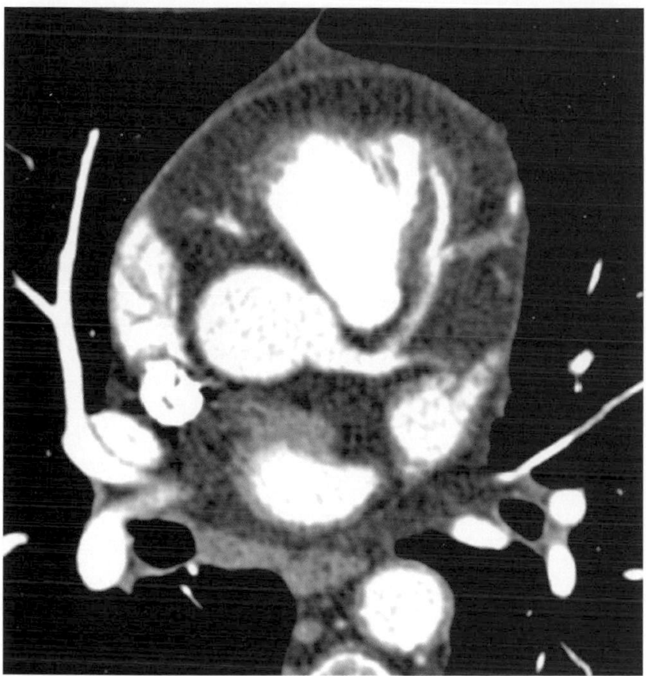

Fig. 5. Irregular, nonhomogenous, and low-density plaques in the left anterior descending coronary artery in a patient with acute coronary syndrome. The lesion most likely corresponds to a thrombus in the coronary artery.

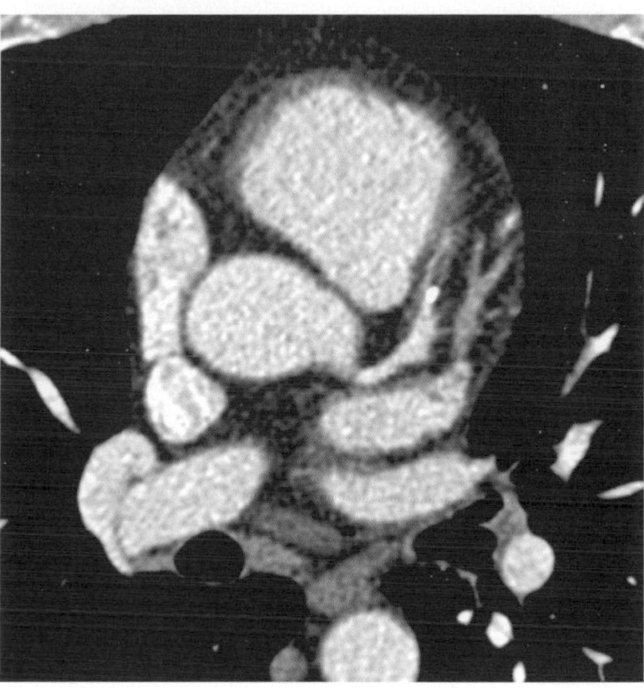

Fig. 6. In a patient with acute coronary syndromes, a calcified nodule may have led to a consecutive thrombus formation (arrow).

coronary death in very rare cases *(7)*. Since atherosclerosis is a continuously ongoing process, different stages of the disease may be found simultaneously in the coronary artery wall. In such cases, coronary calcium may be found together with thrombus formation (Fig. 6).

QUANTIFICATION OF CORONARY ATHEROSCLEROSIS

As already shown in many coronary calcium studies, quantification may have an impact on the risk assessment and follow-up of patients with coronary atherosclerosis. Coronary calcifications can easily be detected and quantified even in the presence of contrast material if the density of calcium (>350 HU) is above the density of the contrast medium in the coronary artery lumen (250–300 HU). The mass of coronary calcifications can best be determined by measuring the volume and density of the plaques. Using correction factors, the mass of calcium can be similarly derived from MDCT angiography studies, as well as from coronary calcium screening studies obtained with no contrast and thicker slices *(8)*.

However, because of partial-volume effects and the close relationship to the myocardium, it is much more difficult to quantify noncalcified plaques and vessel wall changes in the coronary arteries. In addition, with image reconstruction algorithms that are used to visualize the soft tissue in the coronary artery wall, dense material such as calcifications will become exaggerated. In patients with extensive coronary calcifications, noncalcified plaques are rarely found, most likely because the so-called blooming artifact of calcium prevents its assessment. Therefore, the optimal quantification algorithm for determination of the complete amount of noncalcified and calcified atherosclerosis by MDCT is still under development.

CONCLUSION

The newest generation of MDCT scanners now allows for consistently good image quality in patients with regular sinus rhythm and heart rate in the range between 40 and 60 bpm. With targeted administration of contrast medium, an enhancement can be achieved that allows for simultaneous assessment of calcified as well as noncalcified atherosclerotic lesions in the coronary artery wall. Morphologic criteria allow for distinguishing between basic types of atherosclerosis such as thrombus, atheroma, or fibro-calcified plaques. In addition, calibrated HU allows for estimation of the predominant component of lesions. These new features of coronary MDCT angiography may offer the chance to detect, quantify, and follow up vulnerable plaques with a high fraction of lipids. However, partial-volume effects with the myocardium and coronary calcifications may interfere with the detection of these plaques. Therefore, the optimal quantification algorithm is still under development. With these tools, large prospective cohort studies in an asymptomatic population will be necessary to determine the predictive value for future cardiac events and the change over time under therapy of atherosclerosis detected by MDCT.

REFERENCES

1. Schroeder S, Kopp AF, Baumbach A, et al. Noninvasive detection and evaluation of atherosclerotic coronary plaques with multislice computed tomography. J Am Coll Cardiol 2001;37:1430–1435.
2. Fleischmann D. Use of high concentration contrast media: principles and rationale vascular district. Eur J Radiol 2003;45:S88–S93.
3. Nieman K, Cademartiri F, Lemos PA, Raaijmakers R, Pattynama PM, de Feyter PJ. Reliable noninvasive coronary angiography with fast submillimeter multislice spiral computed tomography. Circulation 2002;106:2051–2054.
4. Ropers D, Baum U, Pohle K, et al. Detection of coronary artery stenoses with thin-slice multi-detector row spiral computed tomography and multiplanar reconstruction. Circulation 2003;107: 664–666.
5. Kajinami K, Seki H, Takekoshi N, Mabuchi H. Coronary calcification and coronary atherosclerosis: site by site comparative morphologic study of electron beam computed tomography and coronary angiography. J Am Coll Cardiol 1997;29:1549–1556.
6. Wexler L, Brundage B, Crouse J, et al. Coronary artery calcification: pathophysiology, epidemiology, imaging methods, and clinical implications. A statement for health professionals from the American Heart Association. Circulation 1996;94:1175–1192.
7. Virmani R, Kolodgie FD, Burke AP, Frab A, Schwartz SM. Lessons from sudden coronary death. A comprehensive morphological classification scheme for atherosclerotic lesions. Arterioscler Thromb Vasc Biol 2000;20:1262–1275.
8. Hong C, Becker C, Schoepf UJ, Ohnesorge B, Bruening R, Reiser M. Absolute quantification of coronary artery calcium in nonenhanced and contrast enhanced multidetector-row CT studies. Radiology 2002;223:474–480.
9. Gibbons R, Chatterjee K, Daley J, et al. ACC/AHA/ACP-ASIM guidelines for the management of patients with chronic stable angina: a report of the American College of Cardiology/American Heart Association Task Force on Practice Guidelines (Committee on Management of Patients With Chronic Stable Angina). J Am Coll Cardiol 1999;33:2092–2197.

36 Multidetector-Row CT vs Intravascular Ultrasound for Coronary Plaque Characterization

Axel Kuettner, MD

RATIONALE FOR CORONARY PLAQUE DETECTION

Coronary artery disease (CAD) constitutes a major clinically relevant disease in the Western industrialized world, causing 600,000 deaths annually *(1)*. The underlying pathophysiological mechanism seems to be coronary plaque disruption, subsequent thrombosis, and acute myocardial infarction. Fifty percent of afflicted patients experience this potentially life-threatening condition without experiencing prior symptoms *(2)*. Therefore, direct visualization of epicardial coronary arteries is necessary to assess the focal severity and clinical relevance of the vessel wall alterations. The visualization of plaque has two different clinical focal points. On the one hand, obstructive coronary artery disease causing chronic ischemia to the vessel-dependent myocardial tissue needs to be assessed to determine an adequate revascularization strategy (condition of stable angina pectoris). On the other hand, precursors of the already mentioned unheralded plaque rupture causing unstable angina, myocardial infarction, or sudden death should be assessed to take preventive measures to avoid these acute coronary syndromes.

Evidence suggests that atherosclerotic plaque composition and configuration are important predictors of plaque stability *(3)*. The risk for plaque rupture seems to depend rather on composition rather than on plaque volume *(4,5)*. Most ruptures occur in plaques containing a soft, lipid-rich core that is covered by a thin and inflamed cap of fibrous tissue *(6)*. Small ruptures often remain clinically silent, but more extensive plaque ruptures may cause the onset of unstable angina, myocardial infarction, or sudden death. Thus, the reliable noninvasive detection and classification of coronary lesions would constitute an important step forward in risk stratification of patients with known or suspected coronary artery disease.

The current gold standard to assess the morphological severity of CAD is invasive conventional coronary angiography (CAG). In Germany alone, the total number of conventional CAG has risen by 45%, from 409,000 in 1995 to more than 594,000 annual procedures in the year 2000 *(7)*. However, the fraction of interventional procedures remained constantly low at about 30% *(7)*. Although coronary angiography has become a safe procedure with only a small associated risk, the inconvenience for the patient as well as the economic burden have fuelled the quest to find an alternative, noninvasive method to visualize and assess coronary plaque burden.

From: *Contemporary Cardiology: CT of the Heart: Principles and Applications*
Edited by: U. Joseph Schoepf © Humana Press, Inc., Totowa, NJ

LIMITATIONS OF CONVENTIONAL CAG

Although angiography is still the gold standard used for defining coronary anatomy and to depict CAD, studies have shown that accuracy and reproducibility of this technique can be challenged, and its results are not totally conclusive *(8)*. Visual interpretation of angiograms can exhibit significant observer variability and often correlates poorly with postmortem examination *(9)*. In technical terms, angiography depicts coronary arteries in a two-dimensional projected plane of the contrast-filled lumen. Any angiographic projection may more or less accurately depict the true extent of luminal narrowing. Coronary interventions may increase luminal irregularity, thus further impairing the accuracy of angiography *(10)*. Also, assessment of lesion severity requires the measurement of the intrastenotic minimal luminal diameter as well as a normal segment prior and distal of the lesion. However, postmortem studies demonstrate that CAD constitutes a diffuse disease with no truly normal segments. Remodeling represents another feature of early CAD, making the true assessment of the disease process difficult since true luminal narrowing may be minimal for a long time while plaque enlargement is compensated by outward growth of the vessel. Intravascular ultrasound (IVUS) and multislice CT of the coronaries may be able to overcome these limitations *(11,12)*.

CORONARY PLAQUE IMAGING USING RETROSPECTIVELY GATED MDCT

Since 1999, mechanical multislice spiral computed tomography (MSCT) systems with simultaneous acquisition of four slices and half-second scanner rotation have become available. Multirow acquisition with these scanners allows for considerably improved visualization of the coronary arteries *(13–15)*. Initial experiences have shown that coronary lesions can be detected with acceptable sensitivity and specificity *(16–19)*.

There is evidence that even preclinical atheroma and noncalcified plaque tissue can be identified *(20–22)*. With the introduction of the second generation of multislice spiral scanners with up to 16 detector rows and a gantry rotation time as low as 420 ms, an improved tool to visualize coronary lesion was introduced in 2002 *(18,19)*.

In the following, scanning techniques are described to acquire 4- and 16-slice MSCT data sets suitable for plaque imaging.

In our institution, cardiac MSCT data sets are acquired using 4- and 16-slice CT scanners.

First, a native scan without contrast medium is performed to determine the total calcium burden of the coronary tree (numbers in parenthesis correspond to 16-slice scanning): collimation 2.5 mm (1.5 mm), pitch1.5 (table feed 3.8 mm/rotation), tube current 133 eff. mAs (133 eff. mAs) at 120 kV (120 kV). To determine the circulation time, 20 mL of contrast medium (20 mL at 4 mL/s, 400mg iodine/mL) and a chaser bolus of 20 mL saline is administered in an antecubital vein. The correct scanning delay is established by measuring CT attenuation values in the ascending aorta, using the last slice with maximal contrast as circulation time. By using a dual-head power injector, a total of 150 mL (80 mL) intravenous contrast agent plus a 20-mL chaser bolus is injected (50 mL at 4.0 mL/s, then 100 mL (30 mL) at 2.5 mL/s). CT imaging starts at the diaphragm caudally of all cardiac structures and stops at the aortic root cranial to the coronary ostia: 4 × 1.0-mm collimation (16 × 0.75 mm), pitch 1.5 (table feed 1.5 mm/rotation), tube current 500 eff. mAs at 120 kV for both 4- and 16-slice scanning.

To reconstruct the images, the standard built-in reconstruction algorithm is used. The reconstruction window is set to start at 60% RR interval for all native images as well as for the contrast-enhanced scan. If necessary, a test series is performed ranging from 35% to 75% in 2% steps. That percentage that displayed the least motion artifacts is chosen to reconstruct the entire stack of images of the CT angiography (CTA) scan. Using this reconstruction strategy, sets of images are created that show no substantial motion artifacts.

The calcium score is determined on an offline workstation, based on an Agatston equivalent scoring system as well as expressed in absolute mg calcium-hydroxyapatite.

On the basis of original axial slices, 3D volume-rendering technique (VRT) images as well as thin-sliding maximum intensity projections (MIP), each coronary plaque is assessed. Parameters to describe plaques are density in absolute Hounsfield units (HU), presence or absence of calcifications, length of the lesion, and the degree of luminal narrowing in %.

CORONARY PLAQUE DETECTION USING IVUS: TECHNIQUE AND CLINICAL INDICATIONS

Intravascular ultrasound imaging offers several advantages in the evaluation of CAD. First, as a result of the imaging from inside the vessel, IVUS provides images of the atherosclerotic plaque, not only the lumen. Tomographic orientation of IVUS offers a three-dimensional visualization of the entire circumference of the vessel wall and not just biplanar projections. Also, correct angiographic vessel or stenosis measurements (QCA) require calibration to correct for radiographic magnification, a potential source of errors. IVUS uses an electronically generated scale, performing direct planimetry. The tomographic perspective of ultrasound enables an assessment of vessels that are difficult to image by angiography, including diffusely diseased segments, ostial or bifurcation stenoses, as well as eccentric plaques.

IVUS consists of a catheter incorporating a miniaturized transducer and a console to reconstruct the images. Ultrasound frequencies between 20 and 50 MHz are used, yielding a practical axial resolution of approx 150 μm. Lateral resolution averages 250 μm. Current catheters range from 2.6 to 3.5 French (0.87 to 1.17 mm) and can be placed through a 6-French guiding catheter. Mechanically rotated devices and multielement electronic arrays are available.

Standard techniques for intracoronary catheter delivery are used for intravascular examination. The operator advances or retracts the IVUS device over the wire, recording the data for subsequent analysis. A motorized pullback device is used to withdraw the catheter at a constant speed (0.5 mm/s).

Complication rates of an IVUS exam vary from 1% to 3%, transient spasm being the most common. The complication rate of major dissection or vessel closures is approx 0.5%.

IVUS is accurate in determining the thickness and echogenicity of vessel wall structures, but it is not consistently able to provide actual histology. Validated methods do not yet exist for objective or automated classification of atheromatous lesions. Artifacts may adversely affect ultrasound images. The physical size of ultrasound catheters (currently approx 1.0 mm) constitutes an important limitation in imaging high-grade lesions.

The current clinical application of IVUS is the correct assessment of intermediate lesions and left main artery disease, although no absolute indications exist when the device should be used. In clinical trials, however, IVUS provides an indispensable tool for research. Many important trials that shifted treatment strategies in clinical cardiology used IVUS as reference standard *(23)*.

IVUS AND CT—A COMPARISON STUDY

As mentioned earlier, when MSCT was introduced in 1999, soon evidence was found that even preclinical atheroma and noncalcified plaque tissue could be identified *(20)*. However, these early results had to be confirmed to show whether MSCT was really able to correctly assess not only the severity of the lumen loss, but also plaque composition and plaque configuration. Thus, the purpose of the study was to investigate whether plaque composition as assessed by MSCT corresponds to the gold standard, IVUS.

A total of 15 patients were enrolled in the study who were scheduled for IVUS-guided percutaneous transluminal angioplasty (PTCA). The angiographic criteria for enrolment in the study was a lesion with a stenosis >70% and the absence of severe vessel angulations (>90°) in the proximal vessel segments. Angiographic exclusion criteria were left main artery disease, total occlusions, and vessel diameter <2 mm with bypass lesions. According to the study protocol, all patients

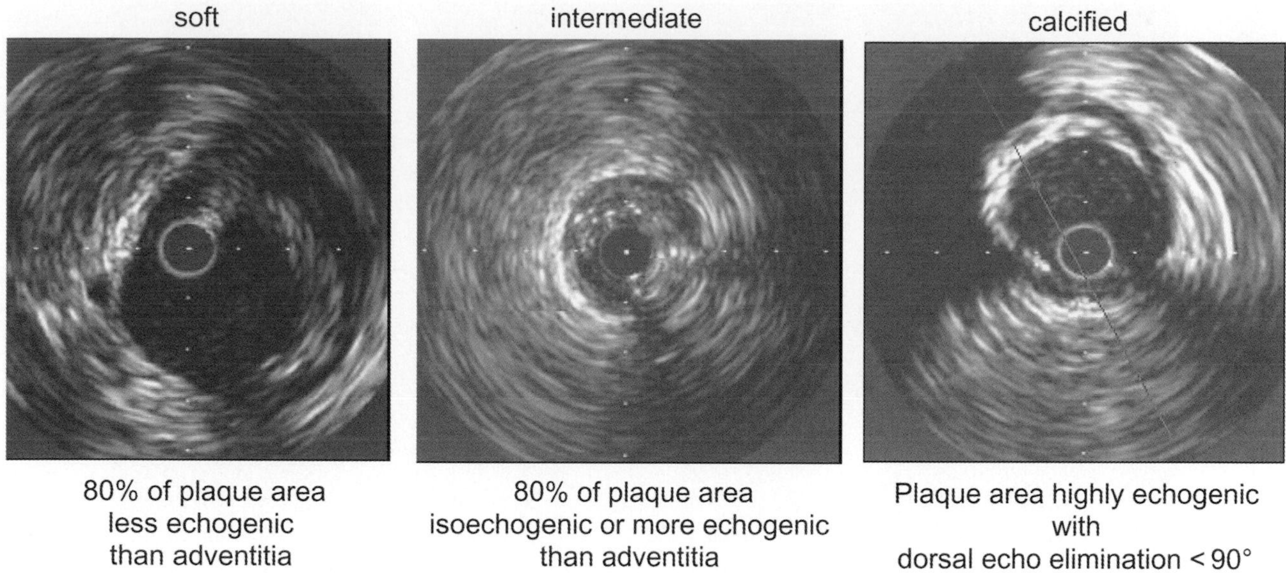

Fig. 1. Intravascular ultrasound criteria for the differentiation of plaque.

were examined by MSCT within 24 h prior to the coronary intervention. The examination protocol used was mentioned earlier in the chapter. Immediately before the intracoronary intervention, IVUS was performed to analyze the vessel configuration proximal to the target lesion and within the lesion. To ensure that identical plaques were assessed by the different techniques and to allow for precise correlations, landmarks such as the origin or side branches and the distance to the target lesion were used.

The assessed plaque configuration was classified according to the following IVUS criteria published by our group and others (Fig. 1):

- Soft plaques: More than 80% percent of the plaque area is composed of tissue with an echogenity of lower than the echogenity of the surrounding adventitia. If calcifications were partially present, the arc of lesion calcium had to be <90%
- Intermediate plaque: More than 80% percent of the plaque area is composed of tissue producing echoes as bright or brighter than those of the surrounding adventitia but without acoustic shadows. If calcifications were partially present, the arc of lesion calcium had to be <90%
- Calcified plaque: This plaque type involves bright echoes with acoustic shadowing accompanying >90° of the vessel wall circumference.

A total of 34 plaques (right coronary artery [RCA] $n = 12$, left anterior descending artery [LAD] $n = 22$) were analyzed by both methods with respect to lesion configuration (Fig. 2). On IVUS, 12 plaques were classified as soft, 5 plaques as intermediate, and 17 plaques as calcified. When comparing these data to MSCT data, the plaques identified by IVUS as soft had a mean density of 14 ± 26 HU, those classified as intermediate had a mean density of 91 ± 21 HU, and calcified plaques had a mean density of 419 ± 194 HU. Calcifications were also found in intermediate plaques; however, only small sprinkles of calcium deposits were found. Interestingly, even with only 34 plaques analyzed, the test for statistical significance was highly positive (Kruskal–Wallis test, $p < 0.0001$) (Figs. 3–5).

Since some patients had up to five plaques, plaque density results had to be tested for independence of the patient itself. First it was tested whether patient groups with either one, two, three, four, or five plaques were significantly different from each other, which was not the case ($p = 0.876$). Also, the independence of patient group and plaque composition was demonstrated ($p = 0.817$).

These data suggest that MSCT is capable of differentiation among different plaque compositions. The density measurements performed by MSCT correlate highly with the well established IVUS criteria (soft, intermediate, and calcified).

There was no overlap in the mean density values among the three groups of plaques. Thus, especially soft plaques with presumably lipid-rich core might be identified by density values <50 HU. Intermediate plaques showed a density ranging from 50 to 119 HU. Lesions with a density >120 HU correlated to calcified plaques in the IVUS study (Fig. 6).

A more precise view by MSCT on plaque configuration by visualizing lipid cores, fibrous caps, or smallest calcified sprinkles is at present restricted because of the limited spatial resolution of the 4-slice MSCT used to perform the study. Further clinical studies are necessary to confirm the relevance of a plaque score that is based on these findings. The impact of 16-slice MSCT will be discussed later in this chapter.

FUTURE DIRECTIONS: 16-SLICE MSCT

With the introduction of the 2nd generation of multislice spiral scanners with up to 16 detector rows and a gantry rotation time as low as 420 ms, an improved tool to visualize coronary lesion was introduced in 2002 *(18,19)*. Thus, a more reliable tool for the visualization of plaques is available. As mentioned earlier, next to a possible prognostic factor of plaque visualization, a keen interest remains whether plaque morphology also is a predictor for the assessment of stenosis.

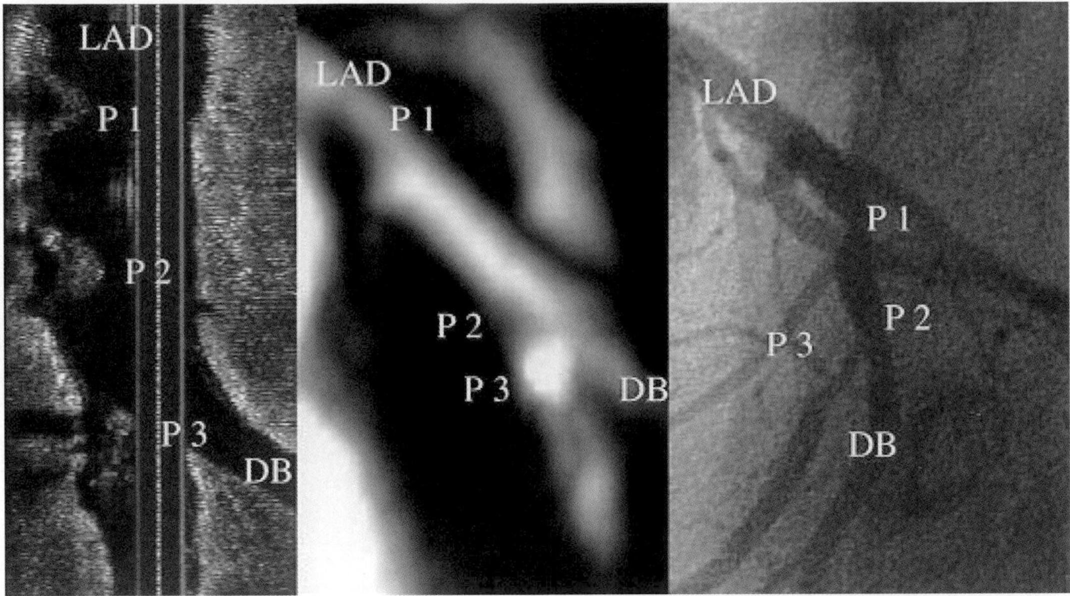

Fig. 2. Comparison between intravascular ultrasound (left), multislice CT (middle), and angiography (right).

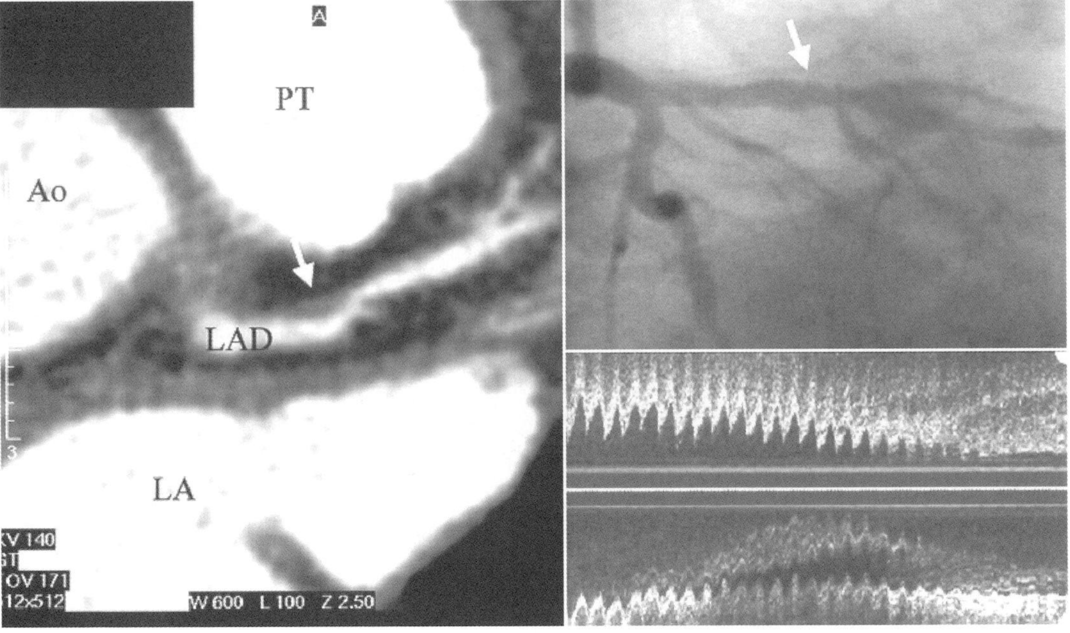

Fig. 3. Multidetector-row CT angiography-criteria soft plaque: hypodense in comparison to vessel filled with contrast, density <50 HU.

A total of 41 patients referred to our institution for conventional CAG were examined also by MDCT according to the protocols given in this chapter.

On the basis of original axial slices, 3D VRT images as well as thin-sliding MIPs, each coronary plaque identified by conventional CAG as a high-grade stenotic lesion or occlusion was assessed.

Depending on the identified plaque composition, each plaque was classified in one of six groups as follows (Fig. 7):

1. Calcified plaque adhered to vessel wall, no vessel obstruction
2. Calcified plaque, CT morphologically complete vessel obstruction
3. Calcified plaque conglomerate
4. Noncalcified plaque
5. Mixed plaque with calcifications predominantly present
6. Mixed plaque with noncalcified tissue predominantly present

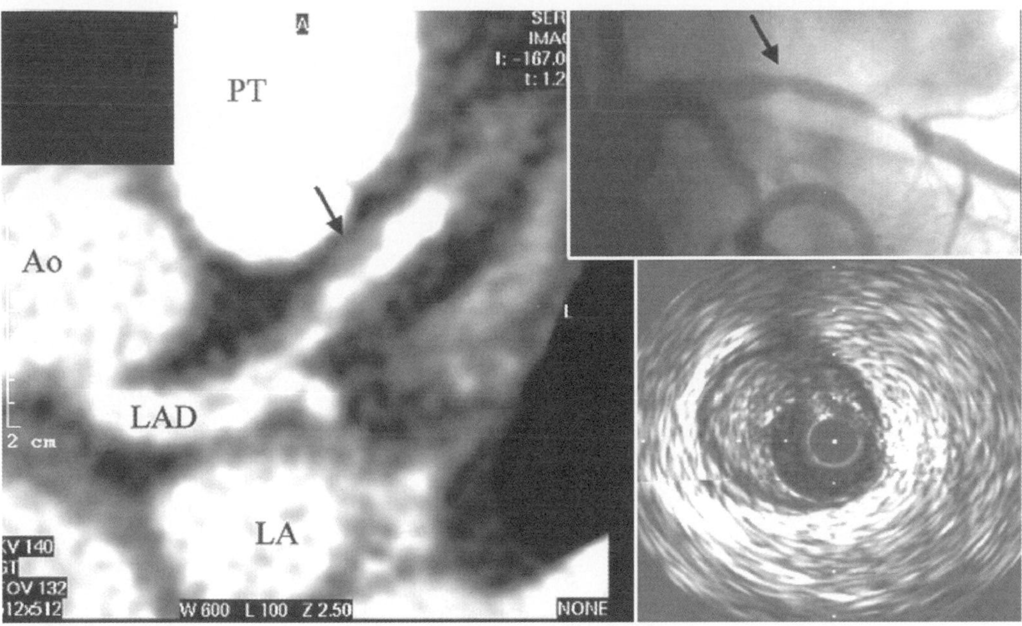

Fig 4. Multidetector-row CT angiography-criteria intermediate plaque: hypodense in comparison to vessel filled with contrast, density 50–120 HU.

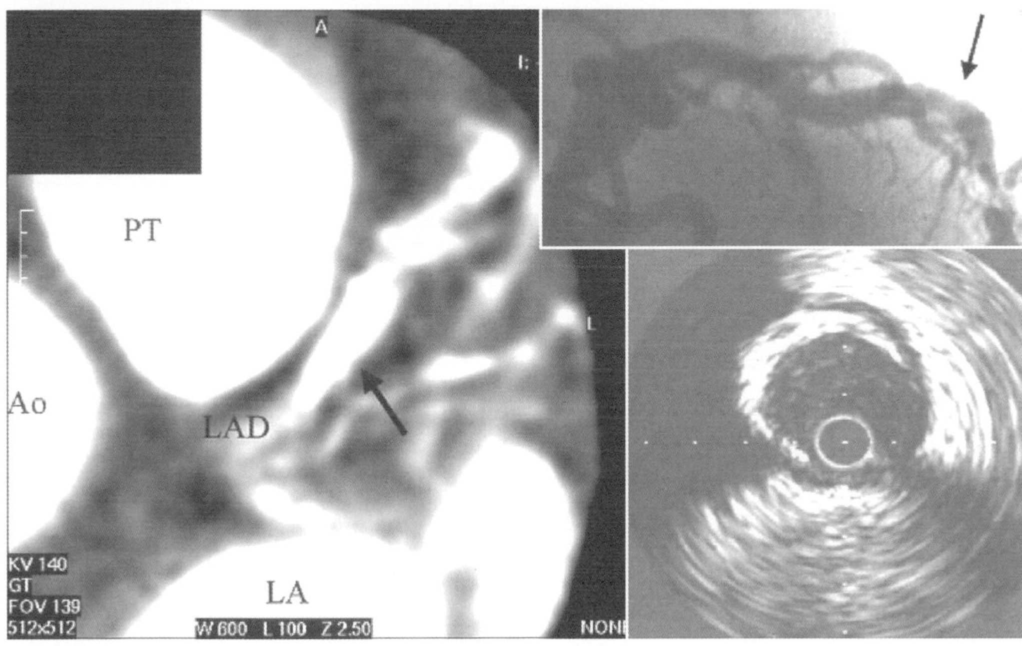

Fig 5. Multidetector-row CT angiography-criteria calcified plaque: hyperdense in comparison to vessel filled with contrast, density >120 HU.

In all patients, coronary angiograms were obtained using 4- and 5-French catheters. The angiograms were evaluated by quantitative coronary analysis. All plaques with an underlying diameter stenosis =70% or total occlusions were documented according to a modified AHA classification *(24)*.

MSCT plaque data were analyzed unblinded to the results of conventional CAG, and each plaque was attributed a group characteristic as described. Next we analyzed which of the plaque groups was predominantly present and whether there were clinically relevant differences between the groups. The primary aim of this pilot study was to principally analyze different types of plaque composition and their predominance in high-grade lesions.

In 533 coronary artery segments scanned, all 69 plaques causing high-grade diameter stenosis or complete occlusion could be detected. These plaques were subclassified according to the defined criteria.

No plaque was attributed group 1 characteristics. 1 plaque was attributed group 2 characteristics, 6 plaques had group 3 characteristics, 20 plaques had group 4 characteristics, 29 plaques were assigned to group 5, and 13 plaques to group 6.

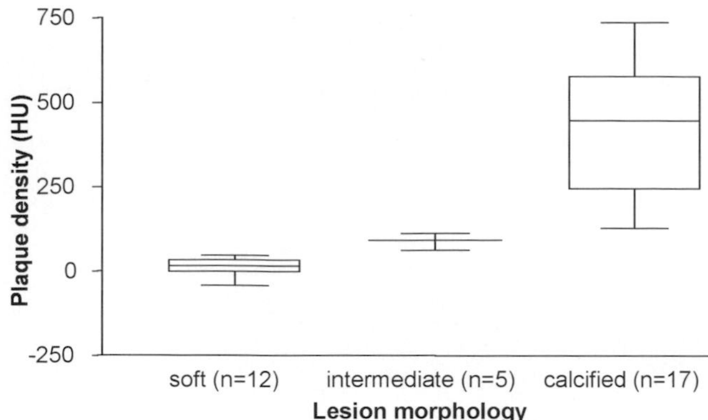

Fig. 6. Density distribution of plaques characterized by intravascular ultrasound as soft, intermediate, and calcified.

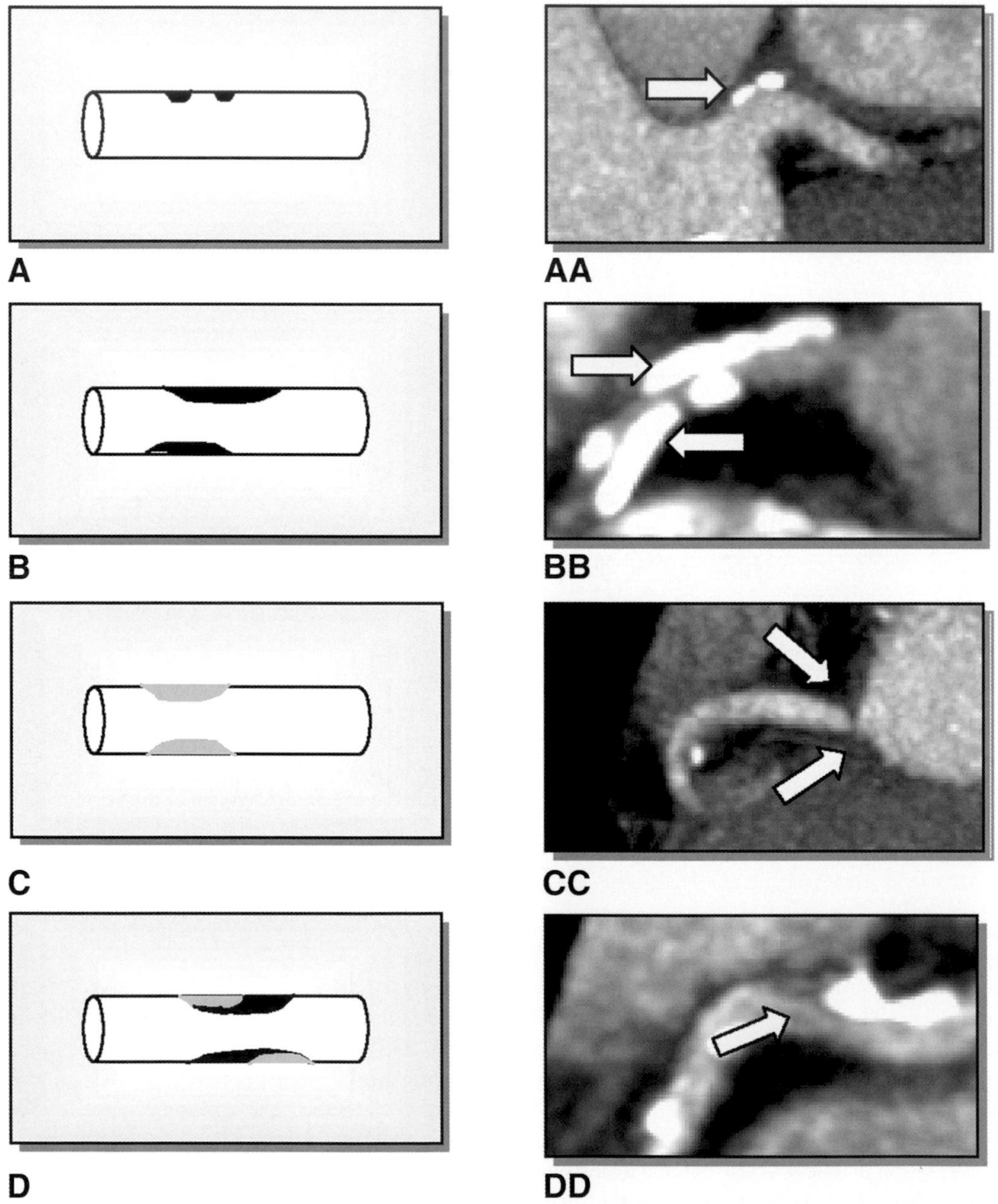

A AA

B BB

C CC

D DD

Fig. 7. Classification of different plaque composition. The first letter represents the plaque scheme, the double letter an actual CT image of the different plaque types. A) + AA): calcified nodule; B) + BB): calcified plaque; C) +CC): soft plaque; D) + DD): mixed plaque.

Conventional coronary angiography revealed a total of 49 high-grade lesions (>70%) and 20 complete occlusions. Of all these lesions, only 9/69 (13%) were caused by calcified plaques. Plaques of group 1 ("calcified nodules") caused no lesion at all; two plaques of group 2 ("vessel obstruction") caused 2/69 (3%) lesions; and six plaques of group 3 ("calcified conglomerate") caused a high-grade lesion (9%); so the total of all calcified plaque types caused only 9/69 (13%) high-grade lesions or occlusions. "Soft plaques" (group 4 plaques) caused 20/69 (29%) high grade lesions, and the majority of all high-grade lesions was caused by mixed plaques (42/69—61%), of which predominantly calcified plaques accounted for 29/69 (42%) lesions and group 6 (predominantly noncalcified plaques) accounted for 13/69 (19%) lesions. All together, 60/69 (87%) of all high-grade lesions or occlusions contain noncalcified plaque tissue. These distribution results are statistically relevant ($p < 0.0001$, Pearsons chi-square test). When analyzing the data with respect to presence of calcified or noncalcified plaque tissue alone, the differences were statistically not relevant (49/69 vs 60/69, $p < 0.2921$).

Intriguingly, the majority of all high-grade lesions and occlusions are not caused by merely calcified plaques but contain noncalcified plaque tissue, which is characteristic for 87% of high-grade lesions in our studied population. Only 13% of the lesions studied were solely calcified plaques.

These data also seem to suggest that a binary decision tree of calcified vs noncalcified plaque tissue is not sufficient to characterize high-grade lesions, since both entities are present in the majority of high-grade lesions. Only the combination yields statistically relevant results.

If these findings can be confirmed in larger studies, this would have a major impact on examination strategies when looking for obstructive CAD using MSCT. These findings suggest that a combination of both exams— the detection of coronary calcifications in combination with a contrast enhanced scan of the coronaries—should be performed to visualize and detect obstructive CAD. Currently, IVUS studies are being performed to verify these data, and preliminary data confirm these findings.

It could be shown that MSCT allows noninvasive determination of plaque morphology, suggesting that high-grade coronary lesions are predominantly caused by mixed plaques. Solely calcified plaques, however, are a less frequent cause of severe lesions.

REFERENCES

1. Wielopolski PA, van Geuns RJ, de Feyter PJ, Oudkerk M. Coronary arteries. Eur Radiol 1998;86:873–885.
2. Falk E. Coronary thrombosis: pathogenesis and clinical manifestations. Am J Cardiol 1991;687:28B–35B.
3. Falk E, Shah PK, Fuster V. Coronary plaque disruption. Circulation 1995;923:657–671.
4. Naghavi M, Libby P, Falk E, et al. From vulnerable plaque to vulnerable patient: a call for new definitions and risk assessment strategies: Part II. Circulation 2003;10815:1772–1778.
5. Naghavi M, Libby P, Falk E, et al. From vulnerable plaque to vulnerable patient: a call for new definitions and risk assessment strategies: Part I. Circulation 2003;10814:1664–1672.
6. Stary HC, Chandler AB, Dinsmore RE, et al. A definition of advanced types of atherosclerotic lesions and a histological classification of atherosclerosis. A report from the Committee on Vascular Lesions of the Council on Arteriosclerosis, American Heart Association. Circulation 1995;925:1355–1374.
7. Mannebach H, Hamm C, Horstkotte D. [18th report of the statistics of heart catheter laboratories in Germany. Results of a combined survey by the Committee of Clinical Cardiology and the Interventional Cardiology and Angiology Working Group for ESC of the German Society of Cardiology-Heart- and Cardiovascular Research 2001]. Z Kardiol 2002; 919:727–729.
8. Zir LM, Miller SW, Dinsmore RE, Gilbert JP, Harthorne JW. Interobserver variability in coronary angiography. Circulation 1976;534:627–632.
9. Grodin CM, Dydra I, Pastgernac A. Discrepancies between cineangiographic and post-mortem findings in patients with coronary artery disease and recent myocardial revascularization. Circulation 1974;49:703–709.
10. Galbraith JE, Murphy ML, de Soyza N. Coronary angiogram interpretation. Interobserver variability. JAMA 1978;240(19): 2053–2056.
11. Kopp AF, Kuttner A, Heuschmid M, Schroder S, Ohnesorge B, Claussen CD. Multidetector-row CT cardiac imaging with 4 and 16 slices for coronary CTA and imaging of atherosclerotic plaques. Eur Radiol 2002;12 Suppl 2:S17–24.
12. Nissen SE, Gurley JC, Grines CL, et al. Intravascular ultrasound assessment of lumen size and wall morphology in normal subjects and patients with coronary artery disease. Circulation 1991;843: 1087–1099.
13. Becker CR, Ohnesorge BM, Schoepf UJ, Reiser MF. Current development of cardiac imaging with multidetector-row CT. Eur J Radiol 2000;362:97–103.
14. Kopp AF, Ohnesorge B, Flohr T, et al. [Cardiac multidetector-row CT: first clinical results of retrospectively ECG-gated spiral with optimized temporal and spatial resolution]. Rofo Fortschr Geb Rontgenstr Neuen Bildgeb Verfahr 2000;1725:429–435.
15. Ohnesorge B, Flohr T, Schaller S, et al. [The technical bases and uses of multi-slice CT]. Radiologe 1999;3911:923–931.
16. Kopp AF, Schroeder S, Kuettner A, et al. Non-invasive coronary angiography with high resolution multidetector-row computed tomography. Results in 102 patients. Eur Heart J 2002;2321: 1714–1725.
17. Nieman K, Oudkerk M, Rensing BJ, et al. Coronary angiography with multi-slice computed tomography. Lancet 2001;3579256: 599–603.
18. Nieman K, Cademartiri F, Lemos PA, Raaijmakers R, Pattynama PM, de Feyter PJ. Reliable noninvasive coronary angiography with fast submillimeter multislice spiral computed tomography. Circulation 2002;106(16):2051–2054.
19. Ropers D, Baum U, Pohle K, et al. Detection of coronary artery stenoses with thin-slice multi-detector row spiral computed tomography and multiplanar reconstruction. Circulation 2003;107(5): 664–666.
20. Becker CR, Knez A, Ohnesorge B, Schoepf UJ, Reiser MF. Imaging of noncalcified coronary plaques using helical CT with retrospective ECG gating. AJR Am J Roentgenol 2000;1752:423–424.
21. Kopp AF, Schroeder S, Baumbach A, et al. Non-invasive characterisation of coronary lesion morphology and composition by multislice CT: first results in comparison with intracoronary ultrasound. Eur Radiol 2001;119:1607–1611.
22. Schroeder S, Kopp AF, Baumbach A, et al. Noninvasive detection and evaluation of atherosclerotic coronary plaques with multislice computed tomography. J Am Coll Cardiol 2001;375:1430–1435.
23. Nissen SE, Yock P. Intravascular ultrasound: novel pathophysiological insights and current clinical applications. Circulation 2001; 103(4):604–616.
24. Austen WG, Edwards JE, Frye RL, et al. A reporting system on patients evaluated for coronary artery disease. Report of the Ad Hoc Committee for Grading of Coronary Artery Disease, Council on Cardiovascular Surgery, American Heart Association. Circulation 1975;51(4 Suppl):5–40.

37 Multidetector-Row CT vs Magnetic Resonance Imaging for Coronary Plaque Characterization

Konstantin Nikolaou, MD, Christoph R. Becker, MD, and Zahi Fayad, MD

INTRODUCTION—IMAGING OF ATHEROSCLEROTIC DISEASE

Reliable noninvasive imaging tools that can detect various stages of atherothrombotic disease in different vessel regions and characterize the composition of the plaques are clinically desirable *(1)*. Such imaging tools would improve our understanding of the pathophysiological mechanisms underlying atherothrombotic processes and allow us to better risk-stratify the disease. Future goals are optimal tailoring of treatment and direct monitoring of the vascular response. Currently available imaging techniques for the diagnosis of coronary artery disease (CAD) are subject to several limitations. Conventional coronary angiography, widely accepted as the gold standard for the detection of coronary artery disease, demonstrates the degree of luminal narrowing, but fails to visualize the coronary artery wall. It has been shown that plaque composition rather than the severity of an actual stenosis predicts the risk of plaque rupture and acute clinical complications of coronary artery disease *(2–4)*. Thus, new imaging techniques that can image the artery wall and characterize different lesion types may allow for identification and follow-up of patients at risk and for selecting appropriate therapeutic strategies *(5)*.

Presently, a number of imaging modalities are employed to study atherosclerosis and to assess luminal diameter, wall thickness, and plaque volume *(6)*. Two noninvasive imaging modalities, computed tomography (CT) and magnetic resonance imaging (MRI), have been introduced for the study of atherothrombosis. Both have been shown to be capable of imaging vessel wall structures and differentiating various stages of atherosclerotic wall changes. The latest generation of multidetector-row computed tomography (MDCT) scanners allow for sufficiently reliable detection of significant proximal coronary stenoses *(7)*, quantitative measurement of atherosclerotic burden including calcified and noncalcified plaques *(8)*, and characterization of the plaque components *(1)*. MRI has been applied in various in-vivo human studies to image atherosclerotic plaques in carotid *(9,10)* and aortic *(11)* arterial disease. In vivo imaging of the coronary artery wall is challenging because of a combination of cardiac and respiratory motion artifacts, and the tortuous course, small size, and location of the vessels. Initial in vivo studies in human coronary arteries have used noninvasive black-blood spin-echo techniques with breath-holding *(12)* or a real-time navigator for respiratory gating *(13)*.

By possibly combining the advantages of both techniques, detecting significant stenoses and describing the plaque composition at the same time, information could be provided that may predict cardiovascular risk, facilitate further study of atherothrombosis progression and its response to therapy, and provide for assessment of subclinical disease.

PLAQUE IMAGING—METHODS

METHODS OF CT PLAQUE IMAGING

In 2002, newly developed 16-row CT systems were clinically introduced, allowing for faster data acquisition with improved spatial resolution *(14)*. Primary requisites for a sufficient delineation and depiction of atherosclerotic calcified and noncalcified plaques are similar to the requirements for a high-quality CT angiography (CTA) of the coronaries—i.e., a high spatial and high temporal resolution at the same time. There are several advantages of a 16-row CT system over a 4-row CT system concerning the depiction of coronary artery plaques. A direct comparison of a 4-row CT and a 16-row CT image clearly demonstrates this advantage (Fig. 1). First, the gantry rotation time in 16-row CT for cardiac investigations is 420 ms, allowing a temporal resolution of =210 ms. This is a gain of about 20% over the temporal resolution of a 4-row CT system. With higher heart rates and multisegment-reconstruction algorithms, the exposure time varies between 105 and 210 ms, depending on the actual heart rate *(15)*. Second, the slice thickness is reduced from 1.25 mm to 0.75 mm, allowing for an improved spatial resolution along the z axis. This way, using 16-row CT, almost isotropic voxels can now be acquired. Based on the improved spatial resolution, "blooming" artifacts of calcium deposits in the vessel wall are reduced as a result of decreased partial-volume effects. This allows for improved depiction and delineation of calcified and noncalcified plaques.

From: *Contemporary Cardiology: CT of the Heart: Principles and Applications*
Edited by: U. Joseph Schoepf © Humana Press, Inc., Totowa, NJ

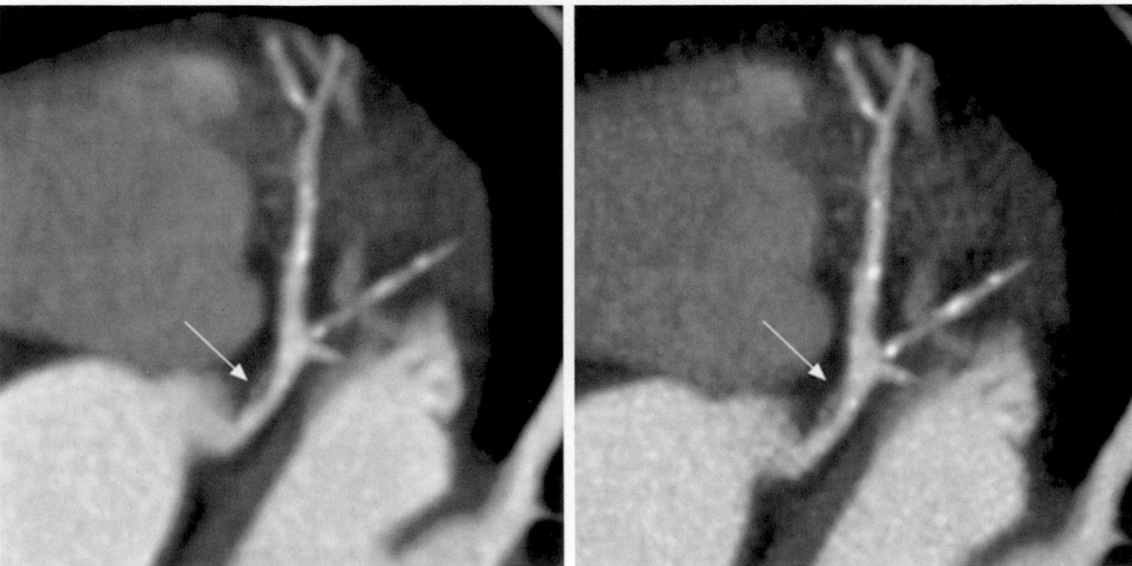

Fig. 1. Comparison of thin maximum intensity projection of a simulated 4-row CT (left) and 16-row CT (right) angiography, depicting a plaque in the left main coronary artery. 4-row CT simulation is based on 16-row CT data set and uses 1.25-mm thick slices. Acquiring thinner, 0.75-mm thick slices with a 16-row CT system (right) clearly improves depiction quality and assessability of the noncalcified plaque (arrows). (Courtesy of T.J. Jakobs, University of Munich.)

Third, and probably most important, the complete heart can now be covered in a significantly shorter breath-hold time of less than 20 s, compared to 35- to 40-s breath-hold time on a 4-row CT. This results in a considerable reduction of motion artifacts and allows for a substantial reduction in contrast volume compared to previously published protocols on 4-row CT. Compared to low-pressure arterial systems such as the pulmonary arteries, where calcifications are absent and the injection rate can be increased to visualize the smallest arterial branches, in coronary arteries the opacification must not exceed approx 300 Hounsfield units (HU) for a reliable depiction and judgment of calcifications. Optimization of vessel contrast-to-noise ratio (CNR) is also mandatory for sufficient visualization of noncalcified plaques, and can be performed either by a test bolus setting (20 mL + 50 mL NaCl) or a bolus tracking. Because nonenhanced blood on CT has attenuation similar (50–70 HU) to that of noncalcified plaques, this type of lesion can be detected only after administration of contrast medium. Therefore, a vessel enhancement significantly above the CT values of noncalcified lesions (150 HU) must be achieved to allow for reliable detection. A target attenuation of 200 HU seems best suited to fulfill this requirement. With this vessel enhancement, calcified coronary lesions remain detectable because their attenuation is significantly higher *(16)*.

METHODS OF MR PLAQUE IMAGING

High-resolution MR has emerged as the potential leading noninvasive in-vivo imaging modality for atherosclerotic plaque characterization. MR differentiates plaque components on the basis of biophysical and biochemical parameters such as chemical composition and concentration, water content, physical state, molecular motion, or diffusion *(17)*. MR provides imaging without ionizing radiation and can be repeated over time. In-vivo MR plaque imaging and characterization have been performed utilizing a multicontrast approach with high-resolution black-blood spin-echo and fast spin echo (FSE) based MR sequences. The signal from the blood flow is rendered black through preparatory pulses (e.g., radiofrequency spatial saturation or inversion recovery pulses) to better image the adjacent vessel wall *(18)*. However, bright blood imaging (i.e., 3D fast time of flight) can be employed in assessing fibrous cap thickness and morphological integrity of the carotid artery plaques *(19)*. This sequence enhances the signal from flowing blood, and a mixture of T2 and proton density contrast weighting highlights the fibrous cap. Atherosclerotic plaque characterization by MR is generally based on the signal intensities and morphological appearance of the plaque on T1-weighted, proton density–weighted, and T2-weighted images as previously validated (*see* references in recent reviews by Fayad et al. *[6]* and Yuan et al. *[20]*).

PLAQUE IMAGING—APPLICATIONS

APPLICATIONS OF CT PLAQUE IMAGING

Noncoronary Plaque Imaging With CT

Several precedent studies in animals and humans in other vascular territories than the coronary arteries have demonstrated the ability of CT to differentiate calcified, fibrous, and lipid-rich plaque components based on CT attenuation (HU). CT is described as an accurate, noninvasive means for studying detailed plaque morphology and composition in the carotid arteries. According to Estes et al. *(21)*, CT accurately defined plaque features containing calcium, fibrous stroma, and lipids in carotid arteries. Using tissue attenuation values, CT distinguished between lipid and fibrous stroma (means 39 ± 12 HU and 90 ± 24 HU, respectively, $p < 0.001$). Oliver et al. *(22)* tried to assess whether features seen at CTA might be used to predict carotid plaque stability by comparing CT angiograms with histopathologic examinations of the carotid artery bifurcation.

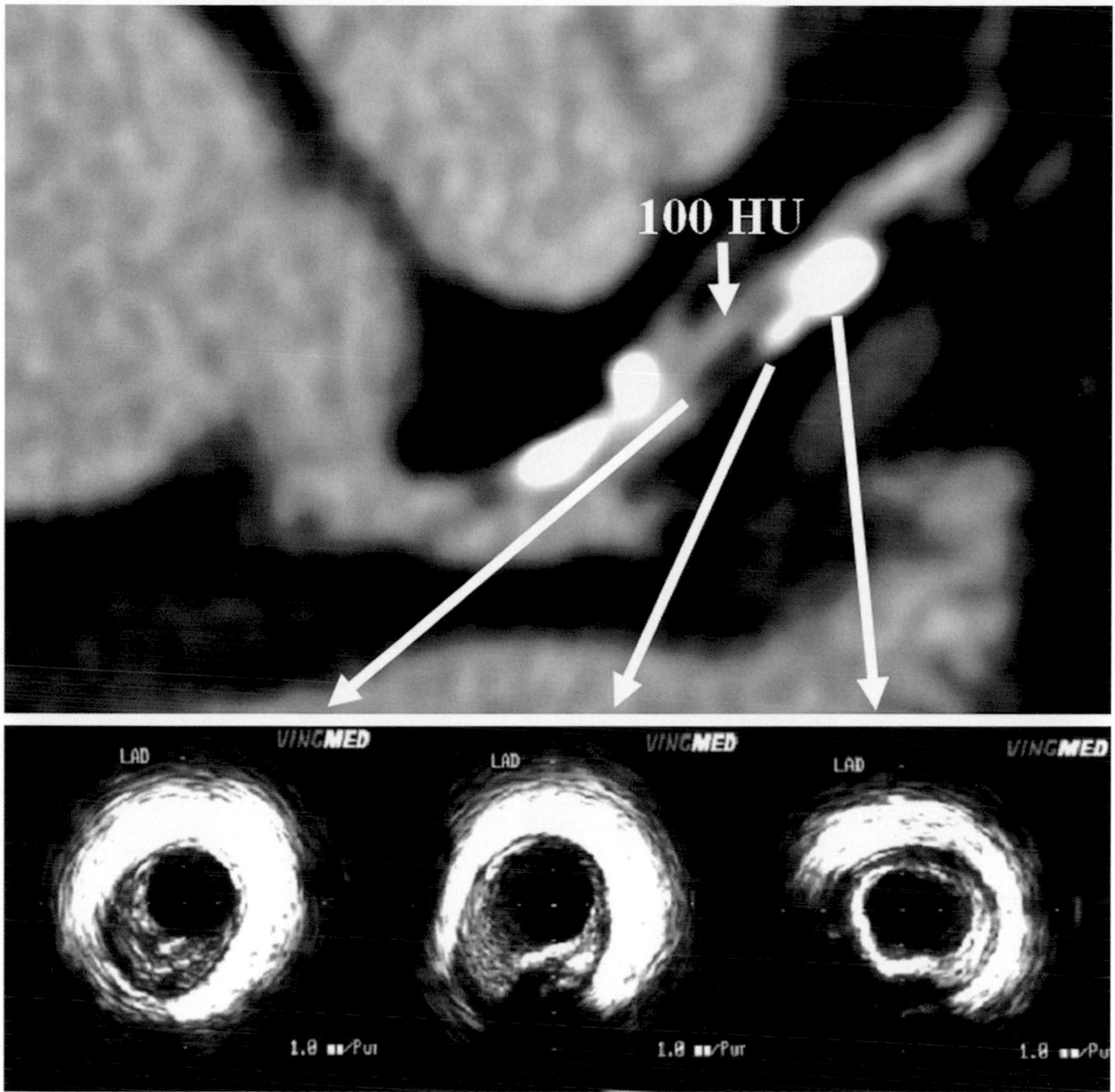

Fig. 2. Mixed fibro-calcified plaque in the proximal left anterior descending coronary artery (LAD), as assessed by multidetector-row CT (MDCT) and intravascular ultrasound (IVUS). Above: MDCT image, maximum intensity projection (MIP), with a fibrous plaque area (100 HU, arrow) next to significant calcifications. Below: IVUS images in cross-sectional views along the course of the plaque, moving from the noncalcified, fibrous plaque area (left) towards the calcifications (middle and right).

That study concluded that CTA is a promising method for assessing the lumen and wall of the carotid artery, and that the apparent correlation between histologic appearance and plaque density on CT angiograms could have important implications for the prediction of plaque stability.

Coronary Plaque Imaging With CT

CT has become an established method for noninvasive and highly sensitive detection of coronary artery calcifications *(23)*. However, calcified plaques are probably the result of repetitive plaque rupture and healing, causing shrinkage of the vessel lumen with subsequent stenosis *(24)*. Earlier stages of atherosclerosis without calcifications might be more prone to rupture, resulting in acute cardiovascular events *(25)*. Yet, this theory does not stand undisputed, as an autopsy study suggested that the degree of calcification was greatest for acute and healed plaque ruptures *(26)*. Recently, it was shown that CT has the potential to identify early, noncalcified plaques in the coronary arteries in vivo *(27,28)*. Various imaging features of noncalcified and calcified plaques depicted with CT correlate well with histopathologic stages of atherosclerosis defined by the American Heart Association (AHA) *(29)*, as demonstrated in a recent ex-vivo study on human hearts *(30)*.

Intravascular ultrasound (IVUS) is the reference standard for invasive detecting and evaluating atherosclerotic plaques in vivo. For plaques with and without signs of calcification detected on intracoronary ultrasound, electron beam CT (EBCT) without contrast enhancement yielded a sensitivity of 97% and 47% and a specificity of 80% and 75%, respectively *(31)*. In an in vivo study on contrast-enhanced MDCT vs IVUS for the accuracy in determining coronary lesion configuration, Schroeder et al. *(16)* reported a good correlation of these two modalities. MDCT was able to differentiate between soft, intermediate, and calcified plaques, as compared to IVUS, with significant differences in CT attenuation values (Fig. 2). In

Table 1
Imaging Parameters for Multidetector-Row CT and Magnetic Resonance Imaging, and Typical Appearance of Different Plaque Types According to the Composition of the Plaque

	Modality				
	CT (HU)	*MR (SI)*			
	C/E	*T1w*	*PDw*	*T2w*	*ToF*
Thrombus	20	+ to ±	– to ±	– to ±	+
Lipids	50	+	+	–	–
Fibrous	100	± to +	+	± to +	– to ±
Calcium	>300	–	–	–	–

HU, Hounsfield units; SI, signal intensities; C/E, contrast-enhanced; T1w, T2w, PDw, ToF, multicontrast MR imaging sequences; –, hypointense; ±, isointense; +, hyperintense.

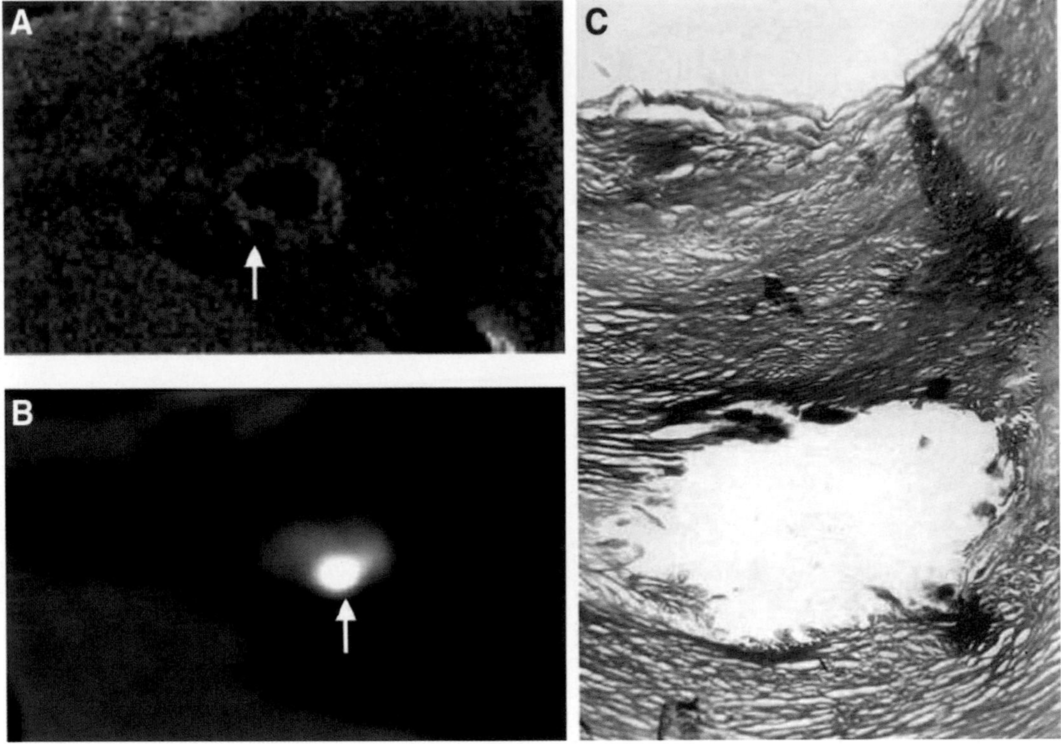

Fig. 3. Magnetic resonance and CT plaque characterization. Coronary artery calcified plaque. (**A**) Cross-sectional ex-vivo T2-weighted MR image of a human left anterior descending artery with a small calcified lesion (arrow) and vessel wall thickening. (**B**) Multislice CT image of the same lesion (arrow), showing the typical blooming effect of calcified lesions in CT images. (**C**) Corresponding histopathologic section; calcium is washed out during the preparation process.

recent studies on MDCT of ex-vivo coronary arteries vs histopathology as the gold standard, again a good correlation was found. Lipid-rich, fibrous, and calcified plaques were differentiated reliably *(30)* (Table 1 and Figs. 3–5). Acute intravascular thrombi can also be detected in vivo, with a typical appearance of the irregular thrombus with typically low attenuation numbers, in the range of 20–30 HU (Fig. 6). Additionally, new image analysis software may enable in-vivo quantification of noncalcified atherosclerotic lesions (Fig. 7) *(8)*.

MDCT possesses a high sensitivity for the detection of calcified plaques, as a result of its inherent high sensitivity for calcifications caused by the high CT attenuation values of these lesions (type Vb lesions). Sensitivity has been reported to be lower for earlier stages of atherosclerosis (type III and IVa plaques), mainly owing to lack of in-plane spatial resolution and to partial-volume effects. Still, heavy coronary calcifications may prevent adequate assessment of complex plaques with calcified and soft plaque components in direct proximity to each other. The reasons for this are considerable beam hardening artifacts and partial-volume effects of calcium on CT. Whereas this effect facilitates the detection of calcium, the same effect hampers the assessment of noncalcified compo-

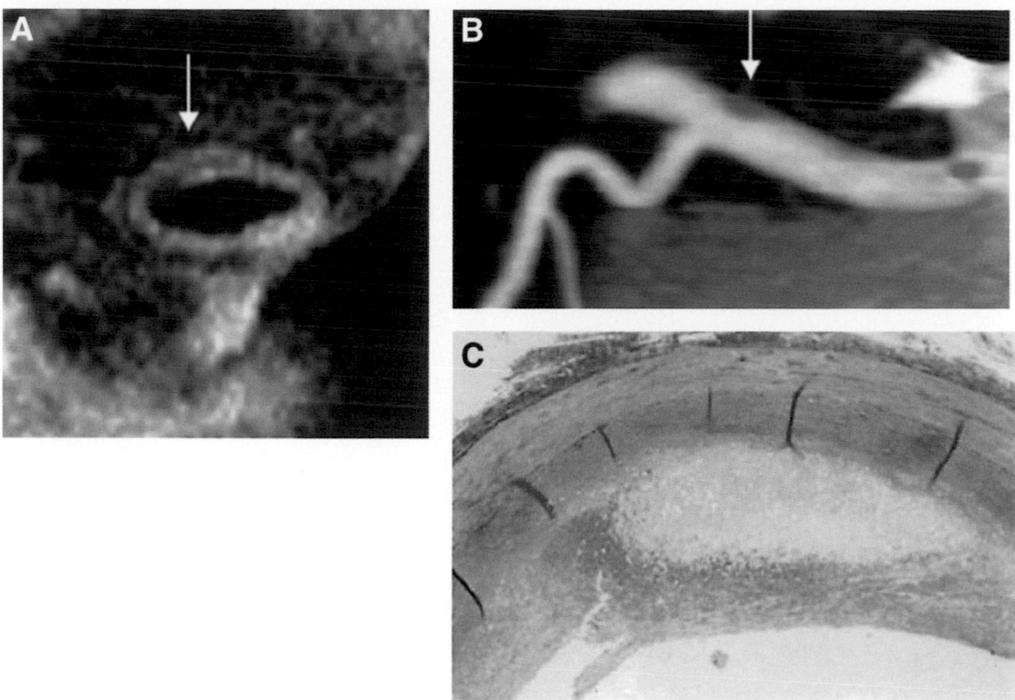

Fig. 4. Magnetic resonance (MR) and CT plaque characterization. Coronary artery lipid-rich plaque. (**A**) Cross-sectional ex vivo T2-weighted MR image of a human left anterior descending artery with a lipid-rich lesion (arrow). (**B**) Multislice CT image of the same lesion (arrow), showing the typical low density of lipid-rich tissue (44 HU). (C) Corresponding histopathologic section with a large extracellular lipid pool.

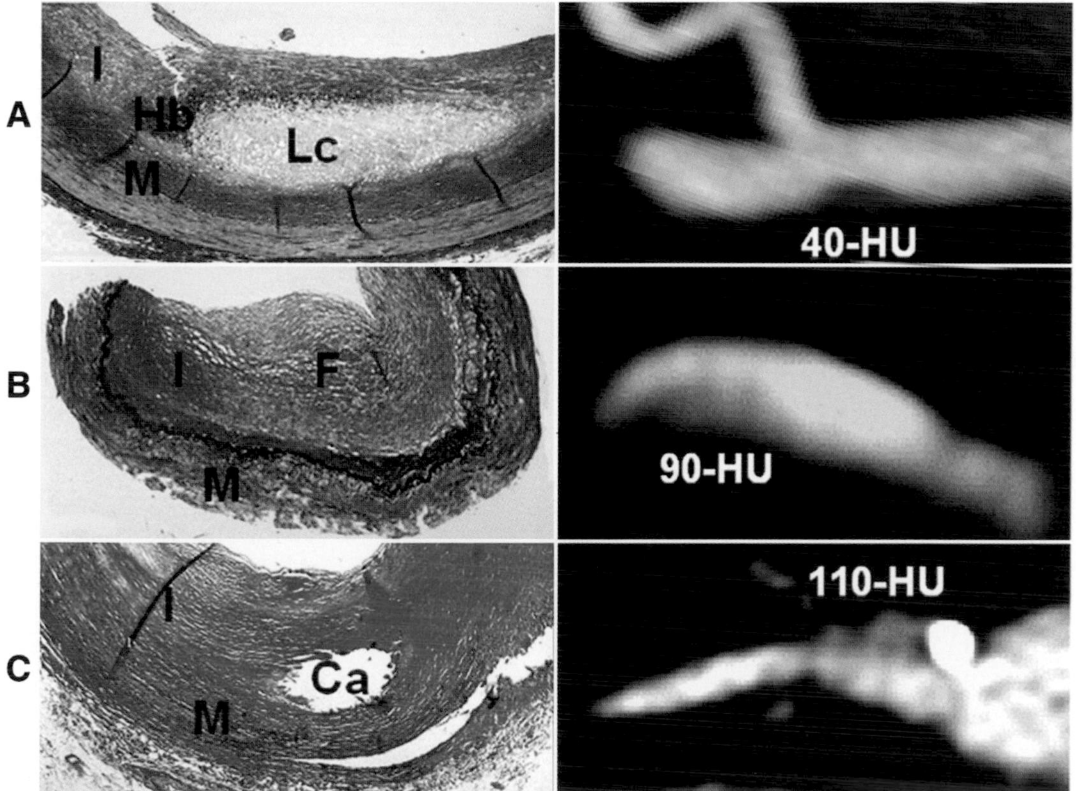

Fig. 5. (**A**) Type VI atherosclerotic lesion with extensive lipid accumulation (Lc = lipid core) and small intra-plaque hemorrhage (Hb) within the atherosclerotic widened intima (I) and media (M) cell layer. Corresponding multidetector-row CT (MDCT) image shows a soft tissue lesion with a mean density of 40 HU. (**B**) In contrast to lipid-rich plaques, purely fibrous (F) plaque (Type Vc) without calcium demonstrate significantly higher attenuation (90 HU) on MDCT. (**C**) "Calcified nodules" or "spotty" lesions contain little pieces of calcium (Ca) that was removed in the process of preparing the slides. On MDCT the calcification can be easily detected and partly covers the adjacent fibrous soft tissue (110 HU). (Courtesy of C.R. Becker, Ludwig-Maximilians-University, Munich, Germany.)

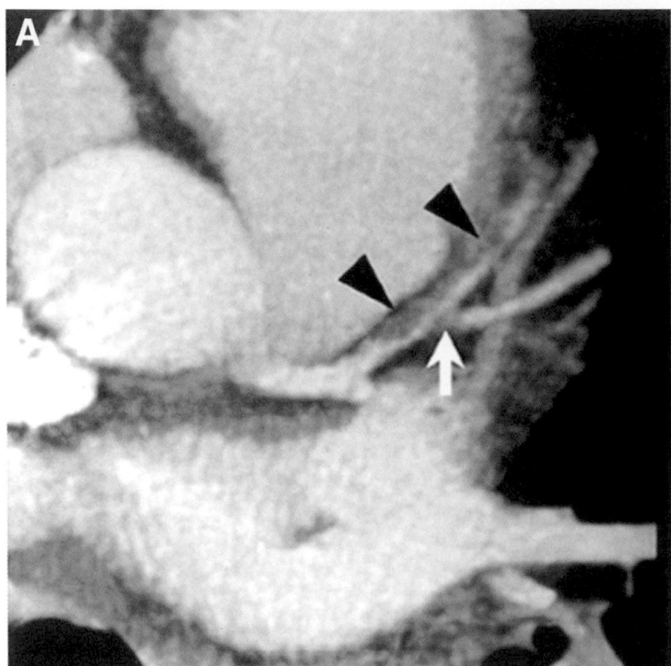

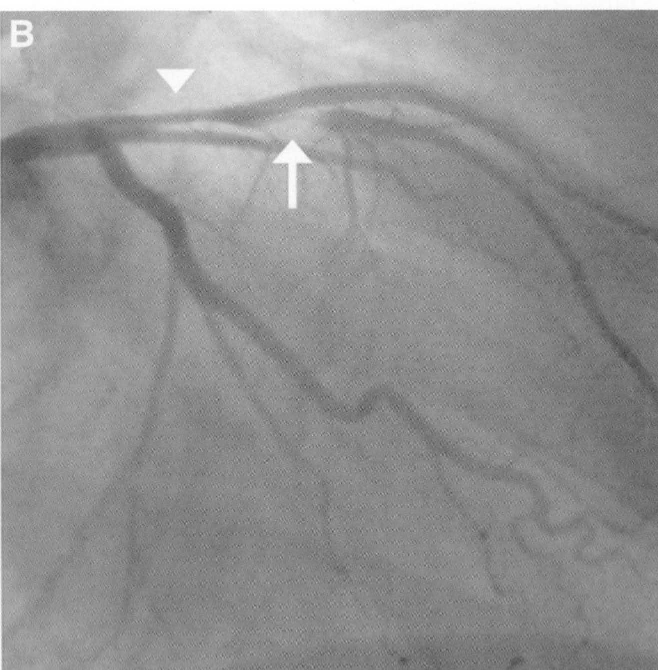

Fig. 6. 41-yr-old man with atypical chest pain. (**A**) Maximum intensity projection of contrast-enhanced helical CT scan reveals lumen obstruction of left anterior descending coronary artery (arrowheads) and first diagonal branch (arrow). A thrombus can be delineated with irregular borders and the typical low CT attenuation. (**B**) Conventional angiogram confirms findings on helical CT scan and also reveals high-grade stenosis of left anterior descending coronary artery (arrowhead) and first diagonal branch (arrow). Modified from ref. *28*.

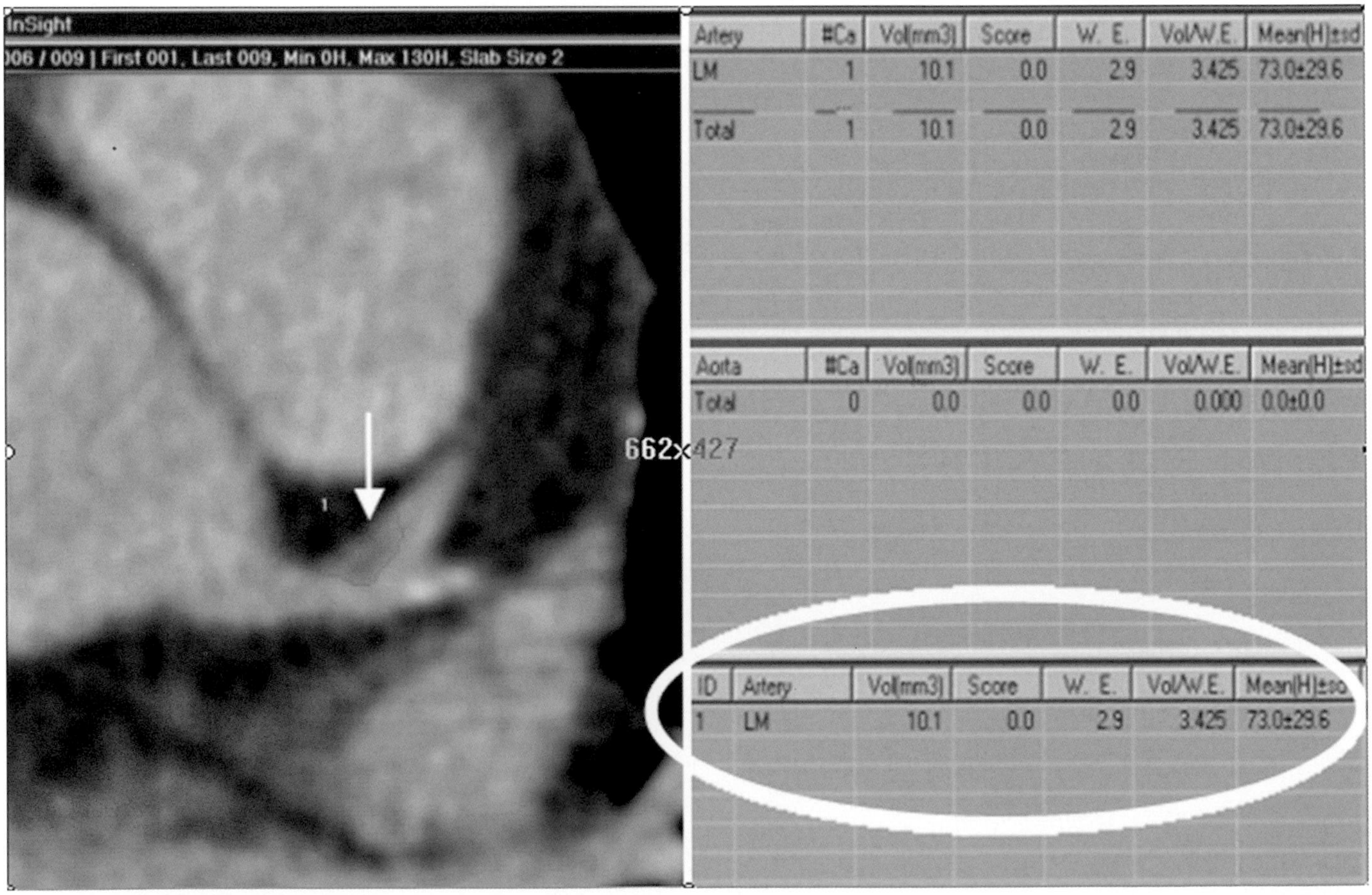

Fig. 7. Quantitative volumetry of noncalcified plaques can be performed on special offline workstations (InSight, NeoImagery, San Francisco, CA). Such volumetry is still conducted semi-quantitatively, segmenting the soft plaque borders by hand (arrow) while the software measures plaque volume automatically according to predefined thresholds (circle).

nents of lesions next to calcified components of the same atherosclerotic plaque. Thus, the soft-tissue components in mixed plaques with a high content of calcium may be unspecific and can resemble any AHA type atherosclerotic lesion on histopathology, although the presence of calcium within the plaque would suggest a classification as AHA type Vb. Yet, the ultimate goal is to detect earlier stage, noncalcified plaques. Calcifications are thought to be more prevalent in advanced stages of atherosclerosis. According to Virmani et al. *(2)*, calcified plaques are likely the result of repetitive plaque rupture and healing, causing shrinkage of the vessel lumen with consequent stenosis. Earlier stages of atherosclerosis without calcifications might be more prone to acute rupture, resulting in acute cardiovascular events *(25)*. Yet, as described above, this presumption does not stand undisputed *(26)*.

APPLICATIONS OF MR PLAQUE IMAGING

Noncoronary Plaque Imaging With MRI

MR has been used to study atherosclerotic plaques in human carotid *(17,32)*, aortic *(18)*, and coronary *(33)* arterial disease. The superficial location and relative absence of motion in carotid arteries presents less of a technical challenge for imaging than the aorta or coronary arteries. Some of the MR studies of carotid arterial plaques include the imaging and characterization of atherosclerotic plaques *(17,32)*, the quantification of plaque size *(34)*, and the detection of fibrous cap "integrity" *(19)*. Typically, the images are acquired with a resolution of $0.25 \times 0.25 \times 2.0$ to $0.4 \times 0.4 \times 3.0$ mm^3 by use of a carotid phased-array coil to improve signal-to-noise ratio and image resolution. In vivo, black-blood MR atherosclerotic plaque characterization of the human aorta has been reported by Fayad et al. *(18)*, who assessed thoracic aorta plaque composition and size with the use of T1-weighted (T1w), T2-weighted (T2w), and proton density–weighted (PDw) images. The acquired images had a resolution of $0.8 \times 0.8 \times 5.0$ mm^3 with a phased-array chest coil. Matched cross-sectional aortic imaging with MR and transesophageal echocardiography showed a strong correlation for plaque composition and mean maximum plaque thickness.

Coronary Plaque Imaging With MRI

With a combination of multicontrast MR imaging sequences, differentiation of fibrocellular, lipid-rich, and calcified regions of the atherosclerotic coronary plaque is feasible, as shown in an ex-vivo study on human coronary arteries in correlation to histopathology *(30)* (Figs. 3 and 4). Calcifications are well defined by signal loss in all sequences (T1w, T2w, PDw), because of the low mobile proton density within the calcified area. Fibrocellular regions are well distinguished by the less dense body of the plaque-containing regions of extracellular lipid deposition on T2w imaging. Fatty lesions are identified as areas of low signal intensity in T2w and intermediate signal intensities in T1w sequences (Table 1).

In vivo studies of coronary artery plaques are obviously more challenging. Preliminary studies in a pig model showed that the difficulties of coronary wall imaging are the result of a combination of cardiac and respiratory motion artifacts, nonlinear course, small size, and location *(35)*. Fayad et al. extended the black-blood MR methods used in the human carotid artery and aorta to the imaging of the coronary arterial lumen and wall (Fig. 8) *(33)*. The method was validated in swine coronary lesions induced by balloon angioplasty *(35)*. High-resolution black-blood MR of both normal and atherosclerotic human coronary arteries was performed for direct assessment of coronary wall thickness and the visualization of focal atherosclerotic plaque in the wall. The difference in maximum wall thickness between the normal subjects and patients (>40% stenosis) was statistically significant. Fig. 8 shows in vivo MR coronary plaque images from two patients. The coronary MR plaque imaging study by Fayad et al. *(33)* was performed during breath-holding to minimize respiratory motion, with a resolution of $0.46 \times 0.46 \times 2.0$ mm^3. To alleviate the need for the patient to hold his or her breath, Botnar et al. *(36)* have combined the black-blood FSE method and a real-time navigator for respiratory gating and real-time slice position correction. A near isotropic spatial resolution ($0.7 \times 0.7 \times 0.8$ mm^3) was achieved with the use of a 2D local inversion and black-blood preparatory pulses *(36)*. This method provided a quick way to image a long segment of the coronary artery wall and may be useful for rapid coronary plaque burden measurements. Future studies need to address these possibilities.

Monitoring of Atherosclerotic Disease With MRI

As shown in animal experimental studies *(37,38)*, MR is also a powerful tool to serially and noninvasively investigate the progression and regression of atherosclerotic lesions in vivo. In asymptomatic, untreated, hypercholesterolemic patients with carotid and aortic atherosclerosis, Corti et al. *(39)* have shown that MR can be used to measure the efficacy of lipid-lowering therapy (statins). Atherosclerotic plaques were assessed with MR at different times after lipid-lowering therapy. Significant regression of atherosclerotic lesions was observed. Despite the early and expected hypolipidemic effect of the statins, changes in the vessel wall were observed after 12 mo of treatment. As with previous experimental studies, there was a decrease in the vessel wall area and no alteration in the lumen area after 12 mo *(37,38)*. A case-controlled study demonstrated substantially reduced carotid plaque lipid content (but no change in overall lesion area) in patients treated for 10 y with an aggressive lipid-lowering regimen, compared with untreated controls *(40)*. Yet, there are no reports so far on longitudinal human in-vivo studies on the alteration of coronary atherosclerotic plaques over time.

POSSIBLE FUTURE IMPROVEMENTS

FUTURE POSSIBILITIES OF CT PLAQUE IMAGING

Next-generation MDCT scanners will most probably allow for even faster gantry rotation and simultaneous acquisition of >16 slices. The breath-hold time may decrease to <10 s, thus reducing the necessary contrast medium (e.g., 60 mL) for sufficient enhancement of the coronary arteries. The temporal and spatial resolution may most likely further decrease to ideally 100 ms and 0.6-mm slice thickness for true isotropic voxel sizes. These enhancements may help in the detection, differentiation, and reliable quantification of calcified and noncalcified coronary artery plaques. Reduction of spatial resolution and new image reconstruction algorithms should further reduce beam hardening artifacts and partial-volume effects caused by calcifications, improving the assessment of complex mixed

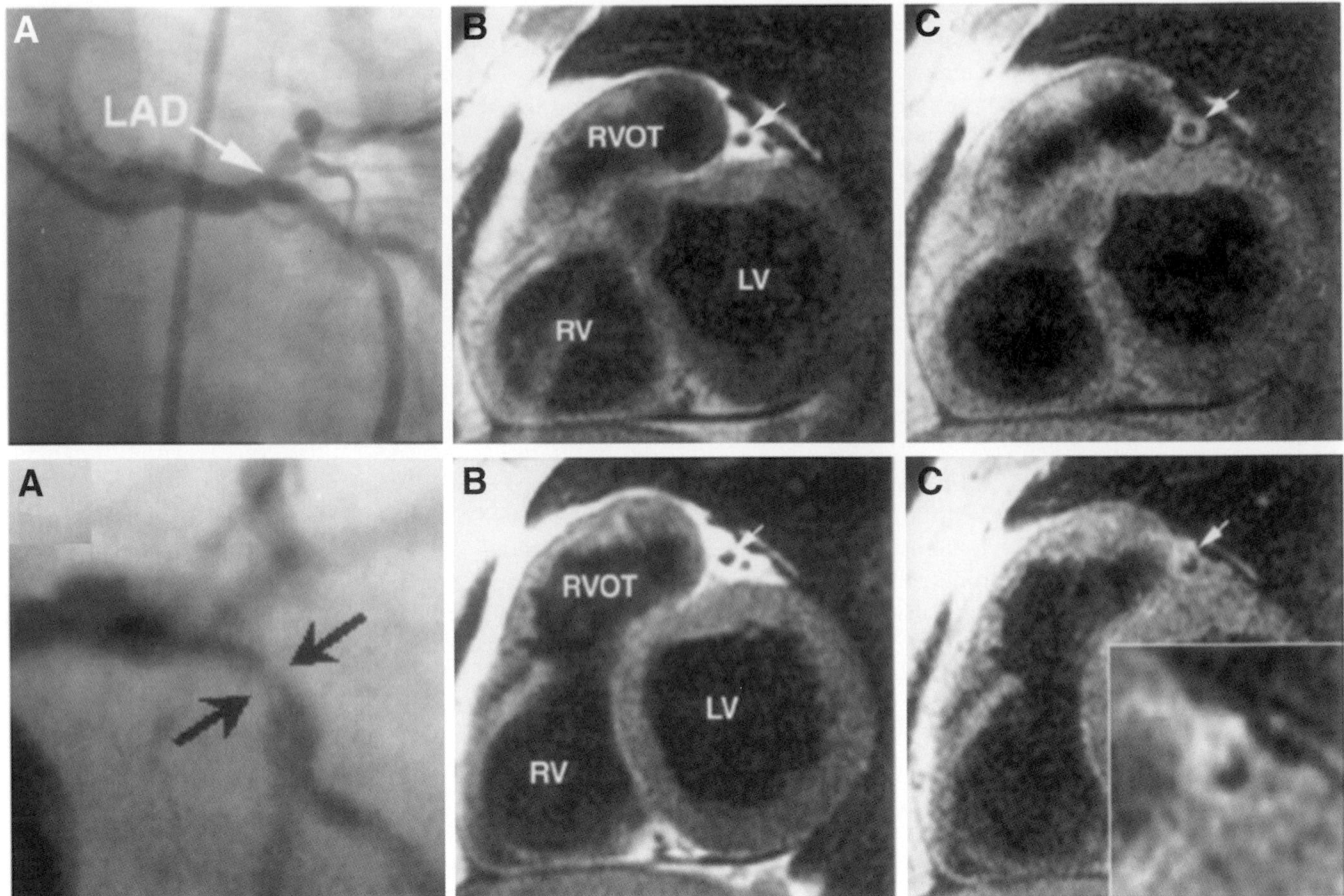

Fig. 8. Upper row: X-ray angiogram from 78-yr-old female patient with mild disease on X-ray angiography in proximal left anterior descending (LAD) artery (arrow, **A**). Black-blood-magnetic resonance (BB-MR) cross-sectional lumen image reveals circular lumen (**B**); wall shows uniformly thickened LAD wall (**B**) with concentric plaque (**C**). Lower row: X-ray angiogram from 76-yr-old male patient shows high-grade stenosis in proximal LAD (arrows, **A**). In vivo cross-sectional BB-MR images of LAD lumen (**B**) shows obstructed lumen (elliptical lumen shape); wall image (**C**) shows large eccentric plaque with heterogeneous signal intensity. (Modified from ref. *12*.)

plaques. Further optimization of multisegmental reconstruction algorithms *(41,42)* yields potential to investigate patients with higher heart rates with a constant image quality.

FUTURE POSSIBILITIES OF MR PLAQUE IMAGING

Thinner slices, such as those obtained with 3D MR acquisition techniques, could further improve artery wall imaging *(36)*. Additional MR techniques, such as water diffusion weighting *(43)*, magnetization transfer weighting *(20)*, steady-state free precession (SSFP) sequences *(44)*, contrast enhancement *(45)*, and molecular imaging *(46,47)* may provide complementary structural information and allow more detailed plaque characterization. New and improved blood suppression methods *(36)* are necessary for accurate plaque imaging, especially in the carotid artery bifurcation.

Contrast-enhanced MR angiography with the use of gadolinium-based contrast agents may provide additional information for plaque characterization by identifying neovascularization in the atherosclerotic plaque, and potentially improve the differentiation between necrotic core and fibrous tissue *(45)*. Furthermore, other nonspecific and specific contrast agents may facilitate accurate plaque constituent characterization and the identification of specific molecular and biological activity *(46,47)*. One promising example is fibrin-specific contrast agents, which allow for reliable detection of thrombotic material and for longitudinal control of thrombus progression or regression *(48)*.

SYNOPSIS

MRI VS MDCT

Both high-resolution MRI and MDCT have specific advantages in the detection and differentiation of atherosclerotic vessel wall changes. Using dedicated MRI techniques, a higher in-plane resolution can be achieved, and in combination with multi-echo sequences, a more detailed analysis of different plaque types and plaque components is feasible. MRI does not suffer from beam-hardening artifacts and partial-volume effects caused by calcifications, allowing superior differentiation of mixed plaques with calcified and noncalcified components. The major disadvantages of MRI are its limitations concerning in vivo application, because the technique suffers from patient movement and breathing artifacts as a result of the comparatively long acquisition times. This is the main reason why, in an in vivo setting, a detailed analysis of coronary artery plaques is hardly feasible yet, and only limited regions of the coronary artery tree can be depicted *(12)*. Also, patients with cardiac pacemakers or other specific metal parts in their body can not undergo MRI.

Currently, MDCT is easier and faster to perform in an in vivo setting, and less sensitive to movement artifacts caused by patient movement or breathing artifacts, despite the relatively long acquisition window of 210 to 250 ms per heartbeat. Modern MDCT scanners with 16 detector rows allow for in-vivo investigation of the entire coronary artery tree with 0.75-mm slice thickness within one short breath-hold, achieving a nearly isotropic submillimeter voxel size, with typically better out-of-plane resolution than MRI. However, MDCT applies a considerable amount of ionizing radiation to the patient, and iodine-containing contrast agents are used.

Another promising technique for noninvasive cardiac imaging and possibly plaque imaging is EBCT. EBCT has mainly been used for accurate quantitation of coronary artery calcium, scanning the entire heart in a single breath-hold from rapid (100 ms) tomographic scans done in synchrony with the heart cycle *(49)*. So far, no reports on the assessment of noncalcified plaque are available using this modality *(50)*.

CT AND MR IMAGING COMBINATION

Cross-sectional modalities—MRI and CT—offer more information than just displays of the patient's coronary vessel lumen. The advantage of MDCT is the potentially complete assessment of the entire coronary artery tree within a very short scan time, and MRI offers excellent soft-tissue contrast. However, because of the limited scan range and long examination time for MRI, MDCT may be used first to localize suspicious CAD lesions in the coronary arteries. With the knowledge of the problematic site in the coronary arteries from MDCT, MRI follow-up may be used for further lesion assessment. Improved CT and MR imaging of the coronaries may in the future allow for better noninvasive evaluation of atherosclerotic plaques. A comprehensive study of atherosclerosis could involve a calcium screening measurement, contrast-enhanced CT for noncalcified plaque burden and stenosis assessment, and multicontrast MR plaque characterization for a detailed analysis and follow-up of the composition of coronary atherosclerotic lesions. The utility of such a noninvasive combined CT and MR approach will have to be tested in future studies.

CONCLUSIONS

CT and MR imaging are emerging as the most promising complementary imaging modalities for coronary atherosclerotic disease detection. They identify flow-limiting coronary stenoses and calcified plaques, directly image the atherosclerotic lesions, measure atherosclerotic burden, and characterize the plaque components. Together, they provide unique information that may predict cardiovascular risk, facilitate further study of the mechanisms of atherosclerosis progression and its response to therapy, and allow for assessment of subclinical disease. However, published studies with relatively small numbers of patients were conducted independently with either CT or MR. These results should be validated in large-scale clinical trials before CT and MR are implemented clinically, outside of research settings, especially for atherosclerotic disease screening. This type of clinical investigation is needed to define the technical requirements for optimal imaging, develop accurate image analysis methods, outline criteria for interpretation, delineate the clinical indications for which CT and MR imaging together should be used as an adjunct to conventional imaging, and address the issue of cost-effectiveness. Finally, imaging may address the high-risk plaque, as described before, but it does not take into account the blood hypercoagulable state or markers of inflammation. Therefore, one of the ultimate goals for clinicians is the identification of the high-risk patient through a combination of strategies such as assessment of conventional risk factors, blood markers, and imaging.

REFERENCES

1. Fayad ZA, Fuster V, Nikolaou K, Becker C. Computed tomography and magnetic resonance imaging for noninvasive coronary angiography and plaque imaging: current and potential future concepts. Circulation 2002;106(15):2026–2034.
2. Virmani R, Kolodgie FD, Burke AP, Farb A, Schwartz SM. Lessons from sudden coronary death: a comprehensive morphological classification scheme for atherosclerotic lesions. Arterioscler Thromb Vasc Biol 2000;20(5):1262–1275.
3. Fuster V, Badimon L, Badimon JJ, Chesebro JH. The pathogenesis of coronary artery disease and the acute coronary syndromes (2). N Engl J Med 1992;326(5):310–318.
4. Fuster V, Badimon L, Badimon JJ, Chesebro JH. The pathogenesis of coronary artery disease and the acute coronary syndromes (1). N Engl J Med 1992;326(4):242–250.
5. Pasterkamp G, Falk E, Woutman H, Borst C. Techniques characterizing the coronary atherosclerotic plaque: influence on clinical decision making? J Am Coll Cardiol 2000;36(1):13–21.
6. Fayad ZA, Fuster V. Clinical imaging of the high-risk or vulnerable atherosclerotic plaque. Circ Res 2001;89(4):305–316.
7. Nieman K, Cademartiri F, Lemos P, Raaijmakers R, Pattynama P, de Feyter P. Reliable noninvasive coronary aniography with fast submillimeter multslice spiral computed tomography. Circulation 2002;106:2051–2054.
8. Nikolaou K, Becker CR, Wintersperger BJ, Sagmeister S, Reiser MF. Assessment of non-calcified vessel-wall changes in the coronary arteries using contrast-enhanced multirow-detector computed tomography. Radiology 2002;225:632.
9. Toussaint J-F, LaMuraglia GM, Southern JF, Fuster V, Kantor HL. Magnetic resonance images lipid, fibrous, calcified, hemorrhagic, and thrombotic components of human atherosclerosis in vivo. Circulation 1996;94(5):932–938.
10. Yuan C, Beach KW, Smith LH, Jr., Hatsukami TS. Measurement of atherosclerotic carotid plaque size in vivo using high resolution magnetic resonance imaging. Circulation 1998;98(24):2666–2671.
11. Fayad ZA, Nahar T, Fallon JT, et al. In vivo magnetic resonance evaluation of atherosclerotic plaques in the human thoracic aorta: a comparison with transesophageal echocardiography. Circulation 2000;101(21):2503–2509.
12. Fayad ZA, Fuster V, Fallon JT, et al. Noninvasive in vivo human coronary artery lumen and wall imaging using black-blood magnetic resonance imaging. Circulation 2000;102(5):506–510.
13. Botnar R, Stuber M, Kissinger K, Kim W, Spuentrup E, Manning W. Noninvasive coronary vessel wall and plaque imaging with magnetic resonance imaging. Circulation 2000;102:2582–2587.
14. Wintersperger BJ, Herzog P, Jakobs TF, Reiser MF, Becker CR. Initial experience with the clinical use of a 16 detector row CT system. Crit Rev Comput Tomogr 2002;43:283–316.
15. Flohr T, Kuttner A, Bruder H, et al. Performance evaluation of a multi-slice CT system with 16-slice detector and increased gantry rotation speed for isotropic submillimeter imaging of the heart. Herz 2003;28(1):7–19.
16. Schroeder S, Kopp AF, Baumbach A, et al. Noninvasive detection and evaluation of atherosclerotic coronary plaques with multislice computed tomography. J Am Coll Cardiol 2001;37(5):1430–1435.

17. Toussaint JF, LaMuraglia GM, Southern JF, Fuster V, Kantor HL. Magnetic resonance images lipid, fibrous, calcified, hemorrhagic, and thrombotic components of human atherosclerosis in vivo. Circulation 1996;94(5):932–938.
18. Fayad ZA, Nahar T, Fallon JT, et al. In vivo MR evaluation of atherosclerotic plaques in the human thoracic aorta: a comparison with TEE. Circulation 2000;101:2503–2509.
19. Hatsukami TS, Ross R, Polissar NL, Yuan C. Visualization of fibrous cap thickness and rupture in human atherosclerotic carotid plaque In vivo with high-resolution magnetic resonance imaging. Circulation 2000;102(9):959–964.
20. Yuan C, Mitsumori LM, Beach KW, Maravilla KR. Carotid atherosclerotic plaque: noninvasive MR characterization and identification of vulnerable lesions. Radiology 2001;221(2):285–299.
21. Estes JM, Quist WC, Lo Gerfo FW, Costello P. Noninvasive characterization of plaque morphology using helical computed tomography. J Cardiovasc Surg (Torino) 1998;39(5):527–534.
22. Oliver TB, Lammie GA, Wright AR, et al. Atherosclerotic plaque at the carotid bifurcation: CT angiographic appearance with histopathologic correlation. AJNR Am J Neuroradiol 1999;20(5): 897–901.
23. Becker CR, Knez A, Jakobs TF, et al. Detection and quantification of coronary artery calcification with electron-beam and conventional CT. Eur Radiol 1999;9(4):620–624.
24. Virmani R, Kolodgie FD, Burke AP, Farb A, Schwartz SM. Lessons from sudden coronary death: a comprehensive morphological classification scheme for atherosclerotic lesions. Arterioscler Thromb Vasc Biol 2000;20(5):1262–1275.
25. Virmani R, Burke AP, Farb A. Sudden cardiac death. Cardiovasc Pathol 2001;10(5):211–218.
26. Burke AP, Taylor A, Farb A, Malcom GT, Virmani R. Coronary calcification: insights from sudden coronary death victims. Z Kardiol 2000;89(Suppl 2):49–53.
27. Becker CR, Knez A, Leber A, Treede H, Haberl R, Reiser MF. [Angiography with multi-slice spiral CT. Detecting plaque, before it causes symptoms]. MMW Fortschr Med 2001;143(16):30–32.
28. Becker CR, Knez A, Ohnesorge B, Schoepf UJ, Reiser MF. Imaging of noncalcified coronary plaques using helical CT with retrospective ECG gating. AJR Am J Roentgenol 2000;175(2):423–424.
29. Stary HC. Natural history and histological classification of atherosclerotic lesions: an update. Arterioscler Thromb Vasc Biol 2000; 20(5):1177–1178.
30. Nikolaou K, Becker CR, Muders M. High-resolution magnetic resonance and multi-slice CT imaging of coronary artery plaques in human ex vivo coronary arteries. Radiology 2001;221:503.
31. Baumgart D, Schmermund A, Goerge G, et al. Comparison of electron beam computed tomography with intracoronary ultrasound and coronary angiography for detection of coronary atherosclerosis. J Am Coll Cardiol 1997;30(1):57–64.
32. Yuan C, Mitsumori LM, Ferguson MS, et al. In vivo accuracy of multispectral magnetic resonance imaging for identifying lipid-rich necrotic cores and intraplaque hemorrhage in advanced human carotid plaques. Circulation 2001;104(17):2051–2056.
33. Fayad ZA, Fuster V, Fallon JT, et al. Noninvasive in vivo human coronary artery lumen and wall imaging using black-blood magnetic resonance imaging. Circulation 2000;102(5):506–510.
34. Yuan C, Beach KW, Smith LH, Jr., Hatsukami TS. Measurement of atherosclerotic carotid plaque size in vivo using high resolution magnetic resonance imaging. Circulation 1998;98(24):2666–2671.
35. Worthley SG, Helft G, Fuster V, et al. Noninvasive in vivo magnetic resonance imaging of experimental coronary artery lesions in a porcine model. Circulation 2000;101(25):2956–2961.
36. Botnar RM, Kim WY, Bornert P, Stuber M, Spuentrup E, Manning WJ. 3D coronary vessel wall imaging utilizing a local inversion technique with spiral image acquisition. Magn Reson Med 2001; 46(5):848–854.
37. McConnell MV, Aikawa M, Maier SE, Ganz P, Libby P, Lee RT. MRI of rabbit atherosclerosis in response to dietary cholesterol lowering. Arterioscler Thromb Vasc Biol 1999;19(8):1956–1959.
38. Helft G, Worthley SG, Fuster V, et al. Progression and regression of atherosclerotic lesions: monitoring with serial noninvasive magnetic resonance imaging. Circulation 2002;105(8):993–998.
39. Corti R, Fayad ZA, Fuster V, et al. Effects of lipid-lowering by simvastatin on human atherosclerotic lesions: a longitudinal study by high-resolution, noninvasive magnetic resonance imaging. Circulation 2001;104(3):249–252.
40. Zhao XQ, Yuan C, Hatsukami TS, et al. Effects of prolonged intensive lipid-lowering therapy on the characteristics of carotid atherosclerotic plaques in vivo by MRI: a case-control study. Arterioscler Thromb Vasc Biol 2001;21(10):1623–1629.
41. Halliburton SS, Stillman AE, Flohr T, et al. Do segmented reconstruction algorithms for cardiac multi-slice computed tomography improve image quality? Herz 2003;28(1):20–31.
42. Flohr T, Kuttner A, Bruder H, et al. Performance evaluation of a multi-slice CT system with 16-slice detector and increased gantry rotation speed for isotropic submillimeter imaging of the heart. Herz 2003;28(1):7–19.
43. Toussaint JF, Southern JF, Fuster V, Kantor HL. Water diffusion properties of human atherosclerosis and thrombosis measured by pulse field gradient nuclear magnetic resonance. Arterioscler Thromb Vasc Biol 1997;17(3):542–546.
44. Coombs BD, Rapp JH, Ursell PC, Reilly LM, Saloner D. Structure of plaque at carotid bifurcation: high-resolution MRI with histological correlation. Stroke 2001;32(11):2516–21.
45. Yuan C, Kerwin WS, Ferguson MS, et al. Contrast-enhanced high resolution MRI for atherosclerotic carotid artery tissue characterization. J Magn Reson Imaging 2002;15(1):62–67.
46. Ruehm SG, Corot C, Vogt P, Kolb S, Debatin JF. Magnetic resonance imaging of atherosclerotic plaque with ultrasmall superparamagnetic particles of iron oxide in hyperlipidemic rabbits. Circulation 2001;103(3):415–422.
47. Flacke S, Fischer S, Scott MJ, et al. Novel MRI contrast agent for molecular imaging of fibrin: implications for detecting vulnerable plaques. Circulation 2001;104(11):1280–1285.
48. Yu X, Song SK, Chen J, et al. High-resolution MRI characterization of human thrombus using a novel fibrin-targeted paramagnetic nanoparticle contrast agent. Magn Reson Med 2000;44(6):867–872.
49. Rumberger JA. Tomographic (plaque) imaging: state of the art. Am J Cardiol 2001;88(2A):66E–69E.
50. Budoff MJ, Raggi P. Coronary artery disease progression assessed by electron-beam computed tomography. Am J Cardiol 2001; 88(2A):46E–50E.

38 Multidetector-Row CT for Detection of Noncalcified and Calcified Coronary Lesions

Clinical Significance

STEPHEN SCHROEDER, MD, PhD

Immediately after the introduction of multidetector-row computed tomography (MDCT) scanners in 1998, one became aware that not only hyperdense but also hypodense areas within contrast-enhanced axial slices could be seen (*see* Fig. 1). The question to be answered was whether these areas are artifacts or atherosclerotic plaques.

As reviewed in Chapters 35 and 36, experimental as well as clinical studies indicate that these lesions correspond with calcified and noncalcified atherosclerotic coronary lesions *(1,2)*. These lesions might be characterized using MDCT by determining tissue density within the plaque area *(2,3)*.

The detection and quantification of coronary calcifications using electron beam computed tomography (EBCT) was introduced in the early 1990s *(4)*. There is evidence by histopathological studies that the calcium score correlates well with the entire atherosclerotic plaque burden, with calcifications accounting for approx 20% *(5)*.

The evaluation of coronary calcifications is no longer limited to EBCT, but might also be performed by new MDCT technology with comparable results and precision *(6,7)*, opening this diagnostic field to more investigators. The predictive value of coronary calcifications on future acute coronary syndromes (ACS) is at present unclear and controversially discussed, because results from large scale cross-sectional studies are still missing *(8)*. However, there is evidence that screening for coronary calcifications in asymptomatic patients with intermediate risk profiles might be helpful in characterizing patients at higher risk for ACS. Just recently, Rich et al. reported in a metanalysis on a risk ratio of 8.7 in patients with positive scans *(9)*.

However, even asymptomatic intermediate risk individuals without coronary calcifications show an elevated risk ratio. Thus far, the exclusion of coronary calcifications is not equivalent with the exclusion of atherosclerotic coronary artery disease (CAD) in this group of patients, and further diagnostic tools for noninvasive risk-stratification appear to be desirable.

From: *Contemporary Cardiology: CT of the Heart: Principles and Applications*
Edited by: U. Joseph Schoepf © Humana Press, Inc., Totowa, NJ

Due to improved spatial and temporal resolution and thin overlapping slices, noncalcified coronary lesions can be visualized on contrast-enhanced axial slices noninvasively, using MDCT technology *(2,3,10,11)*. In a recently published study, we we were able to show that noncalcified plaques might also be present in the absence of coronary calcifications. Thus far, there is growing evidence that contrast-enhanced MDCT scans might be useful in patients with intermediate risk profile to further characterize the individual's risk for ACS. We demonstrated that noncalcified atherosclerotic coronary lesions occur with a prevalence of 10% in this group of patients without coronary calcifications *(12)* (*see* Fig. 2).

The clinical impact of this stepwise approach needs further prospective evaluation to elucidate whether imaging of noncalcified plaques can add additional information to conventional cardiovascular risk factors for defining the individual's risk. There are, however, limitations of methodology, especially in differentiating atherosclerotic plaques from intracoronary thrombi due to similar density attenuation.

Leber et al. recently demonstrated that patients with ACS had a significantly higher number of noncalcified coronary plaques than did patients with stable angina pectoris *(13)*. Their study suggests that the determination of noncalcified plaques might be useful in characterizing patients at higher risk for ACS. However, the number of patients ($n = 24$) was low. Randomized, large-scale prospective studies are needed to determine whether or not the detection of noncalcified plaques is useful for risk stratification in patients with known or suspected CAD.

A major limitation of MDCT for its use as a screening test is the high radiation exposure, approx 5–10 mSv at present *(14,15)*, compared with conventional coronary angiography without the use of intravascular ultrasound (IVUS) (approx 3 msv *[16]*). However, a combination of IVUS and conventional coronary angiography, which would be needed to achieve adequate assessment of vessel lumen and vessel wall morphology, would likely result in a much higher radiation exposure.

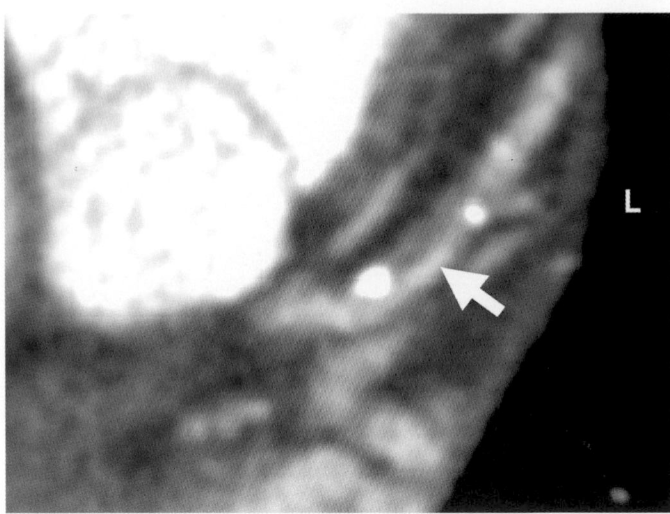

Fig 1. Axial slice image visualizing the contrast-enhanced left anterior descending artery with one hypodense and two hyperdense areas.

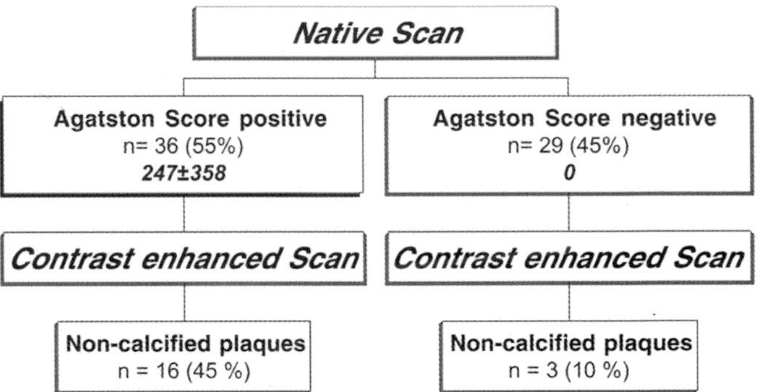

Fig. 2. Prevalence of noncalcified plaques in a study group consting of 68 patients with distinct cardiovascular risk profile but without known coronary artery disease.

Furthermore, improvements of MDCT technology with reduced tube current during systole, reducing radiation exposure by as much as 50% *(17)*, as well as the development of scanners with additional detector slices, allowing for shorter examination times and presumably stabilized image quality, are underway.

Also, the need for iodinated contrast media could be reduced to approx 80 mL per scan, which is in the range of conventional coronary angiography *(16)*.

At present, it is open to speculation whether MDCT might become a useful part of a diagnostic algorithm to further characterize high risk plaques in a combined approach with other imaging modalities, such as magnetic resonance, or whether screening for noncalcified plaques in intermediate or even high-risk patients with or without coronary calcifications might become useful for risk prediction.

REFERENCES

1. Fayad ZA, Fuster V, Nikolaou K, Becker C. Computed tomography and magnetic resonance imaging for noninvasive coronary angiography and plaque imaging: current and potential future concepts. Circulation 2002;106(15):2026–2034.
2. Schroeder S, Kopp AF, Baumbach A, et al. Noninvasive detection and evaluation of atherosclerotic coronary plaques with multislice computed tomography. J Am Coll Cardiol 2001;37(5):1430–1435.
3. Schroeder S, Flohr T, Kopp AF, et al. Accuracy of density measurements within plaques located in artificial coronary arteries by X-ray multislice CT: results of a phantom study. J Comput Assist Tomogr 2001;25(6):900–906.
4. Agatston AS, Janowitz WR, Hildner FJ, Zusmer NR, Viamonte M Jr, Detrano R. Quantification of coronary artery calcium using ultrafast computed tomography. J Am Coll Cardiol 1990;15(4): 827–832.
5. Rumberger JA, Simons DB, Fitzpatrick LA, Sheedy PF, Schwartz RS. Coronary artery calcium area by electron-beam computed tomography and coronary atherosclerotic plaque area. A histopathologic correlative study. Circulation 1995;92(8):2157–2162.
6. Becker CR, Schoepf UJ, Reiser MF. Methods for quantification of coronary artery calcifications with electron beam and conventional CT and pushing the spiral CT envelope: new cardiac applications. Int J Cardiovasc Imaging 2001;17(3):203–211.
7. Becker CR, Kleffel T, Crispin A, et al. Coronary artery calcium measurement: agreement of multirow detector and electron beam CT. AJR Am J Roentgenol 2001;176(5):1295–1298.
8. Rourke RA, Brundage BH, Froelicher VF, et al. American College of Cardiology/American Heart Association Expert Consensus Document on electron-beam computed tomography for the diagnosis and prognosis of coronary artery disease. J Am Coll Cardiol 2000;36:326–340.
9. Rich S, McLaughlin VV. Detection of subclinical cardiovascular disease: the emerging role of electron beam computed tomography. Prev Med 2002;34(1):1–10.
10. Becker CR, Knez A, Ohnesorge B, Schoepf UJ, Reiser MF. Imaging of noncalcified coronary plaques using helical CT with retrospective ECG gating. AJR Am J Roentgenol. 2000;175(2):423–424.
11. Schroeder S, Kopp AF, Baumbach A, et al. Non-invasive characterisation of coronary lesion morphology by multi-slice computed tomography: a promising new technology for risk stratification of patients with coronary artery disease. Heart 2001;85(5): 576–578.
12. Schroeder S, Kuettner A, Kopp AF, et al. Noninvasive evaluation of the prevalence of noncalcified atherosclerotic plaques by multi-slice detector computed tomography: results of a pilot study. Int J Cardiol 2003;92(2–3):151–155.
13. Leber AW, Knez A, White CW, et al. Composition of coronary atherosclerotic plaques in patients with acute myocardial infarction and stable angina pectoris determined by contrast-enhanced multislice computed tomography. Am J Cardiol 2003;91(6):714–718.
14. Achenbach S, Ropers D, Regenfus M, et al. Noninvasive coronary angiography by magnetic resonance imaging, electron-beam computed tomography, and multislice computed tomography. Am J Cardiol 2001;88(2A):70E–73E.
15. Achenbach S, Giesler T, Ropers D, et al. Detection of coronary artery stenoses by contrast-enhanced, retrospectively electrocardiographically-gated, multislice spiral computed tomography. Circulation 2001;103(21):2535–2538.
16. Becker C, Schatzl M, Feist H, et al. [Assessment of the effective dose for routine protocols in conventional CT, electron beam CT and coronary angiography] Rofo Fortschr Geb Rontgenstr Neuen Bildgeb Verfahr 1999;170(1):99–104. German.
17. Jakobs TF, Becker CR, Ohnesorge B, et al. Multislice helical CT of the heart with retrospective ECG gating: reduction of radiation exposure by ECG-controlled tube current modulation. Eur Radiol 2002;12(5):1081–1086.

Index

K

M